FUNCTIONAL LUNG IMAGING

LUNG BIOLOGY IN HEALTH AND DISEASE

Executive Editor

Claude Lenfant
Former Director, National Heart, Lung, and Blood Institute
National Institutes of Health
Bethesda, Maryland

1. Immunologic and Infectious Reactions in the Lung, *edited by C. H. Kirkpatrick and H. Y. Reynolds*
2. The Biochemical Basis of Pulmonary Function, *edited by R. G. Crystal*
3. Bioengineering Aspects of the Lung, *edited by J. B. West*
4. Metabolic Functions of the Lung, *edited by Y. S. Bakhle and J. R. Vane*
5. Respiratory Defense Mechanisms (in two parts), *edited by J. D. Brain, D. F. Proctor, and L. M. Reid*
6. Development of the Lung, *edited by W. A. Hodson*
7. Lung Water and Solute Exchange, *edited by N. C. Staub*
8. Extrapulmonary Manifestations of Respiratory Disease, *edited by E. D. Robin*
9. Chronic Obstructive Pulmonary Disease, *edited by T. L. Petty*
10. Pathogenesis and Therapy of Lung Cancer, *edited by C. C. Harris*
11. Genetic Determinants of Pulmonary Disease, *edited by S. D. Litwin*
12. The Lung in the Transition Between Health and Disease, *edited by P. T. Macklem and S. Permutt*
13. Evolution of Respiratory Processes: A Comparative Approach, *edited by S. C. Wood and C. Lenfant*
14. Pulmonary Vascular Diseases, *edited by K. M. Moser*
15. Physiology and Pharmacology of the Airways, *edited by J. A. Nadel*
16. Diagnostic Techniques in Pulmonary Disease (in two parts), *edited by M. A. Sackner*
17. Regulation of Breathing (in two parts), *edited by T. F. Hornbein*
18. Occupational Lung Diseases: Research Approaches and Methods, *edited by H. Weill and M. Turner-Warwick*
19. Immunopharmacology of the Lung, *edited by H. H. Newball*
20. Sarcoidosis and Other Granulomatous Diseases of the Lung, *edited by B. L. Fanburg*

*The opinions expressed in these volumes do not necessarily represent
the views of the National Institutes of Health.*

FUNCTIONAL LUNG IMAGING

Edited by

David A. Lipson
University of Pennsylvania
Philadelphia, Pennsylvania, U.S.A.

Edwin J. R. van Beek
University of Iowa
Iowa City, Iowa, U.S.A.

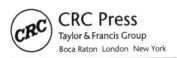

CRC Press
Taylor & Francis Group
Boca Raton London New York

CRC Press is an imprint of the
Taylor & Francis Group, an **informa** business

A TAYLOR & FRANCIS BOOK

CRC Press
Taylor & Francis Group
6000 Broken Sound Parkway NW, Suite 300
Boca Raton, FL 33487-2742

First issued in paperback 2019

© 2005 by Taylor & Francis Group, LLC
CRC Press is an imprint of Taylor & Francis Group, an Informa business

No claim to original U.S. Government works

ISBN-13: 978-0-8247-5427-3 (hbk)
ISBN-13: 978-0-367-39277-2 (pbk)
Library of Congress Card Number 2005041770

Library of Congress Cataloging-in-Publication Data

Functional lung imaging / edited by David Lipson and Edwin van Beek.
   p. cm. -- (Lung biology in health and disease ; v.)
   Includes bibliographical references and index.
   ISBN 0-8247-5427-1 (alk. paper)
   1. Lungs--Imaging. I. Lipson, David. II. Beek, Edwin J. R. van III. Series

RC734.I43F86 2005
616.2'40754--dc22   2005041770

Visit the Taylor & Francis Web site at
http://www.taylorandfrancis.com

and the CRC Press Web site at
http://www.crcpress.com

*I would like to dedicate this volume to my family: Beth, Sarah, and Jeffrey.
Without their love, support, and understanding this volume
would not have been possible.*

David A. Lipson

*I wish to thank my wife (Miriam) and my sons (Andrew and Steven)
for their love, support and understanding. So many things
to catch up on that had to wait for Dad
to finish work ... !*

Edwin J. R. van Beek

Introduction

"Come, come and sit you down. You
shall not budge!
You go not till I set you up a glass
Where you may see the inmost part
of you"
Hamlet
William Shakespeare (1564–1616)

In 1980, the series of monographs *Lung Biology in Health and Disease* introduced volume 16, *Diagnostic Techniques in Pulmonary Diseases*, edited by Marvin A. Sackner a distinguished scientist clinician at the University of Miami School of Medicine. This 941 page volume, published in two parts, included only one section on Radiologic and Radionucleotide Diagnostic Tests. This volume and its contents were the state-of-the-art at the time.

Late in 1990, the series introduced volume 46, *Diagnostic Imaging of the Lung*, edited by Charles E. Putman, Professor of Radiology and Medicine, Duke University School of Medicine. The authors of the last chapter in this volume predicted that "the next frontier will deal with improved characterization, disease processes, identification of the biological status of disease ... and the identification of submacroscopic diseases." In 1997, Charles Putman and his colleague, Caroline Chiles, published *Pulmonary and Cardiac Imaging* as volume 103 in the series.

This field has come a very long way since November 1885 when Wilhelm Roentgen discovered radiography and since the first radiographic imaging of the lung was reported by Francis H. Williams in 1897. It is a clear example where research and application of new technologies are a dynamic and amazingly productive field. As Lord McCauley (1800–1859) said, "Knowledge advances by steps, and not by leaps" but it seems that on the road of imaging, the steps are long and fast.

This is so well demonstrated by the Editors' Preface to this new volume. Indeed, much has happened since volume 103 appeared just a few short years ago. Clinicians, and most importantly the patients, are the beneficiaries of the work presented in this new monograph. Many approaches, each derived from a different technology, are now available to the clinicians who receive real-time information and can witness an accurate and dynamic view of how the lung really works in health or disease. Fatally dangerous inflammatory processes can now be seen and its many manifestations can be differentiated. The emerging field of cellular molecular events, when coupled with dimensional imaging, may permit leaps rather than steps in the understanding of the pathological processes.

Then, surely as Shakespeare said, we will "see the inmost part of you!"

Undoubtedly, the readers of this volume will note that it is the 200th monograph presented by the series, *Lung Biology in Health and Disease*. The first volume appeared in 1976 under the title *Immunologic and Infectious Reactions in the Lung* (Edited by Charles H. Kirkpatrick and Herbert Y. Reynolds). That so many volumes were published in about 30 years is a credit to the international "pulmonary" scientific community whose research has been so productive. In a way, what is so applicable to this new volume, can be said about the entire series of monographs: it has helped clinicians to "see the inmost part of you (the patients)."

Thus, it was indeed a unique opportunity for this series of monographs when Drs. David A. Lipson and Edwin J. R. van Beek agreed to edit this volume *Functional Pulmonary Imaging*. Their own contributions, and those of the many authors from the United States and other continents, result in a unique volume which, like the entire series, will be of value to researchers and clinicians as well. I am grateful to them all for the opportunity to include this landmark volume in the series.

Claude Lenfant, MD
Gaithersburg, Maryland

Foreword

The lung is a highly physiological organ, coordinating regional ventilation and perfusion in carrying out its vitally important role in gas exchange. Nonetheless, until recently progress in pulmonary functional imaging has lagged behind advances in structural imaging of the lungs. Recent years, however, have witnessed an explosive burst of activity in this field. These advances are now providing quantitative visualization of regional lung physiology, moving beyond the spatially-insensitive aggregate measures provided by traditional pulmonary function tests. The contributors to this volume provide an important window into current developments in this emerging field.

Progress in functional lung imaging has been an outgrowth of improvements in scanner technology, combined with new probes to interrogate pulmonary physiology along with advances in computer-based image analysis tools. The spatial and temporal resolution of new generations of clinical multi-slice helical CT scanners provide for breath-hold imaging of the entire lungs with submillimeter slice thickness and isotropic voxels. New CT image acquisition schemes with simultaneous physiological monitoring can capture static images at specified lung volumes, as well as dynamic 4D images at multiple phases of the respiratory cycle. Similarly, the recent advent of parallel processing in MR has greatly improved its temporal and spatial resolution. In addition, micro-CT and micro-PET scanners have provided new opportunities to carry out combined structural-metabolic/molecular imaging of the lungs in small animal models, with morphologic imaging down to the alveolar scale.

A host of new MR-based ventilation agents are being explored; these include the hyperpolarized noble gases (^{3}helium, ^{129}xenon), oxygen, ^{19}fluorine, etc. In addition to providing static and dynamic images of the distribution of these gases, noninvasive MR using these agents can unveil new functional parameters previously inaccessible. These new parameters include: 1) regional alveolar PO_2 concentration, from which the local $\dot{V}/\dot{Q}$ ratio can be indirectly computed; 2) intra-alveolar gas diffusion (apparent diffusion coefficient or ADC), which reflects alveolar microstructure including alveolar size and shape, and is a sensitive tool to detect airspace enlargement in emphysema; and 3) alveolar-capillary gas diffusion (using hyperpolarized ^{129}Xe or oxygen-enhanced MR), which can reflect the thickness of the alveolar-capillary membrane. Interestingly, these functional methods are revealing micro-structural changes which are beyond the spatial resolution of clinical scanners.

Likewise, new methods for MR perfusion scanning have been developed in recent years, including blood-pool gadolinium-based agents, proton perfusion imaging, and arterial spin labeling. The latter two methods do not require administration of any exogenous contrast agents, but quantification is more challenging. Importantly, the development of high-resolution tomographic imaging of ventilation and perfusion has rapidly advanced in the world of functional CT imaging of the lungs, initially with quantitative mapping of perfusion at the microvascular level, and very recently with the introduction of stable xenon-enhanced CT ventilation scans. The latter offer the ability to spatially map ventilation, perfusion, and ventilation/perfusion ratios with sub-millimeter resolution throughout the lungs. These functional CT maps can be integrated with the fine detailed, volumetric, helical-derived structural images. Moreover, these quantitative measures from CT imaging are expected to aid in validating the MR measurements of lung function.

These new scanning techniques, coupled with the growing sizes of the image data sets, have evoked a critical need for computer-based aids to image interpretations. Automated algorithms for segmentation of the lungs, lobes, airway and vascular trees, along with detailed geometric measures of the tracheo-bronchial tree have emerged. Automated co-registration of successive scans provides a means of understanding changes in the lung across time and between interventions. The tools for airway analysis are being used in the assessment of asthma, airway obstructions, and bronchiectasis. Other analysis tools include histogram- and texture-based methods for identification and quantification of emphysema, interstitial lung disease (ILD) and other parenchymal pulmonary disorders. These methods serve to provide highly regionalized measures of lung pathophysiology, which in turn allow for the differentiation of pathologies previously lumped under a few very broad disease categories.

Furthermore, the ability to track the motion of pulmonary structures with changes in lung volumes and pressures provides opportunities to measure and map regional lung mechanics and material properties, including deformation, stress–strain, and lung compliance.

These new methods are not only powerful research tools, but are demonstrating applications to the diagnostic evaluation of patients with chronic obstructive pulmonary disease (emphysema, asthma, and small airways disease), ILD, adult respiratory distress syndrome (ARDS), pulmonary embolism, etc. They have the potential for early disease detection, prior to the advent of image-detectable structural lung changes, as well as for monitoring disease progression and assessing the impact of therapeutic interventions.

These techniques also offer a wide variety of new ways to titrate and optimize therapy. For example, dynamic CT-based mapping of regional alveolar recruitment during the respiratory cycle in patients with ARDS could be used to determine optimal settings for mechanical ventilation. Quantitative CT mapping of regional emphysema has been shown to play an important role in the preoperative evaluation of patients being considered for lung volume reduction surgery. In the National Emphysema Treatment Trial (NETT) image-based measures of emphysema severity and distribution have provided important outcome predictors for success following this surgical intervention. The new airway analysis tools, coupled with assessment of peripheral lung pathologies, are providing guidance for transbronchial and intrabronchial procedures. Examples of the latter include placement of endobronchial valves for the non-surgical approach to lung volume reduction in emphysema, and radiofrequency ablation of airway smooth muscle in the treatment of asthma. Dynamic respiratory-gated CT and MR scans can be used to track the motion of lung tumors during breathing in order to optimize radiation therapy planning. Static and dynamic imaging of the upper airway during wakefulness and sleep have provided important new insights into the pathogenesis of obstructive sleep apnea and clues to novel therapeutic approaches to this disorder.

The functional pulmonary imaging methods described in this book are currently in evolution, and the coming years will undoubtedly witness continued exciting new developments and an expanded clinical role for these physiological imaging techniques. In particular, rapid progress is anticipated in the introduction of molecular reporters for imaging gene expression and gene transfer, tumor, inflammation, and fibrosis. Such molecular imaging will utilize optical, PET, MR, and CT methods for signal detection. In addition, imaging probes for assessing the distribution of drug delivery as well as inhaled particle deposition will likely find increasing applications, e.g., the inhalation of α-1-antitrypsin and other anti-proteases in the treatment of emphysema, and the distribution of gene therapy vectors. The pharmaceutical industry is now turning to imaging to speed the processes of drug discovery, safety testing and outcomes assessment.

The young field of modern functional lung imaging will benefit greatly from the input and wisdom of experienced classical pulmonary physiologists.

Moreover, the combined multi-disciplinary expertise of radiology, pulmonary medicine, anesthesiology, bioengineering, computer science, and molecular biology will be required to assure continued progress and success in this field. Critical to the evolution of these new imaging methods are objective, quantitative tools for image assessment coupled with the traditional experience of the trained observer. The latter faces new challenges in assimilating a growing breadth of both structural and functional detail in image data sets that are expanding exponentially in size as well as richness of information.

Warren B. Gefter, M.D.
Professor of Radiology, University of Pennsylvania
Eric A. Hoffman, Ph.D.
Professor of Radiology and Biomedical Engineering, University of Iowa

Preface

In recent years, the field of medical imaging has rapidly expanded from the morphological into the functional domain. This is due in part to the veritable explosion in raw computing power and to significant advances in imaging hardware. The computer revolution and the development of powerful post-processing techniques have helped to crate a new and emerging medical domain, that of functional imaging.

Functional imaging is a novel field that provides real-time information about anatomic structure and performance of the human body. It is a multidisciplinary field that combines the expertise of radiology, bioengineering, physics, medicine, and surgery. The field is becoming established in the realm of radiology and the neurosciences (where it was first developed), but is unfamiliar territory to the vast majority of clinicians and researchers interested in pulmonary structure and function.

The goal of this volume is to describe the state of the art in the field of functional pulmonary imaging. International leaders in the fields of computed tomography, magnetic resonance, and nuclear medicine will describe advances in lung imaging. Together with respiratory physicians, these authors will translate and apply potential clinical applications of this new technology to various disease states. It is expected that this book will have a very wide audience. Radiologists, chest physicians, physiologists, respiratory therapists, and researchers interested in disease of the chest are but a few of the potential readers. This volume will have an international scope and list of contributors.

Currently, most information about lung function is derived from the use of a battery of pulmonary function tests. Pulmonary function testing presents global information about lung dysfunction, but cannot impart information about anatomic localization of the abnormal lung. Until recently, lung imaging provided only static anatomic information, but functional imaging using computed tomography can yield information about gas distribution, ventilation, vasculature, and ventilation/perfusion ($\dot{V}/\dot{Q}$) relationships. It can quantify and reveal the anatomic distribution of emphysema in the lung as well as provide information about airway size and respiratory mechanics.

Functional lung imaging has also expanded into the field of magnetic resonance with novel sequences in the field of proton magnetic resonance imaging and with the introduction of hyperpolarized noble gas imaging, such as ^{3}He imaging. ^{3}He is a biologically inert, non-radioactive, poorly absorbed gas that is used as a dynamic inhaled contrast agent to provide exquisite images of lung airspaces. When inhaled, dynamic cine images can be created and displayed which demonstrate helium ventilation in the lung. ^{3}He images can be processed mathematically to map the distribution of inhaled gas, the dimensions of distal airspaces, and even the partial pressure of oxygen in the airspaces. Further processes of signal intensity produce three-dimensional images of pulmonary $\dot{V}/\dot{Q}$ ratios. Topical heterogeneity of $\dot{V}/\dot{Q}$ matching may be a particularly sensitive indicator of early lung dysfunction. Clinically, it may be useful in the early detection of obliterative bronchiolitis following lung transplantation, and in the early detection of emphysema. Functional imaging may be particularly useful in guiding surgeons performing lung volume reduction surgery to target areas of diseased lung.

In the field of nuclear medicine, there have been great strides in metabolic imaging using 18F-fluorodeoxyglucose positron emission tomography (FDG-PET) and single proton emission-computed tomography (SPECT). FDG-PET has been shown useful in differentiating benign and malignant processes, and in imaging the activity of various inflammatory lung diseases. FDG-PET may help clinicians determine when to treat various lung diseases.

This book will describe the physiological basis of functional lung imaging and demonstrate its applicability to the study of lung disease. Functional imaging techniques will provide powerful tools in the medical armamentarium to help understand bodily function in health and disease. The field will improve insight in the diagnosis and treatment of various forms of human pathology.

David A. Lipson
Edwin J. R. van Beek

Contributors

Tobias Achenbach, MD   *Department of Radiology, Johannes Gutenberg University Medical School, Mainz, Germany*

Abass Alavi, MD   *Department of Radiology, Hospital of the University of Pennsylvania, Philadelphia, Pennsylvania, USA*

Talissa A. Altes, MD   *Department of Radiology, University of Virginia Health Sciences Center, Charlottesville, Virginia, USA*

Raanan Arens, MD   *Department of Medicine, University of Pennsylvania, Medical Center, Philadelphia, Pennsylvania, USA*

Catherine Beigelman-Aubry, MD   *Service de Radiologie, Hôpital de la Pitié-Salpêtrière, Paris, France*

Yves Berthezéne, MD, PhD   *Hôpital de la Croix Rousse, Service de Radiologie, Lyon, France*

Pietro Biondetti, MD   *UO Radiologia, Fondazione IRCCS—"Ospedale Maggiore Policlinico, Mangiagalli, Regina Elena" di Milano and Università degli Studi di Milano, Milano, Italy*

Harry R. Büller, MD, PhD *Department of Vascular Medicine, Academic Medical Center, Amsterdam, The Netherlands*

Eleonora Carlesso, MSc *Università degli Studi di Milano, Milano, Italy*

Qun Chen, PhD *Department of Radiology, New York University School of Medicine, New York, New York, USA*

Davide Chiumello, MD *Istituto di Anestesia e Rianimazione, Fondazione IRCCS—"Ospedale Maggiore Policlinico, Mangiagalli, Regina Elena" di Milano, Milano, Italy*

Yannick Crémillieux, PhD *Laboratoire de Résonance Magnétique Nucléaire, Domaine Scientifique de la Doua, Villeurbanne, France*

Asger Dirksen, MD, DSc *Department of Respiratory Medicine, Gentofte University Hospital, Hellerup, Denmark*

John Dunning, MB, BCh *Department of Cardiothoracic Surgery, Cambridge University School of Medicine, Cambridge, UK*

Balthasar Eberle, MD *Department of Anesthesiology, University of Berne, Berne, Switzerland*

Christoph Engelke, MD *Klinikum der Technischen Universität München, Munich, Germany*

Catalin Fetita, PhD *Department ARTEMIS, Institut National des Télécommunications, Evry, France*

Stanislao Fichele, PhD *Unit of Academic Radiology, University of Sheffield, Sheffield, UK*

Kevin R. Flaherty MD, MS *Department of Internal Medicine, University of Michigan Health System, Ann Arbor, Michigan, USA*

Luciano Gattinoni, MD, FRCP *Istituto di Anestesia e Rianimazione, Fondazione IRCCS—"Ospedale Maggiore Policlinico, Mangiagalli, Regina Elena" di Milano and Università degli Studi di Milano, Milano, Italy*

Philippe A. Grenier, MD *Service de Radiologie, Hôpital de la Pitié-Salpêtrière, Paris, France*

Naresh Gupta, MD *Department of Radiology, Hospital of the University of Pennsylvania, Philadelphia, Pennsylvania, USA*

Ieneke J. Hartmann, MD *University Medical Center Utrecht, Utrecht, The Netherlands*

Hiroto Hatabu, MD, PhD *Department of Radiology, Beth Israel Deaconess Medical Center and Harvard Medical School, Boston, Massachusetts, USA*

Tae Iwasawa, MD   *Department of Radiology, Kanagawa Cardiovascular and Respiratory Center, Kanazawa-ku, Yokohama, Japan*

Hans-Ulrich Kauczor, MD   *Department of Radiology, Deutsches Krebsforschungszentrum, Heidelberg, Germany*

Robert M. Kotloff, MD   *Department of Medicine, University of Pennsylvania Medical Center, Philadelphia, Pennsylvania, USA*

Justin W. Kung, MD   *Department of Radiology, Hospital of the University of Pennsylvania, Philadelphia, Pennsylvania, USA*

Yasuyuki Kurihara, MD   *Department of Radiology, St. Marianna University School of Medicine, Kanagawa, Japan*

Eduard E. de Lange, MD   *Department of Radiology, University of Virginia Health Sciences Center, Charlottesville, Virginia, USA*

David A. Lipson, MD   *Department of Medicine, University of Pennsylvania Medical Center, Philadelphia, Pennsylvania, USA*

Vu M. Mai, PhD   *Department of Radiology, Evanston Northwestern Healthcare, Evanston, Illinois and Feinberg School of Medicine at Northwestern University, Chicago, Illinois, USA*

Fernando J. Martinez, MD, MS   *Department of Internal Medicine, University of Michigan Health System, Ann Arbor, Michigan, USA*

Jahn Mortensen, MD, DSc   *Department of Clinical Physiology and Nuclear Medicine, Copenhagen University Hospital, Copenhagen, Denmark*

John P. Mugler, III, PhD   *Departments of Radiology and Biomedical Engineering, University of Virginia School of Medicine, Charlottesville, Virginia, USA*

Yoshiharu Ohno, MD, PhD   *Department of Radiology, Kobe University Graduate School of Medicine, Kobe, Japan*

Matthijs Oudkerk, MD, PhD   *Department of Radiology, State University Hospital, Groningen, The Netherlands*

Allan Pack, MB, ChB, PhD   *Department of Medicine, University of Pennsylvania Medical Center, Philadelphia, Pennsylvania, USA*

Mathias Prokop, MD   *University Medical Center Utrecht, Utrecht, The Netherlands*

Lewis J. Rubin, MD   *Pulmonary and Critical Care Medicine, University of California, La Jolla, California, USA*

Michael Salerno, MD, PhD   *Departments of Radiology and Biomedical Engineering, University of Virginia School of Medicine, Charlottesville, Virginia, USA*

Cornelia M. Schaefer-Prokop, MD   *Medical University of Vienna, Vienna, Austria*

Wolfgang G. Schreiber, PhD   *Department of Radiology, Johannes Gutenberg University Medical School, Mainz, Germany*

Richard J. Schwab, MD   *Department of Medicine, University of Pennsylvania, Philadelphia, Pennsylvania, USA*

Maaike Söhne, MD   *Department of Vascular Medicine, Academic Medical Center, Amsterdam, The Netherlands*

Trine Stavngaard, MD   *Department of Clinical Physiology and Nuclear Medicine, Copenhagen University Hospital, Copenhagen, Denmark*

Marije ten Wolde, MD   *Department of Vascular Medicine, Academic Medical Center, Amsterdam, The Netherlands*

Edwin J. R. van Beek, MD, PhD, FRCR   *Department of Radiology, Carver College of Medicine, University of Iowa, Iowa City, Iowa, USA and Unit of Academic Radiology, University of Sheffield, Sheffield, UK*

Jim M. Wild, PhD   *Unit of Academic Radiology, University of Sheffield, Sheffield, UK*

Hongming Zhuang, MD   *Department of Radiology, Hospital of the University of Pennsylvania, Philadelphia, Pennsylvania, USA*

Contents

PART II: COMPUTED TOMOGRAPHY

PART III: MAGNETIC RESONANCE

Part I: Introduction

1

Chest Radiography, Fluoroscopy, Angiography, and Pulmonary Function Testing

EDWIN J. R. VAN BEEK

University of Iowa, Iowa City,
Iowa, USA
University of Sheffield,
Sheffield, UK

DAVID A. LIPSON

University of Pennsylvania Medical Center,
Philadelphia, Pennsylvania, USA

I. Introduction

This book aims to describe the new developments in the assessment of pulmonary ventilatory and vascular disorders. However, it cannot be emphasized enough that the majority of patients with chest diseases are currently managed using fairly basic radiological techniques and lung function tests. This is due to factors such as convenience of access, costs of investigations, and experience with these techniques. This chapter will give a brief review of the most commonly used techniques. It does not aim to be complete, but rather highlights the techniques and their role in the routine care of patients with chest diseases. For the interested reader, excellent textbooks with detailed description of technique and indications for these tests exist (1–3).

II. Chest Radiography

The chest radiograph (CXR) has been available from the early days of the discovery of the Roentgen rays, and could be regarded an antique. That would, however, do the technique injustice, as novel methodologies (digital radiography, e.g.) have developed over the years.

CXRs are the most commonly requested investigations in a radiology department. As an integral part of the physician's armamentarium, it is widely accepted as a good tool to assess the general condition of a patient, whether this is related to cardiac diseases or lung diseases. In the current context of lung diseases, CXRs tend to be the first line investigation in most patients. This will include a wide range of disorders, ranging from the acute to the chronic disorders, from malignant to benign diseases. Given this range of diseases, it is only natural that CXR is not the most sensitive or specific test. However, when it comes to acute diseases, it is a good method to detect, for instance, pneumothorax (Fig. 1.1), pneumonia, and symptomatic lung malignancies. In the chronic disorders, it may be used for the follow-up of patients with chronic obstructive pulmonary disease (Fig. 1.2), lung fibrosis, and asbestosis. Furthermore, the CXR is the method of choice for monitoring of ill patients and the position of essential lines and tubes in the intensive care unit.

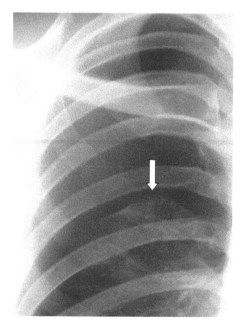

Figure 1.1   Pneumothorax: the arrow points to the superior outline of the right lung.

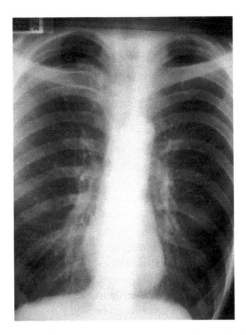

Figure 1.2 Emphysema: the lungs are hyper expanded, the diaphragm has lost its normal curvature and the heart is in a vertical position. Hyperinflation may cause parts of the image to be cut off, requiring repeat imaging.

The CXR may comprise a single postero-anterior projection film with or without lateral view. In debilitated patients, for instance, in the intensive care unit or those that are unable to lie flat, it may be necessary to adjust the basic technique, and anteroposterior views and recumbent or supine views may be required. For the assessment of lung apices, an apical lordotic view, with the beam at an angle of $\sim40°$ cephalad angulation is required.

In this context, it should be remembered that the use of additional films is increasingly being replaced by computed tomography and related techniques. In particular, the development of low-dose multidetector CT has decreased the need for plain radiographs of the chest.

III. Fluoroscopy

The main advantage of fluoroscopy over the plain CXR is its capability to allow the study of the chest while movement takes place. Thus, it can be used to further localize a lesion (e.g., is it in the lung or related to the chest wall), to guide interventions, such as bronchoscopic or transthoracic biopsy procedures, and to study diaphragmatic movement (although this may also be studied using ultrasonography). However, it does not replace CXR, as its inherent spatial resolution is inferior.

Fluoroscopy is increasingly becoming obsolete, as newer imaging techniques, such as ultrasound, CT, and ultrafast MRI, dominate the field. Nevertheless, needle insertion for biopsy or guided aspiration and central line insertion and positioning may still rely on this method.

IV. Angiography

Within the chest, both the pulmonary and the systemic circulation integrally connect. Traditional angiography, as a diagnostic procedure to evaluate large vessel circulatory pathology, is increasingly replaced by CT-angiography (CTA) and MR-angiography (MRA), as these procedures are noninvasive and generally carry a lower radiation burden.

Pulmonary angiography is still seen as the reference method for the diagnosis of pulmonary vascular disorders, such as pulmonary embolism (Fig. 1.3), but its use is increasingly limited due to its poor availability and the lack of trained radiologists to perform this procedure.

Angiography of the other main vessels in the chest has virtually been completely replaced by CTA and MRA. Arch aortography may still be used in acute major trauma victims where a traumatic rupture of the aorta is suspected. However, even this indication has now largely been replaced by multidetector CTA.

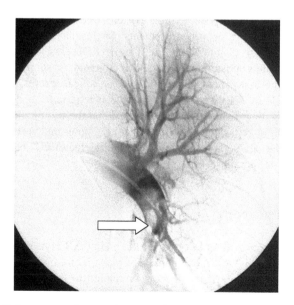

Figure 1.3 Pulmonary angiogram demonstrating central emboli.

V. Pulmonary Function Tests

Pulmonary function tests (PFTs) are a critical set of tools for the physician and physiologist, which yield important *global* information regarding lung function. While the history of respiratory physiology likely dates back to at least the 17th century, modern pulmonary function testing developed its roots in the past half-century with the advent of modern electronics and computing. In a similar way, modern postprocessing and computing have propelled forward the imaging techniques discussed in this book.

Complete pulmonary function testing usually refers to spirometry, before and after bronchodilator administration, measurement of lung volumes, and measurement of diffusion capacity. Respiratory muscle strength may also be evaluated by determination of maximal inspiratory pressures and maximal expiratory pressures.

PFTs quantitate respiratory capacity based on the ability of the subject to move various volumes of air in and out of their lungs. Using a machine called a spirometer, one may measure the forced expiratory volume (FVC), which is the maximum volume of air expelled from the lung following a maximal inspiration. Additionally, it measures the forced expiratory volume in one second (FEV_1), which is the volume expired during the first second of an FVC maneuver. The ratio of FEV_1 to FVC yields important clues regarding underlying airflow obstruction or pulmonary restrictive disease. Evaluation of flow-volume loops can also detect intra-thoracic and extra-thoracic airway obstruction.

There are many indications for performance of spirometry. It may be used to evaluate the severity of lung dysfunction in patients with known pulmonary disease, evaluate pulmonary symptoms such as dyspnea or cough, screen patients at risk for pulmonary disease, or assess pulmonary risk in patients about to undergo surgical procedures (4). It is also commonly performed to evaluate and follow disease progression or useful in widespread epidemiologic studies of lung health and disease (5). Several groups including the American Thoracic Society and the European Respiratory Society have published guidelines on the proper performance of these tests to ensure valid, statistically reproducible measurements (6–8).

Administration of a bronchodilator followed by repeated spirometric measurements is useful in determination of the degree of reversibility of airflow obstruction. An increase in lung volume by at least 12% and ≥ 200 mL indicates significant reversibility.

Divisions of lung volumes and capacities are graphically represented by plotting changes in lung volume while performing various respiratory maneuvers over time (Fig. 1.4) (9). The inspiratory reserve volume (IRV) refers to the maximal volume of air that may be inspired after a normal inspiration. The tidal volume (TV) refers to the volume of air that is inspired during normal, quiet respiration. In contrast, the expiratory reserve volume (ERV) refers to the maximal amount of air that can be expired after end-expiration. The residual

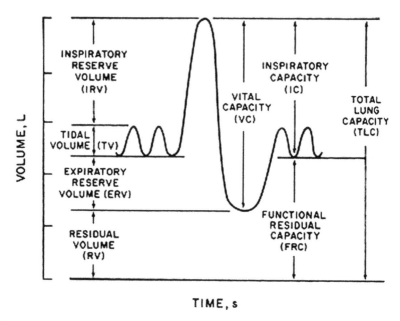

Figure 1.4 Spirometric lung volumes and capacities obtained by graphing changes in lung volume over time while performing respiratory maneuvers. [Adapted from Grippi et al. (9).]

volume (RV) refers to the volume of gas in the thoracic cavity after maximal exhalation. The vital capacity (VC) is the maximal volume of gas exhaled after a maximal inspiration (represented by the sum of IRV, TV, and ERV), whereas the inspiratory vital capacity (IVC) represents the maximal volume of gas that may be inspired following maximal exhalation. The inspiratory capacity (IC) is the volume of air that can be inhaled following a normal exhalation. The IC is the sum of IRV and TV. The functional residual capacity (FRC) refers to the volume of gas in the chest following a quiet exhalation. The FRC is the sum of RV and ERV. Total lung capacity (TLC), as its name implies, is the sum of all the gas volumes in the chest and represents the total amount of gas in the chest following a maximal inspiration.

In practice, there are several ways to determine the TLC of a patient. The helium dilution or nitrogen washout techniques are commonly used, but these may underestimate lung capacity, especially in patients with obstructive lung disease. The most accurate method is performance of body plethysmography. Routine chest X-rays can be used to estimate lung volumes, but this is not often performed in routine clinical practice.

Measurement of diffusion capacity using the single-breath diffusing capacity for carbon monoxide (DL_{CO}) is useful in the evaluation of numerous lung diseases (10). In patients with airflow obstruction, a decrease in the diffusion capacity helps to separate emphysema from other causes of airflow obstruction, such as asthma. Decreased diffusion also helps identify patients at risk for oxyhemoglobin desaturation with exertion, who may benefit from desaturation testing. The DL_{CO} may also identify patients with early pulmonary vascular disease or chronic thromboembolic disease. A low DL_{CO} in combination with a low FEV_1 has also been shown to identify patients at significantly higher risk of mortality following surgical lung volume reduction surgery (11,12).

Despite their utility, PFTs only impart information regarding total lung function, and can yield little *regional* information about lung function. Regional information may yield increased sensitivity to (and detection of) early disease. In future, the imaging techniques that are discussed in the following chapters may help fill in some of the regional information that is lacking in the PFTs of today.

References

1. Armstrong P, Wilson AG, Dee P, Hansell DM, eds. Imaging of diseases of the chest. 2nd ed. St. Louis: Mosby, 1995.
2. Grainger RG, Allison D, Adam A, Dixon AK, eds. Diagnostic radiology—a textbook of medical imaging. 4th ed. London: Churchill Livingstone, 2002.
3. Fraser RS, Müller NL, Colman N, Paré P, eds. Diagnosis of diseases of the chest. Philadelphia: WB Saunders, 1999.
4. Zibrak JD, O'Donnell CR, Marton K. Indications for pulmonary function testing. Ann Int Med 1990; 112:763–771.
5. Crapo RO. Pulmonary function testing. N Engl J Med 1994; 331:25–30.
6. Standardized Lung Function Testing: Official Statement of the European Respiratory Society. Eur Respir J 1993; 6(suppl 16):1–100.
7. American Thoracic Society. Lung function testing: selection of reference values and interpretative strategies. Am Rev Respir Dis 1991; 144:1202–1218.
8. Stocks J, Quanjer PD. Reference values for residual volume, functional residual capacity and total lung capacity: ATS workshop on lung volume measurements. Official Statement of the European Respiratory Society. Eur Respir J 1995; 8:492–506.
9. Grippi MA, Metzger LF, Sacks AV, Fishman AP. Pulmonary function testing. In: Fishman AP, Elias JA, Fishman JA, Grippi MA, Kaiser LR, Senior RM, eds. Fishman's Pulmonary Diseases and Disorders. 3rd ed. New York: McGraw-Hill, 1998.
10. Single breath carbon monoxide diffusing capacity (transfer factor): recommendations for a standard technique: Statement of the American Thoracic Society. Am Rev Respir Dis 1987; 136:1299–1307.
11. National Emphysema Treatment Trial Research Group. Patients at high risk of mortality from lung volume reduction surgery. N Engl J Med 2001; 345:1075–1083.
12. National Emphysema Treatment Trial Research Group. A randomized trial comparing lung-volume—reduction surgery with medical therapy for severe emphysema. N Engl J Med 2003; 348:2059–2073.

Part II: Computed Tomography

2

Computed Tomography: Introduction to CT Imaging

**PHILIPPE A. GRENIER and
CATHERINE BEIGELMAN-AUBRY**

Hôpital de la Pitié–Salpêtrière,
Paris, France

CATALIN FETITA

Institut National des Télécommunications,
Evry, France

I. Introduction

There have been great advances in computed tomography (CT) scanner technology over the past several years. New generation CT scanners, called multislice or multidetector row CT (MDCT), permit multiplanar reformation and 3D reconstruction of the airways, and enhanced image analysis. This has made possible accurate and reproducible quantitative assessment of the airways and lung attenuation at a specific, spirometrically controlled lung volume during CT acquisition, rendering functional CT imaging of the lung a reality. This offers new perspectives for better insight in pathophysiology of obstructive lung disease, particularly asthma and chronic obstructive pulmonary disease (COPD), and to monitor the effects of current and future therapies.

II. Image Acquisition

A. Imaging Principles

CT imaging is based on the principle that the internal structure of an object can be reconstructed from multiple X-ray projections. The CT image is a 2D representation of a 3D cross-sectional slice, the third dimension being the section or slice thickness (collimation) (1). Helical (spiral) CT is a major technical advance that allows continuous scanning while the patient is continuously moved through the CT gantry (2). With this technique, patient translation into the gantry and X-ray source rotation occur simultaneously during data acquisition. Therefore, the X-ray beam traces a helical curve in relation to the patient. Each rotation of the X-ray tube can be considered to generate data, which is specific to an angled plane of section. Cross-sectional images can be reconstructed after these plane specific data are obtained. This mathematical calculation is performed by interpolation of the helical data above and below each plane of section. Most current helical CT scanners reorder the projection data and perform interpolation from views separated by 180° to optimize resolution in the longitudinal axis (3). The position and spacing of these images can be chosen retrospectively for arbitrary table positions and at small increments.

In the early 1990s, the first MDCT scanner was developed by using two rows of detectors. This helical scanner simply placed two single-row detectors side by side, doubling the rate of data acquisition. Owing to the development of multidetector arrays and advances in engineering, in the late 1990s, a new generation of MDCT scanners became available (4). The detector arrays on these scanners are segmented into multiple rows or arcs perpendicular to the longitudinal or *z*-axis. MDCT scanners may have 2, 4, 8, 16, 32, or 64 rows of detectors, permitting the acquisition of 2, 4, 8, or 16 slices per rotation. This technique provides an increased data acquisition speed used either to increase the volume of tissue scanned or to scan the same volume with reduced slice thickness.

B. Slice Thickness

A CT image is composed of multiple picture elements (typically a 512×512 matrix) known as pixels. A pixel is a unit area, that is, each square on the image matrix, which reflects the attenuation of a unit volume of tissue, or voxel (the area of the pixel multiplied by the scan collimation). The X-ray attenuations of the structures within a given voxel are averaged to produce the image. This volume averaging results in loss of spatial resolution: the thicker the slice, the lower the ability of CT to resolve small structures. On the other hand, as section thickness decreases, noise increases, and images are grainer as a result. The optimal effective slice thickness is therefore ≤ 1.25 mm (0.6 or 0.75 mm when using a 16, 32 or 64 detector rows CT scanner) rendering isotropic or near isotropic image reconstruction feasible (1).

C. Radiation Dose

Because of the great natural contrast between the airways, the lung parenchyma and their environment, relatively low kilovoltage (120 kVp) and milliamperage (40–80 mA) may be used in lung CT imaging (5,6). Choi et al. (7) showed recently that image quality of surface rendered 3D images of the central airways is preserved when the tube current decreases from 240 to 50 mA. This resulted in an effective radiation dose of MDCT of the chest of 0.75–1.5 mSv, which is equivalent to the dose of a lateral chest radiograph, $\sim$5–10 pA (8).

D. Rotation Time

The time required to obtain the image (scan time) is determined by the time required for the gantry rotation. In most modern CT scanners, the scan time is on the order of 0.3–0.5 s. A faster scanning speed can be achieved by using electron beam or helical CT. In electron beam CT, the X-ray beam is produced by a focused electron beam that sweeps around a tungsten ring encircling the patient. This technique allows images to be acquired in ≤ 100 ms and has been particularly useful in assessing dynamic changes such as tracheal configuration and cross-sectional area during forced expiration (9).

With MDCT, the entire chest may be completed during a 8 s breath hold while using a 0.6 or 1.25 mm-slice thickness. Faster gantry rotation time decreases the effect of cardiac motion on noncardiac gated acquisitions. The combination of faster gantry rotation time, the simultaneous acquisition of the patient's electrocardiogram, and specialized reconstruction techniques can provide nearly motion-free images during cardiac systole or diastole (10). Cardiac gated images allow the calculation of cardiac volumes and ejection fraction. Cardiac gated reconstruction improves image quality in the great vessels and in structures bordering the heart, particularly, the airways in the right middle lobe and lingula.

E. Lung Volume at Acquisition

Airway imaging is routinely performed at end inspiration during a simple breath hold. Additional scanning is also required during continuous or suspended expiration in patients with either suspected tracheobronchomalacia to assess the degree of abnormal expiratory collapse of the proximal airways at expiration or suspicion of small airway disease to assess the presence and extent of expiratory air trapping. In such cases, a low dose technique (40 mA) is recommended to decrease radiation exposure (11).

The most commonly used technique for the assessment of air trapping by CT is based on postexpiratory CT scans, obtained during suspended respiration following a forced exhalation. Alternatively, dynamic CT acquisition during continuous expiration may be performed (11,12). Motion artifacts, which increase with decreasing temporal resolution, represent the major limitations of continuous expiratory CT. However, a dynamic expiratory maneuver performed during helical CT acquisition may provide good results despite a 0.5 s scanning time per image. The use of 180° linear interpolation algorithms with a 0.5 s rotation time provides images representing scanning periods of ~250 ms. Moreover, motion artifacts are at a maximum during the early phase of expiration and at a minimum during its late phase, which thereby allows good visualization of lobular air trapping with helical CT. Dynamic expiratory maneuvers (called continuous expiratory CT) is performed during helical CT acquisition throughout the last phase of expiration, and may provide reasonable images without significant artifacts (12). Patients can have greater difficulty maintaining the residual volume after a completed exhalation than during an active exhalation, when they have to continue the expiratory effort until the end of the acquisition. The air trapping extent and the relative contrast scores obtained with continuous expiratory CT have proven to be significantly higher than those obtained with suspended end expiratory CT (12). Low dose continuous expiratory MDCT of the chest has become routine in some institutions to depict air trapping (11).

As lung attenuation and airway cross-section areas at CT vary with the volume of the lung during breath hold, quantitative assessment of lung attenuation and airway dimension needs to be performed on images acquired at a selected controlled lung volume. The control of lung volume at CT is obtained by spirometric triggering. During exhalation, the spirometer and the associated microcomputer measure the volume of the gas expired and trigger the CT scanner after the specific volume is reached (13). As the trigger signal is generated, airflow is inhibited by closure of a mechanical occlusion device attached to the spirometer and scanning starts.

F. Field of View

CT scanning should be performed with a field of view large enough to encompass the patient. In general, the commonest matrix available (usually 512 × 512) should be used in image reconstruction to reduce pixel size. Using a field of view of 40 cm and a 512×512 matrix results in a pixel size of 0.78 mm^2. Targeting the image prospectively or retrospectively to a smaller field of view decreases pixel size and increases spatial resolution. For example, targeting the image to a field of view of 13 cm, results in a pixel size of 0.25 mm^2 (14).

G. Image Reconstruction

The continuous nature of CT data acquisition allows true volumetric scanning and the production of multiple overlapping images that result in increased spatial resolution in the longitudinal axis. These overlapping reconstructions allow the production of high-quality multiplanar and 3D reformations without additional radiation exposure. This also eliminates motion artifacts that otherwise degrade image quality.

The CT scan data are reconstructed by using either a standard, soft tissue algorithm that smooths the image and reduces visible image noise, or a high-spatial frequency reconstruction algorithm for optimal assessment of the lung parenchyma. The high-spatial frequency algorithm reduces image smoothing and increases spatial resolution, thereby allowing better depiction of normal and abnormal parenchymal interfaces and thus better visualization of small vessels and bronchi (14,15). The soft tissue algorithm is recommended for quantitative assessment of lung attenuation whereas the high-spatial frequency algorithm is recommended for assessing the airways.

III. Image Visualization and Postprocessing

A. Window Settings

CT numbers in the thorax range from -1000 HU for air in the trachea to $\sim 700 \text{ HU}$ for dense bones. To display the large number of attenuation values (HU) within a limited number of shades of gray, a CT number is selected that corresponds to approximately the mean attenuation value of the tissue being examined. This center CT attenuation value is called the window level. The computer is then instructed to assign one shade of gray to a certain number of CT attenuation values above and below the window level. The range of CT numbers above and below the window level is called the window width. To adequately depict the lungs, a window level of -600 to -700 HU and window width of $1000-1500 \text{ HU}$ are most commonly recommended (16) [Fig. 2.1(a)]. However, for quantitative assessment of the airways, a window level of -450 to -500 HU and a window width of $1000-1500 \text{ HU}$ are recommended (16) [Fig. 2.1(b)].

B. Cine Viewing

Visualization of the overlapped thin axial images sequentially in a cine-mode allows the bronchial divisions to be followed from the segmental origin to the

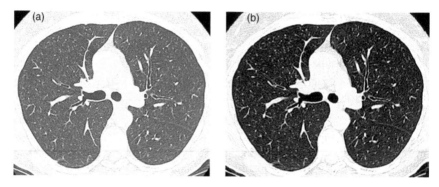

Figure 2.1 Axial 1.25 mm CT scan at the anatomic level including the right and left main bronchi, after MDCT acquisition at suspended full inspiration. (a) Normal appearance of bronchi, vessels and lung parenchyma at −600 HU window level and 1600 HU width. (b) Normal appearance of bronchi, vessels and lung parenchyma at −400 HU level and 1200 HU width.

distal bronchial lumens down to the smallest bronchi that can be identified on thin section images. This viewing technique helps to indicate the segmental and sub-segmental distribution of any airway lesion and may serve as a roadmap for the endoscopist. Moving up and down through the volume at the monitor has become an alternative to film-based review. Image processing includes multiplanar reformations and techniques that produce 3D images, such as minimum intensity projection (mIP) or 3D surface shaded display and volume rendering (17) (Fig. 2.2). The in-plane resolution is defined by the reconstruction kernel and field of view, whereas the through-plane or z-axis resolution is defined by the collimator width, pitch, and interpolation algorithm. Therefore, as the angle of the reformation plane increases relative to the plane of acquisition, spatial resolution decreases.

C. Multiplanar Reformations

These are the easiest reconstructions to generate, usually interactive in real time at the console or workstation. They permit the creation of images in the plane oriented along the long axis of any airway [Fig. 2.2(b)]. Whereas the thickness of the displayed planar image is 0.6–0.8 mm, depending on the dimension of the field of view, multiplanar volume reconstruction (MPVR) consists of a slab with a thickness of several pixels and results in a less noisy reformation (18) [Fig. 2.2(e)]. MPVR may be associated with the use of the intensity projection techniques. A section of the reformation plane may be chosen from the 3D reconstructed image of the airways (19).

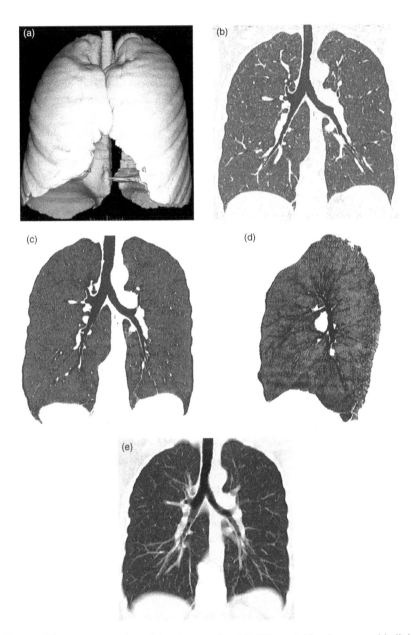

Figure 2.2 Reconstruction of the airways after MDCT acquisition in a normal individual. (a) 3D surface reconstruction of airways and lung parenchyma. (b) Coronal oblique reformated image of the airways (0.6 mm thick curvilinear plane). (c) MPVR–mIP image (10 mm thick slab) in a coronal view. (d) MPVR–mIP image in a sagittal slab perpendicular to the right hilum. (e) MPVR (10 mm thick slab) in a coronal view permitting a good assessment of the relationships between vessels and airways.

D. Minimum Intensity Projection (mIP)

mIP imaging is a simple form of volume rendering that is able to project the tracheobronchial air column into a viewing plane. It is usually applied to a selected volume of the thorax containing the airways under evaluation (sliding thin slab or MPVR–mIP technique) [Fig. 2.2(c) and (d)]. Pixels encode the minimum voxel value encountered by each ray. Airways are visualized because air contained within the tracheobronchial tree is lower in attenuation than surrounding pulmonary parenchyma, with a small density difference between pulmonary parenchyma and airways of 50 and 150 HU (20).

E. 3D Surface Rendering Technique with Shaded Display (3D-SSD)

Another method is the 3D surface rendering technique with shaded display (3D-SSD) [Fig. 2.2(a)]. In this technique, the surface of the volume of air contained in the airways is isolated from the initial volume data by thresholding segmentation (18,19,21). Shading the surface obtained from depth encoding optimally renders the impression of depth. The major limitation of this technique is related to thresholding range. The result of reconstruction is also sensitive to volume partial artifacts, stair step artifacts, and motion-related artifacts (19). In addition, voxels fractionally composed of the tissue and air are not integrated in the final image (18).

F. CT Bronchography

CT bronchography is a new functionality consisting segmentation of the lumen–wall interface of the airways. Rémy-Jardin et al. (22) used a continuous rim of peripheral voxels and a volume rendering algorithm. This technique has proven to be of particular interest in diagnosing mild changes in airway caliber and understanding complex tracheobronchial abnormalities (23). Using the same concept, Fetita et al. (24) developed a fully automatic method for 3D bronchial tree reconstruction based on bronchial lumen detection within the thoracic volume data set obtained from thin multidetector CT acquisition and thin collimation during breath hold. It provides a specific visualization modality relying on an energy-based 3D reconstruction of the bronchial tree up to the sixth to seventh-order subdivisions with a semi-transparent volume rendering technique (25) (Fig. 2.3). In addition, automatic delimitation and indexation of anatomical segments making possible local and reproducible analysis at a given level of the bronchial tree, and an automatic extraction of the central axis of the bronchial tree, which simplifies the interactivity during the navigation within CT bronchography or virtual endoscopy modes. These tools can also be used for quantitative assessment of the wall and lumens of the airways on cross-section images of the bronchi reconstructed perpendicular to their central axis.

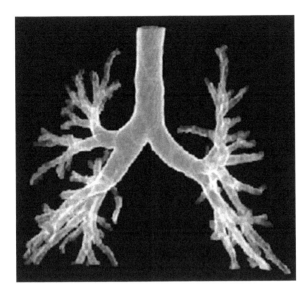

Figure 2.3 CT bronchogram in a normal individual after MDCT acquisition in a frontal view.

G. Virtual Bronchoscopy

Virtual bronchoscopy provides an internal rendering of the tracheobronchial walls and lumen. Owing to a perspective rendering algorithm, this simulates an endoscopist's view of the internal surface of the airways (Fig. 2.4). The observer may interactively move through the airways. This technique may be obtained from both 3D surface rendering and volume rendering techniques. The volume rendering technique is less sensitive to partial volume effects than surface rendering. Powerful computers permit realtime rendering (15–25 images/s) making virtual "flying" within the airways possible. Virtual endoscopy is applicable to the central airways including the subsegmental bronchi. The technique allows accurate reproduction of major endoluminal abnormalities with an excellent correlation with fiberoptic bronchoscopy results regarding the location, severity, and shape of airway narrowing (25). Virtual bronchoscopy is also able to visualize the bronchial tree beyond an obstructive lesion, and thus, one may perform a "retroscopy" by looking back at the distal part of the stenosis. Despite these appreciable abilities, virtual endoscopy remains very sensitive to the partial volume averaging effect and motion artifacts. Discontinuities in the walls of airways can be artifactually created and structures typically appear irregular due to the polygonal modeling applied to the surfaces (20,26). In addition, virtual endoscopy is unable to identify all causes of bronchial obstruction (17). Mild stenosis, submucosal infiltration, and superficial spreading tumors are not well identified (18).

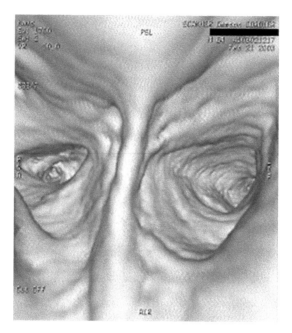

Figure 2.4 Virtual bronchoscopy in a patient with COPD. Descending view from the trachea showing abnormal thickening of the carina and irregularities of the mucosal surface.

IV. Image Analysis

A. Bronchi and Vessel Appearances

The appearance of bronchi and vessels depends on their orientation: when imaged along their long axes, they appear as cylindrical structures that taper as they branch; when imaged at an angle to their longitudinal axes, they appear as rounded structures if perpendicular to the plane of the CT, or as elliptical structures when oriented obliquely (Fig. 2.1). The outer walls of pulmonary vessels form smooth and sharply defined interfaces with the surrounding lung. Central pulmonary vessels can be readily recognized as arteries by their location adjacent to bronchi (Fig. 2.1). Central pulmonary veins can be identified as they course toward the left atrium. The outer diameter of a bronchus is approximately equal to that of the adjacent pulmonary artery. However, the apparent bronchial wall thickness and the diameter of bronchi and vessels are markedly influenced by the display parameters. According to three studies based on phantoms (27,28) and inflated-fixed lung specimens (29), the window and width levels that provide the most accurate measurement of bronchial caliber and wall thickness are −450 to −500 and 1000–1500 HU, respectively. When an incorrect parameter is used, the error in estimating the thickness or size of a structure is related to its actual thickness or size: greater fractional overestimates or under-estimates are made for smaller structures.

The pulmonary artery-to-outer bronchial diameter ratio, measured in a study of 30 patients without cardiopulmonary disease on thin collimation scans was 0.98 ± 0.14 (range, 0.53–1.39) (30). The measurement was influenced by altitude, presumably as a result of the combination of hypoxic vasoconstriction and bronchodilatation. In one investigation of 17 normal, nonsmoking subjects living at 1600 m and 16 living at sea level, the mean bronchoarterial ratio was 0.76 at altitude and 0.62 at sea level (31).

Although the mean internal bronchial diameter-to-pulmonary arterial diameter and the mean outer bronchial diameter-to-pulmonary artery diameter ratios at sea level are approximately 0.65 and 1, respectively, there is considerable variation in these ratios within a given segment or lobe (32). Anatomically, the normal bronchial wall thickness is usually equivalent to ~10–15% of the bronchial diameter (33). This measure is slightly overestimated on CT because of inaccuracies in boundary detection, the CT measurement including the surrounding peribronchial interstitium. In one study of 502 normal subsegmental bronchi in 30 patients, the mean inner-to-outer bronchial diameter ratio was found to be 0.66 ± 0.06 (range, 0.51–0.86) (30). This ratio corresponds to a mean bronchial wall thickness equivalent to 17% of the luminal diameter with a range of 7–25%. In another investigation in six healthy men, bronchial wall area and percent wall area were assessed by thin collimation CT (34). Bronchial wall area was 14 mm^2 for airways 2–4 mm in diameter, 25 mm^2 for airways 4–6 mm in diameter and 43 mm^2 for airways >6 mm in diameter. The relative airway wall area increased as the size of the airway decreased, the percent wall area increasing from 55% in airways >6 mm in diameter to 81% in airways <2 mm in diameter. Because of pixel size and the spatial resolution of CT, it is difficult to obtain accurate measurements of airways measuring <2 mm in diameter.

B. Quantitative CT Assessment of Airways

Airway lumen and airway wall areas may be quantitatively assessed on CT images by using specific techniques that must be reproducible as well as accurate in order to compare the airways pre and postintervention (bronchoprovocation, bronchodilatation, and therapeutic response) and to carry out longitudinal studies of airway remodeling. Airway lumen and wall areas measured on axial images depend on the lung volume, and angle between the airway central axis and the plane of section. Volumetric acquisition at controlled lung volume is required in order to precisely match the airways of an individual on repeated studies.

Measurements of airway lumen and wall area have to be restricted to airways that appear to have been cut in cross-section based on the apparent roundness of the airway lumen. Measuring airway lumen and airway walls when they are not perpendicular to the scanning plane may lead to significant errors, the magnitude of which will depend on how acutely the airways are angled, the collimation, and the field of view. The larger the angle and field of view and the thicker the collimation, the greater the overestimation airway wall area. Most of the airways examined in axial CT slices are also more likely to be running obliquely to the plane of the section, rather than perpendicularly, owing to the anatomy of the lung. With MDCT, it becomes possible to acquire a volume of lung with slice thickness $\leq 0.6-0.75$ mm and to reconstruct axial images every 0.6 mm or less by interpolation; in such a maneuver, the CT voxels may be converted into cubic dimension (isotropic voxels). Segmentation of the bronchial lumens and reconstruction of the airways in 3D then allow determination of the central axis of the airways, and reconstruction of the airway cross-section in a plane perpendicular to this axis [Fig. 2.5(a) and (b)]. This analysis technique overcomes the major limitation to the use of high-resolution computed tomography (HRCT) in quantitative analysis, which is that accurate or true airway lumen and airway wall area can only be measured from airways which are oriented approximately perpendicular to the plane of scanning [Fig. 2.5(c) and (d)].

Different image analysis techniques have been developed to make measurements of airway dimensions on CT scans. McNamara et al. (28) modified a method developed by Webb et al. (27) on the basis of visual analysis of photographed images. They found that it was crucial to use a window level of -450 HU. Amirav et al. (35) developed a computerized algorithm for measuring airway lumen area, based on an edge detection method using the full width at half maximum principle that has advantages of less subjectivity and greater speed than the method of McNamara et al. (28). With Prêteux et al. (36) we developed an automatic method for segmentation and calculation of airway lumen areas based on mathematical morphology theory, marking techniques derived from the concept of connection cost, and conditional watershed segmentation [Fig. 2.5(e)]. Wood et al. (37) developed an algorithm to measure airway lumens and the airway angle of orientation using 3D reconstruction of the lung. This technique allowed cross sectional images of the airways to be generated irrespective of airway of orientation. King et al. (38) more recently developed an automatic computed tomographic image analysis algorithm to measure not only the airway lumen areas but also the wall areas and angle of orientation of airways. Perot et al. (39) had a different approach with similar results as King et al. (38). These results proved to be more accurate than those obtained with manual methods. All these analysis algorithms have been validated using data from phantom studies (28,35–38) and excised animal lungs (38,39), or by developing a realistic modeling of airways and pulmonary arteries included in CT scans of animal lungs obtained *in vivo* (36). Their accuracy in measuring the airways lumen (28,35,36,38) and wall (38,39) areas was only acceptable for bronchi measuring at least 2 mm in diameter. These techniques have been used to quantify the magnitude and distribution of airway narrowing in excised and

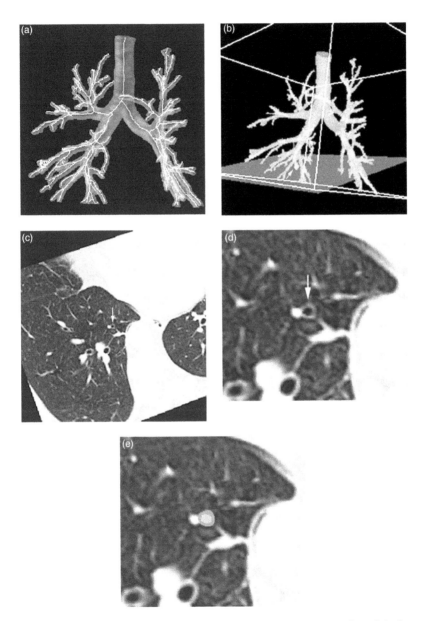

Figure 2.5 Quantitative assessment of the airways. (a) 3D reconstruction of the bronchial tree and its central axis. (b) Positioning of a reformatted plane strictly perpendicular to the central axis of the airway, in a point selected on a subsegmental bronchus of the paracardiac segment of the right lower lobe. (c) Reformatted oblique CT slice perpendicular to the bronchus selected in b. (d) Targeting on the selected bronchial cross-section. (e) Segmentation of the inner and outer contours of the selected bronchial cross-section to calculate the bronchial wall area.

in vivo animal lungs, and in normal and asthmatic subjects (28,35,40–42). Although they have been used almost exclusively for research purposes, they likely will, with continued refinements, eventually be of benefit in the clinical practice of radiology (43–46).

C. Lung Parenchyma

Attenuation of lung parenchyma is determined by the relative proportions of blood, gas, extravascular fluid, and pulmonary tissue in the image (47). Normal lung parenchyma has a fairly homogeneous attenuation that is slightly greater than that of air. However, a gradient is normally present, the attenuation being greater in the dependent than in the nondependent regions (47,48) (Fig. 2.6). The gradient is also larger at the lung bases than at the lung apices, though the attenuation gradient is usually relatively small (on the order of 50–100 HU) (32). The anteroposterior increase in attenuation is not homogeneous. For example, there is typically a discontinuity at the major fissure, with the posterior aspect of the upper lobes having greater attenuation than the anterior aspect of the lower lobes (49) (Fig. 2.7). In some normal individuals, the lingula and superior segments of the lower lobes have relatively low attenuation when compared with other lung regions (49). As lung gas volume is reduced, lung attenuation increases, the increase being greatest in the dependent portions of the lung (49–51).

Normal lung attenuation is also influenced by the degree of inflation (lung volume), capillary blood volume, and varies considerably between lung regions at different times in the normal respiratory cycle. The dependent and nondependent gradient of attenuation is significantly greater at a lung volume of 10% vital capacity than at a volume of 90% vital capacity in both the supine and prone positions. To obtain accurate and reproducible measurements of lung attenuation, it is necessary to use spirometrically gated CT. This procedure allows the selection

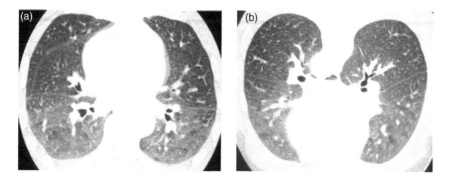

Figure 2.6 Normal thin collimation CT scan acquired at suspended full expiration in supine (a) and prone (b) positions. In expiration, lung attenuation and the dependent-nondependent attenuation gradient increases, while lung cross-section area decreases.

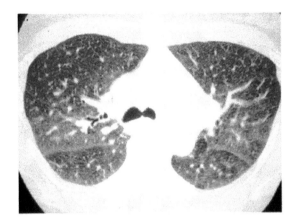

Figure 2.7 Axial CT scan at the level of the upper lobes obtained at maximum suspended expiration in supine position. The dependent–nondependent attenuation gradient has a lobar component. Lung attenuation within the upper segment of the lower lobe behind the fissure appears lower than the posterior part of the upper lobe before the fissure.

of a specific point in the respiratory cycle at which flow can be interrupted by closing a valve in the spirometer and CT can be obtained (51,52). With this technique, the mean lung attenuation in a normal subject has been shown to be approximately -760 HU at 20% vital capacity, -835 HU at 50% vital capacity, and -860 HT at 80% vital capacity (52). By linear extrapolation it has been estimated that the mean lung attenuation away from visible vessels at 0% and 100% vital capacity would be -730 and -895 HU, respectively, which corresponds to a change in lung density of 0.27–0.105 g/mL (51). In a study, in which thin collimation CT was performed in 42 healthy subjects who were examined at maximum of inspiration, the mean lung attenuation was found to be -866 HU, which corresponds to a mean lung density of 0.134 g/mL (53).

Although the mean attenuation values within any given area of lung show a relatively smooth gradient from the apical to the caudal regions and from the nondependent to the most dependent regions, there is a wide range of attenuation values within any unit volume or pixel. In one study, frequency distribution analysis demonstrated that $\sim$13% of the lung had attenuation values < -900 HU, 57% had attenuation values between -899 and -800 HU, 17% had attenuation values between -799 and -700 HU, and 13% had attenuation values > -699 HU (54).

During the respiratory cycle, in normal individuals, there is a significant correlation between the decrease in cross-sectional area and the increase in lung attenuation in each of the lung zones. There is no significant difference in mean attenuation values between men and women. There is also no significant correlation between mean lung density and age, although there is slight correlation between age and the percentage of lung attenuation values < -950 HU (53).

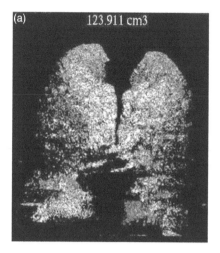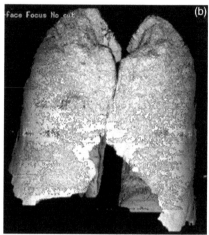

Figure 2.8 Quantitative assessment of emphysema by the "density mask" technique. (a) All the pixels having an attenuation value lower than -950 HU are segmented, counted and displayed in a 3D coronal projection. The volume of emphysema is calculated. (b) The pixels of emphysema are superimposed to the 3D surface reconstruction of the lungs providing a good display of the distribution of emphysema within the lungs.

Although measurements of lung attenuation usually have a limited role in clinical assessment of lung parenchyma, there are some exceptions. Attenuation values are useful to determine the presence, distribution, and extent of emphysema (55–57) (Fig. 2.8). They are also useful in the quantitative assessment of expiratory air trapping on CT scans performed at full expiration (58,59), and helpful in the assessment of the presence of inflammation in the small airways of smokers (60) and in patients with mild intermittent asthma (42).

References

1. Fraser RS, Muller NL, Colman N, Pare PD. Methods of radiologic investigation. In: Fraser RS, Muller NL, Colman N, Pare PD, eds. Diagnosis of Diseases of the Chest. Vol. 1. 4th ed. Philadelphia: Saunders, 1999:299–338.
2. Kalender WA, Seissler W, Klotz E, Vock P. Spiral volumetric CT with single-breath-hold technique, continuous transport, and continuous scanner rotation. Radiology 1990; 176:181–183.
3. Poliacin A, Kalender WA, Marchal G. Evaluation of section sensitivity profiles and image noise in spiral CT. Radiology 1992; 185:29–35.
4. Rydberg J, Buckwalter KA, Caldemeyer KS, Phillips MD, Conces DJ Jr, Aisen AM, Persohn SA, Kopecky KK. Multisection CT: scanning techniques and clinical applications. Radiographics 2000; 20:1787–1806.

5. Naidich DP, Marshall CH, Gribbin C, Arams RS, McCauley DI. Low-dose CT of the lungs: preliminary observations. Radiology 1990; 175:729–731.

6. Zwirewich CV, Mayo JR, Muller NL. Low-dose high-resolution CT of lung parenchyma. Radiology 1991; 180:413–417.

7. Choi YW, McAdams HP, Jeon SC, Park CK, Lee SJ, Kim BS, Kim JI, Hahm CK. Low-dose spiral CT: application to surface-rendered three-dimensional imaging of central airways. J Comput Assist Tomogr 2002; 26:335–341.

8. Geleijns J, Broerse JJ, Julius HW, Vrooman HA, Zoetelief J, Zweers D, Kool LJ. AMBER and conventional chest radiography: comparison of radiation dose and image quality. Radiology 1992; 185:719–723.

9. Stern EJ, Graham CM, Webb WR, Gamsu G. Normal trachea during forced expiration: dynamic CT measurements. Radiology 1993; 187:27–31.

10. Ohnesorge B, Flohr T, Becker C, Kopp AF, Schoepf UJ, Baum U, Knez A, Klingenbeck-Regn K, Reiser MF. Cardiac imaging by means of electrocardiographically gated multisection spiral CT: initial experience. Radiology 2000; 217:564–571.

11. Gotway MB, Lee ES, Reddy GP, Golden JA, Webb WR. Low-dose, dynamic, expiratory thin-section CT of the lungs using a spiral CT scanner. J Thorac Imaging 2000; 15:168–172.

12. Lucidarme O, Grenier PA, Cadi M, Mourey-Gerosa I, Benali K, Cluzel P. Evaluation of air trapping at CT: comparison of continuous-versus suspended expiration CT techniques. Radiology 2000; 216:768–772.

13. Grenier PA, Beigelman-Aubry C, Fetita C, Preteux F, Brauner MW, Lenoir S. New frontiers in CT imaging of airway disease. Eur Radiol 2002; 12:1022–1044.

14. Mayo JR, Webb WR, Gould R, Stein MG, Bass I, Gamsu G, Goldberg HI. High-resolution CT of the lungs: an optimal approach. Radiology 1987; 163:507–510.

15. Zwirewich CV, Terrif B, Muller NL. High-spatial frequency (bone) algorithm improves quality of standard CT of the thorax. AJR Am J Roentgenol 1989; 153:1169–1173.

16. Webb WR, Muller NL, Naidich DP. High Resolution CT of the Lung. 3rd ed. New York: Lippincott-Williams and Wilkins, 2001.

17. Ferretti GR, Bricault I, Coulomb M. Virtual tools for imaging of the thorax. Eur Respir J 2001; 18:381–392.

18. Remy-Jardin M, Remy J, Deschildre F, Artaud D, Ramon P, Edme JI. Obstructive lesions of the central airways: evaluation by using spiral CT with multiplanar and three-dimensional reformations. Eur Radiol 1996; 6:807–816.

19. Remy J, Remy-Jardin M, Artaud D, Fribourg M. Multiplanar and three-dimensional reconstruction techniques in CT: impact on chest diseases. Eur Radiol 1998; 8:335–351.

20. Rubin GD. Techniques of reconstruction. In: Remy-Jardin M, Remy J, eds. Medical Radiology Spiral CT of the Chest. Berlin: Springer Verlag, 1996:101–127.

21. Kauczor HU, Wolcke B, Fischer B, Mildenberger P, Lorenz J, Thelen M. Three-dimensional helical CT of the tracheobronchial tree: evaluation of imaging protocols and assessment of suspected stenoses with bronchoscopic correlation. AJR Am J Roentgenol 1996; 167:419–424.

22. Remy-Jardin M, Remy J, Artaud D, Fribourg M, Naili A. Tracheobronchial tree: assessment with volume rendering—technical aspects. Radiology 1998; 208:393–398.

23. Remy-Jardin M, Remy J, Artaud D, Fribourg M, Duhamel A. Volume rendering of the tracheobronchial tree: clinical evaluation of bronchographic images. Radiology 1998; 208:761–770.
24. Fetita CI, Preteux F, Beigelman-Aubry C, Grenier PA. 3D bronchoview: a new software package for investigating airway diseases. Eur Radiol 2002; 12:394 (abstract).
25. Hopper KD, Iyriboz TA, Mahraj RPM, Wise SW, Kasales CJ, Ten-Have TR, Wilson RP, Weaver JS. CT bronchoscopy: optimization of imaging parameters. Radiology 1998; 209:872–877.
26. Summers RM, Shaw DJ, Shelhamer JH. CT virtual bronchoscopy of simulated endobronchial lesions: effect of scanning, reconstruction, and display settings and potential pitfalls. AJR Am J Roentgenol 1998; 170:947–950.
27. Webb WR, Gamsu G, Wall SD, Cann CE, Proctor E. CT of a bronchial phantom. Factors affecting appearance and size measurements. Invest Radiol 1984; 19:394–398.
28. McNamara AE, Muller NL, Okazawa M, Arntorp J, Wiggs BR, Pare PD. Airway narrowing in excised canine lungs measured by high-resolution computed tomography. J Appl Physiol 1992; 73:307–316.
29. Bankier AA, Fleischmann D, Mallek R, Windisch A, Winkelbauer FV, Kontrus M, Havelec L, Herold CJ, Hubsch P. Bronchial wall thickness: appropriate window settings for thin-section CT and radiologic-anatomic correlation. Radiology 1996; 199:831–836.
30. Kim SJ, Im JG, Kim IO, Cho ST, Cha SH, Park KS, Kim DY. Normal bronchial and pulmonary arterial diameters measured by thin section CT. J Comput Assist Tomogr 1995; 19:365–369.
31. Kim JS, Muller NL, Park CS, Lynch DA, Newman LS, Grenier P, Herold CJ. Bronchoarterial ratio on thin-section CT: comparison between high-altitude and sea level. J Comput Assist Tomogr 1997; 306:21–311.
32. Fraser RS, Muller NL, Colman N, Pare PD. The normal lung: computed tomography. In: Fraser RS, Muller NL, Colman N, Pare PD, eds. Diagnosis of Diseases of the Chest. Vol. 1. 4th ed. Philadelphia: Saunders, 1999:281–295.
33. Webb WR, Müller NL, Naidich D. High-resolution CT of the Lung. 2nd ed. New York: Lippincott-Raven, 1996.
34. Okazawa M, Muller NL, McNamara AE, Child S, Verburgt L, Pare PD. Human airway narrowing measured using high resolution computed tomography. Am J Respir Crit Care Med 1996; 154:1557–1562.
35. Amirav I, Kramer SS, Grunstein M, Hoffman EA. Assessment of methacholine-induced airway constriction with ultrafast high-resolution computed tomography. J Appl Physiol 1993; 75:2239–2250.
36. Prêteux F, Fetita CI, Capderou A, Grenier P. Modeling, segmentation, and caliber estimation of bronchi in high resolution computerized tomography. J Electron Imaging 1999; 8:36–45.
37. Wood SA, Zerhouni EA, Hoford JD, Hoffman EA, Mitzner W. Measurement of three-dimensional lung tree structures by using computed tomography. J Appl Physiol 1995; 79:1687–1697.
38. King GG, Muller NL, Whittall KP, Xiang QS, Pare PD. An analysis algorithm for measuring airway lumen and wall areas from high-resolution computed tomographic data. Am J Respir Crit Care Med 2000; 161:574–580.

39. Perot V, Desberat P, Berger P, Begueret H, Elias J, Laurent F. Nouvel algorithme d'xtraction des paramètres géométriques des bronches en TDMHR. J Radiol 2001; 82:1213 (abstract).

40. Brown R, Georakopoulos I, Mitzner W. Individual canine airway responsiveness to aerosol histamine and methacholine *in vivo*. Am J Respir Crit Care Med 1998; 157:491–497.

41. Brown R, Mitzner W, Bulut Y, Wagner E. Effect of lung inflation *in vivo* on airways with smooth-muscle tone or edema. J Appl Physiol 1997; 82:491–499.

42. Beigelman-Aubry C, Capderou A, Grenier PA, Straus C, Becquemin MH, Similowski T, Zelter M. Mild intermittent asthma: CT assessment of bronchial cross-sectional area and lung attenuation at controlled lung volume. Radiology 2002; 223:181–187.

43. King GG, Muller NL, Pare PD. Evaluation of airways in obstructive pulmonary disease using high-resolution computed tomography. Am J Respir Crit Care Med 1999; 159:992–1004.

44. Niimi A, Matsumoto H, Amitani R, Nakano Y, Mishima M, Minakuchi M, Nishimura K, Itoh H, Izumi T. Airway wall thickness in asthma assessed by computed tomography. Relation to clinical indices. Am J Respir Crit Care Med 2000; 162:1518–1523.

45. Nakano Y, Muro S, Sakai H, Hirai T, Chin K, Tsukino M, Nishimura K, Itoh H, Pare PD, Hogg JC, Mishima M. Computed tomographic measurements of airway dimensions and emphysema in smokers. Am J Respir Crit Care Med 2000; 162:1102–1108.

46. Nakano Y, Muller NL, King GG, Niimi A, Kalloger SE, Mishima M, Pare PD. Quantitative assessment of airway remodeling using high-resolution CT. Chest 2002; 122(suppl):271S–275S.

47. Hedlund LW, Vock P, Effmann EL. Computed tomography of the lung: densitometric studies. Radiol Clin North Am 1983; 21:775–788.

48. Rosenblum LJ, Mauceri RA, Wellenstein DE, Thomas FD, Bassano DA, Raasch BN, Chamberlain CC, Heitzman ER. Density patterns in the normal lung as determined by computed tomography. Radiology 1980; 137:409–416.

49. Webb WR, Stern EJ, Kanth N, Gamsu G. Dynamic pulmonary CT: findings in healthy adult men. Radiology 1993; 186:117–124.

50. Robinson PJ, Kreel L. Pulmonary tissue attenuation with computed tomography: comparison of inspiration and expiration scans. J Comput Assist Tomogr 1979; 3:740–748.

51. Verschakelen JA, Van Fraeyenhoven L, Laureys G, Demedts M, Baert AL. Differences in CT density between dependent and nondependent portions of the lung: influence of lung volume. AJR Am J Roentgenol 1993; 161:713–717.

52. Kalender WA, Rienmuller R, Seissler W, Behr J, Welke M, Fichte H. Measurement of pulmonary parenchymal attenuation: use of spirometric gating with quantitative CT. Radiology 1990; 175:265–268.

53. Gevenois PA, Scillia P, de Maertelaer V, Michils A, De Vuyst P, Yernault JC. The effects of age, sex, lung size, and hyperinflation on CT lung densitometry. AJR Am J Roentgenol 1996; 167:1169–1173.

54. Rienmuller RK, Behr J, Kalender WA, Schatzl M, Altmann I, Merin M, Beinert T. Standardized quantitative high resolution CT in lung diseases. J Comput Assist Tomogr 1991; 15:742–749.

55. Kinsella M, Muller NL, Abboud RT, Morrison NJ, DyBuncio A. Quantitation of emphysema by computed tomography using a "density mask" program and correlation with pulmonary function tests. Chest 1990; 97:315–321.
56. Müller NL, Staples CA, Miller RR, Abboud RT. "Density mask": an objective method to quantitate emphysema using computed tomography. Chest 1988; 94:782–787.
57. Gevenois PA, de Maertelaer V, de Vuyst P, Zanen J, Yernault JC. Comparison of computed density and macroscopic morphometry in pulmonary emphysema. Am J Respir Crit Care Med 1995; 152:653–657.
58. Gevenois PA, de Vuyst P, Sy H, Scillia P, Chaminade L, de Maertelaer V, Zanen J, Yernault JC. Pulmonary emphysema: quantitative CT during expiration. Radiology 1996; 199:825–829.
59. Newman KB, Lynch DA, Newman LS, Ellegood D, Newell JD Jr. Quantitative computed tomography detects air trapping due to asthma. Chest 1994; 106:105–109.
60. Wollmer P, Albrechtsson U, Brauer K, Eriksson L, Johnson B, Tylen B. Measurement of pulmonary density by means of X-ray computerized tomography. Relation to pulmonary mechanics in normal subjects. Chest 1986; 90:387–391.

3

CT Ventilation Imaging: Technical Background and Impact in Acute Lung Injury and ARDS Management

LUCIANO GATTINONI and DAVIDE CHIUMELLO

Istituto di Anestesia e Rianimazione, Fondazione IRCCS—"Ospedale Maggiore Policlinico, Mangiagalli, Regina Elena" di Milano and Università degli Studi di Milano, Milano, Italy

PIETRO BIONDETTI

UO Radiologia, Fondazione IRCCS—"Ospedale Maggiore Policlinico, Mangiagalli, Regina Elena" di Milano and Università degli Studi di Milano, Milano, Italy

ELEONORA CARLESSO

Università degli Studi di Milano, Milano, Italy

I. Introduction

Rommelsheim et al. (1), to our knowledge, were the first to report the use of computed tomography (CT) scan in acute respiratory distress syndrome (ARDS) patients in 1983. Unfortunately, their observations did not have impact on the scientific and clinical communities as their report appeared in a German journal. Three years later, Maunder (2) and our group independently described the appearances of ARDS on CT scans and its response to positive end-expiratory pressure (PEEP) ventilation (3). This technique completely changed our vision and interpretation of the syndrome. What was considered as a homogeneous involvement of the lung parenchyma, due to a widespread alteration of lung capillaries' permeability, on CT scan appeared inhomogeneous with prevalent involvement of the caudal and dependent lung regions. This pattern raised relevant clinical issues: Is the ARDS lung composed of healthy and diseased regions, as it appears at first sight? What is the nature of the observed densities? How can these findings change our approach to the mechanical ventilation of acute lung injury (ALI)/ARDS patients? Moreover, the widespread use of the CT scan led the clinicians to recognize clinical problems, as localized pneumothorax, pleural effusions, bronchial and tracheal alterations, not revealed on chest radiographs. In this chapter, we would like to integrate the knowledge derived by the use of the CT scan in the general framework of ARDS, in its physiological, pathological, and clinical aspects. We also refer to the dedicated chapter on ARDS (Chapter 19).

II. ARDS Morphology

A. Terminology

We have adopted the following descriptors proposed by the Fleischner Society Nomenclature Committee (4).

1. *Ground-glass opacification*: a hazy increase in lung attenuation, with preservation of bronchial and vascular margins.
2. *Consolidation*: a *homogeneous* increase in lung attenuation that obscures bronchovascular margins in which an air-bronchogram may be present.
3. *Reticular pattern*: innumerable interlacing line shadows, which may be fine, intermediate, or coarse.

Before attempting to correlate these descriptors with their possible anatomical–pathological equivalent, it is worth to briefly discuss the "resolution" limits of the CT scan, that is, which are the smallest anatomical structures that the CT scan can discriminate.

B. Anatomical Equivalents

The "CT pulmonary units," the voxel, may have different dimensions. In most ARDS studies, the standard 10 mm axial thickness was used (matrix size 256×256), which corresponds to a voxel volume of $22.5 \, mm^3$ (i.e., $1.5 \times 1.5 \times 10 \, mm^2$). This matches to the volume of the pulmonary unit, the acinus, at functional residual capacity. In fact, the dimensions of a normal acinus at end-expiration is in the range of $16–22 \, mm^3$, and each includes about 2000 alveoli. Approximately 10% of this volume is represented by the tissue, consisting of the fiber cytoskeleton, the interstitial space, and the alveolar and endothelial cells (5). It follows that if the acinus is gasless, its representative volume is $\sim 2 \, mm^3$, and one standard voxel comprises about 10 acini (20,000 alveoli). At maximal lung inflation (total lung capacity), corresponding to a transpulmonary pressure of $\sim 30 \, cmH_2O$ (difference between intraalveolar and pleural pressure), one voxel includes the structures of only half of an acinus, that is, 1000 alveoli.

Recent new CT multislice technology allows one to acquire several lung slices simultaneously (from 2 to 40), during each $360°$ gantry rotation of the helical volumetric scan. This technique decreases both scan time and slice thickness, while significantly increasing the spatial resolution along the vertical axis of the scanned patient (Z-direction).

With a 16 slice CT scanner, it is possible to acquire the entire volume of the thorax in less than a breath hold (<10 s) with a slices thickness of 0.4–0.7 mm. With this kind of acquisition, the imaged volume consists of cubic voxels which have virtually equal sizes in all 3 directions and a volume of 0.216–0.343 mm^3 (so called "isotropic spatial resolution"). This implies that at FRC, a voxel only includes 1% of an acinus, that is, the structure of approximately 20 alveoli. As CT inherently measures tissue density, which is made up of the ratio between tissue mass and total volume (tissue mass + volume of gas), it become evident that standardization of the imaging protocol is essential to compare the findings. Parameters that need to be uniform include slice thickness, scan acquisition time, and phase of mechanical ventilation (end-expiration or end-inspiration). All, in fact, may markedly affect the morphological pattern seen on CT.

C. Structure/Morphology Relationship

In ALI/ARDS, the ground-glass opacification is a reflection of increased tissue mass, which is the result of the inflammatory process and incomplete aeration of the alveolar spaces (6). This process should involve both the interstitia, with increased thickening of the alveolar wall and/or (incomplete) filling of the alveolar space with neutrophils, macrophages, cellular debris, and edema. Consolidation, on the other hand, should represent a similar process but at higher level of severity, with complete loss of aeration of the air spaces. The consolidation, otherwise called "dense parenchymal opacification," may be patchy or diffuse. In ALI/ARDS, it is more prevalent in the caudal regions and in the most dependent areas of the lung (3,6,7). In this setting, the distinction between consolidation due to edema/inflammatory cells from atelectasis is extremely difficult. A total collapse of potentially recruitable units results in a similar morphological picture. It is likely, however, that both edema and collapse coexist in ALI/ARDS (6).

The reticular pattern consists of discrete and recognizable thickening of the interstitium. This may occur acutely (edema or interstitial inflammation) or may be a chronic phenomenon (fibrosis) (6). In fibrosis, however, the lines are more sharply defined, and parenchyma is usually destroyed, although there is evidence of traction on surrounding tissues, such as traction bronchiectasis.

D. Pulmonary and Extrapulmonary ARDS Morphology

ALI and ARDS may be caused by a direct pulmonary injury (through the airway, pulmonary ARDS) or by inflammatory mediators released from an extrapulmonary focus, as in peritonitis (extrapulmonary ARDS) (8). These two different mechanisms may lead to different morphological patterns. In pulmonary ARDS, the primary lesions are within the alveolar space and the primary morphological equivalent should be either patchy or diffuse consolidation, depending on the severity of the insult. If the compartmentalization of the infection is lost, and inflammatory mediators are released through the blood stream, endothelial cell permeability is affected with consequent interstitial pulmonary edema (9). The morphological equivalent is ground-glass opacification. Furthermore, because both consolidation and ground-glass opacification effectively lead to an increase in tissue mass (and weight), this is the primary determinant of compression atelectasis in the dependent lung regions.

Pulmonary ARDS is mainly characterized by patchy consolidation associated with ground-glass opacification (due to the loss of compartmentalization), whereas extrapulmonary ARDS is primarily characterized by the ground-glass opacification (10). Moreover, both should also present coexisting gravity dependent compression atelectasis, which is commonly associated with pleural effusions. Goodman et al. (11) prospectively compared the morphological findings of pulmonary ARDS with extrapulmonary ARDS. They found that pulmonary ARDS tended to be asymmetric with a mixture of dense parenchymal opacification and ground-glass opacification, whereas extrapulmonary ARDS was characterized by symmetric ground-glass opacification and dorsal consolidation. Similar findings were obtained by Desai et al. (12,13). Winer-Muram et al. (14) demonstrated that more homogeneous and dependent densities were prevalent in extrapulmonary ARDS. Rouby et al. (15) reached similar conclusions, using different morphological descriptors (i.e., lobar, diffuse, or patchy attenuation).

Unfortunately, the authors who investigated the possible relationship between the CT morphology and the pathogenetic pathway did not use identical protocols and/or descriptive terms. For instance, the CT scans in the studies were taken at different degrees of inflation, and the studies were limited in size. Furthermore, extrapulmonary ARDS group often included patients after cardiac surgery, in which the left lower lobe collapse is a frequent finding. In addition, direct and indirect insults may coexist (i.e., one or more lobes with the direct insult and both lungs with the indirect insult), making the morphological pattern difficult to interpret (9,11,16). Clinically, it is unclear if making a distinction between pulmonary or extrapulmonary ARDS affects outcome.

III. Time Evolution

A. Late ARDS

ALI and ARDS are dynamic processes, which follow a variable course. Some patients show a clinical resolution within 1 week, whereas others have a more protracted course or show progression to death. Imaging reflects both the normal evolution of the underlying pathology and the additional damages due to the mechanical ventilation, which are usually referred as "ventilator-induced lung injury". The two processes may be so strictly associated that the effects and end-results become undistinguishable.

The natural course of the inflammation is remodeling of the lung structure, which starts with a fibrotic reaction. This may cause, with time, an extensive modification of the lung shape with distortion of the interstitium and bronchovascular bundles. An example of the interaction between the underlying pathology and the possible damages induced by mechanical ventilation is the dramatic increase, with time, of subpleural cysts and bullae (17). These emphysematous cysts or pneumatoceles vary in size from a few millimeters to several centimeters (18). It is known that high pressure and/or high volume mechanical ventilation may induce similar damages in healthy lungs. In fact, this type of ventilation induces excessive stress and strain on the fiber cytoskeleton, which will ultimately lead to rupture (19). On the other hand, the natural course of the disease may cause similar lesions, for instance, following cavitation due to an abscess or due to a pulmonary infarction. There are some conflicting reports about the location of the bullae. Some authors found a primary location in the nondependent lung zones (18,20,21), whereas others found a higher prevalence in the dependent lung zones (22). It is possible that the bullae, if originating from the cavitation of abscess, simply follow the random distribution of the intraparenchymal infection. However, if it is due to the mechanical ventilation, two distinct patterns may occur, depending on the ventilator setting used. If the PEEP is adequate to prevent the end-expiratory lung collapse, the nondependent lung regions will undergo the greatest stress and strain, and the bullae should be primarily located in those regions (23). However, if PEEP is inadequate, the dependent lung regions undergo intratidal collapse and re-expansion. This causes relevant shear forces, leading to rupture and bullae formation. Indeed, the apparently contradictory results in the literature may be simply due to different ventilator strategies, but this remain speculative, as the ventilator setting used in the patients in whom the bullae were found was not reported.

B. Follow-Up

From the perspective described earlier, it is of interest to consider the morphological changes observed at the follow-up of ALI/ARDS patients. It has been consistently reported that these patients present a reticular pattern in the nondependent lung regions (10). As previously discussed, this is suggestive of lung fibrosis occurring in the lung regions least affected by the original disease process (24,25). This pattern has been found to correlate with the length of mechanical ventilation and with the use of inverse ratio ventilation (12). We believe that as for the bullae, the location of fibrosis depends on the exposure to mechanical ventilation and on the kind of ventilation used. With inverse ratio ventilation, the collapsing and re-expanding phenomena are unlikely, because the end-expiratory pressure is usually sufficient to prevent it. On the other hand, the densely opacified regions (the most dependent) not ventilated are protected from high FiO$_2$ and pressures. Accordingly, a negative correlation was noted between the extent of reticular pattern on the follow-up of CT scan and the extent of intense opacification on initial CT scan. The bulk of available data suggests that fibrosis mainly occurs in the regions more exposed to mechanical ventilation, whereas the truly consolidated and nonventilated lung regions are somewhat protected from the ventilator-induced lung injury.

IV. Quantitative CT Analysis

A. Physical Principles of CT Scan

The CT scanner produces a digital image that consists of a square matrix of picture elements, that is, the pixel. Each pixel in the matrix represents a voxel (volume element of the tissue). What the CT scan measures is the linear attenuation coefficient (μ), which is the reduction of the radiation intensity upon passage through matter, resulting from all types of interactions. Traversing from one side of the patient to the other side, the X-ray beam will be attenuated by all the voxels through which it has passed. The intensity of the emerging X-ray is described by the Lambert law of absorption, that is,

$$I = I_0 \ e^{\int \mu dl}$$

By measuring the intensities I and I_0, the CT calculates the integral over the function μ of the attenuation coefficient along the X-ray beam, then through a different mathematical algorithm (usually filtered back projection), a given attenuation number μ is assigned to each voxel. The attenuation number depends on the energy of the X-ray photons and on the both density and atomic number (Z) of the material scanned. For CT imaging, a high kilovolt (in the range 120–140 kV) and heavy beam filtration is used. These technical arrangements minimize the X-ray matter interactions, which are influenced by the Z of material. Therefore, the attenuation is primarily determined by the density of the tissue. After measuring the attenuation coefficients, the CT scanner converts the measured μ of the voxel to CT numbers. Indeed, for a given voxel, the CT number is expressed as (Fig. 3.1)

$$CT = 1000^*(\mu I - \mu_{water})/\mu_{water}$$

It is evident from the earlier formula that the CT number of water is 0, because anything subtracted from itself is zero and zero multiple for anything is zero. The factor scale of 1000 is used to magnify the small differences of the attenuation coefficient of the different tissues. Indeed, for practical purposes, the CT number is a measure of density, that is, the ratio of mass to the volume.

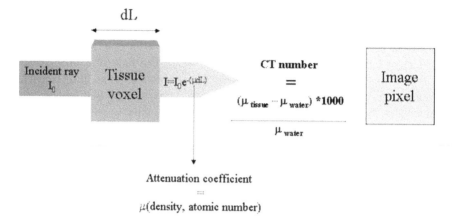

Figure 3.1   The incident ray I_0 traversing the tissue voxel is attenuated according to the Lambert law of absorption. By a mathematical algorithm, the CT calculates the attenuation coefficient μ of each voxel, which is function of the density and of the atomic number of the scanned material. The measured μ of the voxel is converted to CT numbers. The image is an array of pixels.

However, we must always remember that several factors may lead to under or overestimation of the attenuation coefficient of a given voxel (26,27).

B.   CT Scanning and X-ray Exposure

Although CT is only 4% of all medical X-ray examinations, it represents 40% of the collective radiation dose. The growth of CT is dramatic: from 2.8 million CT exams in 1981 to 20 million CT exams in 1995. There is no consensus about the connection between low level radiation and cancer. However, on the basis of the data on the excess relative risk for cancer mortality in Japanese atomic bomb survivors of all ages, followed for 40 years (1957–1990), the fatal cancer risk to population per dose of 10 mSv (sievert: unit of absorbed effective dose), which is in the range of body CT X-ray per dose, is 1/2000 (national individual risk: 1/4–1/5). Indeed, when CT scan is indicated, great attention has to be paid to the technical protocol, to keep the X-ray exposure as low as reasonably possible (28). This is especially true for volumetric multislice CT scanners, where, due to the speed and ease of use, significant X-ray doses can be delivered to patients.

To illustrate this issue, let us assume that a CT is required for ALI/ARDS. Two different approaches can be used: volumetric high resolution scan and single high resolution slices acquired every 2 cm to sample the entire lungs. If a 16 slice multidetector CT scanner is considered, and using 0.6 mm slice thickness, 140 kV, 250 mA, and pitch of 1.5, the volumetric approach implies an X-ray dose of 7.5 mSv compared with 0.5 mSv using the simple slice approach. In this example, the advantages of a volumetric acquisition have to be compared with an approximately 15 times increase in X-ray dose delivered to the patient. It is obvious that for most patients in this scenario, a single slice technique should be employed.

C. Computation of Gas and Tissue Volume

The quantitative analysis of ALI/ARDS lungs consists of the estimate of the gas and tissue volume of each voxel in the region-of-interest. The tissue volume, in a given voxel, is computed as:

$$\text{Volume of tissue} = \left(1 - \frac{\text{CT}}{-1000}\right) \times \text{total volume}$$

Considering the specific weight of tissue equal to 1, it is possible to compute the lung weight in a region-of-interest. As shown in Fig. 3.2, the earlier formula allows the computation of tissue and gas in the whole lung, the whole slice, and the regions along the vertical or longitudinal axis. Knowing the actual tissue mass and the expected normal tissue mass, it is possible to compute the excess tissue mass, which should represent primarily edema.

$$\text{Excess tissue mass} = \text{actual tissue mass} - \text{expected tissue mass}$$

In animal experiments, it is possible to precisely quantify the excess tissue mass as the baseline lung CT scan before the insult is usually available. In patients, this is impossible. To estimate the hypothetical "normal tissue" of a given patient, it is possible to estimate the expected FRC (in supine position, with sedation) and to assign an "average" normal CT. For FRC, we used the Ibanez formula (29), which refers to supine patients, and for average CT, we used −654 HU, as derived in normal subjects (30). Indeed, the expected tissue mass is computed

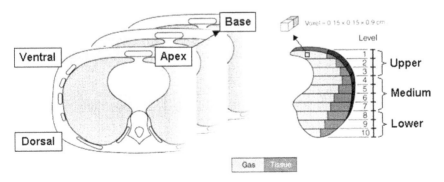

Figure 3.2 A diagrammatic representation of regional quantitative CT analysis.

as follows:

$$\text{Expected tissue mass} = \frac{\text{gas volume} \times (-1000 - \overline{\text{CT}})}{\overline{\text{CT}}}$$

where gas volume is the expected normal gas volume, and $\overline{\text{CT}}$ is the average normal CT.

D. Hydrostatic Pressures Through the Lung: The Concept of Superimposed Pressure

This analysis assumes that the hydrostatic pressures are transmitted throughout the lung parenchyma as in a fluid (fluid-like model). Consequently, at any given lung level, the pressure is defined as $P = \rho g h$. Accordingly, the superimposed pressure at any given lung level is equal to:

$$P_{\text{level}} = \left(1 - \frac{\text{CT}}{-1000}\right) * \text{Height} + P_{\text{above level}}$$

As $(1 - (\text{CT}/-1000))$ is the tissue mass, its increase directly influences the superimposed pressure. In a normal lung in supine position, with a vertical height of 12 cm and a normal density of 0.25 Kg/dm^3, the superimposed pressure in the most dependent regions would be 3 cmH$_2$O. In experiments, in normal subjects, we found that superimposed lung pressure at a given lung height (h) is $0.178(\pm 0.012)hL + 0.008(\pm 0.0006)hL^2$, whereas in ARDS patients, it was two to three times greater (30) (Fig. 3.3).

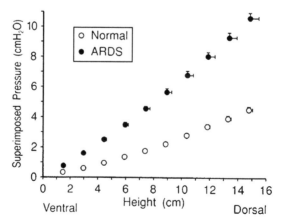

Figure 3.3 The estimated superimposed pressure as a function of ventral-to-dorsal lung height in normal subjects (open circles, 24 lungs) and patients with ARDS (solid circles, 34 lungs). The data (mean $\pm$ SEM) of both normal patients with ARDS fit the general quadratic equation: SPL $= a \times hL + b \times hL^2$. [From Pelosi et al. (30).]

The superimposed pressure (i.e., the lung weight), together with the lung and the thoracic cage shape, is a key variable in dictating the regional inflation (31–37). This inflation depends on the local transpulmonary pressure (P_L), based on the following equation:

$$P_L = P_{aw} - P_{pl}$$

where P_{aw} is the pressure inside the alveoli and P_{pl} is the local pleural pressure. In normal lung, the superimposed pressure increases the pleural pressure along the vertical axis, and this accounts for the decrease of the regional inflation. In ARDS, due to the two or threefold increase of superimposed pressure, this phenomenon is magnified, accounting for the tendency of ARDS lung to collapse in the most dependent regions. This has been shown directly in animal experiments, in which the changes of superimposed pressure (computed with the CT scan) in an oleic acid dog model were linearly associated with the changes in pleural pressure measured directly in the pleural space (38). Indeed, we may conclude that the increase of superimposed pressure is a key variable in dictating the tendency of the ARDS lung to collapse, with relevant consequences on the choice of ventilator setting and body position.

E. Lung Compartments

Definition and quantification of lung compartments based on their degree of inflation allows us to better investigate the relationship between the lung structure and function. On the basis of the CT number frequency distribution of normal subjects (Fig. 3.4), we arbitrarily defined four lung compartments: normal, poorly aerated, nonaerated, and overinflated lung (39). The threshold CT values we used were either adopted or modified by others (Table 3.1).

Two different methods have been used for quantification of these compartments. The approach we used was to compute the amount of tissue of the compartment (39), whereas others computed the total volume (i.e., tissue + gas) (40–42).

In mathematical form, for a given compartment:

Volume of compartment = number of voxels × volume of voxel

It is evident that the tissue compartment equals its volume only in the nonaerated compartment where the average CT = 0. The estimates of the aerated compartments are largely different. As an example, in a study assessing the overinflation induced by PEEP in ALI/ARDS, the volume of the overinflated compartment (i.e., tissue + gas), at total lung capacity in the healthy volunteers was ~30% (41). However, the tissue of the overinflated compartment was only ~9% of the baseline lung tissue. We believe that referring to tissue, instead of volume, presents several advantages, as it is the lung tissue, and not volume, which is strained and stressed by mechanical ventilation. Knowing the amount

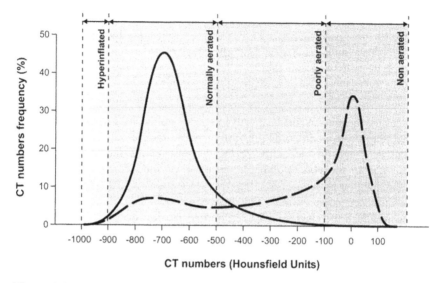

Figure 3.4 The lung compartments, as defined by CT numbers, in normal condition (solid line) and in typical ALI/ARDS (dashed line). [From Gattinoni et al. (54).]

of tissue in a compartment allows, in our opinion, a better understanding of the changes induced by different ventilator settings, as PEEP, or plateau pressures. Moreover, the total tissue is a precise reference, as it does not change with the inflation.

The modeling of lung parenchyma into compartments requires further explanation. It is important to point out that these compartments relate only to the gas/tissue ratio. Indeed, the hyperinflated compartments, as an example, only refer to the overfilling of the acini with gas and not necessarily to its "over-distension or overstretching," which refers to alveolar wall tension. The poorly aerated compartment (which is approximately the quantitative equivalent of the ground-glass pattern) refers to a gas/tissue ratio, which is also present in normal subjects, at least at end-expiration (6), but is more extensive in ALI/ARDS. In most cases, the nonaerated compartment includes the voxels between − 100 and 0 HU, that is, with a gas/tissue ratio from 1/100 down to zero. This takes into account that in small airway collapse, some gas is left in the collapsed alveoli.

Table 3.1 The Threshold CT Numbers to Define the Lung Compartments

Hyperinflated	Normally aerated	Poorly aerated	Nonaerated	References
—	− 1000 to − 500	− 500 to − 100	− 100 to 100	(7,34)
—	− 900 to − 500	− 500 to 100	− 100 to 100	(39,89)
− 1000 to − 800	—	− 800 to − 150	− 150 to 100	(42)
− 1000 to − 900	− 900 to − 500	− 500 to − 100	− 100 to 100	(40,41)

Indeed, when comparing the results of different authors that used the same terminology to define the compartments, it is essential to know the different cutoff values used (Table 3.1), and, perhaps more importantly to understand whether the compartments were quantified as total volume or as tissue volume (Table 3.2).

V. Physiological Insight

A. Modeling of ALI/ARDS Lung: The "Baby" Lung and the "Sponge" Lung

ALI and/or ARDS usually presents with a near-normal aeration in the nondependent regions, ground-glass opacification in the middle regions, and consolidation in the most dependent regions. This is the "classical picture" of the diffuse ARDS, which on pathology reveals diffuse alveolar damage. It has also been suggested that ARDS may present as "lobar" ARDS, usually involving the lower left lobe, particularly in patients following cardiac or major vascular surgery (15). We may question whether this picture may represent a "true" ARDS, which, by definition, should represent a generalized inflammation of the pulmonary parenchyma leading to a noncardiogenic pulmonary edema.

Whatever the morphology, however, quantitative analysis of CT scans reveals that in most patients, part of the lung is normally aerated. The amount of tissue of this compartment may be very low (on the order of 200–300 g in an adult with an expected normally aerated tissue mass of ~1000 g). This led to the concept of the "baby lung," which we initially considered as an anatomical entity, usually located in nondependent lung regions. The early CT scan studies describing the structure/functional relationships in ALI/ARDS showed that the amount of nonaerated tissue was correlated with lower PaO_2, increased right–left shunt, and increased dead space and that the excess tissue mass was correlated with the increase of pulmonary pressure (43).

However, the most striking result of these early studies was to recognize that the ARDS lung is small (instead of "stiff") and that the respiratory system compliance was correlated with the dimensions of the baby lung (instead of

Table 3.2 Quantification of Compartments According to the Hounsfield Unit

Quantifications	References
Tissue weight	(39,40)
Percentage of each compartment surface area respect to the total surface area	(42)
Lung volumes (gas + tissue)	(7,40,41)
Gas volume	(40)
Volume lung tissue	(40)

the amount of nonaerated tissue) (44). In this view, the respiratory compliance is virtually a direct "measure" of how the "well the lung is."

As soon as we observed that the nondependent regions were usually normally aerated, it was hypothesized that by prone positioning the patient, the "baby lung" (in the dependent position) would become better perfused, thus increasing oxygenation (45). Although oxygenation did increase in most patients, we also demonstrated through prone CT imaging that the densities re-distributed from dorsal to ventral, clearly showing that an "anatomical" baby lung does not exist (46). To understand the density re-distribution, the regional characteristics of the ALI/ARDS lung along the ventral sternovertebral axis were analyzed (30). The most consistent finding was that the edema was evenly distributed from ventral to dorsal, without any gravitational distribution (46), as previously observed in patients and in experimental animals (47,48).

These observations led to a different model, the "sponge lung," which proposes that edema is evenly distributed in ALI/ARDS (49). However, due to the increased mass (and increased superimposed pressure), the gas is squeezed out of the most dependent regions, leading to the classical CT appearance of gasless dependent regions. A further support to this model was provided by construction of a gas/tissue pressure curve at end-expiration (50). This analysis clearly showed that the pressure at which the lung collapses along the sternovertebral axis was dependent on the superimposed pressure. Animal studies, with oleic acid induced ARDS, further supported this hypothesis (38).

The sponge lung model, in which the progressive de-aeration along the ventral–dorsal axis, is primarily explained by the increased superimposed pressure has been recently challenged. Wilson et al. (51), on the basis of previous experimental works (52), in which regional volumes were measured by markers, proposed the following model: in the edematous lung, the pressure first causes the air–fluid interface to penetrate the mouth of the alveoli (airway pressure $\sim$20 cmH$_2$O), then the air–fluid interface is inside the alveoli and the lung becomes compliant. The basic difference between the two views is that in the sponge model, the edema is believed to be primarily in the interstitium (causing alveolar collapse volume effect and compression), whereas in the air–fluid interface model, the edema is predominantly in the alveoli. In both models, the total lung volume is near normal. We have to consider, however, that models may not be able to completely explain a complex syndrome such as ALI/ARDS.

B. Recruitment and De-recruitment

Potential for Recruitment

"Recruitment," in medical language, should generally define the involvement of increasing number of units in a given status/function in response to increasing strength of a stimulus. If we accept this broad definition, the difficulty of defining "recruitment" in ALI/ARDS is evident. First, we need to define the "pulmonary unit," and, second, the status and/or function to which the unit is recruited.

It is convenient to refer to the acinus (2000–3000 alveoli) as functional pulmonary unit (5). The key issue, however, is to define at which status and function the pulmonary units are recruited. The "pulmonary unit status" may be defined by its degree of inflation (23). Indeed, we may recruit pulmonary units from a degree of inflation of zero (nonaerated compartment) to any degree of inflation. In this case, the recruitment is defined as:

$$\text{(Grams of nonaerated tissue)}_{\text{Paw1}} - \text{(Grams of nonaerated tissue)}_{\text{Paw2}}$$

where Paw1 and Paw2 are the "stimuli," that is, the applied airway pressure. Accordingly, the potential for recruitment may be defined as the difference of nonaerated tissue measured at highest pressure (usually 45 cmH$_2$O) and lowest pressure (usually 0 or 5 cmH$_2$O).

Using oleic acid animal models (38,53), the huge potential for recruitment (i.e., at highest pressure the nonaerated tissue is near zero) has been demonstrated. More importantly, it showed that recruitment, as previously defined, is an inspiratory phenomenon as it occurs continuously along the inspiratory volume pressure curve (54) (Fig. 3.5), which may be considered as

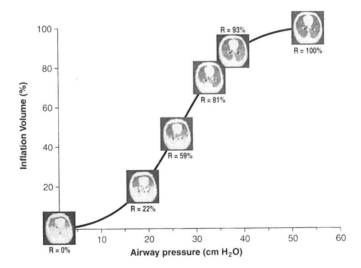

Figure 3.5 Recruitment in an experimental ARDS model (oleic acid in dogs), as a function of the applied airway pressures. Recruitment occurs along the entire volume–pressure curve, even after the upper inflection point. "*R*" indicates the percentage of recruitment occurring at the corresponding airway pressure. The data were fitted with a sigmoid function. Similar results were obtained in patients. [From Gattinoni et al. (54).]

"recruitment pressure curve." The sigmoid shape of the recruitment pressure curve indicates a gaussian distribution of opening pressure in a range from 0 to 45 cmH$_2$O (55) (Fig. 3.6). This phenomenon was observed in models with high potential for recruitment, but the same rules apply to patients in which the potential for recruitment was very low (only 5% of the nonaerated tissue was "opened" at 45 cmH$_2$O). Despite this, similar recruitment pressure curves and distribution have been observed.

However, the recruitment concept may be applied not only to the changes from the gasless status to the aeration, but also to the changes to any intermediate status. Indeed, some authors defined the "recruitment" as the differences between the sum of nonaerated and poorly aerated volumes (not tissue) as follows (40):

$$\text{Recruitment} = [\text{nonaerated volume} + \text{poorly aerated volume}]_{Paw2}$$
$$- [\text{nonaerated volume} + \text{poorly aerated volume}]_{Paw1}$$

where Paw1 and Paw2 are the two different stimuli. In this way, the recruitment is the measure of gas entering the nonaerated and poorly aerated compartment. As the poorly aerated compartment usually is not modified, this computation primarily reflects the changes of the nonaerated compartment. We believe that the most straightforward definition of recruitment is the change between the gasless status to aeration, which also allows the definition of the corresponding opening pressures and avoids the mixing of tissue and volume concepts (Fig. 3.7).

The ideal definition of recruitment should be the involvement of new pulmonary units to a normal function, that is, to a normal gas exchange. Unfortunately, CT can only give a rough estimate of ventilation (as change of inflation status), and not the regional perfusion, although new technologies (CT with Xenon inhalation) appear promising (56,57). We also refer to the chapter on hyperpolarized 3-helium MRI (Chapter 7).

De-recruitment and Positive End-Expiratory Pressure

De-recruitment is defined as the transition from aerated to gasless status, but this pathway is different from that of recruitment (38,55). The closing pressures leading to collapse are in a lower range than the opening pressures (Fig. 3.8).

After lung opening (recruitment), there are three possible causes for the lung collapse (58):

- low arterial V_A/Q of some pulmonary units
- surfactant alterations
- superimposed pressure higher than closing pressure

With the CT scan, it is possible to show only the importance of the compressive forces due to the increased lung mass in causing de-recruitment. In ALI/ARDS, the expiratory inflection zone (i.e., the pressure at which the lung collapse) increased progressively from frontal to dorsal lung regions in a

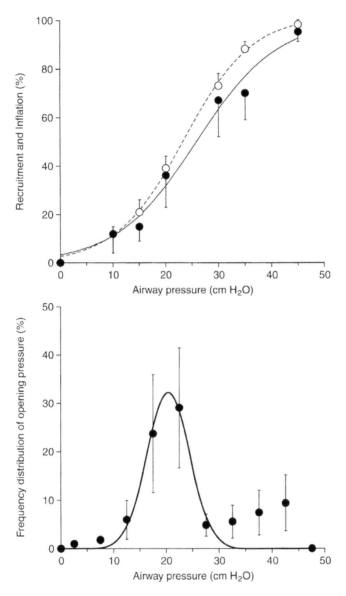

Figure 3.6 *Upper panel*: Recruitment as a function of airway pressure. Solid circles and solid line refer to fractional recruitment of the potential for recruitment ($r = 0.99$, $P = 0.0002$); open circles and dashed line refer to fractional inflation of the lung CT slice ($r = 0.99$, $P < 0.0001$). *Lower panel*: Frequency distribution of estimated threshold opening pressures as a function of aiway pressure ($r = 0.9$, $P < 0.01$). Each point has been computed at 5 cmH$_2$O pressure intervals from the fitted recruitment pressure curve obtained in each patient. Thus, these points are not experimental but an estimate of the threshold opening pressures. Data are expressed as mean $\pm$ SEM. [From Crotti et al. (55).]

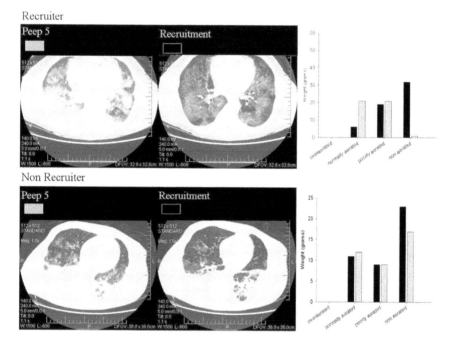

Figure 3.7 CT showing an high potential for recruitment (upper panel) and low potential for recruitment (lower panel). The corresponding amount of hyperinflated, normally aerated, poorly aerated, and nonaerated tissues at 5 cmH$_2$O PEEP (gray column) and at 45 cmH$_2$O (black column) is shown on the right.

supine position. Moreover, the collapse pressure was linearly correlated with the superimposed pressure at that height (50) (Fig. 3.9).

Animal models have demonstrated by CT that this form of collapse may be prevented, if PEEP is equal or greater than the applied compressive forces. When the compressive forces were greater than the applied PEEP, the collapse was several orders of magnitude greater than when PEEP was higher than the compressive force (38). There is, however, an unavoidable consequence. When PEEP greater than the compressive forces in the most dependent regions is applied, there is hyperinflation of the nondependent lung regions, where the compressive forces are nil.

Overinflation

Hayhurst et al. (59) reported that emphysema patients had a clear shift of the CT number frequency distribution towards the -900 to -1000 HU range, "the hyperinflated compartment." CT is well suited for detection of hyperinflation.

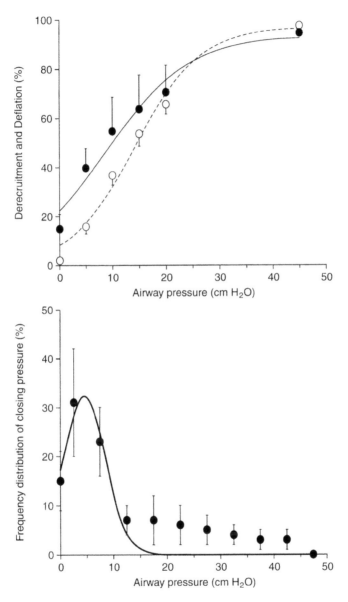

Figure 3.8 *Upper panel*: De-recruitment as a function of airway pressure. Solid circles and solid line refer to the fractional derecruitment of the potential for recruitment ($r = 0.98$, $P < 0.01$); open circles and dashed line refer to the fractional deflation of the lung CT slice ($r = 0.99$, $P < 0.01$). *Lower panel*: Frequency distribution of estimated threshold closing pressures as a function of airway pressure ($r = 0.91$, $P < 0.001$). Each point has been computed at 5 cmH$_2$O pressure intervals from the fitted de-recruitment pressure curve obtained in each patient. Thus, these points are not experimental, but an estimate of the threshold closing pressures. Data are expressed as mean $\pm$ SEM. [From Crotti et al. (55).]

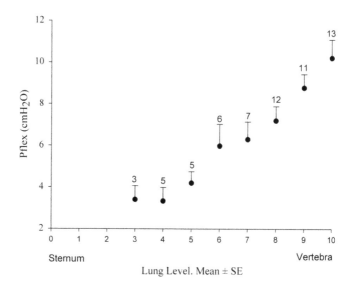

Figure 3.9 Inflection point pressure (Pflex) of the biphasic gas/tissue ratio PEEP curves as a function of the lung levels. The numbers above the plotted points refer to the number of data points. [From Gattinoni et al. (50).]

In normal man, at functional residual capacity, the hyperinflated compartment represents only a minimal fraction of the whole lung (2–3%) (43). However, at total lung capacity in normal patients, this compartment increases up to ~30% (41). In ALI/ARDS patients, Dambrosio et al. (42) found that above the upper inflection point of the volume–pressure curve, the number of voxels between -1000 and -800 HU increased by 10%. (*Note*: The cutoff of -800 HU is higher than the commonly used cutoff of -900 HU.) Vieira et al. (41) showed that an increase in pressure ventilation increased the hyperinflated compartment in six patients with ALI/ARDS. Hence, these authors concluded that CT is a useful tool to detect "overdistention" in patients with ALI/ARDS. Others have found that at PEEP of 15 cmH2O the -1000 to -900 HU compartment in ALI/ARDS was only 4% (43). These apparently contradictory results may be merely due to semantics. Hyperinflation should refer to gas overfilling (i.e., the voxels of a given pulmonary unit that composed of all gas or gas/tissue ratio of greater than 9/1), whereas overdistension or overstretching refers to increased alveolar wall tension. In normal lung, or in ALI, in which at least part of the lung is near normal, the increase in pressure and the increase of gas filling are parallel phenomena, and hyperinflation and overdistension occur simultaneously. On the contrary, in severe ARDS, in which the whole lung has an increased mass, the increase of pressure may result in overdistension without reaching the critical number of -900 HU to be considered hyperinflated.

C. Ventilation

Distribution of Ventilation

With modern, fast speed CT scanners, it is possible to investigate the dynamics of ventilation, and this has been studied in experimental models (60–62). Similar results, however, have been obtained in patients, in which the "ventilation" was computed in static conditions as the difference, in a given lung region, between the volume of gas at end-inspiration and at end-expiration (23). These studies have clearly indicated that the ventilation, in subjects lying supine during anesthesia/paralysis, distributes preferentially to the nondependent regions when PEEP is low (0–5 cmH$_2$O). These findings confirmed other studies in which the ventilation distribution was estimated with X-rays (63). However, increasing the PEEP, it has been found that the ventilation distributes more evenly between the nondependent and dependent lung regions, and, at PEEP 15–20 cmH$_2$O, the ratio between dependent and nondependent ventilation was close to 1/1. This was attributed to the PEEP-induced decrease of compliance in the nondependent regions (already open) associated with an increased compliance (recruitment) in the most dependent regions. Independent of recruitment, more homogeneous ventilation distribution is usually associated with better oxygenation, and this may explain the beneficial effect of PEEP on oxygenation in late ALI/ARDS, where the compressive atelectasis is unlikely to occur (22).

Inspiratory–Expiratory Interaction and Recruitment Maneuvers

The CT scan also allowed to investigate and to clarify the interaction between end-inspiration and end-expiration, which may be clinically relevant. Both in animal models and in patients, the amount of collapse at end-expiration is linearly related with the amount of collapse at end-inspiration (38,55). In other words, at the same PEEP, the amount of collapse depends on the previous inspiratory pressure. This phenomenon is easily understandable considering the distribution range of opening pressure in ALI/ARDS. If the inspiratory pressure is insufficient to open some lung regions, PEEP cannot act to keep these open at end-expiration. These findings are relevant in the context of low tidal ventilation and recruitment maneuvers.

There is sufficient evidence that low tidal volume ventilation results in better survival than high tidal volume ventilation (64). However, it has been shown that low tidal volume ventilation may lead to further decreased lung volume, likely due to atelectasis (65). This is probably caused by progressive atelectasis due to the low V_A/Q ratio of some lung regions (re-absorption atelectasis) (58). If this occurs, the inspiratory pressure is insufficient to re-open the lung, increasing hypoxemia. On the basis of the CT scan studies and previous observations, there are two possibilities to prevent/resolve these kinds of complications. First, it has been shown that infrequent (1–2 per min) delivery of higher tidal volume may prevent re-absorption atelectasis (58,66). Secondly, the recruitment maneuvers, that is, the controlled inflations at 40–45 cmH$_2$O, may provide sufficient inspiratory pressure to re-open the stitch atelectasis, characterized by elevated opening pressures (67,68).

VI. CT Scan and Position

Prone positioning was suggested several years ago, on theoretical and clinical basis, to improve oxygenation in ALI/ARDS (69–71). After initial CT studies in ALI/ARDS, which showed the "baby lung" in the independent lung regions, patients were studied prone to improve perfusion of the "dependent" baby lung. However, as discussed earlier, the CT scan in prone position showed density re-distribution from dorsal to ventral, leading to concept of "sponge model." The CT scan regional analysis of ALI/ARDS patients in supine and prone position, as well as of normal subjects, revealed that the density re-distribution of prone position is not just reversed to supine, as it would be if solely function of the gravitational forces but, instead, that it is more "flat" in prone (46). This indicates that the regional inflation is more homogeneous in prone when compared with that in supine.

Oxygenation improvement was also related to the increased homogeneity of the gas/tissue distribution (72). Thus, forces other than gravity [as heart weight (73,74), abdominal pressure, and the lung/thoracic cage interaction] play a substantial role in making the prone position more advantageous in ALI/ARDS. Moreover, there is now consistent experimental evidence that prone positioning is somewhat protective from the lung ventilation injury (75–77), likely because the more homogeneous distribution of the inflation decreases the stress/strain maldistribution caused by mechanical ventilation in supine position (19).

VII. CT Scan and Abdominal Pressure

A proportion of patients with ALI/ARDS present with an abnormal abdominal pressure (78). This may be due to anthropometric characteristics, sedative drugs, or more frequently, to abdominal disease, as peritonitis or intestinal infarction, which may cause extrapulmonary ARDS. We already discussed the effects of increased abdominal pressure on chest wall mechanics, and, in turn, on lung distension. Here, however, we would like to describe the effects of acute abdominal hypertension (20 cmH$_2$O, a value often recorded in critically ill) on lung edema. In a model of oleic acid, increasing the abdominal pressure led to two to threefold increase of pulmonary edema (53). This was likely due to blood shift from abdomen to the thorax, which in turn causes the edema to increase. Moreover, the increase of pleural pressure induced by the increased abdominal pressure may impair the edema clearance. Although data on patients are lacking, it is possible that in ALI/ARDS, a sudden increase of abdominal pressure may induce not only a decrease of gas content, but also an increase of pulmonary edema, as documented by CT scan.

VIII. Clinical Use of the CT Scan

Soon after the application of CT to ALI/ARDS patients, it became evident that the information gained on CT frequently alters patient management (17,79). The largest published study on the clinical impact of CT scanning is a retrospective review of 74 ALI/ARDS patients (80). Not surprisingly, it showed that pleural effusions, lobar atelectasis, lung abscesses, bullae, occult pneumothoraces, occult barotruama, and unsuspected tube malpositions were seen more often and more definitely on CT than on chest X-ray. In total, the CT yielded additional information in 66% of patients and had a direct influence on patient treatment in 22%. The advantages of CT, however, must be balanced against the potential risks of transporting critically ill patients, the additional cost, and the additional radiation. Desai and Hansell (81) indicate that CT is best used to detect occult complications in patients who are deteriorating or not improving at the expected rate, to quantify the extent of lung involvement in ALI/ARDS, to resolve contradictory radiographic, clinical, or physiologic signs, and to demonstrate significant areas of dependent atelectasis.

In summary, the indications for the use of CT in clinical practice are not totally clear but, in our practice, we have two essential indications:

1. *Patients in early phase of ARDS.* Early in the course of the ALI/ ARDS patients, CT is helpful in assessing the nature of the patients' infiltrates and their response to mechanical ventilation. We limit the CT scan to two or three slices, repeating the same slices at different ventilator settings (e.g., end-inspirations and at different PEEP levels). By imaging only a few levels, we are able to keep the total X-ray exposure at an acceptable level, while acquiring the relevant information. The use of different pressures helps to distinguish between areas of alveolar collapse and consolidation providing helpful information about the potential for recruitment and mechanical ventilation parameters.

2. *Assessment of comorbid conditions and occult complication.* The CT is helpful in assessing comorbid conditions (lung laceration, abscess, etc.) in early ALI/ARDS. Beyond the initial phases, CT is particularly helpful in explaining discrepancies between the chest X-ray and various clinical and physiologic parameters or when there is physio-logic deterioration without obvious reason. In these cases, occult pneu-mothorax, pneumomediastinum, pneumatocele formation, abscesses, septic emboli, and effusions may be revealed that require immediate therapeutic intervention such as CT-guided catheter drainage (82,83). Pulmonary emboli are another cause of hypoxia or hemodynamic

instability in the face of an unchanging chest X-ray. In this patient population, they may be best studied with contrast-enhanced helical CT, because the lung scan is often inconclusive, and pulmonary angiography is invasive, potentially hazardous, and not always available (84–87). Fast scanning is also valuable in the evaluation of great vessel catastrophies (aortic dissection and leaking aneurysm) and tracheobronchial diseases (stenosis, malacia, or obstruction).

Indeed, the bulk of data strongly suggests that despite the difficulties of transporting critically ill patients for CT, the X-ray exposure, and significant cost, the use of CT scan justified owing to the rate of detection on unsuspected thoracic alterations, whereas bedside X-ray examinations fails to explain adequately the clinical findings (88).

References

1. Rommelsheim K, Lackner K, Westhofen P, Distelmaier W, Hirt S. Respiratory distress syndrome of the adult in the computed tomography. Anasth Intensive Ther Notfallmed 1983; 18:59–64.
2. Maunder RJ, Shuman WP, McHugh JW, Marglin SI, Butler J. Preservation of normal lung regions in the adult respiratory distress syndrome. Analysis by computed tomography. JAMA 1986; 255:2463–2465.
3. Gattinoni L, Mascheroni D, Torresin A, Marcolin R, Fumagalli R, Vesconi S, Rossi GP, Rossi F, Baglioni S, Bassi F. Morphological response to positive end expiratory pressure in acute respiratory failure. Computerized tomography study. Intensive Care Med 1986; 12:137–142.
4. Austin JH, Muller NL, Friedman PJ, Hansell DM, Naidich DP, Remy-Jardin M, Webb WR, Zerhouni EA. Glossary of terms for CT of the lungs: recommendations of the Nomenclature Committee of the Fleischner Society. Radiology 1996; 200:327–331.
5. Weibel E. The Pathway for Oxygen. Structure and Function in the Mammalian Respiratory System. Cambridge: Harvard University Press, 1984.
6. Remy-Jardin M, Remy J, Giraud F, Wattinne L, Gosselin B. Computed tomography assessment of ground-glass opacity: semiology and significance. J Thorac Imaging 1993; 8:249–264.
7. Puybasset L, Cluzel P, Chao N, Slutsky AS, Coriat P, Rouby JJ. A computed tomography scan assessment of regional lung volume in acute lung injury. The CT Scan ARDS Study Group. Am J Respir Crit Care Med 1998; 158:1644–1655.
8. Gattinoni L, Pelosi P, Suter PM, Pedoto A, Vercesi P, Lissoni A. Acute respiratory distress syndrome caused by pulmonary and extrapulmonary disease. Different syndromes? Am J Respir Crit Care Med 1998; 158:3–11.
9. Tutor JD, Mason CM, Dobard E, Beckerman RC, Summer WR, Nelson S. Loss of compartmentalization of alveolar tumor necrosis factor after lung injury. Am J Respir Crit Care Med 1994; 149:1107–1111.
10. Muller-Leisse C, Klosterhalfen B, Hauptmann S, Simon HB, Kashefi A, Andreopoulos D, Kirkpatrick CJ, Gunther RW. Computed tomography and

histologic results in the early stages of endotoxin-injured pig lungs as a model for adult respiratory distress syndrome. Invest Radiol 1993; 28:39–45.

11. Goodman LR, Fumagalli R, Tagliabue P, Tagliabue M, Ferrario M, Gattinoni L, Pesenti A. Adult respiratory distress syndrome due to pulmonary and extrapulmonary causes: CT, clinical, and functional correlations. Radiology 1999; 213:545–552.

12. Desai SR, Wells AU, Rubens MB, Evans TW, Hansell DM. Acute respiratory distress syndrome: CT abnormalities at long-term follow-up. Radiology 1999; 210:29–35.

13. Desai SR, Wells AU, Suntharalingam G, Rubens MB, Evans TW, Hansell DM. Acute respiratory distress syndrome caused by pulmonary and extrapulmonary injury: a comparative CT study. Radiology 2001; 218:689–693.

14. Winer-Muram HT, Steiner RM, Gurney JW, Shah R, Jennings SG, Arheart KL, Eltorky MA, Meduri GU. Ventilator-associated pneumonia in patients with adult respiratory distress syndrome: CT evaluation. Radiology 1998; 208:193–199.

15. Rouby JJ, Puybasset L, Cluzel P, Richecoeur J, Lu Q, Grenier P. Regional distribution of gas and tissue in acute respiratory distress syndrome. II. Physiological correlations and definition of an ARDS Severity Score. CT Scan ARDS Study Group. Intensive Care Med 2000; 26:1046–1056.

16. Spragg RG, Levin D. ARDS and the search for meaningful subgroups. Intensive Care Med 2000; 26:835–837.

17. Goodman LR. Congestive heart failure and adult respiratory distress syndrome. New insights using computed tomography. Radiol Clin North Am 1996; 34:33–46.

18. Rouby JJ, Lherm T, Martin DL, Poete P, Bodin L, Finet JF, Callard P, Viars P. Histologic aspects of pulmonary barotrauma in critically ill patients with acute respiratory failure. Intensive Care Med 1993; 19:383–389.

19. Gattinoni L, Carlesso E, Cadringher P, Valenza F, Vagginelli F, Chiumello D. Physical and biological triggers of ventilator-induced lung injury and its prevention. Eur Respir J Suppl 2003; 47:15s–25s.

20. Treggiari MM, Romand JA, Martin JB, Suter PM. Air cysts and bronchiectasis prevail in nondependent areas in severe acute respiratory distress syndrome: a computed tomographic study of ventilator-associated changes. Crit Care Med 2002; 30:1747–1752.

21. Churg A, Golden J, Fligiel S, Hogg JC. Bronchopulmonary dysplasia in the adult. Am Rev Respir Dis 1983; 127:117–120.

22. Gattinoni L, Bombino M, Pelosi P, Lissoni A, Pesenti A, Fumagalli R, Tagliabue M. Lung structure and function in different stages of severe adult respiratory distress syndrome. JAMA 1994; 271:1772–1779.

23. Gattinoni L, Pelosi P, Crotti S, Valenza F. Effects of positive end-expiratory pressure on regional distribution of tidal volume and recruitment in adult respiratory distress syndrome. Am J Respir Crit Care Med 1995; 151:1807–1814.

24. Nobauer-Huhmann IM, Eibenberger K, Schaefer-Prokop C, Steltzer H, Schlick W, Strasser K, Fridrich P, Herold CJ. Changes in lung parenchyma after acute respiratory distress syndrome (ARDS): assessment with high-resolution computed tomography. Eur Radiol 2001; 11:2436–2443.

25. Finfer S, Rocker G. Alveolar overdistension is an important mechanism of persistent lung damage following severe protracted ARDS. Anaesth Intensive Care 1996; 24:569–573.

26. Drummond GB. Computed tomography and pulmonary measurements. Br J Anaesth 1998; 80:665–671.

27. Mull RT. Mass estimates by computed tomography: physical density from CT numbers. Am J Roentgenol 1984; 143:1101–1104.

28. Kalra M, Maher M, Saini S. CT radiation exposure: rationale for concern and strategies for dose reduction. Applied Radiology 2003; 45–54 (Online Supplement).

29. Ibanez J, Raurich JM. Normal values of functional residual capacity in the sitting and supine positions. Intensive Care Med 1982; 8:173–177.

30. Pelosi P, D'Andrea L, Vitale G, Pesenti A, Gattinoni L. Vertical gradient of regional lung inflation in adult respiratory distress syndrome. Am J Respir Crit Care Med 1994; 149:8–13.

31. Hogg JC, Nepszy S. Regional lung volume and pleural pressure gradient estimated from lung density in dogs. J Appl Physiol 1969; 27:198–203.

32. Agostoni E. Mechanics of the pleural space. In: Maklem P, ed. Handbook of Physiology. The Respiratory System. Bethesda: Am Physiol Soc, 1986:531–559.

33. Milic-Emili J. Static distribution of lung volumes. In: Maklem P, ed. Handbook of Physiology. The Respiratory System. Bethesda: Am Physiol Soc, 1986:561–574.

34. Milic-Emili J, Henderson JA, Dolovich MB, Trop D, Kaneko K. Regional distribution of inspired gas in the lung. J Appl Physiol 1966; 21:749–759.

35. Glaister DH. Distribution of pulmonary blood flow and ventilation during forward (plus Gx) acceleration. J Appl Physiol 1970; 29:432–439.

36. Bryan AC, Milic-Emili J, Pengelly D. Effect of gravity on the distribution of pulmonary ventilation. J Appl Physiol 1966; 21:778–784.

37. Michels DB, West JB. Distribution of pulmonary ventilation and perfusion during short periods of weightlessness. J Appl Physiol 1978; 45:987–998.

38. Pelosi P, Goldner M, McKibben A, Adams A, Eccher G, Caironi P, Losappio S, Gattinoni L, Marini JJ. Recruitment and derecruitment during acute respiratory failure: an experimental study. Am J Respir Crit Care Med 2001; 164:122–130.

39. Gattinoni L, Pesenti A, Avalli L, Rossi F, Bombino M. Pressure–volume curve of total respiratory system in acute respiratory failure. Computed tomographic scan study. Am Rev Respir Dis 1987; 136:730–736.

40. Malbouisson LM, Muller JC, Constantin JM, Lu Q, Puybasset L, Rouby JJ. Computed tomography assessment of positive end-expiratory pressure-induced alveolar recruitment in patients with acute respiratory distress syndrome. Am J Respir Crit Care Med 2001; 163:1444–1450.

41. Vieira SR, Puybasset L, Richecoeur J, Lu Q, Cluzel P, Gusman PB, Coriat P, Rouby JJ. A lung computed tomographic assessment of positive end-expiratory pressure-induced lung overdistension. Am J Respir Crit Care Med 1998; 158:1571–1577.

42. Dambrosio M, Roupie E, Mollet JJ, Anglade MC, Vasile N, Lemaire F, Brochard L. Effects of positive end-expiratory pressure and different tidal volumes on alveolar recruitment and hyperinflation. Anesthesiology 1997; 87:495–503.

43. Gattinoni L, Pesenti A, Bombino M, Baglioni S, Rivolta M, Rossi F, Rossi G, Fumagalli R, Marcolin R, Mascheroni D. Relationships between lung computed tomographic density, gas exchange, and PEEP in acute respiratory failure. Anesthesiology 1988; 69:824–832.

44. Gattinoni L, Pesenti A, Baglioni S, Vitale G, Rivolta M, Pelosi P. Inflammatory pulmonary edema and positive end-expiratory pressure: correlations between imaging and physiologic studies. J Thorac Imaging 1988; 3:59–64.

45. Langer M, Mascheroni D, Marcolin R, Gattinoni L. The prone position in ARDS patients. A clinical study. Chest 1988; 94:103–107.
46. Gattinoni L, Pelosi P, Vitale G, Pesenti A, D'Andrea L, Mascheroni D. Body position changes redistribute lung computed-tomographic density in patients with acute respiratory failure. Anesthesiology 1991; 74:15–23.
47. Jones T, Jones HA, Rhodes CG, Buckingham PD, Hughes JM. Distribution of extravascular fluid volumes in isolated perfused lungs measured with H215O. J Clin Invest 1976; 57:706–713.
48. Hales CA, Kanarek DJ, Ahluwalia B, Latty A, Erdmann J, Javaheri S, Kazemi H. Regional edema formation in isolated perfused dog lungs. Circ Res 1981; 48:121–127.
49. Bone RC. The ARDS lung. New insights from computed tomography. JAMA 1993; 269:2134–2135.
50. Gattinoni L, D'Andrea L, Pelosi P, Vitale G, Pesenti A, Fumagalli R. Regional effects and mechanism of positive end-expiratory pressure in early adult respiratory distress syndrome. JAMA 1993; 269:2122–2127.
51. Wilson TA, Anafi RC, Hubmayr RD. Mechanics of edematous lungs. J Appl Physiol 2001; 90:2088–2093.
52. Martynowicz MA, Minor TA, Walters BJ, Hubmayr RD. Regional expansion of oleic acid-injured lungs. Am J Respir Crit Care Med 1999; 160:250–258.
53. Quintel M, Pelosi P, Caironi P, Meinhardt JP, Luecke T, Herrmann P, Taccone P, Rylander C, Valenza F, Carlesso E, Gattinoni L. An increase of abdominal pressure increases pulmonary edema in oleic acid-induced lung injury. Am J Respir Crit Care Med 2004; 169:534–541.
54. Gattinoni L, Caironi P, Pelosi P, Goodman LR. What has computed tomography taught us about the acute respiratory distress syndrome? Am J Respir Crit Care Med 2001; 164:1701–1711.
55. Crotti S, Mascheroni D, Caironi P, Pelosi P, Ronzoni G, Mondino M, Marini JJ, Gattinoni L. Recruitment and derecruitment during acute respiratory failure: a clinical study. Am J Respir Crit Care Med 2001; 164:131–140.
56. Kreck TC, Krueger MA, Altemeier WA, Sinclair SE, Robertson HT, Shade ED, Hildebrandt J, Lamm WJ, Frazer DA, Polissar NL, Hlastala MP. Determination of regional ventilation and perfusion in the lung using xenon and computed tomography. J Appl Physiol 2001; 91:1741–1749.
57. Simon BA. Non-invasive imaging of regional lung function using X-ray computed tomography. J Clin Monitor Comput 2000; 16:433–442.
58. Pelosi P, Cadringher P, Bottino N, Panigada M, Carrieri F, Riva E, Lissoni A, Gattinoni L. Sigh in acute respiratory distress syndrome. Am J Respir Crit Care Med 1999; 159:872–880.
59. Hayhurst MD, MacNee W, Flenley DC, Wright D, McLean A, Lamb D, Wightman AJ, Best J. Diagnosis of pulmonary emphysema by computerised tomography. Lancet 1984; 2:320–322.
60. Neumann P, Berglund JE, Mondejar EF, Magnusson A, Hedenstierna G. Effect of different pressure levels on the dynamics of lung collapse and recruitment in oleic-acid-induced lung injury. Am J Respir Crit Care Med 1998; 158:1636–1643.
61. Markstaller K, Kauczor HU, Weiler N, Karmrodt J, Doebrich M, Ferrante M, Thelen M, Eberle B. Lung density distribution in dynamic CT correlates with oxygenation in ventilated pigs with lavage ARDS. Br J Anaesth 2003; 91:699–708.

62. Markstaller K, Eberle B, Kauczor HU, Scholz A, Bink A, Thelen M, Heinrichs W, Weiler N. Temporal dynamics of lung aeration determined by dynamic CT in a porcine model of ARDS. Br J Anaesth 2001; 87:459–468.

63. Froese AB, Bryan AC. Effects of anesthesia and paralysis on diaphragmatic mechanics in man. Anesthesiology 1974; 41:242–255.

64. Anonymous. Ventilation with lower tidal volumes as compared with traditional tidal volumes for acute lung injury and the acute respiratory distress syndrome. The Acute Respiratory Distress Syndrome Network. N Engl J Med 2000; 342:1301–1308.

65. Richard JC, Brochard L, Vandelet P, Breton L, Maggiore SM, Jonson B, Clabault K, Leroy J, Bonmarchand G. Respective effects of end-expiratory and end-inspiratory pressures on alveolar recruitment in acute lung injury. Crit Care Med 2003; 31:89–92.

66. Pelosi P, Bottino N, Chiumello D, Caironi P, Panigada M, Gamberoni C, Colombo G, Bigatello LM, Gattinoni L. Sigh in supine and prone position during acute respiratory distress syndrome. Am J Respir Crit Care Med 2003; 167:521–527.

67. Valente Barbas CS. Lung recruitment maneuvers in acute respiratory distress syndrome and facilitating resolution. Crit Care Med 2003; 31:S265–S271.

68. Bugedo G, Bruhn A, Hernandez G, Rojas G, Varela C, Tapia JC, Castillo L. Lung computed tomography during a lung recruitment maneuver in patients with acute lung injury. Intensive Care Med 2003; 29:218–225.

69. Douglas W, Rehder K, Froukje M, Sessler A, Marsh H. Improved oxygenation in patients with acute respiratory failue: the prone position. Am Rev Respir Dis 1974; 115:559–566.

70. Douglas WW, Rehder K, Beynen FM, Sessler AD, Marsh HM. Improved oxygenation in patients with acute respiratory failure: the prone position. Am Rev Respir Dis 1977; 115:559–566.

71. Phiel M, Brown R. Use of extreme position changes in acute respiratory failure. Crit Care Med 1976; 4:13–14.

72. Gattinoni L, Pelosi P, Valenza F, Mascheroni D. Patient positioning in acute respiratory failure. In: Tobin M, ed. Priciples and Practice of Mechanical Ventilation. New York: McGraw-Hill, 2004:1067–1076.

73. Malbouisson LM, Busch CJ, Puybasset L, Lu Q, Cluzel P, Rouby JJ. Role of the heart in the loss of aeration characterizing lower lobes in acute respiratory distress syndrome. CT Scan ARDS Study Group. Am J Respir Crit Care Med 2000; 161:2005–2012.

74. Albert RK, Hubmayr RD. The prone position eliminates compression of the lungs by the heart. Am J Respir Crit Care Med 2000; 161:1660–1665.

75. Du HL, Yamada Y, Orii R, Suzuki S, Sawamura S, Suwa K, Hanaoka K. Beneficial effects of the prone position on the incidence of barotrauma in oleic acid-induced lung injury under continuous positive pressure ventilation. Acta Anaesthesiol Scand 1997; 41:701–707.

76. Nishimura M, Honda O, Tomiyama N, Johkoh T, Kagawa K, Nishida T. Body position does not influence the location of ventilator-induced lung injury. Intensive Care Med 2000; 26:1664–1669.

77. Broccard A, Shapiro RS, Schmitz LL, Adams AB, Nahum A, Marini JJ. Prone positioning attenuates and redistributes ventilator-induced lung injury in dogs. Crit Care Med 2000; 28:295–303.

78. Malbrain ML, Chiumello D, Pelosi P, Wilmer A, Brienza N, Malcangi V, Bihari D, Innes R, Cohen J, Singer P, Japiassu A, Kurtop E, De Keulenaer BL, Daelemans R, Del Turco M, Cosimini P, Ranieri M, Jacquet L, Laterre PF, Gattinoni L. Prevalence

of intra-abdominal hypertension in critically ill patients: a multicentre epidemiological study. Intensive Care Med 2004; 30:822–829.

79. Snow N, Bergin KT, Horrigan TP. Thoracic CT scanning in critically ill patients. Information obtained frequently alters management. Chest 1990; 97:1467–1470.

80. Tagliabue M, Casella TC, Zincone GE, Fumagalli R, Salvini E. CT and chest radiography in the evaluation of adult respiratory distress syndrome. Acta Radiol 1994; 35:230–234.

81. Desai SR, Hansell DM. Lung imaging in the adult respiratory distress syndrome: current practice and new insights. Intensive Care Med 1997; 23:7–15.

82. Chon KS, van Sonnenberg E, D'Agostino HB, O'Laoide RM, Colt HG, Hart E. CT-guided catheter drainage of loculated thoracic air collections in mechanically ventilated patients with acute respiratory distress syndrome. Am J Roentgenol 1999; 173:1345–1350.

83. Boland GW, Lee MJ, Sutcliffe NP, Mueller PR. Loculated pneumothoraces in patients with acute respiratory disease treated with mechanical ventilation: preliminary observations after image-guided drainage. J Vasc Interv Radiol 1996; 7:247–252.

84. Goodman LR, Lipchik RJ, Kuzo RS, Liu Y, McAuliffe TL, O'Brien DJ. Subsequent pulmonary embolism: risk after a negative helical CT pulmonary angiogram—prospective comparison with scintigraphy. Radiology 2000; 215:535–542.

85. Goodman LR, Lipchik RJ. Diagnosis of acute pulmonary embolism: time for a new approach. Radiology 1996; 199:25–27.

86. Schoepf UJ, Bruening R, Konschitzky H, Becker CR, Knez A, Weber J, Muehling O, Herzog P, Huber A, Haberl R, Reiser MF. Pulmonary embolism: comprehensive diagnosis by using electron-beam CT for detection of emboli and assessment of pulmonary blood flow. Radiology 2000; 217:693–700.

87. Qanadli SD, Hajjam ME, Mesurolle B, Barre O, Bruckert F, Joseph T, Mignon F, Vieillard-Baron A, Dubourg O, Lacombe P. Pulmonary embolism detection: prospective evaluation of dual-section helical CT versus selective pulmonary arteriography in 157 patients. Radiology 2000; 217:447–455.

88. Mirvis SE, Tobin KD, Kostrubiak I, Belzberg H. Thoracic CT in detecting occult disease in critically ill patients. Am J Roentgenol 1987; 148:685–689.

4

Imaging Respiratory Mechanics

HANS-ULRICH KAUCZOR

Deutsches Krebsforschungszentrum,
Heidelberg, Germany

I. Introduction

The lung, pleura, chest wall, and diaphragm constitute a joint mechanical system, whose elasticity, viscosity, and musculature work together to enable respiration. Elasticity, a component of this system, is a vector with a certain size and direction. The lung itself has an inward vector aimed at diminution, whereas the thorax, with the lung expanded, has an outward vector aimed at extension. This interrelation can be described by Eq. (4.1)

$$\Delta p = E \times \frac{\Delta V}{V_0} \qquad (4.1)$$

where Δp is the pressure change at the lung surface, E is the elasticity module, V_0 is the starting lung volume, for example, functional residual capacity, and ΔV is the lung volume change, for example, tidal volume.

From here, two important indices can be derived:

$$\text{Elastance} = \frac{E}{V_0} = \frac{\Delta p}{\Delta V} \ (\text{kPa/L})$$

$$\text{Compliance} = C = \frac{V_0}{E} = \frac{\Delta V}{\Delta p} \ (\text{L/kPa})$$

If the elasticity model of the lung were constant, a linear correlation between trans-pulmonary pressure and lung volume as shown by the pressure–volume (PV) curve would be observed. However, even for small changes of lung volume, for example, tidal breathing, this is not the case. Airway resistance results in a pressure difference between inspiration and expiration, altering lung compliance $(\Delta V/\Delta p)$ and contributing to hysteresis observed in the PV curve. Larger volume changes, as encountered in deep inspiration or expiration, lead to reduced compliance when the maximum or minimum distensibility of the lung is approached. Various diseases also alter compliance. In pulmonary emphysema, there is a loss of lung elasticity that increases compliance. In pulmonary fibrosis, the lung is stiffened and the compliance is reduced. In addition to compliance, the trans-pulmonary pressure can describe the strength of pulmonary retraction in deep inspiration (1). The study of respiratory mechanics is very complex, and the role of imaging in this field is just beginning. The field can be divided into the mechanics of the diaphragm, chest wall, and the pulmonary parenchyma on a macro- and microscopic level. The imaging approaches toward the mechanical properties of these two levels are different and will be discussed separately.

II. Parenchymal Mechanics

Imaging has been limited in the study of lung parenchymal mechanics because of its complicated nature and because it is not within the mainstream of morphological CT scanning. Until recently, CT only examined macromechanical structure, essentially ignoring the even more difficult field of micromechanics. Applications of MRI toward pulmonary mechanics have been even less frequent. Before the advent of imaging in the field of respiratory mechanics, researchers had started to elucidate the mechanical properties of the lung with the measurement of the PV curve. Obviously, the PV curve only provides global information about the mechanics of lung parenchyma. This information is limited because it is based on the simplest model, which describes the parenchyma as a uniform isotropic material that is uniformly inflated. However, in reality, the lung does not expand uniformly, but different regions of the lung will open and empty asynchronously. Such heterogeneous patterns cannot be detected adequately by a global test such as the PV curve but by a modality which will allow for depiction of regional inhomogeneities, such as imaging. The weight of the lungs is a cause for nonuniform lung expansion, as it produces distortions and strain on the supporting elements of the lung. Thus, the weight of the lung requires a higher pleural pressure at the bottom of the lung than at the top. This gradient in pleural pressure, and hence trans-pulmonary pressure, can be located in different regions and corresponds to different points on the PV curve. Since lung compliance increases as trans-pulmonary pressure decreases, the base of the lung, where the trans-pulmonary pressure is smaller, is more compliant at the beginning of expiration than the apex and reaches residual volume earlier. Thus, the base contributes more to expiration at the beginning, and the apex more towards the end of expiration. Studies using radioactive xenon showed the predicted vertical gradient of pleural pressure as well as the differences in regional expansion that were consistent with these predictions (2).

The weight of the lung and the associated nonuniformities of the transpulmonary pressure are not the only cause for nonuniform lung expansion. Further evidence has been obtained by studies of regional lung volumes in supine dogs by parenchymal markers, which had been implanted in the lower lobes of open-chest supine dogs and tracked by biplane video fluoroscopy (3). During deflation from total lung capacity, regional rates of emptying were found to vary by ± 10% from the mean. In the supine dog, an anterior–posterior gradient of regional emptying was observed, but this accounted for only 30% of the total variability (3). Presumably, nonuniform parenchymal expansion is caused by nonuniformities in the volume densities of connective tissue and surface area (2). Further measurements have examined the lung at regional tidal volumes of ~20% of total lung capacity, which were tracked within samples of lung parenchyma during sinusoidal volume oscillations. Frequencies of 1–40 breaths/min were used before and after methacholine challenge. The volumes of tetrahedrons with apexes at the four markers were computed. Sine waves were fit to the data for volume vs. time for each tetrahedron. The ratio of mean regional volume to mean airway pressure decreased by 10–45% after methacholine challenge. Dynamic lung elastance and resistance of the constricted lungs were larger than controls, and both were frequency dependent. Regional elastance and resistance varied considerably among tetrahedrons, and these were also frequency dependent. The data were fit by a model in which tissue elastance was uniform and nearly equal to elastance in the control state, but small airway resistance was high and variable. It was concluded that the lung contracts under bronchoconstriction but the increased dynamic elastance and resistance of the constricted lung may be primarily the result of nonuniform increased airway resistance at the level of the terminal bronchioles (4).

The properties of the different compartments in respiratory mechanics have been studied using imaging and by the application of various models. The pleural membrane as well as the geometry and mechanical properties of the bronchial tree and the acinus have been a major focus. However, there is only a very limited amount of information about the structure of the lung between the scale of the lobe and the scale of the acinus.

III. Interaction Between Airways and Parenchyma

One may examine the interaction between changes of bronchial diameters and the ventilatory state and the deformation of the corresponding and surrounding alveolar space. If bronchi expanded similarly to the lung and their diameters increased proportionally with the cube root of lung volume, the parenchyma surrounding the bronchi would expand uniformly. As the stress carried by the parenchyma is approximately equal to the trans-pulmonary pressure, parenchymal attachments would exert a tensile stress of approximately the same amount on the outer surface of the bronchus. The sum of this tensile stress and the stress exerted by alveolar gas pressure would then equal pleural pressure. In that case, peribronchial pressure would equal pleural pressure and the transmural pressure that expands the bronchus would equal trans-pulmonary pressure. In the normal lung, bronchial diameters increase nearly proportionally with lung volume, and peribronchial pressure is nearly equal to pleural pressure (5).

More useful information about pulmonary macromechanics can be derived from CT studies in different ways. One way is to investigate the correlation of lung area or volume with lung density, the other is to correlate between these characteristics and the area or diameter of the large airways (6). Ideally, data would have been obtained during continuous dynamic scanning during the whole respiratory cycle. As the acquisition of dynamic images at full inspiration and full expiration is very difficult to obtain in CT imaging, it is widely accepted to evaluate at least two important points during the respiratory cycle (7,8).

An important step in elucidating pulmonary macromechanics is the correlation between lung area and lung density. The changes of mean lung density and the cross-sectional area of the lung from inspiration to expiration showed a high correlation with a correlation coefficient of $r = 0.82$ (6). This indicates a clear dependency between the air content of the lung (inflation state) and the air/tissue ratio (lung volume). In normal subjects, both are the major contributors to lung attenuation and cross-sectional lung area (Fig. 4.1) (9). The correlation of the changes between inspiration and expiration indicates the dependency of the decreasing air content which causes an increase of mean lung density and the reduced gas volume which leads to a decrease of the cross-sectional lung

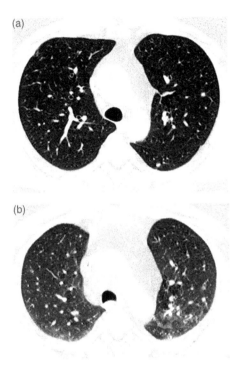

Figure 4.1 54-year-old woman with rectal carcinoma. (a) CT at full inspiration shows normal lung attenuation and a normal cross-sectional area of the trachea and the lung. (b) CT at full expiration shows a normal increase in lung density with some subtle areas of air trapping in the left lung as well as a normal decrease of both cross-sectional area of the trachea and the lung. Also, note the physiological difference in lung attenuation between the apex of the superior segment of the left lower lobe (low density) and the left upper lobe with higher density in the regions adjacent to the fissure. [Reprinted with permission from Ederle et al. (6).]

area (6). These correlations were also observed in patients with obstructive or restrictive ventilatory impairment. The relative changes between inspiration and expiration are related to the behavior of both airways and parenchymal mechanics. Such correlations allow for estimation of their properties. They are more or less valid regardless of the underlying type of ventilatory impairment. Thus, small airways and parenchymal mechanics have parallel effects on the CT parameters density and area. In obstructive ventilatory impairment at full inspiration, lung density is low and lung area is high. At full expiration, density will still be low and area high because of expiratory collapse of small airways and air trapping, which are caused by increased compliance and impaired parenchymal mechanics (Fig. 4.2). In restrictive impairment at full inspiration, lung density is high and lung area is small. At full expiration, density will be even higher

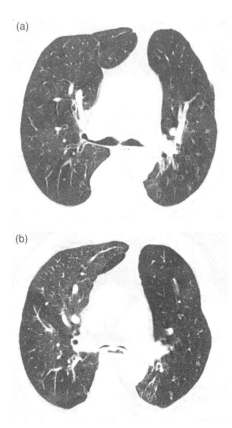

Figure 4.2 72-year-old patient with bronchiectasis. (a) CT at full inspiration shows inhomogeneous lung attenuation due to hypoxic vasoconstriction and mosaic perfusion, an increase of lung area, and a normal diameter of the main bronchi. (b) CT at full expiration more obviously shows inhomogeneous lung attenuation indicative of air trapping in the whole left lung and parts of the right lung. There is only a minor decrease in lung area, but a massive reduction of the diameter of the main bronchi. [Reprinted with permission from Ederle et al. (6).]

and area even smaller owing to traction bronchiolectasis, constriction of small airways, and decreased compliance and impaired parenchymal mechanics in fibrosis (6). Such results show effects of properties of the small airways and parenchymal mechanics indirectly assessed by CT.

Characteristics of the lung parenchyma are correlated with descriptors of the large airways. The cross-sectional area of the trachea and the diameter of the main stem bronchi have been selected to represent the large airways and then compared with the cross-sectional area of the lung as well as the mean lung density (6). There are significant correlations between the inspiratory–expiratory changes of mean lung density and the cross-sectional area of the trachea with a correlation coefficient of $r = 0.61$ (Fig. 4.1). At the same time, mean lung density highly correlates with the diameter of the main bronchi ($r = -0.52$). Also, the cross-sectional areas of lung and trachea exhibited a significant correlation ($r = 0.67$). Correlations with the diameter of the main bronchi are lower and less meaningful as they are limited by the two-dimensional approach, although disturbances by spatial volume effects are supposed to be minimal in strict anterior–posterior direction. It is important to recognize that the correlations between the lung parenchyma and the large airways are significantly affected by disease. When affected by disease, the optimized adjustments between lung volumes, air/tissue ratio, and airway dimensions are impaired. In obstructive ventilatory impairments, the air content increases to a larger extent than the size of the central airways (Fig. 4.2), where an increase can be regarded as a sign of advanced disease. Additionally, the airways in obstructive ventilatory impairments are prone to collapse, especially upon expiration, resulting in air trapping (Fig. 4.2). In restrictive lung disease, the relationship reverses: decreased air content and air/tissue ratio are associated with an increase of airway size. It is speculated that in advanced fibrosis with decreased compliance, the central airways try to adapt by increasing their lumen to facilitate gas movement (6).

To further elaborate on the relationship between lung PV behavior, bronchial pressure–diameter behavior, and parenchymal shear modulus, a dedicated method was developed (5). The method was applied to predict changes in intraparenchymal bronchial diameter that occurred when lobe PV behavior and parenchymal shear modulus (see what follows) were markedly changed by inducing air trapping in isolated dog lobes. The predictions agreed with actual measurements, thereby supporting the general hypothesis. Measured values for the shear modulus were approximately 0.7 times the trans-pulmonary pressure for the control state. Estimated values for the peribronchial pressure difference from pleural pressure during a deflation PV maneuver for trans-pulmonary pressures below $12 \, cmH_2O$ were small, approximately $\pm 1 \, cmH_2O$. They can be positive or negative, depending on whether the bronchus was dilated or constricted at the beginning of the procedure (5).

IV. Malacia of Airways

Cine CT, which is confined to imaging of a single slice, can be used as an alternative to dynamically follow changes in airway caliber over the respiratory cycle. When looking at the severity of bronchial or tracheal collapse in bronchomalacia, cine CT is significantly more sensitive compared with an assessment based on spiral CT scans acquired in full inspiratory and expiratory position because cine CT shows an expiratory reduction in cross-sectional lumen of 44 instead of 28%. As a consequence, a pathological collapse of more than 50% of maximum cross-sectional area was found significantly more frequent in cine CT (38%) compared with paired spiral CT (13%) (10). The use of cine CT can significantly improve the evaluation of respiratory collapse in localized tracheal instability (Fig. 4.3). Tailored functional studies of the trachea can also be performed using dynamic MRI with high temporal resolution (Fig. 4.4). It has been shown that COPD patients exhibit a significantly larger median collapse of the upper trachea (64%) than healthy volunteers (43%). This finding indicates a loss of elastic fibers in the tracheal wall of COPD patients (11) which might also be similar to the bronchial walls.

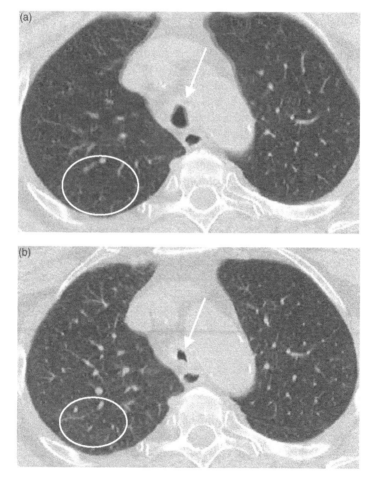

Figure 4.3 CT images taken from a dynamic cine series representing the maximum (= inspiratory) (a) and minimum (= expiratory) (b) diameter of the trachea showing a significant decrease (arrow) as well as the corresponding increase in lung attenuation in expiration (ellipse). [Reprinted with permission from Ley et al. (35).]

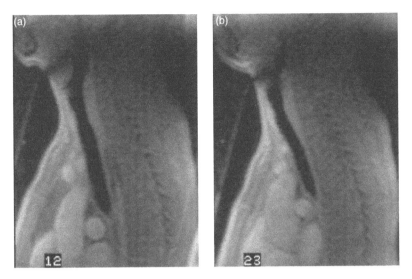

Figure 4.4 Sagittal MR images taken from a dynamic series representing the maximum (= inspiratory) (a) and minimum (= expiratory) (b) diameter of the trachea showing a normal decrease in expiration. [Reprinted with permission from Ley et al. (35).]

V. Bulk and Shear Modulus

Models of the lung as an elastic continuum undergoing small distortions from a uniformly inflated state have been used to describe many lung deformation problems. Adequate lung stress–strain material properties are needed for such a model. Two elastic models have been introduced: the bulk modulus, which describes a uniform inflation and the shear modulus, which describes an isovolumetric deformation. Both bulk modulus and shear modulus of human lungs obtained at autopsy have been measured at several fixed trans-pulmonary pressures. The bulk modulus was obtained from small PV perturbations on different points of the deflation PV curve. The shear modulus was obtained from indentation tests on the lung surface. The results indicate that, at a constant trans-pulmonary pressure, both bulk and shear moduli increase with age, and the increase was greater at higher trans-pulmonary pressure values. The micromechanical basis for these changes still remains to be elucidated (12).

VI. Gravitational Effects

Interest in the gravitational distortion of the lung led to a number of questions about the mechanics of lung distortion. In the upright or standing position, the lung distorts under its own weight; the alveoli at the base of the upright lung are relatively compressed compared with the apical alveoli. At the same time, strain and stress on interstitial tissue will be highest at the apex of the erect lung because of gravity (13,14). Because poorly expanded lung is more compliant, ventilation increases at the base of the upright human lung. Thus, the changes in ventilation are in the same direction as those for blood flow, but the magnitude of the inequality of ventilation is less. A striking change in the regional distribution for ventilation occurs at low lung volumes because the basal airways close. Thus, under these conditions, the normal pattern of ventilation is reversed with the apex being ventilated best. The weight of the lung is supported to a large extent by the rib cage and diaphragm. As a result of the downward-acting weight force, the pressure is less negative at the bottom of the lung than at the top. Just as the relative overexpansion of the lung is associated with very low intrapleural pressures, it also causes large mechanical parenchymal stress. Because of technical difficulties these have not been measured directly, but the pattern of stress distribution has been analyzed by finite element techniques (14). Stresses are greatest in the vertical direction or—more specific—in the direction of gravity. Interestingly, lateral stresses are almost as great as those in the vertical direction. Higher lateral stresses result, because, as the lung sags down, it must expand laterally to fill the expanding chest cage (14). Thus, expanding stresses in the lung periphery are much greater than in the middle of the lung, making the periphery more vulnerable to mechanical failure if the supporting connective tissue is weakened (15). The higher stresses near to the apex may explain, at least in part, the pattern of development and distribution of several diseases, including centrilobular emphysema, spontaneous pneumothorax, ankylosing spondylitis, and the cavities in postprimary tuberculosis and pulmonary infarction (16). Besides the vertical-lateral stress gradient throughout the lung, a similar gradient may be present in the individual lobes, for example, centrilobular emphysema has a predilection for the apex of the superior segment of the lower lobe when compared with a corresponding region of the middle or upper lobe at the same horizontal level (17). Calculations suggest that as a consequence of the major fissure, the tip of the superior segment of the lower lobe behaves like the apex of the upper lobe and is a region of high expanding stress (13,16).

A major limitation of both the cross-sectional imaging studies, using either CT or MRI, is that they are performed in lying, either supine or prone, position, which obviously is not the normal human erect position that is routinely used for pulmonary function tests. Thus, "normal" conditions cannot be assessed adequately while using the available CT or MRI scanners. This general limitation has to be taken into account when interpreting the data.

VII. Anterior–Posterior Gradients in Imaging

In multiple studies, an anterior–posterior gradient in lung density, pulmonary perfusion, and ventilation has been described. Additionally, an anterior–posterior gradient in regional emptying was observed as lung volume decreased from total lung capacity (4). Surprisingly, this anterior–posterior gradient was not anatomically reversed when the animal or human is rotated to the prone posture. In the prone posture, regional emptying was much more uniform. Imaging studies using CT have confirmed these results. Measurements of mean tissue density at different anterior–posterior levels of canine lungs have been performed in the supine and prone postures. At total lung capacity, the tissue density is uniform at both postures, indicating that the lung is uniformly expanded. As lung volume decreases, tissue density increases. However, in the supine posture, density increases more rapidly in the more posterior, gravity-dependent levels than in the more anterior levels. This implies that the "posterior-dependent" regions empty more rapidly than the "anterior-independent" regions (Figs. 4.1 and 4.3). In the prone position, tissue density decreases at the same rate at all anterior–posterior levels. These results have also been confirmed with a highly sophisticated CT technique, the so-called "dynamic spatial reconstructor" (18). This technique was used to study *in vivo* lung geometry and function. The lungs of three dogs were replaced with potato flakes and ping-pong balls of known air content. Scanning of these realistic phantoms revealed the estimated accuracy of lung density to be within 7% together with a high ($\pm 3\%$, standard error) internal consistency (relative density within dogs). Change in total lung air content (y) as calculated from CT volume imaging of anesthetized dogs matched the known inflation steps (x) to within 7% [range was $1-7\%$ with a mean of $3 \pm 0.5\%$ (standard error)]. An anterior–posterior gradient of decreasing percent lung air content was measured at functional residual capacity in the supine position ($y = 3.3\%$ air content/cm lung height $+ 46.5\%$ air content; $r = 0.9$). Regional lung air content change with lung inflation was greatest in the dependent lung regions. In contrast, regional lung air content at functional residual capacity was approximately uniform [it was $66 \pm 0.6\%$ (standard error)] along the anterior–posterior direction with the dog in the prone position. Anterior–posterior gradients in lung air content measured within an isogravimetric plane of the dogs in the left or right lateral decubitus position suggest that regional differences in lung air content cannot be explained solely on the basis of a direct gravitational effect on the lung (18). A possible role of the intrathoracic position of the mediastinal contents in determining these lung air content distributions has been proposed (18).

VIII. Differences Between Supine and Prone Posture

The fact that the anterior–posterior gradient of regional volume is different in the prone and supine postures implies that lung deformation cannot simply be a gravitational deformation of the lung within a rigid chest wall. The deformation must be the result of both the direct effect of gravity on the lung and a deformation in response to a change of chest wall shape. Both effects have been included in an analysis of lung deformations (19). Experimental data on chest wall shape obtained from CT scans were used as the boundary conditions in a finite-element analysis of lung deformations. It was also assumed that the lung was uniformly expanded at total lung capacity. A hypothetical chest wall shape was constructed, which was similar to the shape at total lung capacity, but with a volume reduced to volume at functional residual capacity. Boundary displacements were defined as the difference between the hypothetical and measured chest wall shapes at functional residual capacity, and the deformation of the lung caused by both the gravitational force on the lung and the boundary displacements was computed. In prone dogs, only minor variations were found in fractional volume along the cephalocaudal axis. In transverse planes, opposing deformations were caused by the change of shape of the transverse section and the gravitational force on the lung, and the resultant fractional volume and pleural pressure distributions were nearly uniform. In supine dogs, there was a small cephalocaudal gradient in fractional volume, with lower fractional volume caudally. In transverse sections, the heart and abdomen extended farther dorsally at functional residual capacity, squeezing the lung beneath them. The gradients in fractional volume and pleural pressure caused by shape changes were in the same direction as the gradients caused by the direct gravitational force on the lung, and these two factors contributed about equally to the large resultant vertical gradients in fractional volume and pleural pressure. In the prone position, the heart and upper abdomen rested on the rib cage, whereas in the supine posture, much of their weight was carried by the lung (19). Data on the shape of the chest wall of dogs at total lung capacity and functional residual capacity in the prone and supine postures were obtained by Margulies and Rodarte (20). They found that the shape of the rib cage remains similar as lung volume decreases, but, because the volumes of the heart and abdomen do not decrease, the shape of the lung at functional residual capacity is not similar to its shape at total lung capacity. They determined the shape of the passive chest wall of six anesthetized dogs at total lung capacity and functional residual capacity in the prone and supine body positions by use of volumetric CT images. The transverse cross-sectional areas of the rib cage, mediastinum, and diaphragm were calculated every 1.6 mm along the length of the thorax. The changes in the volume and the axial distribution of transverse area of the three chest wall components with lung volume and body position were evaluated. The decrease of the transverse area within the rib cage between total lung and functional residual capacity, as a fraction of the area at total lung capacity, was uniform from the apex of the thorax to the base. The volume of the mediastinum increased by 14% of its volume at total lung capacity in supine and 20% in prone position, squeezing the lung between it and the rib cage. In the transverse plane, the heart was positioned in the midthorax and moved little between inspiration and expiration. The shape, position, and displacement of the diaphragm were described by contour plots. In both postures, the diaphragm was flatter at functional residual capacity than at total lung capacity, because of larger displacements in the dorsal than in the ventral region of the diaphragm. Rotation from the prone to supine body position produced a lever motion of the diaphragm, displacing the dorsal portion of the diaphragm cephalad and the ventral portion caudad (20).

IX. "Air Trapping"

The cause of nonuniform volume expansion at small scale is unknown. Presumably, the compliance of the lung is nonuniform because the density of connective tissue and surface area is nonuniform. Nonetheless, it may be worthwhile to point out that the anatomy of the intersegmental septa and the connections between the pleural membrane and the bronchial tree have not been thoroughly investigated and that these components of the connective tissue skeleton of the lung, which presumably play a role in the expansion of the passive bronchial tree, may provide a coupling between bronchoconstriction and lung recoil. Changes from the normal relationship between lung recoil and the passive properties of the bronchi can result in trapped air, which (to a mild degree) can be regarded as a physiological phenomenon. Such air trapping has been the focus of a series of CT studies.

Expiration leads to a homogeneous increase in lung density with respect to gravity- and nongravity-dependent gradients. When heterogeneities are revealed, focal areas of low attenuation are called focal air trapping (Fig. 4.1) (21). Focal air trapping includes the occasional secondary lobule as well as extensive disease-involving multiple secondary lobules and larger subsegmental areas. The evaluation of focal air trapping as an early sign of impaired pulmonary parenchymal mechanics and small airway disease must respect findings already existing on inspiratory scans to exclude any pre-existing heterogeneities that could be caused by centrilobular emphysema, pneumonia, hypoxic vasoconstriction in advanced airway disease, or vascular obstruction such as in chronic thromboembolic pulmonary hypertension (mosaic perfusion).

Widespread focal air trapping is a hallmark of obstruction or collapse of small airways (bronchioles), which only become evident at expiration. Bronchiolitis is among the main causes and associated with many diseases: a history of dust or fume exposure, smoking, postinfection, connective tissue disease, sarcoidosis, or idiopathic diseases. A local decrease or loss of compliance is involved in most cases. In a nonselected patient population, undergoing CT focal air trapping has a prevalence of up to 80% (21). This high prevalence of focal air trapping supports the theory that focal air trapping may occur physiologically. This physiological phenomenon seems to be unrelated to age and gender. Physiological heterogeneities in ventilation are usually mild, whereas disorders of ventilation distribution due to bronchiolitis will be widespread and severe. Focal air trapping occurs predominantly in the posterior and caudal lung regions because of supine position and larger absolute volume changes. If patients are scanned in the prone position, the antero-posterior gradient is reversed, and focal air trapping is observed more easily and frequently in the anterior portions (22). Quantitative evaluation of lung density changes between corresponding inspiratory and expiratory CT exhibited high and significant correlations with intrathoracic gas volume, residual volume, and forced expiratory volume in 1 s/vital capacity as measured by pulmonary function tests (7).

The ratio of the quantitative CT lung density measured on scans, which were obtained in full inspiration and full expiration (E/I ratio), is another helpful parameter to characterize the functional impairment in cigarette smokers. The E/I ratio reflected hyperinflation and airway obstruction components regardless of the functional characteristics of emphysema (23).

In 40% of patients, a lower expiratory increase in density can be observed in the superior segment of the lower lobe with predominance in the apical part of this segment (Figs. 4.1 and 4.5). In this case, local gradients probably caused by differences in elastic recoil and mechanical stress along the fissures most likely result in high pressures which may hinder early expiration and lead to physiologic air trapping as it has been described for the development of emphysema in this region (16).

X. Parenchymal Mechanics in Different Lung Diseases

In pulmonary emphysema, CT scans of the whole lung with supine patients breathing at functional residual capacity can be used to investigate the effects of emphysematous destruction on the apex-to-base gradient of lung density and lung mass as well as their correlation with pulmonary function. Regional lung density was lower in patients with low lung mass due to both lung hyperinflation and tissue loss, whereas in patients with high or normal lung mass the reduction of lung density was only caused by hyperinflation (24). In emphysema, a good correlation between the reduction of the CO diffusion constant and reduced lung density on CT has been described (25). Both parameters closely reflect the extent of emphysema. However, reduced lung density did not correlate with the maximal static elastic recoil pressure and the exponential constant (K) of the PV curve (25). Thus, using static CT acquired at full inspiratory position the elastic properties of lung tissue cannot be predicted.

Airway hyper-responsiveness, such as in asthma, is characterized by an increase in airway sensitivity and excessive airway narrowing upon exposure to inhaled bronchoconstrictive stimuli. There is experimental evidence that maximal airway narrowing is related to lung elasticity in normal and asthmatic subjects. When using spirometrically gated CT and quantitative evaluation, lung density correlated with the maximal response to methacholine challenge in patients suffering from alpha-1-antitrypsin deficiency (26). These findings suggest that the level of maximal airway narrowing increases with the loss of

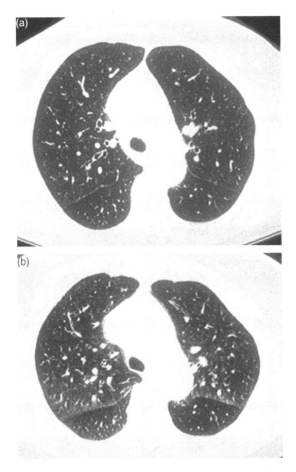

Figure 4.5 70-year-old female patient with normal pulmonary function. (a) Paired inspiratory and (b) expiratory CT shows a large relatively hypodense zone in the superior segment of the left lower lobe indicating physiological air trapping caused by regional differences in elastic recoil and mechanical stress along the fissure. [Reprinted with permission from Kauczor et al. (21).]

lung elasticity, which is associated with reduction in diffusing capacity and reduced lung density (26).

Chronic obstructive pulmonary disease and emphysema increase lung compliance by promoting the destruction of the alveolar framework. Fibrosis stiffens the lung via an idiopathic increase in parenchymal connective tissue, thus leading to a reduction of compliance. The ability to quantify lung deformation is useful in characterizing the changes brought on by these diseases. MR techniques, such as the application of two-dimensional bands of inverted magnetization directly onto the pulmonary parenchyma, are able to evaluate local mechanical properties of the lung (27). These measurements allowed for quantification of local pulmonary tissue deformation, or strain, throughout the respiratory cycle by applying finite strain definitions from continuum mechanics. The dynamics of lung deformation are exemplified by a series of motion and strain tensor maps. The magnitude of strain was maximal at the base and the apex of the lung, but it was curtailed at the hilum, the site with the poorly mobile bronchial and vascular insertions. In-plane shear strain mapping showed mostly positive shear strain, predominant at the apex throughout inhalation. As it was expected from physiology, it also increased with expanding volume. Anisotropy mapping showed that vertical strain was greater than horizontal strain at the apex and base, whereas the opposite was true for the middle lung field (27).

Acute respiratory distress syndrome (ARDS) is another disease which reveals important information about the correlation of CT data and respiratory mechanics (28). For a long time, it was a common belief that the ARDS lung was stiff because of the low compliance of the respiratory system. However, it is thought that respiratory compliance was not related to the amount of non-aerated or poorly aerated tissue, but it closely associated with the amount of normally aerated tissue, which receives most of the insufflated gas during ventilation. Thus, respiratory compliance in early ARDS appears to be a direct measure of normally aerated tissue. This suggests that in ARDS, the aerated lung is not stiff but, small in volume. In ARDS, this concept is referred to as the "baby lung" hypothesis (28). In patients suffering from acute lung injury, including ARDS, requiring mechanical ventilation, the different inspiratory flow patterns and inspiratory-to-expiratory ratios applied may alter lung strain. When different ventilation regimens, that is, pressure-controlled, volume-controlled, and pressure-controlled inverse ratio ventilation, were compared in 18 acute lung injury patients, there was no difference in static mechanics, oxygenation, or hemodynamics. However, an index of nonlinear elastic behavior, calculated by multiple linear regression analysis of dynamic airway pressure and airflow, using a volume-dependent single compartment model, was least with pressure-controlled ventilation followed by volume-controlled ventilation, and pressure-controlled inverse ratio ventilation had the greatest value. Higher values for the nonlinear elastic behavior showed a correlation with hyperinflation detected by dynamic CT at a subcarinal level (29).

XI. Diaphragm and Chest Wall

The various inspiratory muscles, including the diaphragm and the various components of the rib cage, constitute the respiratory pump, which applies expanding forces to the lungs and thus induces alveolar ventilation. As such, the respiratory pump represents one of the most important components in the act of breathing. Studies of structure and function of the respiratory pump are very difficult to perform due to the complex geometry of active and passive elements.

Cross-sectional imaging, especially MRI, is extremely helpful in elucidating structure–function relationships (30).

The diaphragm and chest wall are best assessed by three-dimensional analysis, which should consist of the shape of diaphragm and rib cage, the volumes displaced during the respiratory cycle, and the relationship between the two (Figs. 4.6 and 4.7). For simplicity, the anatomy of the diaphragm can be divided in two zones, the diaphragmatic dome and the apposition zone (30). The diaphragmatic dome is roughly horizontal and abuts on the lung above and the abdomen below. The apposition zone is roughly vertical and abuts on the chest and abdominal wall. The definition of the rib cage is straightforward. After triangulation of object

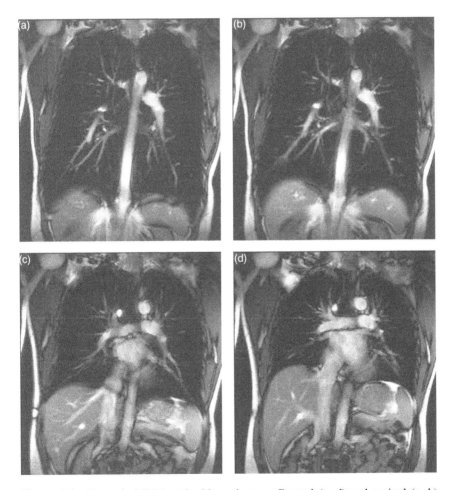

Figure 4.6 Dynamic MRI in a healthy volunteer. Coronal (a–d) and sagittal (e–h) images obtained during the respiratory cycle demonstrate homogeneous motion of lung, diaphragm, and chest wall.

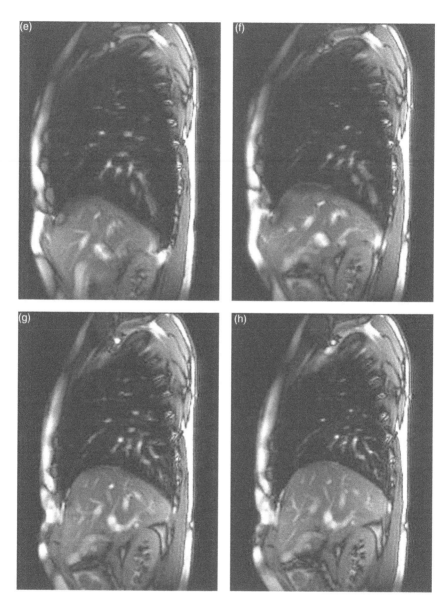

Figure 4.6 *Continued.*

contours, a three-dimensional reconstruction of the diaphragm can be performed
(30). From there, total diaphragmatic length, length of the apposition zone and the
diaphragmatic dome can be calculated along predefined coronal and sagittal
planes. Additionally, diaphragmatic surface areas, such as total, dome, and apposition area, can be calculated. The shape of the diaphragm changes markedly along

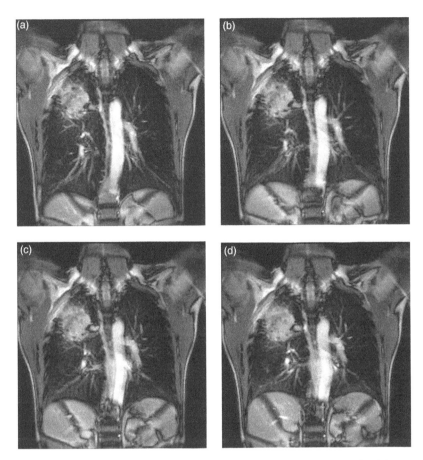

Figure 4.7 Dynamic coronal MRI (a–d) in a patient with lung cancer in the right upper lobe and chest wall infiltration shows heterogeneous motion due to reduced mobility of the tumor-bearing right upper lobe.

coronal and sagittal planes with lung inflation (30,31). At full inspiration, there is a significant length reduction of the human diaphragm, which leads to an entire elimination of the apposition zone of the diaphragm (30). Area variations estimated with MRI confirm the remarkable shortening of relaxed human diaphragm fibers (55 $\pm$ 11%) at vital capacity. MRI is also well suited to measure the volume displaced by diaphragmatic motion directly, which amounts to ~60% of the inspired volume over a vital capacity maneuver (30). Complete analysis of diaphragmatic mechanics must consider the relationships among tension, transdiaphragmatic pressure, muscle fiber length, thickness, and shape for various conditions of load and of activation of muscle fibers, for example, in sitting position, the diaphragm loses its effectiveness as a pressure generator as lung volume increases (32). At a volume close to total lung capacity, the diaphragm is still able to generate a trans-diaphragmatic pressure but it becomes less efficient at converting this into a useful inspiratory pressure.

Chest wall motion is nonuniform. Because of the axis of the rotation of the ribs about the spine, the anterior chest wall sweeps up and out in a longer arc than does the posterior chest wall. An outward excursion of the lateral chest wall also occurs, which is less than that of the anterior but more than that of the posterior

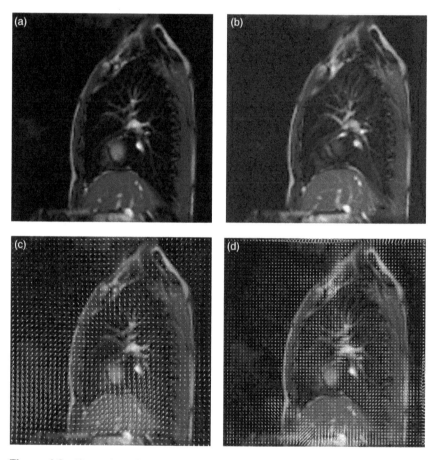

Figure 4.8   Illustration of the estimated lung motion between two frames in a sequence of MR images (a, b). The registration transformation between the images, represented as a field of displacement vectors, is shown superimposed on the first image (c), where the vectors indicate the corresponding locations in the second image and thus provide a direct, quantitative measure of the lung motion between the images. The strain induced by the motion is also shown (d), where each strain tensor is depicted using an ellipse with major and minor axes directed along its eigenvectors and scaled by the corresponding principal strain values. [Reprinted with permission from Gee et al. (33).]

chest wall (16). Because the lung must follow the motion of the chest wall, disparities in lung excursion occur. Dynamic MRI is capable of describing the motion of diaphragm, the chest wall, and the lungs. When the diaphragm rises, the lung volume decreases from total lung capacity to residual volume, and at the same time the posterior portion of the lung displaces superiorly, whereas the anterior portion is displaced posteriorly and superiorly (Fig. 4.8). Regional parenchymal strain vectors appear to be oriented towards the hilum (Fig. 4.8) with strain magnitude maximal at the midcycle of expiratory phase (33).

All these factors have to be taken into consideration in a mechanical model of the respiratory pump, which should also include the effects of stress and strain onto the lung on a regional basis. It is adequate to directly relate human anatomical data obtained from MRI with the parameters of a mathematical model permitting numerical simulations (34). Such a two-compartmental model, which also includes an elastic membrane representing the diaphragm can be further improved by splitting the system in kinematic, constitutive, and force balance equations, and the behavior of the respiratory pump can be simulated in a straightforward manner. In such a model, muscles are represented physiologically realistic by active, elastic, and viscous components. After validation of the model through a series of numerical simulations (34), it offers the potential of predicting the behavior of the respiratory pump even in diseases which will affect its mechanical or geometrical characteristics. The prediction of the results of functional surgery, such as lung volume reduction surgery in emphysema, is certainly one of the more attractive applications.

XII. Conclusion

The lung, diaphragm, and chest wall represent three structures with highly different mechanical properties which are joined together to generate our most vital function, breathing. Given the many inter-related properties of the system and the fact that it can be affected by disease in a variety of ways, this complex system has been very difficult to unravel. Cross-sectional imaging offers some excellent tools to explore respiratory mechanics, and provide new physiological insights for fundamental research and promising clinical applications.

References

1. Smidt U, Schulz V, Ferlinz R. Physiologie und Pathophysiologie. In: Ferlinz R, ed. Pneumologie in Praxis und Klinik. Stuttgart, New York: Georg Thieme Verlag, 1994:25–65.
2. Wilson T. Parenchymal macromechanics. In: Hlastala M, Robertson H, eds. Complexity in Structure and Function of the Lung. New York: Marcel Dekker Inc., 1998:75–98.

3. Hubmayer R, Walters B, Chevalier R, Rodarte J, Olson L. Topographical distribution of regional lung volume in anesthetized dogs. J Appl Physiol 1983; 54:1048–1056.

4. Hubmayr R, Hill M, Wilson T. Nonuniform expansion of constricted dog lungs. J Appl Physiol 1996; 80:522–530.

5. Lai-Fook S, Hyatt R, Rodarte J. Effect of parenchymal shear modulus and lung volume on bronchial pressure-diameter behavior. J Appl Physiol 1978; 44:859–868.

6. Ederle J, Hast J, Heussel C, Fischer B, van Beek E, Ley S, Thelen M, Kauczor H-U. Evaluation of changes in central airway dimensions, lung area and mean lung density at paired inspiratory/expiratory high-resolution computed tomography. Eur Radiol 2003; 13(11):2454–2461.

7. Kauczor H-U, Hast J, Heussel C, Schlegel J, Mildenberger P, Thelen M. Densitometry of paired inspiratory/expiratory high resolution CT: comparison with pulmonary function tests. Eur Radiol 2002; 12:2757–2763.

8. Tanaka N, Matsumoto T, Suda H, Miura G, Matsunaga N. Paired inspiratory–expiratory thin-section CT findings in patients with small airway disease. Eur Radiol 2001; 11:393–401.

9. Robinson PJ, Kreel L. Pulmonary tissue attenuation with computed tomography: comparison of inspiration and expiration scans. J Comput Assist Tomogr 1979; 3:740–748.

10. Heussel C, Hafner B, Lill J, Schreiber W, Thelen M, Kauczor H-U. Paired inspiratory/expiratory spiral-CT and continuous respiration cine-CT in the diagnosis of tracheal instability. Eur Radiol 2001; 11:982–989.

11. Heussel CP, Ley S, Biedermann A, Rist A, Gast KK, Schreiber WG, Kauczor H-U. Respiratory lumenal change of pharynx and trachea in normal subjects and COPD patients: assessment by cine-MRI. Eur Radiol 2004; 14:2188–2197.

12. Lai-Fook S, Hyatt R. Effects of age on elastic moduli of human lungs. J Appl Physiol 2000; 89:163–168.

13. West J. Distribution of mechanical stress in the lung, a possible factor in localization of pulmonary disease. Lancet 1971; 1:839–841.

14. West J, Matthews F. Stresses, strains, and surface pressure in the lung caused by its weight. J Appl Physiol 1972; 32:332–345.

15. Goddard PR, Nicholson EM, Laszlo G, Watt I. Computed tomography in pulmonary emphysema. Clin Radiol 1982; 33:379–387.

16. Gurney JW. Cross-sectional physiology of the lung. Radiology 1991; 178:1–10.

17. Thurlbeck W. The incidence of pulmonary emphysema, with observations on the relative incidence of spatial distribution of various types of emphysema. Am Rev Respir Dis 1963; 87:206–215.

18. Hoffman EA. Effect of body orientation on regional lung expansion: a computed tomographic approach. J Appl Physiol 1985; 59:468–480.

19. Liu S, Margulies S, Wilson T. Deformation of the dog lung in the chest wall. J Appl Physiol 1990; 68:1979–1987.

20. Margulies S, Rodarte J. Shape of the chest wall in the prone and supine anesthetized dog. J Appl Physiol 1990; 68:1970–1978.

21. Kauczor H-U, Hast J, Heussel C, Schlegel J, Mildenberger P, Thelen M. Focal airtrapping at expiratory high-resolution CT: comparison with pulmonary function tests. Eur Radiol 2000; 10:1539–1546.

22. Verschakelen JA, Scheinbaum K, Bogaert J, Demedts M, Lacquet LL, Baert AL. Expiratory CT in cigarette smokers: correlation between areas of decreased lung attenuation, pulmonary function tests and smoking history. Eur Radiol 1998; 8:1391–1399.

23. Kubo K, Eda S, Yamamoto H, Fujimoto K, Matsuzawa Y, Maruyama Y, Hasegawa M, Sone S, Sakai F. Expiratory and inspiratory chest CT and pulmonary function tests in smokers. Eur Respir J 1999; 13:252–256.

24. Diallo M, Guenard H, Laurent F, Carles P, Giron J. Distribution of lung density and mass in patients with emphysema as assessed by quantitative analysis of CT. Chest 2000; 118:1566–1575.

25. Baldi S, Miniati M, Bellina C, Battolla L, Catapano G, Giustini D, Giuntini C. Relationship between extent of pulmonary emphysema by HRCT and lung elastic recoil in patients with COPD. Am J Respir Crit Care Med 2001; 164:585–589.

26. Cheung D, Schot R, Zwinderman A, Zagers H, Dijkman J, Sterk P. Relationship between loss in parenchymal elastic recoil pressure and maximal airway narrowing in subjects with alpha-1-antitrypsin deficiency. Am J Respir Crit Care Med 1997; 155:135–140.

27. Napadow V, Mai V, Bankier A, Gilbert R, Edelman R, Chen Q. Determination of regional pulmonary parenchymal strain during normal respiration using spin inversion tagged magnetization MRI. J Magn Reson Imaging 2001; 13:467–474.

28. Gattinoni L, Caironi P, Pelosi P, Goodman L. What has CT taught us about the ARDS? Am J Respir Crit Care Med 2001; 164:1701–1711.

29. Edibam C, Rutten A, Collins D, Bersten A. Effect of inspiratory flow pattern and inspiratory to expiratory ratio on nonlinear elastic behavior in patients with acute lung injury. Am J Respir Crit Care Med 2003; 167:702–707.

30. Cluzel P, Similowski T, Chartrand-Lefebvre C, Zelter M, Derenne J-P, Grenier P. Diaphragm and chest wall: assessment of the inspiratory pump with MR imaging—preliminary observations. Radiology 2000; 215:574–583.

31. Cassart M, Genevois P, Estenne M. Rib cage dimensions in hyperinflated patients with severe chronic obstructive pulmonary disease. Am J Respir Care Med 1996; 154:800–805.

32. Smith J, Bellemare F. Effect of lung volume on in vivo contraction characteristics of human diaphragm. J Appl Physiol 1987; 62:1893–1900.

33. Gee J, Sundaram T, Hasegawa I, Uematsu H, Hatabu H. Characterization of regional pulmonary mechanics from serial MRI data. Acad Radiol 2003; 10(10):1147–1152.

34. Basso-Ricci S, Cluzel P, Constantinescu A, Similowski T. Mechanical model of the inspiratory pump. J Biomech 2002; 35:139–145.

35. Ley S, Mayer D, Brook B, van Beek E, Heussel C, Rinck D, Hose R, Markstaller K, Kauczor H-U. Radiological imaging as the basis for a simulation software of ventilation in the tracheo-bronchial tree. Eur Radiol 2002; 12:2218–2228.

5

Pulmonary CT Angiography

MATHIAS PROKOP and
IENEKE J. HARTMANN

University Medical Center Utrecht,
Utrecht, The Netherlands

CORNELIA M. SCHAEFER-PROKOP

Medical University of Vienna,
Vienna, Austria

CHRISTOPH ENGELKE

Klinikum der Technischen Universität
  München,
Munich, Germany

I. Introduction

Since its introduction in 1992 (1), computed tomography angiography (CTA) of the pulmonary arteries has become the main diagnostic test for the evaluation of pulmonary embolism (PE). Pulmonary CTA, however, is not limited to evaluating embolism but can be used for a multitude of other diseases of the pulmonary vascular bed. It is a relatively simple technique that can rapidly solve a vast number of clinical questions. It is even able to detect extravascular reasons for a patient's complaints because it always includes the information from the surrounding structures as well.

With the advent of multislice scanning, CTA has gained substantially in spatial resolution. Modern 16-slice scanners can cover the whole chest in <10 s with submillimeter resolution. Consequently, the required amount contrast material can be reduced to 50–80 mL. Improvements in scanning technique have allowed for reduction in radiation dose as well (depending on the size of the patient), with an effective dose in the range of 1–2 mSv for a non-obese individual.

Still, it is necessary to pay attention to optimizing scanning technique and contrast injection in order to obtain studies of uniformly high quality. There are a few sources of misinterpretation that should be known, especially when CTA is performed for ruling out PE.

II. Acquisition Technique

The choice of scanning parameters varies with the available scanner equipment. For best results, one should strive for using thin sections and achieving a high and homogenous enhancement of the pulmonary vessels. At the same time, one has to consider whether the patient is dyspneic and can sustain the required breath-hold phase. This yields the following consequences for protocol design.

A. Inspiratory Breath-hold

In cooperative patients without dyspnea the scan is performed during an inspiratory breath-hold. It is helpful to have the patients hyperventilate briefly before each scan, that is, have them take a deep breath and breathe in and out several times. Proper training is crucial for achieving good results. The technologists should instruct the patients carefully and perform a trial breath-hold for the required scan duration. By watching the surface of the abdomen, they can determine whether the patient can properly suspend respiration. Breath-hold duration can be increased by supplemental oxygen.

Toward the end of the scan, some patients tend to "gasp for air" internally against the closed glottis. Such involuntary diaphragmatic movements lead to motion artifacts but can be suppressed if the patient is instructed accordingly. Such diaphragmatic movements can also be detected by watching the abdomen.

Finally, it is important to train the technologists not to start the scans too early. The patients require at least 4 s, in most cases 6 s, between the breath-hold command and the actual scan before they have fully suspended diaphragmatic motion. If the start delay is too short and the scan is performed in a caudo-cranial direction, substantial movement artifacts may occur.

In our experience, which is similar to that of other institutions, ~90% of patients evaluated for suspected PE can successfully suspend respiration given proper training (2).

B. Dyspneic Patients

In the ~10% of patients who are uncooperative or dyspneic, breath-holding should not be attempted because markedly increased artifacts will result as these patients resume breathing during data acquisition. Shallow respiration is a good alternative that results in minimum artifacts and substantially better image quality. Consequently, the computed tomography (CT) technologists should instruct those patients that could not hold their breath sufficiently during the trail breath-holds to hyperventilate (i.e., take three to four deep breaths) prior to the exam and then to breathe as shallowly as possible during the scan.

Only with multislice scanners is it possible to attempt a short breath-hold in dyspneic patients. Using a 4 × 2.5 mm collimation and reducing the scan range (aortic arch to diaphragms) will allow scan durations of <5 s. With 16-slice scanners, even thinner collimation is possible at very short scan durations (e.g., 16 × 1.5 at 3.3 s for a 24 cm scan range). Proper patient instruction, however, is again mandatory for good results.

C. Scan Range

Scan length is not a limiting factor for multislice CTA, but it is critical for spatial resolution in single-slice CTA. Keeping the range to a minimum reduces scan time, allows for thinner collimation and thus better spatial resolution, reduces motion-related artifacts, contrast material requirements, and patient dose. Because of the limited ability of (older) CTA techniques to reveal peripheral emboli, the scan range excludes the most cranial and most caudal sub-subsegmental arteries because the likelihood of successfully detecting an isolated, peripheral pulmonary embolus in these vessels is exceedingly small. Up to now, no significant change in diagnostic accuracy has been reported when increasing the scan range to include the whole chest. Depending upon the spatial resolution of the chosen scan technique, the scan range can be limited from the lower hemidiaphragm (at least 2 cm below the orifice of the lowest pulmonary veins) to 2–4 cm above the aortic arch. The scan length thus can be limited to some 16–24 cm, which reduces radiation exposure and scan duration by 20–45% compared with a full chest scan of 30 cm (Fig. 5.1). Such a limited scan range had been first suggested for single-slice CT (1) but also can be used for multislice CT if larger sections have to be used for data reconstruction (effective section width ≥2 mm).

Only with multislice scanning using a section collimation below 1.5 mm does it make some sense to expand the scan range to include the whole chest because this technique has enough spatial resolution to detect emboli even in small peripheral arteries in the cranial and caudal regions of the lungs (3,4). Even then, the most cranial and caudal portions of the lungs may be excluded from the scan range because small vessels in these regions will rarely be enhanced enough to allow for evaluation. Consequently, the scan range may be limited to some 24 cm even for multislice CT (see Table 5.1).

D. Scan Direction

Most institutions now prefer a caudo-cranial scanning direction rather than a cranio-caudal data acquisition because breathing artifacts are substantially less disturbing in the upper portions of the lung compared with the lower portions, if the patient resumes breathing during the final phase of data acquisition.

However, as already pointed out, sufficient time (4–6 s) should be allowed for the patient to breathe in and hold the breath before actually staring the data acquisition.

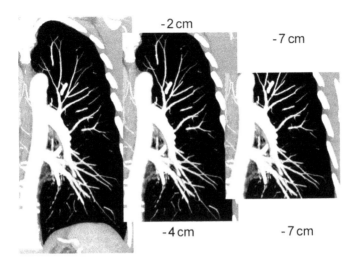

Figure 5.1 Comparison of scan ranges for CTA of the pulmonary arteries. The MIP display demonstrates that almost none of the visible arteries are lost when the range is reduced from 30 to 24 cm. Even if the rage is reduced to 16 cm, only small peripheral arteries are lost.

E. Scanning Parameters

Scanning parameters strongly depend on the available scanner technology and the time that the patients can hold their breath (Table 5.1).

With 1 s single-slice scanners, a 3 mm collimation and 5 mm table feed (pitch 1.7) is recommended as the standard scanning technique. It can cover a range of 16 cm from the dome of the diaphragm to the aortic arch within some 32 s and yields an effective section width of 3.6 mm. By increasing the pitch to 2, the scan duration can be reduced to 27 s but image quality is slightly impaired (section width 3.9 mm). With subsecond single-slice scanners (0.75 s rotation time), a 2 mm collimation and 4 mm table feed (pitch = 2) can be chosen, which improves the effective section width to 2.6 mm and can cover the same scan range in 30 s. It has been shown that this technique improves detection of more peripheral arteries (5). For all single-slice techniques, images are reconstructed with a 2 mm reconstruction increment to gain overlapping sections for improved detection of abnormalities.

With four-slice scanners, $4 \times 1-1.25$ mm collimation and a table feed of 6–8 mm is employed in patients who can hold their breath for some 20 s. Images are reconstructed at 0.7–1 mm intervals. This protocol yields a section width of only 1.25–1.5 mm and allows for evaluation of fifth- to eighth-order branches. In patients who can hold their breath for <10 s, the scan range can be limited to the central 20 cm of the pulmonary vasculature and a $4 \times 2-2.5$ mm collimation is used. This allows for completing the scan within some 7 s with an effective section width of 2.5–3.0 mm. Images should be reconstructed at

Table 5.1 Scanning Parameters

Scan range	Single-slice CT	Lower hemidiaphragm (2–3 cm below pulmonary veins) to just above aortic arch
	Multislice CT	Lung bases to lung apex (24 cm scan range usually suffices for cooperative patients)
		Lower hemidiaphragm to just above aortic arch (dyspnoic patients)
Scan direction		Cranio-caudal
Tube voltage	Standard	120 kVp
	Low-dose	80–100 kVp
$CTDI_{vol}$	Standard	5–14 mGy (depending on patient size)
	Low-dose	1.5–4 mGy (depending on patient size)
		Dose reduction by adaptive tube current modulation (if available)
Section thickness	Single-slice CT	2–3 mm
	4-slice scanners	4×1–1.25 mm (4×2–2.5 mm in dyspnoic patients)
	8-slice scanners	8×1–1.25 mm (8×2–2.5 mm in dyspnoic patients)
	16-slice scanners	16×0.75–1.5 mm (depending on dyspnoea and scanner type)
Pitch		1.35–2 (depending on specific scanner properties)
Reconstructed thickness	Single-slice CT	Not applicable
	Multislice CT	1.0–1.5 mm (standard)
		2 mm (obese patients)
		2.5–3 mm (dyspnoic patients, 4–8×2.5 mm)
Reconstruction increment	Single-slice CT	2 mm
	Multislice CT	0.7–1.5 mm
Scan duration	Single-slice CT	30 s
	4-slice scanners	16–30 s (5 s for dyspnoic patients: 4×2.5 mm, reduced range)
	8-slice scanners	8–15 s (3 s for dyspnoic patients: 8×2.5 mm, reduced range)
	16-slice scanners	4–8 s (4 s for dyspnoic patients)
Window/level		Adjust to maximum contrast enhancement

1.5 mm intervals. Image quality is still superior than with single-slice scanning because of less pulsation and reduced risk of breathing artifacts. If patients cannot hold their breath, shallow respiration and the $4 \times 1-1.25$ mm protocol are suggested.

With 16-slice scanners, $16 \times 0.75-1.25$ mm collimation and a pitch of $1.2-1.75$ are used for patients who can hold their breath for some 10 s. Within this time, the whole chest can be covered with an effective section width of between 1.0 and 1.5 mm. For shortest scan duration, the maximum rotation speed of the tube should be chosen ($0.37-0.5$ s). If the next thicker collimation is used ($16 \times 1.5-2$ mm), the scan duration can be cut in half. In GE scanners, 16×1.25 mm serves as the technique of choice in all cases (scan duration 5.5 s for a pitch of 1.375 and 4.2 s for a pitch of 1.75). Images are reconstructed at $0.7-1$ mm intervals using the thinnest available section width. No results are published yet, but image quality appears consistently high and allows for evaluation of very small peripheral arteries.

In very obese patients, image noise may become excessive and can interfere with image interpretation. In such cases, using a smoothing reconstruction filter and reconstructing $2-3$ mm thick sections from the same raw data set can decrease image noise and yield a diagnostic exam. However, this comes at the expense of reduced detail in peripheral arteries and thus a lower detection rate for peripheral emboli (Fig. 5.2).

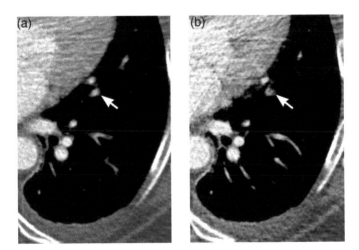

Figure 5.2 Multislice CT with 4×1 mm collimation and 6 mm table feed. Comparison of a 3 mm thick section (a) reconstructed from the same raw data set as an adjacent 1.25 mm thick sections at the same anatomic level (b). The embolus is not seen on the 3 mm sections while it is clearly visible on the 1.25 mm section. Note the diagnostic quality despite markedly increased noise in this obese patient scanned at 80 kVp and $CTDI_{vol} < 3$ mGy.

F. Dose Issues

The peripheral pulmonary arteries are the most challenging vessels for pulmonary CTA because they are located in the lung periphery and are thus subject to substantial partial volume effects. Reducing these partial volume effects requires the choice of thin sections (effective section width) and a high vascular contrast enhancement. The resulting "signal" (CT numbers of a specific peripheral pulmonary artery) is balanced by the image noise that is increased at thin collimation. Thus, there is a delicate balance between dose reduction, acceptable image noise, and vessel contrast.

Most authors suggest 120 kVp and $\sim$100 mAs as the standard exposure parameters for pulmonary CTA. The resulting CT dose index ($CTDI_{vol}$) will vary between scanners but is in the range of 7–14 mGy, which is in the same dose range as that found for evaluation of PE in a national survey in Germany (6). The resulting effective dose depends very much on the chosen scan length and the patient's sex. For a total chest CTA (30 cm), the effective dose E is $\sim$40% of the $CTDI_{vol}$ for males and amounts to $\sim$50% of the $CTDI_{vol}$ in females (7). If the scan range can be reduced, the effective dose decreases proportionally, for example, by one-third if the scan range is limited to 20 cm. As a consequence, effective dose may vary substantially despite the fact that the same mAs and kVp settings had been chosen. For example, a 20 cm scan covering the central pulmonary vessels in a male patient scanned at 100 mAs and 120 kVp with a scanner that yields 7 mGy $CTDI_{vol}$ at these settings will result in an effective dose of $\sim$1.9 mSv. If the same mAs and kVp settings are used to scan the whole chest (30 cm) in a female patient using a scanner that yields 14 mGy $CTDI_{vol}$, then the effective dose will amount to 7 mSv. That these numbers are realistic is underlined by a recent comparative study between multislice CTA and pulmonary DSA that found a mean effective dose of 4.2 mSv (range 2.2–6.0 mSv) for CTA and 7.1 mSv (range 3.3–17.3 mSv) for DSA (8).

We suggest ignoring mAs setting but rather focusing on the $CTDI_{vol}$ that is displayed on the user interface of most modern CT scanners. For standard size patients (70 kg, 170 cm), a $CTDI_{vol}$ of 5–7 mGy is sufficient. If no dose modulation is available, one should adapt the dose to the patient's size. As a rule of thumb, the $CTDI_{vol}$ has to be increased by a factor of two every 4 cm of additional fat layer. Adaptive tube current modulation (e.g., Smart-mA, GE; DoseRight, Philips; C.A.R.E. dose, Siemens; and Real EC, Toshiba) can compensate for the increased dose requirements in obese patients as well as for varying dose requirements between different body cross-sections such as the shoulder regions and the air-filled chest. At a constant image quality, adaptive tube current modulation can reduce the dose by some 10–30%, depending on the body region (shoulders, central chest, diaphragm). Because of a better detector efficiency at thin collimation, 16-slice scanners require some 20–30% less dose than four-slice scanners for similar image quality.

Increasing the contrast of the pulmonary vessels may be used to increase the signal and thus to be able to accept an increased image noise at the same signal-to-noise ratio. Increasing the vascular contrast can be achieved by optimizing the injection protocol or by increasing the X-ray absorption of iodine. The fact that the radiation attenuation of iodine increases at lower X-ray energies can thus be used for dose reduction.

For CTA of the pulmonary arteries, the use of 100 instead of 140 kVp will, on an average, increase vascular opacification by some 80–100 HU for identical injection parameters, and thus allow for scanning the chest with a reduced $CTDI_{vol}$ of 3–4 mGy for a non-obese individual (Fig. 5.3) (9). The resulting effective dose will be in the range of 1.5–2 mSv. A tube voltage of 80 kVp holds an even higher potential for dose savings in slim individuals and children, with a $CTDI_{vol}$ of 1.5–3 mGy and an effective dose under 1.5 mSv. In obese patients, the increased absorption of lower energy radiation in the body leads to a disproportional increase in image noise, which makes a low kVp technique not feasible with present scanners.

Using such low-kVp scan protocols, CTA in pregnant women has a substantially lower uterine radiation exposure than V/Q scanning. Lower kVp settings also improve vascular enhancement especially of small arteries that suffer most from partial volume effects. Together with a narrow collimation of 3 mm for 1 s single-slice scanners, 2–3 mm for 0.75 s scanners, and 1–2 mm for dual and multislice scanners, the number of subsegmental arteries that can be evaluated grows substantially and should further improve the diagnostic accuracy of CTA for the detection of acute embolism.

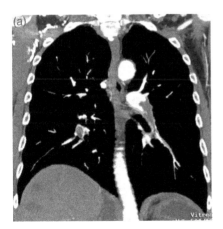 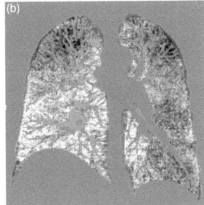

Figure 5.3 **(See color insert)** Low-dose scan at 80 kVp scan in a patient with recurrent PE. Note the excellent contrast even in very small peripheral vessels despite a $CTDI_{vol}$ of <3 mGy (a). Color map of the variations in pulmonary density in the same patient (b). Note that hypoperfused regions are darker.

III. Contrast Material Injection

For evaluation of suspected pulmonary embolism, optimum vascular opacification is mandatory. For the evaluation of peripheral pulmonary arteriovenous malformations, on the other hand, contrast material is only required for detecting thrombosed portions and therefore is less crucial.

A. Venous Access

A sufficiently large-bore intravenous catheter (18-gage) should be placed in a cubital vein to enable a high flow rate for contrast injection. The injected arm should be stationary and well extended to prevent catheter kinking and reduce venous compression effects. Right cubital venous access is preferred for pulmonary CTA because this will avoid streak artifacts caused by the approximately horizontal course of the left brachiocephalic vein.

Some authors prefer positioning the left arm above the head and the right arm parallel to the body and using right cubital venous access for the contrast injection (1). This technique reduces compression effects in the area where the brachiocephalic vein crosses the ribs.

Central venous lines should be avoided unless they are large bore catheters such as for dialysis or hemofiltration. It is always advisable to test catheters or check with manufacturers to determine the maximum flow rate that is still safe. For most central venous lines, a flow rate of 2 mL/s should not be exceeded.

B. Injection Parameters

Contrast material should be administered using a power injector. Nonionic contrast media are preferred because of less allergic reactions and less patient discomfort at high injection speeds. High flow rates ensure better contrast opacification, which in turn enhances visualization of small, more peripheral vessels and thus improves the overall sensitivity of the technique. Most authors nowadays suggest flow rates of 3–5 mL/s. Biphasic injections may improve the uniformity of contrast enhancement over the whole duration of the scan (10) but is less important with the short scan durations obtained with modern multislice units. As a general rule, the volume of contrast material should be chosen so that the duration of contrast injection is approximately equal to the scan duration. For very short scan durations, one has to increase the injection time by some 4–5 s to allow for contrast buildup in peripheral pulmonary arteries. Table 5.2 gives an overview of contrast injection parameters depending on the scan duration.

C. Scan Delay

The time interval between the application of contrast material and the start of data acquisition, the scan delay, should be chosen according to the patient's clinical

Table 5.2 Contrast Material Injection

Contrast	120 mL (20–30 s scan duration)
material	80 mL (10–20 s scan duration)
volume	60 mL (3–10s scan duration)
Saline flush	40 mL (immediately following the contrast material)
Injection rate	4 mL/s
Start delay	20 s (fixed delay, >20 s scan duration)
	5–8 s (bolus triggering in pulmonary artery, >10 s scan duration)
	8–10 s (bolus triggering in pulmonary artery, 3–10 s scan duration)

status. In patients who have no history, signs and symptoms of pulmonary arterial hypertension, right ventricular failure, or overall cardiac failure, a scan delay of 20 s is sufficient to allow for optimum vessel opacification (11). A recent study has shown that such a standard 20 s scan delay provides an opacification of pulmonary arteries that is equally good as with an individually determined scan delay using a test bolus injection.

Individual adaptation of scan delay, however, should be considered in patients with known pulmonary arterial hypertension, right heart failure, or overall cardiac failure because starting too early will result in inadequate opacification of the pulmonary arteries on the first images. On the other hand, there may not be enough contrast material left towards the end of the scan if the start delay is too long. This may be the case in young individuals with a high cardiac output.

Bolus triggering techniques monitor contrast enhancement at a predefined site [e.g., a region of interest (ROI) in the pulmonary trunk] during the early stages of contrast medium injection and start image acquisition automatically when a desired level of enhancement (trigger level) is reached. Care has to be taken to choose the trigger ROI on a scan that was acquired during quiet breathing or mid-inspiration because otherwise the trigger ROI might move in and out of the target region as the patient continues breathing quietly during the trigger scans. In addition, there will have to be some 4–6 s after the trigger level is reached in order to allow for the patient to breathe in and hold the breath. Bolus triggering techniques are mandatory with multislice scanners if the amount of contrast is adapted to the scan duration.

D. Saline Flush

The injected contrast material can be used to better advantage if the injection veins are flushed by a bolus of normal saline, injected immediately after the contrast material using similar flow rates (12,13). Such a saline flush pushes the contrast material forward and thus increases the length of the contrast plateau. It can also be used to save contrast material without jeopardizing vascular contrast, and to increase vascular opacification if combined with higher flow rates. It is particularly important when small amounts of contrast material are injected, and therefore becomes essential for short multislice CT acquisitions. In addition, a saline flush will reduce the amount of artifacts in the superior vena cava and brachiocephalic injection veins when pulmonary CTA acquisitions are obtained in a caudo-cranial scanning direction.

Dual-barrel injectors are presently entering the market and make a saline flush technique much easier to perform; no refill is necessary between patients, and preparation of contrast injection is much faster. In addition, such injectors allow for multiphasic injection protocols.

It is not yet clear how much saline has to be injected for optimum results. On the basis of our clinical experience, we suggest 40–60 mL. When determining the proper scan delay, any saline that is left in the injection lines has to be taken into account. This is no problem when bolus triggering techniques are used but may be problematic when scan delay is derived from a test bolus injection.

IV. CT Venography

CTA also offers a "one-stop shop" approach for evaluation of thrombembolic disease by adding a venous phase scan of the abdomen and lower extremities (see Fig. 5.17) (14,15). With a delay of 120–180 s after pulmonary CTA is completed, the lower extremity is scanned from the iliac crest to the popliteal fossa using the already injected contrast material. This technique can detect peripheral venous thrombi at least as well as ultrasound. Low-dose scanning should be mandatory and may be achieved by thick sections and low mAs and $CTDI_{vol}$ settings (16). Discontinuous scanning, for example, with 4–5 mm sections every 2 cm is also acceptable (e.g., using 4×1–1.25 mm collimation merged to 4–5 mm thick sections).

However, substantial numbers of patients have to be exposed to radiation (97% of scanned patients in a large study) to detect those individuals in whom clinical consequences arise (15). For the evaluation of the deep venous system, duplex ultrasound should probably be preferred.

V. Image Evaluation and Postprocessing

Depending on the clinical imaging task, evaluation of pulmonary CTA is primarily based on axial sections (pulmonary embolism) or on various 3D displays (pulmonary vascular anomalies). Image interpretation is typically performed using both soft tissue (mediastinum) and pulmonary parenchymal windows. This side-by-side analysis of images may help in differentiating pulmonary arteries that accompany the bronchi from venous structures, which, in the early phase of scanning, may be unenhanced. In addition, cine-mode viewing provides a dynamic impression of the pulmonary arteries and is generally considered helpful in the evaluation of acute PE.

A. Axial Sections

Evaluation of axial sections requires an interactive cine mode because of the large number of sections, which are in the range of 150 for single-slice CTA, and around 300–450 images for multislice CTA. The reconstruction increment, but not the number of detector rows, determines the number of images produced. The number, therefore, should not become larger as newer scanners with more detector rows are introduced. The reviewing workstation must allow for rapid scrolling through these large data sets rapidly. Scrolling speed should be intuitively and interactively adjustable so that fine detail can be evaluated more slowly while large ranges can be covered rapidly. Not all current systems are equally suited for this task, especially when large multislice data sets are involved.

B. Multiplanar Planar Reformations

Added multiplanar reformations are rarely necessary for acute PE. They may aid inexperienced viewers to distinguish between a central clot and a mediastinal lymph node or may be helpful for distinguishing between pulsation artifacts and real emboli (17). In chronic pulmonary embolism, coronal and sagittal reformations may help to better delineate the (organized) thrombotic material along the vessel wall (see Fig. 5.3) For arteriovenous malformations (AVMs) and pulmonary anomalies, various 3D displays are better suited. Curved planar reformations are rarely useful for pulmonary CTA.

C. Maximum Intensity Projections

Maximum intensity projections (MIPs) are an excellent tool for providing angiography-like images of the peripheral pulmonary arteries. Best results are obtained with thin-section multislice acquisitions if interactive sliding thin-slab MIPs are used. This technique uses MIPs of 5–20 mm thickness that can be interactively moved through the data set, thereby allowing for superior delineation of small peripheral vessels (see Fig. 5.6). Small peripheral clots will appear as vessel segments that are less enhanced (i.e., have soft-tissue density) than neighboring vessels of the same size. Thin-slab MIPs are particularly helpful in chronic pulmonary embolism to demonstrate peripheral stenoses that can easily be missed on axial images. No prior data editing is required with thin-slab MIPs.

A "paddle wheel reconstruction" consists of MIPs from thin slabs of 10–20 mm thickness that rotate around a horizontal axis set approximately to the level of the pulmonary arteries. This type of reconstruction has been suggested because it is better adapted to the natural course of the pulmonary arteries (18). It requires profound anatomic knowledge to begin with, but may then be quite effective for detecting and displaying pathologic findings. Since the pulmonary arteries are not leaving the mediastinum at the same level, the paddle wheel reconstruction does not always yield ideal longitudinal displays of both sides of the pulmonary arterial system and has therefore not entered clinical practice on a large scale.

D. Volume Rendering

Volume rendering techniques (VRTs) are excellent for display of complex pathology such as pulmonary arterial anomalies or AVMs (see Fig. 5.24). In patients with chronic PE, VRT may provide an overview of dilated and stenotic segments. Prior editing of the chest wall is not mandatory if thin-slab techniques are used, but provides superior results if an overview of the pulmonary vasculature is to be gained. Most modern workstations allow for semi-automated bone removal, which substantially reduces the time to obtain images of diagnostic quality.

E. Lung Density Maps

Color-coded displays of the density of the lung parenchyma can be used to increase the sensitivity towards small density differences such as in segmental PE or chronic thromboembolic disease. This can be achieved by using a rainbow spectrum as the color map for thin-slab volume rendering [Fig. 5.3(b)] or by using special software that first extracts the pulmonary parenchyma, smoothes the data, and projects it back over the original image (19).

VI. Acute Pulmonary Thromboembolism

The main indication for pulmonary CTA is suspected acute PE. Acute PE is characterized by a partial or complete obstruction of central or peripheral pulmonary arteries by thromboembolic material. Acute PE is a potentially life-threatening complication of peripheral deep venous thrombosis (DVT) but can also occur in conjunction with thromboses of other systemic veins or thrombotic appositions on venous catheters. Untreated PE is associated with a mortality risk of up to 30% (20). It is estimated that some 10% of patients do not survive the initial event, and that the diagnosis is missed or delayed in 70% of survivors (21). Table 5.3 provides a clinical and pathophysiologic classification scheme for grading the severity of acute PE (22). Substantial numbers of patients with acute massive PE do not undergo any imaging because they die before the diagnosis is suspected or they are treated on suspicion and are too unstable for off-site diagnostic procedures necessitating transportation. Since the clinical symptoms as well as laboratory and ECG findings are frequently unspecific (23), imaging plays a central role in the diagnostic workup of acute PE.

Risk factors for DVT are also risk factors for acute PE. Immobilization, for example, during car or airplane travel, extensive surgery, or manifest DVT increase the risk of acute PE. Other risk factors include pneumonia, vasculitis, coagulation disorders, or malignant disease. Up to 90% of thrombi arise from the deep venous system of the legs. Thrombi in the proximal veins of the thigh

Table 5.3 Clinical Grading of the Severity of Acute PE

Grade	Finding	Clinical symptoms	Therapy
Acute massive (3–5%)	Sudden obstruction of pulmonary artery by ≥50% (<50% with preexistent cardiorespiratory insufficiency)	10% lethal within first hours; massive dyspnea, cyanosis, angina pectoris, pathological ECG, shock, circulatory failure	Thrombolysis, thrombectomy
Acute submassive	Proximal emboli	Dyspnea and tachycardia, signs of right heart failure but no circulatory failure	Thrombolysis, heparin
Acute nonmassive	Mainly peripheral (sub)segmental emboli	Infarct with pleurisy and hemoptysis, no hypoxemia, no signs of right heart failure	Heparin

have a higher risk for PE than thrombi in the lower legs. Other sources of emboli include neck and arm veins, pelvic veins, the inferior and superior vena cava, the right atrium and ventricle, as well as the valves of the right heart.

The thromboembolic occlusion of a pulmonary artery causes a bronchial constriction with formation of atelectasis and reduction of gas exchange. Depending on the extent of the embolism, the pressure in the pulmonary arteries and right heart rises and may ultimately lead to right heart dilatation and acute right heart failure. In 15% of cases, a lung infarction is seen with concomitant hemorrhage or hemorrhagic necrosis.

Clinical symptoms include sudden onset of dyspnea and tachypnea in a patient without pre-existent pulmonary disease and an acute deterioration of pulmonary symptoms in patients with known pulmonary disease. PE is considered to be the cause of 5–15% of cases of "sudden death" (23). Acute massive embolism (Table 5.3) may cause circulatory failure and systemic hypotension, usually caused by occlusion of large central pulmonary arteries. Pleuritic chest pain is commonly the result of a pulmonary infarct caused by peripheral emboli. Acute PE, however, is not necessarily accompanied by clinical symptoms, and incidental findings are known from CT scans of asymptomatic patients that were examined because of other reasons (commonly malignancies) (24). The extent of embolism is only loosely correlated with clinical symptoms.

Patients who are referred for imaging have to be in a sufficiently stable clinical condition. The role of imaging is to confirm or rule out the diagnosis of acute PE, and, if possible, to establish an alternative diagnosis. This is important because up to 60% of patients have a false positive clinical suspicion of PE. In addition, DVT cannot be ruled out clinically because less than one-third of patients with DVT of the lower extremity are symptomatic.

Blood tests such as D-dimer have a high negative predictive value although they do not completely rule out PE. The literature describes sensitivities for new ELISA techniques in the range of 92–100% while older techniques are associated with sensitivities of as low as 77–78% (25). D-dimer tests are rather unspecific, with published specificities in the range between 29% and 75% (25). Positive results may be associated with a host of diseases that are associated with clotting activity. The D-dimer may be increased because of venous thrombosis, infection, malignant disease, cardiac failure, acute myocardial infarction, stroke, collagen diseases, renal insufficiency, liver disease, pregnancy, trauma, or a postoperative state. Thus, D-dimer is mainly used to rule out PE: a negative D-dimer test is considered sufficient for stopping further evaluation if clinical pretest probability is low to moderate (26). Various scoring systems for determining such a pretest probability have been suggested. Table 5.4 provides the Wells score as an example for such a classification (27). In patients with a high pretest probability, the D-dimer plays a lesser role and even normal D-dimer values will require further workup of the patients. A positive D-dimer on the other hand will always necessitate further studies to differentiate between PE and other reasons for a positive test result. For diagnostic purposes, various imaging modalities have been considered in the evaluation in the last few decades.

A. Other Imaging Techniques

Chest radiography is normal in many patients with PE or may just demonstrate mild effusion and plate-like atelectasis. Pulmonary infarction is rare and may

Table 5.4 Clinical Pretest Probability for the Presence of Acute PE [Modified Scoring System According to Wells (27)]

Symptom	Score
Clinical symptoms of deep venous thrombosis	3
No probable other diagnosis except PE	3
Tachycardia >100/min	1.5
Immobilization in last 4 weeks	1.5
History of earlier thrombosis or PE	1.5
Hemoptysis	1
Neoplasm within previous 6 months	1
Sum score	*Pretest probability*
<2	Low
2–6	Moderate
>6	High

occur in only 10–15% of cases. Direct signs of PE, such as narrowed vessels in the affected segments, are rare and not very reliable. Chest radiography, therefore, mainly plays a role in establishing alternative diagnoses, such as pneumonia or pneumothorax, and in deciding upon which further diagnostic tests to perform (28).

Transthoracic or transesophageal echocardiography is used in suspected massive PE (unstable patients) for the detection of acute right heart overload (29). They are not commonly used to diagnose PE in stable patients because they lack the sensitivity to rule out peripheral emboli.

Doppler ultrasound of the peripheral venous system has superseded X-ray phlebography for ruling out DVT in the legs and has become an integral part of clinical schemes for evaluating patients with suspected PE (26). However, its ability to rule out thrombi in the pelvic and abdominal veins is limited.

Pulmonary angiography is considered the radiological gold standard for the diagnosis of PE (30,31). However, despite excellent sensitivity and specificity, the method has not gained widespread acceptance because it is invasive and clinicians are reluctant to expose patients, who often may have unstable cardiovascular conditions, to a potentially risky procedure. This explains the results of a study in a large academic hospital that revealed that 92% of patients with low-probability V/Q scans and 70% of patients with inconclusive V/Q scans were not further investigated with pulmonary angiography or other imaging modalities (32). This study showed that a large number of patients were treated on the basis of the "best clinical guess" method. Other studies found a lower interobserver agreement for the presence of PE than with CTA (32). In addition, animal studies suggest that the sensitivity and specificity of pulmonary angiography is similar to high-quality CTA for detecting the presence of pulmonary emboli (33). Using pulmonary angiography as a gold standard in clinical studies, therefore, may underestimate the true accuracy of other techniques such as CTA.

V/Q scintigraphy used to be the noninvasive procedure of choice for the assessment of patients with suspected PE. V/Q scanning provides probability estimates for the presence of acute PE. A normal or near-normal V/Q scan exclude embolic disease with a high likelihood (>90%), while a high-probability/ abnormal result indicates PE in the context of corresponding clinical symptoms (>95%) (34,35). An intermediate or low-probability (inconclusive) result on V/Q scans specifies the need for additional imaging, because the percentage of positive pulmonary angiograms has been shown to be as high as 33% for intermediate results and 16% for low-probability results (34). Large studies in an unselected population demonstrated that the number of high-probability positive or negative findings is quite low (in the 30–35% range in total) (34,36). Even modern scintigraphic techniques could only slightly improve these numbers. As a consequence, most clinicians would treat according to their clinical judgment and not based on imaging findings.

Far better results are obtained in that subgroup of patients who were previously healthy and without signs of cardiopulmonary disease on chest radiographs. High-probability results are achieved in >80% of such patients (37). Because most of these ventilation scans are normal, perfusion (Q) scanning alone suffices and provides a good diagnostic option in this patient group. Conversely, the number of high-probability results in patients with known cardiopulmonary disease or pathologic abnormalities on chest radiographs is extremely low (37). This is the group that profits most from alternative imaging techniques such as CTA.

Gadolinium-enhanced magnetic resonance (MR) angiography has been suggested as a test for acute PE (38,39). It offers direct visualization of emboli without invasiveness or ionizing radiation. The accuracy was reported to be high but large patient studies are not yet available. Potential drawbacks are the limited access to the (potentially unstable) patient, the higher susceptibility to breathing artifacts, an examination volume that usually does not cover the whole chest, and the lack of display of the surrounding parenchyma for establishing potential alternative diagnoses.

B. Findings at CTA

Emboli within the pulmonary arteries can be directly visualized with CTA. Acute pulmonary thromboemboli can be seen as hypoattenuating intraluminal filling defects, partly or completely surrounded by opacified blood, or as a complete filling defect that leaves the respective vessel totally unopacified (Figs. 5.4–5.7). CTA can also help detect indirect signs of PE such as pleural-based densities, linear densities, or plate-like atelectases, central or peripheral dilatation of pulmonary arteries, and pleural effusions (28).

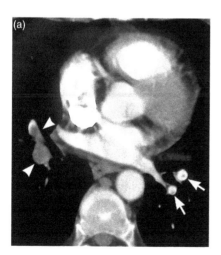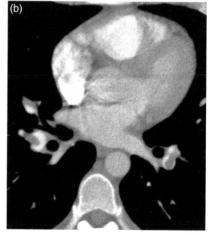

Figure 5.4 Typical emboli can occur as intraluminal filling defects (arrows) or complete occlusion (arrowheads) (a). The affected vessel may enlarge before complete occlusion occurs (arrow) (b). Compare with the corresponding contralateral vessel.

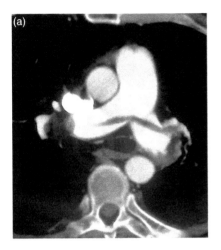

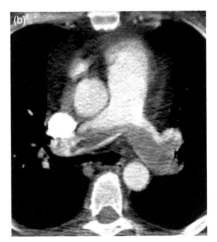

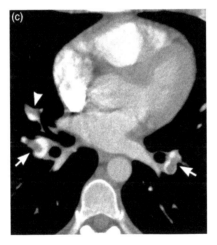

Figure 5.5 Riding emboli may occur at the pulmonary bifurction (a, b) but can also be seen at segmental or further distal branching points (arrows) (c). Note also the embolus in the middle lobe artery (arrowhead).

Rarely, acute emboli may be seen on nonenhanced chest CT images performed for other reasons as hyperattenuating material within the pulmonary arteries (40).

Acute emboli get trapped either at pulmonary artery bifurcations (riding emboli) or in peripheral arteries that are smaller than the embolus (Fig. 5.5). Such riding emboli may not only occur at the pulmonary artery bifurcation but also at the segmental or subsegmental level. Long emboli from peripheral veins may involve more than one artery, may coil up in a larger vessel, or may become fragmented and lead to a shower of small emboli into multiple lung

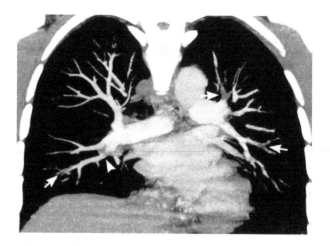

Figure 5.6   Thin-slab MIP excellently display small peripheral arterial occlusions (arrows). Central emboli, however, may be hard to detect (arrowhead). Note that this MIP was part of a "paddlewheel reconstruction" rotating around the axis of the main pulmonary arteries.

segments. The diameter of the embolus, and thus the level of vascular obstruction, corresponds to its site of origin.

More peripheral emboli tend to partially or completely occlude the affected vessel. Such emboli can often be better evaluated with thin-slab MIP because a longer portion of a peripheral vessel is displayed so that the boundary of contrast enhancement is more easily appreciated (Fig. 5.6) (8). The effect requires thin-section imaging and high intravascular contrast, which is more easily achieved with multislice techniques (4).

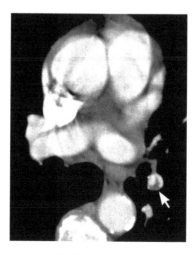

Figure 5.7   Older emboli are wall-adherent and have partially concave contours as a sign of beginning resorption.

Complete occlusion of a vessel by fresh emboli is possible but residual perfusion in the periphery is more usual. Secondary thrombosis of this residual lumen may occur, leading to a moderate enlargement of the vessels with secondary thrombosis of a distal portion of the artery [Fig. 5.4(b)]. In such a case, mosaic perfusion with reduced attenuation in the affected segment will occur. Mosaic perfusion may also be secondary to high-grade obstruction because of vasoconstriction (Euler–Liliestrand effect) of the affected pulmonary artery segment [see Fig. 5.8(b)]. The mosaic pattern is more easily appreciated in the pulmonary parenchymal phase some 30 s after the start of contrast injection and 5–15 s after opacification of the pulmonary arteries. Color-coded density maps can improve detection of such abnormalities (19).

In a matter of days, the clot usually adheres to the vascular wall and shows signs of resorption (Fig. 5.7) (41). Early segmental arterial vasoconstriction distal to the site of embolism can persist to the chronic phase as segmental or subsegmental vascular asymmetry. Normal bronchial arteries take over the blood supply to the embolized lung areas immediately. Pulmonary infarcts, which can complicate various pulmonary vascular disorders including PE, can occur after hours if the collateral supply by bronchial arteries is insufficient. The CT morphology reflects the appearance on the conventional radiograph (28,42): ground-glass opacity can precede the typically wedge-shaped segmental consolidation. Larger infarcts may contain varying amounts of air [Fig. 5.8(a)]. Regions within non-aerated lung that are suspicious for infarction display lack of contrast

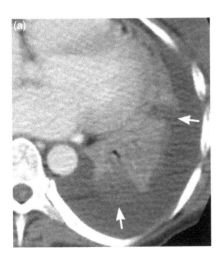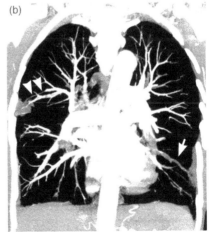

Figure 5.8 Pulmonary infarcts. Infarcts (arrows) in atelectatic lung (a). Peripheral emboli displayed on a thin-slab MIP (b). Note the lack of enhancement of the subsegmental artery leading to the infarct in the left lower lobe (arrow) and the enhancing artery leading to the infarct in the right upper lobe. This artery contains a central embolus and appears to be recanalized. There is a small, constricted vessel with abrupt caliber change leading to the infarcted area as well (arrowheads).

enhancement while atelectatic lung usually has ample contrast enhancement [Fig. 5.8(b)]. Within the infracted areas no vascular enhancement is seen [Fig. 5.8(c)]. Infarcts occur in up to 15% of acute PE cases. Cavitation is frequently observed in septic infarcts, rarely in bland infarcts, but cavitation may develop in the late stage of bland infarcts as well. Occasionally, pulmonary infarcts are associated with pneumothorax.

An enlarged right ventricle (RV/LV diameter >1.3), septal bulging (flattened contour of the septum or bulging to the left), a dilated coronary sinus, or dilated pulmonary artery (greater than the aortic diameter) are signs of acute right heart failure (43). However, this can only be used if there is no preexistent pulmonary hypertension, such as in patients with chronic thromboembolic pulmonary hypertension, which can be detected by looking at the thickness of the right ventricular wall. In acute right heart failure it remains thin while it is thickened in chronic situations (Fig. 5.9).

C. Artifacts and Pitfalls

The commonest factors leading to false positive and false negative results of CTA are summarized in Table 5.5. Common interpretation errors occur with subsegmental PE, suboptimal image quality, motion artifacts, hilar lymph nodes, and partial opacification of the pulmonary veins (1,2,44,45). In addition, pulmonary artery segments that are oblique to the imaging plane, for example, the lingula and middle lobe, may not be demonstrated adequately by single-slice CTA. Knowledge of bronchovascular anatomy is mandatory and training and

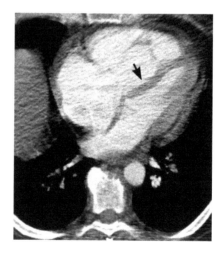

Figure 5.9 Right ventricular dilatation in acute PE. Note the thin right ventricular wall, the increased RV/LV ratio and the septal bulging (arrow) that indicate acute right heart decompensation.

Table 5.5 Pitfalls in CTA for Acute PE

False positive findings
   Breathing artifacts
   Pulsation artifacts
   Partial volume effects
   Differential enhancement of arterial territories
   Hilar lymph nodes
   Unenhanced pulmonary veins
False negative findings
   Poor vascular enhancement
   Breathing artifacts
   Pulsation artifacts
   Inadequate scanning parameters
   High-contrast artifacts
   Isolated subsegmental PE

experience in the interpretation of CT scans for detecting PE further improves observer agreement and performance of CTA.

Technically inadequate or indeterminate single-slice CTA examinations are found in 2–10% of the cases and are mainly related to inadequate vascular opacification poor signal-to-noise ratio and/or and severe dyspnea. In comparison, in the PIOPED study, 4% of the pulmonary angiograms were considered inadequate or were incomplete.

Breathing is the single most important factor that can render a CTA of the pulmonary arteries useless. Breathing can abruptly decrease vascular contrast and should not be mistaken for intraluminal filling defects (Fig. 5.10). Breathing artifacts may be hard to identify with a soft-tissue window setting but they are readily apparent as distortion of anatomic structures with a lung window setting. Breathing may decrease the density of obliquely oriented vessels to an extent that makes them impossible to evaluate (47).

Pulsation predominantly affects the lung parenchyma of the lingula and left lower lobe. It aggravates partial volume effects in obliquely oriented vessels. Pulsation appears as double contours, decreased enhancement simulating thrombus, or vessel beading (Fig. 5.11). False negative findings may be the result of inconsistent visualization of smaller arteries in the affected segments.

Partial volume effects make the apparent enhancement of a vessel decrease as the vessel becomes smaller in the periphery. Vessels with a more horizontal course are more susceptible to these effects (48). Mistaking such partial volume artifacts for a real embolus will lead to false positive findings. However, comparing the density of a vessel to its more distal portions or to a vessel of similar size and orientation will allow a more confident diagnosis to be made. In addition may lymphatic tissues at vessel bifurcations appear as intraluminal clots (Fig. 5.12). Differentiation is again possible by comparison with distal portions of the

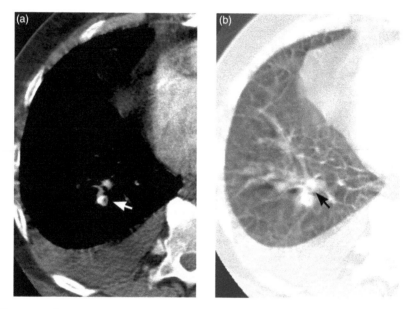

Figure 5.10 Breathing may simulate an embolus on soft tissue window settings (a) but can be differentiated by the presence of movement artifacts with lung window settings (b). [With permission from Prokop and Engelke (46).]

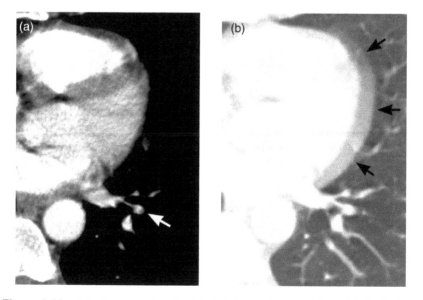

Figure 5.11 Pulsation may also simulate intraluminal filling defects (a). In the lung window setting a double contour of the heart can be appreciated with decreasing density towards the anterior portions (arrows) (b).

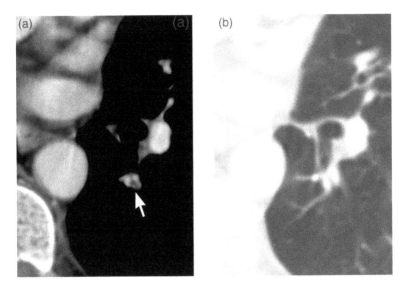

Figure 5.12 Partial volume effect at an arterial bifurcation simulates an intraluminal clot (a). The branching point can be better appreciated on the lung window setting (b).

vessel and by using a lung window for better display of the vessel course. Partial volume effects are also responsible for lack of visualization of more peripheral artery branches and therefore may cause false negative diagnosis. Too thick a collimation will substantially impair the diagnostic accuracy of CTA. For good quality MPR, the collimation should not exceed 2 mm.

Poor vascular enhancement aggravates the problems with other artifacts, in particular partial volume and breathing effects, and may result in nondiagnostic examinations. The main reasons are a low injection rate, wrong bolus timing, or too low a contrast volume [Fig. 5.13(a)]. Valsalva maneuvers during the course of the scan lead to a sudden drop of venous inflow via the brachiocephalic veins and may cause variations in arterial enhancement that varies with table position [Fig. 5.13(b)]. Proper patient instruction is crucial to avoid these effects. Vascular enhancement can be substantially improved by using low kVp settings, high flow rates (>3 mL/s), and a saline flush to optimize utilization of contrast material (see Fig. 5.3).

Differential enhancement of the arterial lumen between various segments of the pulmonary arterial tree can be seen even at identical table positions. It occurs when there is increased flow due to peripheral abnormalities, or decreased outflow, and may even be seen sporadically without apparent reason. It is most frequently encountered in early scans, especially when (fast) multislice scanning is employed. Usually, however, the density of the affected vessel is higher than that of soft tissue, making it easy to distinguish it from a true embolus.

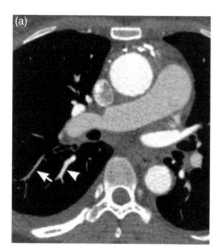
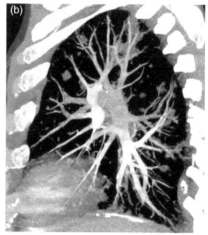

Figure 5.13 Problems with contrast injection can lead to inhomogenous enhancement of the pulmonary vascular system. Scanning too late may lead to loss of enhancement in the arteries (arrow) while the veins are still strongly enhancing (arrowhead) (a). If the patient performs a Valsalva maneuver during the scan there may be a rapid drop-off in enhancement of the inflowing blood (b). Note that the arteries in the basal portions of this caudo-cranial scan are well enhanced, followed by enhancement of the veins in the central portions and lack of enhancement in the lung apex. Scan duration was <10 s (16 × 0.75 mm).

High-contrast artifacts from the injection veins may make evaluation of arteries in or close to the mediastinum difficult. Artifacts can be reduced with caudo-cranial scanning direction and the use of a saline flush. Contrast delivery through catheters that are positioned in the pulmonary artery (*Swan–Ganz catheters*) will cause major artifacts and will leave one lung without sufficient contrast enhancement.

Anatomic pitfalls include *lymph nodes* that are seen in typical locations at the origin of upper lobe vessels, alongside lower lobe arteries, and at the origin of branching segmental arteries and can be mistaken for central emboli [Fig. 5.14(a)]. If in doubt, coronal or sagittal MPR will help. Isolated wall-adherent thrombi at these positions are rare in acute PE. With caudocranial scanning, the enhancement of the *pulmonary veins* can be lower than in the pulmonary arteries and may be mistaken for intraluminal clots [Fig. 5.14(b)]. The veins can be differentiated from the arteries using their anatomic position (medial to the lower lobe arteries), their continuity to the left atrium, and their lack of proximity to the bronchi. *Mucous plugging* within the bronchial system may be mistaken for pulmonary emboli on soft-tissue windows but following the structures on lung windows usually makes differentiation easy [Fig. 5.14(c)].

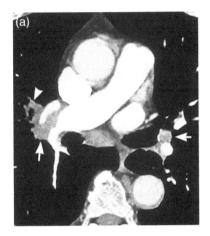
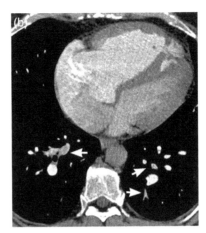

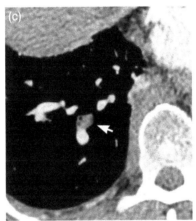

Figure 5.14 Normal anatomy may simulate emboli. Differentiating hilar lymph nodes (arrows) from emboli (arrowhead) may be difficult (a). Veins may not yet be enhanced (b). Intrabronchial mucous plugs may simulate a nonenhancing vessel (c).

D. Results of CTA

Single-slice CTA provides excellent results for the detection of emboli located in the main, lobar, and segmental pulmonary arteries; but where emboli are limited to subsegmental and more peripheral arteries, the sensitivity of single-slice CTA is limited (2,33,47–53). Initial experience with multislice CT indicates that this method will further refine the CT approach to PE, particularly in the diagnosis of small subsegmental emboli (Table 5.6) (54,55). In the first study by Remy-Jardin et al. (1), there was an average of more than six emboli within the pulmonary arterial system in patients with proven PE. This study and other larger series indicate that the prevalence of isolated subsegmental pulmonary embolism is low.

Table 5.6 Performance of CTA for the Diagnosis of Acute PE

Author	Scanner	n	Sensitivity (%)	Specificity (%)
Goodman et al., 1995 (49)	Single-slice	20[a]	63	89
Remy-Jardin et al., 1996 (48)	Single-slice	75	91	78
van Rossum et al., 1996 (2)	Single-slice	149	94	82
Mayo et al., 1997 (47)	Single-slice	142	87	95
Van Rossum et al., 1998 (50)	Single-slice	123	75	90
ESTIPEP 1999 (51)	Single-slice	401	88	94
Kim et al., 1999 (52)	Single-slice	110	92	96
ANTELOPE 1999 (53)	Single-slice	617	69	84
Qanadli et al., 2000 (54)	Dual-slice	157	90	94
Choche et al., 2003 (55)	Four-slice	94	96	98

[a]All patients with intermediate probability results of V/Q scintigraphy.

In addition, the incidence of PE in a given patient cohort influences the reported accuracy for spiral CT (47,48,52).

Another important consideration is whether pulmonary angiography should be the gold standard against which CTA is measured. Significant variation in interobserver agreement related to embolus size was observed for pulmonary angiography (30,56,57). In the PIOPED study, the interobserver agreement on the presence or absence of subsegmental PE was found to be 66% as compared with 98% and 90% on lobar and segmental PE, respectively (30). This suggests that subsegmental PE may even be difficult to diagnose by pulmonary angiography. Baile et al. (33) compared spiral CTA and pulmonary angiography for the detection of subsegmental-sized PE by using a methacrylate cast of porcine pulmonary vessels as an independent gold standard. They found no difference between thin-section CTA and angiography for the detection of small emboli, which supports the use of CTA as stand-alone imaging modality for PE diagnosis.

Since pulmonary angiography may not be an adequate gold standard for PE diagnosis, the true accuracy of spiral CT in patients with suspected PE cannot be determined. However, there are other measures of the reliability of a test such as inter- and intraobserver agreement. As shown for pulmonary angiography, interobserver agreement per artery is better for main and lobar PE ($\kappa = 0.75-0.95$) than for segmental emboli ($\kappa = 0.47-0.88$) (58–60). Since most patients have multiple thrombi, the observed per-patient interobserver agreement including subsegmental PE is better: $\kappa = 0.77-0.97$ (2,61). In a prospective study in 142 patients, Mayo et al. (47) compared single-slice CTA with V/Q scintigraphy and found not only better interobserver agreement with CTA ($\kappa = 0.85$ vs. 0.61) but also greater sensitivity (87% vs. 65%). Others found single-slice CTA not only to be more sensitive (65% and 75% vs. 20% and 49%) but also to be more specific (90% and 97% vs. 47% and 52%) than V/Q scintigraphy (62,63).

Single-slice CTA is considered unable to reliably detect PE when emboli are limited to subsegmental or smaller vessels. However, the development of multislice techniques as well as optimizing the contrast medium injection and scanning protocols have improved the visualization of the pulmonary tree and appear to enable detection that approaches that of pulmonary angiography (4,64). Reduction of scanning time to <10 s will further reduce motion artifacts and improve spatial resolution, and can lead to further improvement of the image quality (65). Reduction of slice thickness has been shown to improve the ability to visualize the vascular tree adequately, enhancing the interpretation of the scan and improving observer agreement (4,5). It can be expected that an improved overall image quality associated with the use of these new techniques will lead to a better accuracy of spiral CT in detecting PE.

E. Role of CTA

Because of the disadvantages of the traditional diagnostic methods, and on the basis of the evidence that CTA can depict pulmonary emboli with good sensitivity and specificity, it seems reasonable to incorporate this modality into clinical practice.

Considering the current knowledge about the accuracy of different methods in the assessment of PE, and the heterogeneity in method availability and acceptance, it is clear that, for the near future, several different diagnostic strategies and algorithms will coexist. In addition, it seems that CTA will play an increasingly important role. At this point, CTA has already been incorporated into the clinical routine in many institutions. CTA is already used as a primary screening test for PE where nuclide lung imaging is unavailable, and in this context, CTA can be regarded as sensitive and specific enough to diagnose or rule out relevant PE.

CTA, combined with V/Q scanning, is more acceptable to clinicians than a strategy involving pulmonary arteriography, and thus reduces the potentially dangerous "best clinical guess" approach (32). A diagnostic strategy suggested by Gottschalk (37) uses conventional radiographs to exclude major pulmonary or cardiovascular abnormalities (e.g., atelectasis, infiltrates, congestion, and major emphysema). Patients with normal or near-normal chest radiographs then can safely undergo V/Q scanning because diagnostic yield will be much higher than in an unselected group (well above 80% definite diagnoses). In patients with abnormal chest radiographs, V/Q sans rarely yield high-probability results and therefore should be avoided. CTA is feasible even for critically ill or intubated patients, and CTA is now the imaging method of choice at our institution for intensive care patients with suspected PE. In addition, spiral CT can be useful for monitoring patients who undergo thrombolytic therapy. In these patients, CTA allows the visualization of embolic material without the need for a central venous puncture.

In many institutions, CTA is now the most frequently used technique for the evaluation of stable patients with suspected PE (66). It is the first-line modality in patients with an abnormal chest radiograph or history of cardi-opulmonary disease (Fig. 5.15), and can be used as an alternative to perfusion scanning for all other patients. Interobserver agreement is substantially higher than for V/Q scanning or pulmonary angiography (2,47,58–63). The number of indeterminate diagnoses is <10%. Specificity is well above 80% for single-slice CTA, while sensitivity varies depending on the study design and the patient group examined (Table 5.6). False negative findings are frequently due to breathing artifacts and peripheral emboli, which are beyond the resolution of single-slice scanners. Isolated peripheral emboli are rare in a general patient group (3–7%) but are more frequent in patients with indeterminate V/Q scans (30%) (30,49). Their clinical importance is a matter of controversy. Multislice CTA with 1 mm sections substantially improves detection rates of subsegmental emboli and evaluation of more distal pulmonary arteries. It yields higher interobserver agreement than with thicker sections.

One of the biggest advantages of CTA, however, is that it can establish an *alternative diagnosis* in up to 30% of patients with suspected PE (Fig. 5.16). It allows for direct visualization of the thrombotic material as well as of signs of right heart overload. It has the potential of distinguishing massive from nonmassive PE. Two-thirds of patients who initially had a clinical suspicion of having PE do not have this disease. The combination of V/Q scintigraphy and pulmonary angiography does not provide an explanation for the symptoms of patients who eventually do not have PE. CTA enables the concurrent visualization of the pulmonary parenchyma, pleura, and mediastinum and there is evidence that spiral

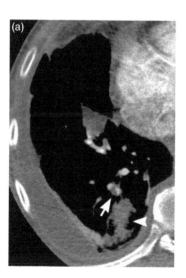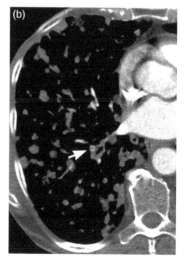

Figure 5.15 CTA is usually successfully detecting emboli (arrows) even in pre-existent lung disease: pleural effusion and infarct (arrowhead) (a) and extensive metastatic disease (b).

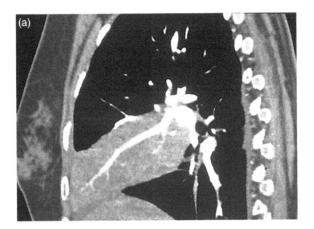

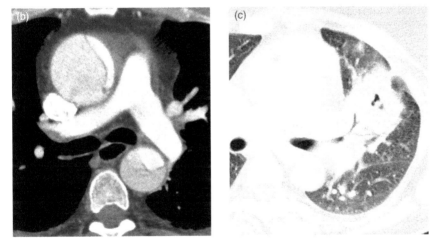

Figure 5.16 Alternative diagnoses include lobar pneumonia (a), acute aortic dissection (here: type A) (b), or bronchogenic cancer (c).

CT provides important information pertinent to alternative diagnoses in the absence of PE (47,61,67–69). Alternative diagnosis that have been found include pneumonia, cardiovascular disease, and malignancy and were found in up to 67% of patients without PE (52).

Single-slice CTA also seems to be a *cost-effective* method, as reported in a study by van Erkel et al. (70), who investigated different combinations of tests to diagnose PE. The authors showed that the five strategies with the lowest cost per life saved (and the five strategies with the lowest mortality) all included spiral CT angiography of the pulmonary arteries.

Clinical outcome in patients in whom no PE was found at CTA is quite favorable, despite the fact that the negative predictive values is not yet as good as the best values described for angiography or scintigraphy that the published patient numbers are not yet high enough to make definitive statements (71–74). Ferretti et al. (72) followed a group of 164 patients with clinically suspected PE, intermediate probability at V/Q scanning, and a negative result at CTA. Of the 164 patients with negative CTA and initially negative results at Duplex ultrasound of the leg, three were found to have clots in the calf veins at short-term follow-up, and were categorized as initially false negative on CTA. These authors concluded that in patients with negative CTA, clinical outcome was comparable to that in patients with negative V/Q scintigraphy or negative pulmonary angiography. In our institution, a study of patients who underwent spiral CT angiography for suspected PE between 1993 and 1995 showed that in 260 cases with negative spiral CT angiography, in which anticoagulation was withheld, one recurrent PE (0.4%) was documented (73). Goodman et al. followed patients who had negative imaging results and who were not anticoagulated for 3 months. Subsequent PE was found in two (1%) of 198 patients with negative CT scans in comparison with none of 188 patients with negative V/Q scans (74).

Patients with signs of right heart failure or a large amount of intravascular clot have a substantially reduced prognosis. Quantification of clot burden has been tried using various techniques (75). The PE index suggested by Qanadli et al. (76) has been shown to have a good correlation with patient outcome. With a PE index <60%, all patients recovered from the embolic event, while five of six patients (83%) with a PE index ≥60% died (77). The index is derived by first attaching a "D-score" to each segmental pulmonary artery (10 on either side), where $D = 1$ for a partial obstruction and $D = 2$ for a complete occlusion of the vessel. If a clot is located proximal to the segmental level, each of the segments arising from this artery is treated as if it also contained a clot of the same degree of obstruction (e.g., partial obstruction of the right pulmonary artery will yield a PE score of 10 segments $\times$ 1 = 10, complete occlusion of an additional segmental branch on the same side will increase the score by 1). The maximum PE score for both lungs would be 40, which is converted into a percentage to yield the PE index.

F. Diagnostic Algorithms

Diagnostic algorithms for the clinical and imaging workup of acute PE are highly disputed and undergo frequent revisions depending on new technical developments and on the clinical subspecialty that are issuing them. When designing a diagnostic algorithm, one has to keep the following facts in mind:

- Clinical and imaging tests will depend on the severity of the symptoms of PE.
- In patient with signs of acute massive PE (see Table 5.3) transthoracic or transesophageal echo may be used to detect signs of right heart failure, which may prompt immediate therapy.

- In clinically stable patients with signs of acute massive PE or acute sub-massive PE, CTA will have a very high sensitivity because proximal clots are expected. CTA may be considered the technique of choice in such patients.
- In patients with signs of acute nonmassive PE, more peripheral emboli can be expected, and the performance of CTA depends strongly on the available scanning technique. In this setting, the pretest probability plays a major role in further patient workup.
- In general, clinical pretest probability will influence the interpretation of a positive of negative test result (D-dimer/imaging). In case of concordance between the test and pretest probability, no further test may be necessary, while more sensitive or specific tests may become necessary in case of discrepancies.
- The D-dimer test (ELISA) can be used to rule out PE if clinical pretest probability is low to moderate (26). It is not useful in patients with a high pretest probability. Positive D-dimer warrants further diagnostic workup.
- Perfusion scintigraphy may be considered in patients with near-normal chest radiographs or if (D-dimer is positive and) pretest probability is low to moderate. It is not helpful in patients with abnormal chest radiographs (37).
- Ultrasound of the lower extremity veins can be considered in stable patients (examination time and access to the legs may be a limiting factor in sick patients). If positive, no further imaging is needed (26).
- A negative CTA together with a low pretest probability is considered sufficient to withhold anticoagulation. A negative CTA in a setting of moderate to high pretest probability should require further testing if no alternative diagnosis can be made based on CT findings (26). Such further tests include leg ultrasound or CT venography (treatment if such test are positive), and angiography if discrepancies remain. If CTA was performed on a multislice scanner and a high image quality was obtained, no further testing may be required.
- In intensive care patients or patients with abnormal chest radiographs, D-dimer is unspecific and CTA may be considered as the primary test to demonstrate PE.

G. CT Venography

Recently, studies have been published that combined spiral CT of the chest with scanning of pelvic and leg veins which can demonstrate DVT without the need for additional contrast medium injection (14–16,78,79).

Several studies revealed that indirect CT venography is as accurate as ultrasound in the detection of DVT in the femoropopliteal system (14,15). In addition, indirect CT venography can depict DVT in iliac veins and vena cava (Fig. 5.17),

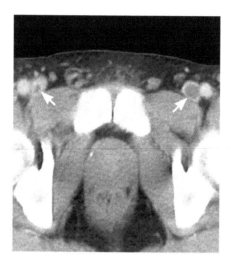

Figure 5.17 CT venography demonstrates a small thrombus in the right and a nearly occluding thrombus in the left femoral veins (arrows).

vessels that are poorly shown on sonography. The interobserver agreement, however, may be lower that the agreement for pulmonary spiral CT (78).

In a large study, Loud et al. (14) found PE in 91 of their 541 patients. Of these 91 patients with PE, 29 patients also had DVT. Only 16 patients had DVT without PE and thus also required treatment. These 16 patients amount to only 3% of the whole scanned population, which means that 97% are exposed to radiation without clinical consequences.

These data need to be validated in further studies, and cost-effective analyses are warranted to consider the true value of this technique in the diagnostic workup for PE.

VII. Chronic Thromboembolic Pulmonary Hypertension

Within 6 weeks to several months, 60–65% of all acute pulmonary emboli will resolve or recanalize (25–30%) (41). Some 15% of patients with incomplete resolution of thrombus after 10 months will develop secondary chronic thrombembolic pulmonary arterial hypertension (CTEPH). CTEPH develops if a sufficiently large cross-sectional area of the pulmonary arteries is occluded or suffers from reduced perfusion due to vasoconstriction.

The clinical diagnosis of chronic thrombembolic pulmonary hypertension is difficult owing to nonspecific symptoms and lung function tests. Progressive occlusion of the pulmonary vascular bed will cause pulmonary hypertension. Often the patients present with pulmonary hypertension after progressive occlusion of the pulmonary vascular bed caused by medial hypertrophy, intimal fibrosis, and arterialization of pulmonary arterioles. Most patients have a substantial right ventricular hypertrophy and may even suffer from secondary tricuspid incompetence due to dilatation of the ventricle and the valvular ring.

Causative treatment is possible if central thrombotic material in the pulmonary arteries can be removed by pulmonary arterial thrombendarterectomy. CTA plays a crucial role in differentiating CTEPH from other causes of pulmonary hypertension and in defining the presence of wall-adherent material in the proximal pulmonary arteries (80). Single-slice CTA is always complemented by pulmonary arteriography but multislice CTA has the potential to become the sole diagnostic modality for this patient group.

A. Findings at CTA

The presence of wall-adherent intraluminal thrombotic material is virtually diagnostic for CTEPH. In CTEPH, the central pulmonary vessels enlarge, while more peripheral recanalized vessels may have a reduced size with eccentric, smoothly marginated residual thrombus adhering to the vessel wall (Fig. 5.18). MPR may be helpful to distinguish lymphatic tissue from thrombus (Fig. 5.19). Thrombotic material can display dystrophic calcification. Peripheral stenoses may form during recanalization of vessels [Fig. 5.20(a)]. They are best appreciated on volume-rendered views or thin-slab MIP. Intraluminal webs can be found as a residuum of emboli [Fig. 5.20(b)]. Chronically occluded vessels have a substantially reduced size and are associated with mosaic oligemia (80,81).

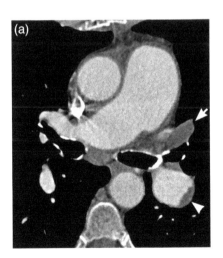 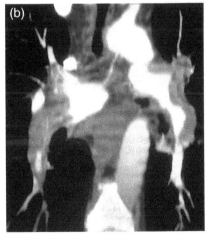

Figure 5.18 Chronic thromboembolic pulmonary hypertension with wall-adherent apposition thrombus (arrowhead) and occlusion of the lingula artery (arrow) (a). Coronal reformation in another patient with large amounts of wall-adherent thrombotic material in the main pulmonary arteries (single-slice CT) (b).

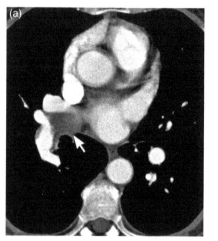 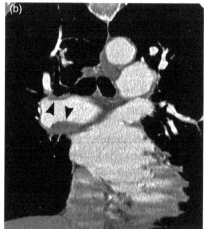

Figure 5.19 Differentiation between wall-adherent thrombi and lymphatic tissue may be difficult to appreciate on axial scans (arrow) (a). On coronal MPR the thrombus is easily seen (arrowheads) (b).

Mosaic oligemia (mosaic perfusion) is a typical feature of chronic PE and is characterized by areas of reduced lung attenuation and reduced vessel diameter due to hypoperfusion and the vasoconstriction effect (Fig. 5.21). Noninvolved areas appear denser than hypoperfused areas and may be mistaken for areas

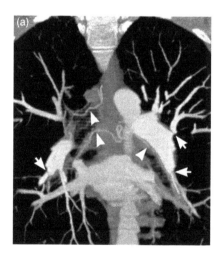 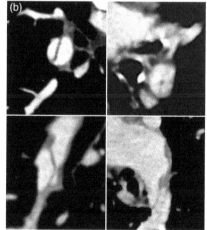

Figure 5.20 Peripheral stenoses (arrows) in CTEPH can better be appreciated on thin-slab MIP than on axial sections. Also note the hypertrophied bronchial arteries (arrowheads) (a). Intraarterial webs are typical residue of embolic material in CTEPH (b). [With permission from Prokop and Engelke (46).]

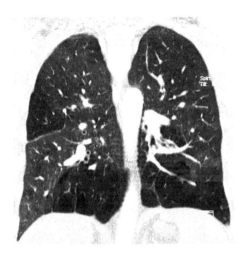

Figure 5.21 Mosaic perfusion is characterized by geometric areas of ground glass attenuation representing well-perfused lung regions and often wedge-shaped regions with hypoattenuation and small vessels, representing perfusion deficit after chronic embolism. [Compare also to the color map in Fig. 5.3(b) in color plate section.]

of pathologic ground-glass opacity. Mosaic oligemia is virtually diagnostic of chronic pulmonary embolism, even without additional demonstration of intra-arterial thrombus. Lung areas with normal perfusion pattern do not exclude the presence of proximal intravascular embolic material in the supplying artery. The pattern is best appreciated on color-coded images.

Scars or nodular masses may be seen as a consequence of old *pulmonary infarction.* Such old infarcts may present as a cavitating nodule. Plexiform lesions are rarely seen in CTEPH.

Bronchial arteries frequently hypertrophy in chronic PE and can often be seen running alongside the occluded artery, especially when thin-section scanning is performed [Fig. 5.20(a)] (81,82). However, bronchial artery aneurysms and extensive chest wall or infradiaphragmatic collateralization, as in pulmonary artery interruption, have not been reported in PE.

The *right heart* is dilated and shows signs of hypertrophy consisting of a thickened wall and increased trabeculation. Secondary tricuspid valve insufficiency can be suspected if the right atrium is dilated and the tricuspid valvular ring is substantially wider than the mitral valvular ring [Figs. 5.9(b) and 5.22]. Reflux of (cubitally injected) contrast material into the hepatic veins can be seen in patients with chronic right heart failure [Fig. 5.22(b)].

B. Differential Diagnosis

Table 5.7 gives an overview of criteria that can be used to distinguish morphologically between acute PE and CTEPH.

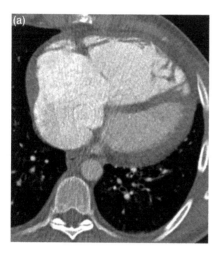
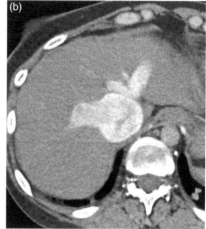

Figure 5.22 Right ventricular hypertrophy in CTEPH is characterized by a dilated ventricle with a thickened wall and increased trabeculation. Also note the dilated tricuspid ring representing an indirect sign of tricuspid insufficiency (a). Right heart failure is frequently associated with reflux of contrast material through the right atrium into the inferior vena cava and into dilated liver veins (b).

Wall-adherent apposition thrombus may form in the central pulmonary arteries of extreme cases of primary pulmonary hypertension or Eisenmenger's syndrome because of slow or turbulent flow in these arteries. In such cases, however, there is massive enlargement of the central pulmonary arteries

Table 5.7 CT Criteria for Differentiating Acute PE from CTEPH

Acute PE	CTEPH
Central intraluminal thrombotic material	Wall-adherent thrombus
	Cacified thrombus
	Intraluminal webs
Normal size vessels in subtotal occlusion	(Markedly) reduced vessel size
Dilated vessels in secondary thrombosis	Peripheral stenoses
Reduced vessel size in proximal obstruction	
Wedge-like consolidations:	Peripheral consolidation of varying shape and size
A telectases (enhancement)	
Infarcts (no enhancement)	Cavernating lesions possible
No or minimal mosaic perfusion pattern	Substantial mosaic perfusion pattern
No dilation of bronchial arteries	Dilated bronchial arteries
Right heart dilatation with normal myocardial thickness	Right heart dilatation with increased myocardial thickness

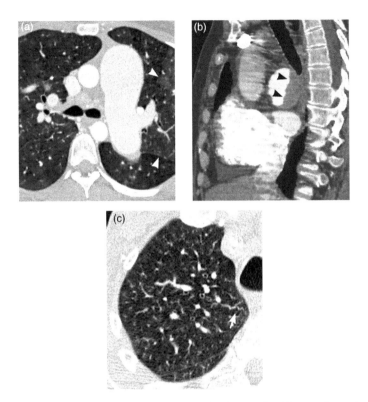

Figure 5.23 Primary pulmonary hypertension is characterized by massive pulmonary arterial dilatation. Also note the ground glass opacities (arrowheads) in this patient with hemoptysis (a). Apposition thrombus may form in these patients if the main pulmonary arteries are strongly dilated and flow is low and turbulent (b). Small tortuous vessels are frequently found in the lung periphery may be due to plexogenic arteriopathy (arrow) (c).

(see Fig. 5.23). Pulmonary artery sarcomas may also present as wall-adherent masses but they show contrast enhancement of variable degree [see Fig. 5.29(a)].

Moderate mosaic perfusion may also be seen in other causes of pulmonary hypertension. It usually is less pronounced than in CTEPH.

VIII. Other Causes of Pulmonary Hypertension

Pulmonary hypertension can be the result of a large number of disease entities. CTA is particularly important for identifying individuals with recurrent PE and CTEPH, who can be successfully treated by thromboendarterectomy. CTA and high-resolution computed tomography (HRCT) can be used to differentiate between the various disorders that cause pulmonary hypertension. The diagnosis of *primary pulmonary hypertension* (PPH) is made by excluding any clinical or radiological alternative etiologies.

Plexogenic arteriopathy is a vascular hyperplasia that affects small to medium-sized pulmonary arteries. It is one of several responses of the pulmonary arteries to continued stress from chronic severe pulmonary arterial hypertension. The vascular lesions have no significant connections to pulmonary veins that would allow for arteriovenous shunting. Plexogenic arteriopathy can occasionally be detected on CT.

A. Findings on CTA

Regardless of the presence and nature of an underlying pathology, the basic radiological pattern of chronic pulmonary arterial hypertension includes central pulmonary arterial dilatation, tapering of peripheral pulmonary arteries, and right heart hypertrophy. The correlation of the *pulmonary artery diameter* on CTA to the degree of pulmonary hypertension is nonlinear. A main pulmonary artery diameter of ≥ 29 mm at its widest point has a positive predictive value $>95\%$, and a distal pulmonary artery trunk exceeding the diameter of the ascending aorta has a positive predictive value $>90\%$. The distal vessels may be large, normal, or reduced in caliber.

Massive enlargement of the central pulmonary arteries is found in PPH [Fig. 5.23(a)]. The turbulent flow in these arteries may lead to formation of apposition thrombus that can be hard to differentiate from CTEPH [Fig. 5.23(b)]. Mosaic perfusion, however, is usually much less in PPH than with CTEPH.

In patients with *secondary pulmonary hypertension*, a variety of CTA and HRCT features can provide information about primary disorders and facilitate their differential diagnosis. Table 5.8 lists the CT-morphological criteria that aid in the exclusion of PPH and the differential diagnosis of disorders with secondary pulmonary hypertension.

Plexogenic arteriopathy is characterized by dilated small tortuous peripheral arteries without evidence of a large AV shunt as in pulmonary AVMs [Fig. 5.23(c)].

IX. Arteriovenous Shunting

Pulmonary AVMs are commonly associated with hereditary hemorrhagic telangiectasia (Osler–Weber–Rendu disease). Many pulmonary AVMs are discovered incidentally in adulthood. Patients are frequently asymptomatic and present with a suspicious nodule or abnormal vessel on chest radiographs. Untreated or occult pulmonary AVM can increase in size over time, with increasing shunt volumes inducing hypoxemia, together with an increased risk of pulmonary hemorrhage, stroke, or AVM-rupture. CTA has an important role in screening for pulmonary AVM, with a sensitivity $>95\%$. CTA provides 3D rendering of complex malformations and thus facilitates planning of transarterial

Table 5.8 CT Criteria that Aid in Differential Diagnosis of
Chronic Pulmonary Arterial Hypertension

Wall-adherent material
  CTEPH
  Severe PPH (apposition thrombus)
  Pulmonary artery sarcoma
Intraluminal calcifications
  CTEPH
  Very longstanding severe pulmonary hypertension
  Eisenmenger's syndrome
  Idiopathic infantile arterial calcification (IIAC)
Dilated central and peripheral vessels
  Increased pulmonary blood flow with L–R shunt
Dilated pulmonary veins, intestinal or alveolar edema
  Mitral stenosis
  Mediastinal fibrosis or tumor mass
  Pulmonary vein stenosis
  Pulmonary veno-occlusive disease
Peripheral pulmonary AV shunting
  Hepatopulmonary syndrome
  Chronic pulmonary schistosomiasis
Diffuse or focal decreased lung attenuation
  Chronic obstructive lung disease
  Pulmonary emphysema
  Cavitating lesions in granulomatous infections
  Vasculitis
Signs of interstitial lung disease or granulomatous infections
  Interstitial fibrosis
  Sarcoidosis
  Granulomatous infections
  Pneumoconiosis
  Vasculitis
  Alveolar capillary dysplasia
  Pulmonary capillary hemangiomatosis
  Venoocclusive disease.

Source: Adapted from Prokop and Engelke (46).

embolization. CTA is especially helpful in complex malformations with more than one feeding vessel. A diameter of the feeding artery of ≥ 3 mm is regarded as an indication for embolization.

Diffuse pulmonary arteriovenous shunting can occur in pregnancy, Osler–Weber–Rendu disease, complex cardiac malformations, proximal pulmonary artery interruption, polysplenia syndrome, liver disease, and chronic schistosomiasis. The patients present with severe hypoxemia and commonly have a history of systemic embolism with neurological complications. Spontaneous regression after pregnancy has been reported. DSA is required to assess the morphology and flow characteristics prior to coil embolization of larger communications. Contrast-enhanced echocardiography or labeled microsphere or red-cell nuclear imaging can provide information about the shunt volume during rest and exercise. The role of CTA is not yet defined.

A. Findings on CTA

Spiral scanning without the use of intravenous contrast material may already be able to demonstrate the pulmonary malformation, which consists of a, frequently tortuous, feeding artery and an enlarged draining vein. Aneurysms are common in the region of the actual AV shunt (Fig. 5.24). Pulmonary AVM enhances simultaneously with the pulmonary arteries. Complex AVMs have more than one feeding artery or draining vein and are best evaluated by SSD or VRT (83).

Multiple AVMs are a common finding. In order to not miss these small lesions, thin-slab MIP or volume-rendered images (after removal of the chest wall) are particularly helpful. In addition, the cine viewing of axial or multiplanar sections demonstrates disproportionably large vessels in the lung periphery, or vessels with an increased tortuosity. Demonstration of an AV shunt in these regions confirms the diagnosis of AVM.

Shunts between the *bronchial arteries* and pulmonary veins are extremely rare causes of pulmonary hemorrhage. Such findings are very hard to demonstrate

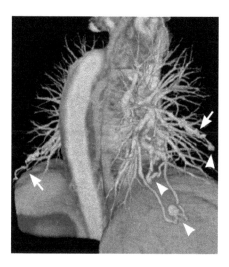

Figure 5.24 Pulmonary AVM in a patient with Osler's disease (volume rendering after chest wall removal). There was successful embolization of a pulmonary AVM in the left lower lobe and a partially successful one with residual perfusion and aneurysm on the right (arrows). Note the other, not yet embolized pulmonary AVMs in the right lower lobe (arrowheads).

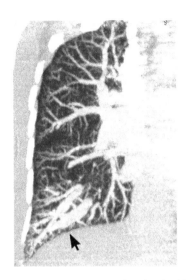

Figure 5.25 Diffuse pulmonary arteriovenous shunting in this young pregnant woman is characterized by massively dilated veins in the lower lobe without visible AV shunt. The exam was performed at ultralow dose (80 kVp, $CTDI_{vol} = 0.6$ mGy).

but may be approached by thin-section multislice scanning and thin-slab MIP or volume rendering.

Bleeding typically presents as areas of patchy to lobular ground-glass opacities in patients with hemoptysis, through to consolidation in patients with massive hemorrhage.

Diffuse pulmonary AV shunting appears as massively dilated veins (Fig. 5.25), sometimes associated with conglomerate areas of small web-like dilated arteries including the lung periphery.

X. Pulmonary Aneurysms

Congenital aneurysms are typically located in the central pulmonary artery system (84). They may be induced by systolic jets from a stenotic pulmonary valve. Other pulmonary or cardiovascular abnormalities including pulmonary vascular stenoses may be present.

Infection is an important pathogenetic factor in (peripheral) pulmonary artery pseudoaneurysm formation (85). It occurs with pulmonary aspergillosis and rarely with tuberculosis (Rasmussen aneurysm) or syphilis. Once demonstrated on CTA, early treatment is indicated because rupture is usually fatal.

Primary vasculitic pulmonary artery aneurysms are found in giant cell arteritis, polyarteritis nodosa, Behçet's disease, and the Hughes–Stovin syndrome. Distal pulmonary thromboembolism caused by the aneurysm can induce pulmonary infarcts and aneurysmal rupture (86).

Pulmonary artery aneurysms may also develop in patients with cystic media necrosis and Marfan's syndrome.

Bronchial artery aneurysms can be idiopathic or occur in association with pulmonary artery aplasia, Ehlers–Danlos syndrome, trauma, infection, silicosis, and vasculitis including Behçet's disease, Hughes–Stovin syndrome, and polyarteritis nodosa.

Iatrogenic pulmonary artery pseudoaneurysms, commonly induced by Swan–Ganz catheters, are prone to rupture and, like infectious aneurysms, require early treatment (by embolization).

Postoperative pulmonary artery aneurysms can be due to anastomotic leaks or suboptimal correction of the pathological hemodynamics at the pulmonary outflow. They do not always require immediate correction.

A. Findings on CTA

CTA in *congenital aneurysms* demonstrates a fusiform dilatation of a central portion of the pulmonary arteries. Associated peripheral pulmonary artery stenoses may be present. If caused by a stenotic pulmonary valve, the aneurysm involves the most anterior portion of the pulmonary trunk or the proximal left main pulmonary artery.

Infectious pseudoaneurysms may be found within an area of consolidation representing pneumonia. They may develop rapidly and are prone to rupture as the pneumonia resolves. Aneurysms may be multiple and care has to be taken to look for further lesions by using an MIP display (Fig. 5.26).

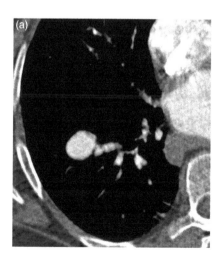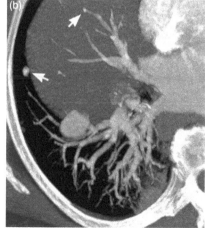

Figure 5.26 Pulmonary pseudoaneurysm that developed within 1 week after catheter-induced septicemia (a). On the thin-slab volume rendered image, multiple additional smaller aneurysms were seen (arrows) (b).

Massive hemorrhage can cause consolidation but there are usually other morphologic signs of pulmonary hemorrhage present in the periphery of such a consolidation (centrilobular and geometric ground-glass opacities, sometimes with a gravity-dependent density gradient), and the patient will complain of hemoptysis.

Other causes of peripheral pulmonary aneurysms may be hard to differentiate. *Thrombosis* of the aneurysm can occur in vasculitic syndromes, which can be complicated by distal embolism and pulmonary infarction. Small peripheral aneurysms may present as small enhancing nodules on thin-section CTA.

Bronchial artery aneurysms are readily identified when involving the mediastinal portions of the bronchial arteries (Fig. 5.27). In the lung periphery they are generally hard to differentiate from pulmonary artery aneurysm.

XI. Vasculitis

Takayasu arteritis and *granulomatous* (*temporal* or *giant cell*) *arteritis* can affect the central pulmonary artery system. In the acute stage there is inflammatory wall thickening; in the chronic stage, smooth fibrotic narrowing or occlusion with arterial thrombosis and distal pulmonary infarction may occur (87). CTA is excellently suited to demonstrate not only the luminal but also wall changes. Low-dose examination techniques are generally sufficient.

Various vasculitic diseases of intermediate and small-size vessels may affect the pulmonary arteries. These include among others, polyarteritis nodosa, Microscopic polyangitis, Wegener's disease, Churg–Strauss syndrome, and systemic lupus erythematosus (88). They are not evaluated by CTA but by HRCT and are not discussed here.

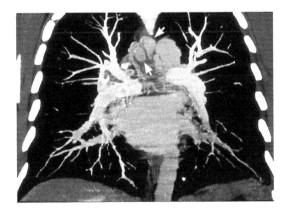

Figure 5.27   Thin-slab MIP of multiple bronchial artery aneurysms in a patient with Ehlers–Danlos syndrome (arrows).

A. Findings on CTA

Takayasu arteritis and granulomatous arteritis cannot be distinguished based on morphological findings at CT. Arterial wall thickening indicates vasculitic activity and usually disappears with a chronic course of the disease or in response to immunosuppressive therapy. Stenosis of the affected pulmonary segments induces peripheral pulmonary perfusion asymmetry (Fig. 5.28) and leads to thinning of peripheral vessels that can be excellently demonstrated by thin-slab MIP or volume rendering (87). Complete obstruction with distal arterial thrombosis may be a complication in more extensive disease. Nonenhancing, linear or wedge-shaped peripheral consolidation may be seen as a consequence of distal pulmonary infarction. Very rarely, pulmonary granulomatous arteritis may cause aneurysms that are prone to rupture.

XII. Tumors Involving the Pulmonary Vessels

Leiomyosarcoma or *angiosarcoma* of the pulmonary arteries generally develops in the main or central pulmonary arteries, often in close relationship to the pulmonary valve. The tumor can extend to the contralateral pulmonary artery or into the right ventricle. Secondary thromboembolic events are common and frequently cause the presenting clinical features. CT and MR are well suited to demonstrate both the endoluminal as well as extraluminal tumor components.

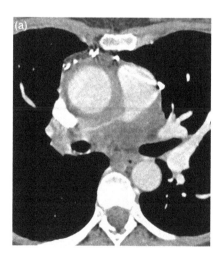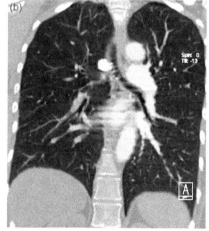

Figure 5.28 Arteritis of the right pulmonary artery with substantial wall thickening and a thread-like stenosis (a). Coronal reformation after 6 months demonstrates substantial asymmetry in the enhancement of the pulmonary vessels and absence of a patent right main pulmonary artery (b).

Although central pulmonary artery *tumor invasion* can occasionally be seen in stage IV bronchogenic cancer or in metastatic disease, the preoperative identification of arterial wall infiltration presents a major diagnostic problem. Intravascular or transesophageal ultrasound is probably superior to CTA.

Pulmonary veins are frequently involved by bronchogenic cancer or metastatic tumor invasion, which will increase the risk of systemic metastatic spread. In advanced cases segmental obstruction of central pulmonary drainage can occur, which can be complicated by retrograde thrombosis.

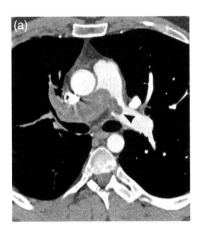
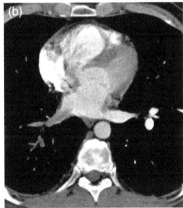
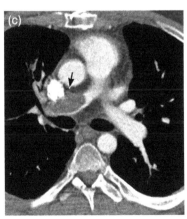

Figure 5.29 Pulmonary sarcoma with near occlusion of the right pulmonary artery. Note the enhancement of the intraluminal mass and the small nonenhancing apposition thrombus on the left (arrowhead) (a). There is no visible enhancement of peripheral arteries and delayed opacification of the right-sided pulmonary veins (b). One year after resection of the tumor there is recurrence with sings of mediastinal invasion (arrow) (c).

A. Findings on CTA

Pulmonary artery sarcomas appear as a lobulated mass within the vessel lumen that may be distinguished from thromboembolism by the presence of contrast uptake in the tumor [Fig. 5.29(a)] (89,90). In ~50% of cases, pulmonary artery sarcomas spread endoluminally to the periphery with a centrifugal growth pattern. Such endoluminal tumor growth may lead to hematogenic metastases to the lungs as well as to arterial obstruction with pulmonary oligemia and delayed enhancement of the pulmonary veins [Fig. 5.29(b)]. Complete obstruction may be complicated by secondary pulmonary artery thrombosis. The tumor may locally invade the mediastinum or the lungs [Fig. 5.29(c)].

Extrinsic compression of the *pulmonary arteries* is frequently observed in advanced stages of bronchogenic carcinoma or other malignancies infiltrating the hila or mediastinum. Circumferential tumor encasement of the pulmonary artery is associated with a higher wall infiltration rate.

CTA can directly demonstrate involvement of *pulmonary veins* with compression, intraluminal filling defects or total venous occlusion. Signs of venous obstruction with segmental or lobar edema (Fig. 5.30) and altered contrast dynamics can be indicators of secondary pulmonary venous thrombosis, which is demonstrated on CTA by the failure of the venous lumen to opacify.

XIII. Summary

Pulmonary CTA has become a standard technique for the evaluation of acute PE. With the advent of multislice CT scanning, image quality has improved

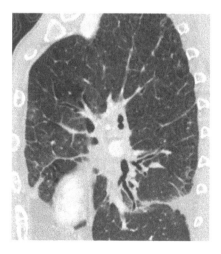

Figure 5.30   Hilar vascular encasement in a patient with bronchogenic cancer. Note the reduced size of the vessel cross-sections and the signs of peripheral venous congestion with thickened interlobular septa.

substantially and now allows also for evaluation of peripheral arteries. In many institutions, multislice CTA has now become the primary, and frequently the only, modality for the evaluation of acute pulmonary embolism. Multislice CTA has the potential to reduce the need to perform invasive arterial angiography of the pulmonary arteries in the diagnostic workup of CTEPH. It may be able to provide all the anatomic information needed to distinguish between patients suited for surgical thromboendarterectomy and those requiring conservative treatment. The three-dimensional capabilities of CTA make it an attractive technique for evaluating other entities as well, including pulmonary AVM or aneurysms. In pulmonary large vessel vasculitis, such as Takayasu or giant cell arteritis, CTA is not only able to demonstrate luminal abnormalities but also inflammatory wall thickening. Since CTA also provides all the information from a standard chest CT, it is excellently suited for evaluating tumor involvement of the pulmonary vessels. Alternative techniques, however, should be considered in patients with reduced renal function given the contrast load, or young individuals in whom multiple scans may lead to unacceptably high radiation exposure.

References

1. Remy-Jardin M, Remy J, Wattinne L, Giraud F. Central pulmonary thromboembolism: diagnosis with spiral volumetric CT with the single-breath-hold technique–comparison with pulmonary angiography. Radiology 1992; 185:381–387.
2. van Rossum AB, Pattynama PM, Ton ER et al. Pulmonary embolism: validation of spiral CT angiography in 149 patients. Radiology 1996; 201:467–470.
3. Remy-Jardin M, Mastora I, Remy J. Pulmonary embolus imaging with multislice CT. Radiol Clin North Am 2003; 41:507–519.
4. Schoepf UJ, Holzknecht N, Helmberger TK et al. Subsegmental pulmonary emboli: improved detection with thin-collimation multi-detector row spiral CT. Radiology 2002; 222:483–490.
5. Remy-Jardin M, Remy J, Artaud D, Deschildre F, Duhamel A. Peripheral pulmonary arteries: optimization of the spiral CT acquisition protocol. Radiology 1997; 204:157–163.
6. Galanski M, Nagel HD, Stamm G. CT radiation exposure risk in Germany. Rofo 2001; 173:R1–R66.
7. Prokop M. [Optimizing dosage in thoracic computerized tomography] Radiologe 2001; 41(3):269–278.
8. Kuiper JW, Geleijns J, Matheijssen NAA, Teeuwisse W, Pattynama PMT. Radiation exposure of multi-row detector spiral computed tomography of the pulmonary arteries. Comparison with digital subtraction pulmonary angiography. Eur Radiol 2003; 13:1496–1500.
9. Weidekamm C, Schaefer-Prokop C, Prokop M. CT Angiography for the evaluation of pulmonary embolism: improvement of vascular enhancment by low kVp settings. Radiology 2005. In press.

10. Fleischmann D, Rubin GD, Bankier AA, Hittmair K. Improved uniformity of aortic enhancement with customized contrast medium injection protocols at CT angiography. Radiology 2000; 214(2):363–371.
11. Hartmann IJ, Lo RT, Bakker J, de Monye W, van Waes PF, Pattynama PM. Optimal scan delay in spiral CT for the diagnosis of acute pulmonary embolism. J Comput Assist Tomogr 2002; 26:21–25.
12. Hopper KD, Mosher TJ, Kasales CJ, TenHave TR, Tully DA, Weaver JS. Thoracic spiral CT: delivery of contrast material pushed with injectable saline solution in a power injector. Radiology 1997; 205(1):269–271.
13. Haage P, Schmitz-Rode T, Hubner D, Piroth W, Gunther RW. Reduction of contrast material dose and artifacts by a saline flush using a double power injector in helical CT of the thorax. AJR 2000; 174(4):1049–1053.
14. Loud PA, Grossman ZD, Klippenstein DL, Ray CE. Combined CT venography and pulmonary angiography: a new diagnostic technique for suspected thromboembolic disease. AJR 1998; 170:951–954.
15. Cham MD, Yankelevitz DF, Shaham D et al. Deep venous thrombosis: detection by using indirect CT venography. The Pulmonary Angiography-Indirect CT Venography Cooperative Group. Radiology 2000; 216:744–751.
16. Rademaker J, Griesshaber V, Hidajat N, Oestmann JW, Felix R. Combined CT pulmonary angiography and venography for diagnosis of pulmonary embolism and deep vein thrombosis: radiation dose. J Thorac Imaging 2001; 16:297–299.
17. Remy-Jardin M, Remy J, Cauvain O, Petyt L, Wannebroucq J, Beregi JP. Diagnosis of central pulmonary embolism with helical CT: role of two-dimensional multiplanar reformations. AJR 1992; 165:1131–1138.
18. Simon M, Chiang EE, Boisille PM. Paddle-wheel multislice CT display of pulmonary vessels and lung structures. Radiol Clin N Am 2003; 41:617–626
19. Wildberger JE, Niethammer MU, Klotz E, Schaller S, Wein BB, Gunther RW. Multi-slice CT for visualization of pulmonary embolism using perfusion weighted color maps. Rofo 2001; 173(4):289–294.
20. Dalen JE, Alpert JS. Natural history of pulmonary embolism. Prog Cardiovasc Dis 1975; 17:257–270.
21. Anderson FA Jr, Wheeler HB, Goldberg RJ et al. A population-based perspective of the hospital incidence and case-fatality rates of deep vein thrombosis and pulmonary embolism. The Worcester DVT Study. Arch Intern Med 1991; 151:933–938.
22. Hampson NB, Culver BH. Clinical aspects of pulmonary embolism. Semin Ultrasound CT MR 1997; 18:314–322.
23. Miniati M, Prediletto R, Formichi B et al. Accuracy of clinical assessment in the diagnosis of pulmonary embolism. Am J Respir Crit Care Med 1999; 159:864–871.
24. Gosselin MV, Rubin GD, Leung AN, Huang J, Rizk NW. Unsuspected pulmonary embolism: prospective detection on routine helical CT scans. Radiology 1998; 208(1):209–215.
25. Frost SD, Brotman DJ, Michota FA. Rational use of D-dimer measurement to exclude acute venous thromboembolic disease. Mayo Clin Proc 2003; 78:1385–1391.
26. Perrier A, Roy PM, Aujesky D et al. Diagnosing pulmonary embolism in outpatients with clinical assessment, D-Dimer measurement, venous ultrasound, and helical computed tomography: a multicenter management study. Am J Med 2004; 116:291–299.

27. Wells PS, Ginsberg JS, Anderson DR, Kearon C, Gent M, Turpie AG, Bormanis J, Weitz J, Chamberlain M, Bowie D, Barnes D, Hirsh J. Use of a clinical model for safe management of patients with suspected pulmonary embolism. Ann Intern Med 1998; 129(12):997–1005.
28. Coche E, Verschuren F, Hainaut P, Goncette L. Pulmonary embolism findings on chest radiographs and multislice CT. Eur Radiol 2004; 14:1241–1248.
29. Pruszczyk P, Torbicki A, Kuch-Wocial A, Szulc M, Pacho R. Diagnostic value of transoesophageal echocardiography in suspected haemodynamically significant pulmonary embolism. Heart 2001; 85(6):628–634.
30. Stein PD, Athanasoulis C, Alavi A et al. Complications and validity of pulmonary angiography in acute pulmonary embolism. Circulation 1992; 85:462–468.
31. van Beek EJ, Brouwerst EM, Song B, Stein PD, Oudkerk M. Clinical validity of a normal pulmonary angiogram in patients with suspected pulmonary embolism—a critical review. Clin Radiol 2001; 56(10):838–842.
32. Schluger N, Henschke C, King T, Russo R, Binkert B, Rackson M, Hayt D. Diagnosis of pulmonary embolism at a large teaching hospital. J Thorac Imaging 1994; 9:180–184.
33. Baile EM, King GG, Muller NL et al. Spiral computed tomography is comparable to angiography for the diagnosis of pulmonary embolism. Am J Respir Crit Care Med 2000; 161:1010–1015.
34. The PIOPED investigators. Value of the ventilation/perfusion scan in acute pulmonary embolism. Results of the prospective investigation of pulmonary embolism diagnosis (PIOPED). JAMA 1990; 263:2753–2759.
35. Blachere H, Latrabe V, Montaudon M et al. Pulmonary embolism revealed on helical CT angiography: comparison with ventilation-perfusion radionuclide lung scanning. AJR 2000; 174:1041–1047.
36. Miniati M, Pistolesi M, Marini C et al. Value of perfusion lung scan in the diagnosis of pulmonary embolism: results of the Prospective Investigative Study of Acute Pulmonary Embolism Diagnosis (PISA-PED). Am J Respir Crit Care Med 1996; 154(5):1387–1393.
37. Gottschalk A. New criteria for ventilation-perfusion lung scan interpretation: a basis for optimal interaction with helical CT angiography. Radiographics 2000; 20(4):1206–1210.
38. Oudkerk M, van Beek EJ, Wielopolski P, van Ooijen PM, Brouwers-Kupyer EM, Bongaerts AH, Berhout A. Comparison of contrast-enhanced magnetic resonance angiography and conventional pulmonary angiography for the diagnosis of pulmonary embolism: a prospective study. Lancet 2002; 359:1643–1647.
39. van Beek EJ, Wild JM, Fink C, Moody AR, Kauczor HU, Oudkerk M. MRI for the diagnosis of pulmonary embolism. J Magn Reson Imaging 2003; 18(6):627–624.
40. Kanne JP, Thoongsuwan N, Stern EJ. Detection of central pulmonary embolism on computed tomography densitometry images before computed tomography pulmonary angiography. J Comput Assist Tomogr 2003; 27(6):907–910.
41. Remy-Jardin M, Louvegny S, Remy J, Artaud D, Deschildre F, Bauchart J-J, Thery C, Duhamel A. Acute central thromboembolic disease: Posttherapeutic follow-up with spiral CT angiography. Radiology 1997; 203:173–180.
42. Coche EE, Mueller NL, Kim K, Wiggs B, Mazo J. Acute pulmonary embolism: ancillary findings at spiral CT. Radiology 1998; 207:753–758.
43. Contractor S, Maldjian PD, Sharma VK, Gor DM. Role of helical CT in detecting right ventricular dysfunction secondary to acute pulmonary embolism. J Comput Assist Tomogr 2002; 26(4):587–591.

44. Aviram G, Levy G, Fishman JE, Blank A, Graif M. Pitfalls in the diagnosis of acute pulmonary embolism on spiral computer tomography. Curr Probl Diagn Radiol 2004; 33(2):74–84.
45. Beigelman C, Chartrand Lefebvre C, Howarth N, Grenier P. Pitfalls in diagnosis of pulmonary embolism with helical CT angiography. AJR 1998; 171:579–585.
46. Prokop M, Engelke C. Vascular system. In: Prokop M, Galanski M, eds. Spiral CT and Multislice CT of the Body. New York: Thieme Medical Publishers, 2003:825–928.
47. Mayo JR, Remy Jardin M, Muller NL et al. Pulmonary embolism: prospective comparison of spiral CT with ventilation-perfusion scintigraphy. Radiology 1997; 205:447–452.
48. Remy-Jardin M, Remy J, Deschildre F et al. Diagnosis of pulmonary embolism with spiral CT: comparison with pulmonary angiography and scintigraphy. Radiology 1996; 200:699–706.
49. Goodman LR, Curtin JJ, Mewissen MW et al. Detection of pulmonary embolism in patients with unresolved clinical and scintigraphic diagnosis: helical CT versus angiography. AJR 1995; 164:1369–1374.
50. van Rossum AB, van Erkel AR, van Persijn van Meerten EL, Ton ER, Rebergen SA, Pattynama PMT. Accuracy of helical CT for acute pulmonary embolism: ROC analysis of observer performance related to clinical experience. Eur Radiol 1998; 8:1160–1164.
51. The ESTIPEP investigators. Prospective evaluation of pulmonary embolism: Diagnostic performance of spiral CT angiography in the ESTIPEP trial. Radiology 1999; 213(P):126.
52. Kim K, Müller NL, Mayo JR. Clinically suspected pulmonary embolism: Utility of spiral-CT. Radiology 1999; 210:693–697.
53. van Strijen MJ, de Monyé W, Kieft GJ, Bloem JL. Diagnosis of pulmonary embolism with spiral CT: a prospective cohort study in 617 consecutive patients. Radiology 1999; 213(P):127.
54. Qanadli SD, Hajjam ME, Mesurolle B et al. Pulmonary embolism detection: prospective evaluation of dual-section helical CT versus selective pulmonary arteriography in 157 patients. Radiology 2000; 217:447–455.
55. Coche E, Verschuren F, Keyeux A et al. Diagnosis of acute pulmonary embolism in outpatients: comparison of thin-collimation multi-detector row spiral CT and planar ventilation-perfusion scintigraphy. Radiology 2003; 229(3):757–765.
56. Diffin DC, Leyendecker JR, Johnson SP, Zucker RJ, Grebe PJ. Effect of anatomic distribution of pulmonary emboli on interobserver agreement in the interpretation of pulmonary angiography. AJR 1998; 171:1085–1089.
57. Quinn MF, Lundell CJ, Klotz TA et al. Reliability of selective pulmonary arteriography in the diagnosis of pulmonary embolism. AJR 1987; 149:469–471.
58. Chartrand Lefebvre C, Howarth N, Lucidarme O, Beigelman C, Cluzel P, Mourey Gerosa I et al. Contrast-enhanced helical CT for pulmonary embolism detection: inter- and intraobserver agreement among radiologists with variable experience. AJR 1999; 172:107–112.
59. Domingo ML, Marti-Bonmati L, Dosda R, Pallardo Y. Interobserver agreement in the diagnosis of pulmonary embolism with helical CT. Eur J Radiol 2000; 34:136–140.
60. Herold CJ, Hahne J, Ghaye B et al. Prospective evaluation of pulmonary embolism: diagnostic performance of spiral CT in the ESTIPEP trial (abstr). Radiology 1999; 213(P):126–127.

61. Remy-Jardin M, Remy J, Baghaie F, Fribourg M, Artaud D, Duhamel A. Clinical value of thin collimation in the diagnostic workup of pulmonary embolism. AJR 2000; 175:407–411.

62. Teigen CL, Maus TP, Sheedy PF et al. Pulmonary embolism: diagnosis with contrast-enhanced electron-beam CT and comparison with pulmonary angiography. Radiology 1995; 194:313–319.

63. van Rossum AB, Pattynama PM, Mallens WM, Hermans J, Heijerman HG. Can helical CT replace scintigraphy in the diagnostic process in suspected pulmonary embolism? A retrolective-prolective cohort study focusing on total diagnostic yield. Eur Radiol 1998; 8:90–96.

64. Schoepf UJ, Costello P. CT angiography for diagnosis of pulmonary embolism: state of the art. Radiology 2004; 230:329–337.

65. Raptopoulos V, Boiselle PM. Multi-detector row spiral CT pulmonary angiography: comparison with single-detector row spiral CT. Radiology 2001; 221:606–613.

66. Trowbridge RL, Araoz PA, Gotway MB, Bailey RA, Auerbach AD. The effect of helical computed tomography on diagnostic and treatment strategies in patients with suspected pulmonary embolism. Am J Med 2004; 116(2):84–90.

67. van Strijen MJ, de Monye W, Schiereck J et al. Advances in New Technologies Evaluating the Localisation of Pulmonary Embolism Study Group. Single-detector helical computed tomography as the primary diagnostic test in suspected pulmonary embolism: a multicenter clinical management study of 510 patients. Ann Intern Med 2003; 138(4):307–314.

68. Garg K, Sieler H, Welsh CH, Johnston RJ, Russ PD. Clinical validity of helical CT being interpreted as negative for pulmonary embolism: implications for patient treatment. AJR 1999; 172:1627–1631.

69. Cross JJ, Kemp PM, Walsh CG, Flower CD, Dixon AK. A randomized trial of spiral CT and ventilation perfusion scintigraphy for the diagnosis of pulmonary embolism. Clin Radiol 1998; 53:177–182.

70. van Erkel AR, van Rossum AB, Bloeum JL et al. Spiral CT angiography for suspected pulmonary embolism: cost-effectiveness analysis. Radiology 1996; 201:29–36.

71. Lomis NNT, Yoon HC, Moran AG, Miller FJ. Clinical outcomes of patients after a negative spiral CT pulmonary arteriogram in the evaluation of acute pulmonary embolism. J Vasc Intervent Radiol 1999; 10:707–712.

72. Ferretti GR, Bosson JL, Buffaz PD et al. Acute pulmonary embolism: role of helical CT in 164 patients with intermediate probability at ventilation-perfusion scintigraphy and normal results at duplex US of the legs. Radiology 1997; 205:453–458.

73. Krestan CR, Klein N, Kreuzer S, Minar E, Janeta J, Herold CJ. Value of a negative spiral-CT angiography in patients with suspected acute PE: Retrospective analysis of PE recurrence and outcome. Eur Radiol 1999; 9(suppl 2):878.

74. Goodman LR, Lipchik RJ, Kuzo RS et al. Subsequent pulmonary embolism: risk after a negative helical CT pulmonary angiogram—prospective comparison with scintigraphy. Radiology 2000; 215:535–542.

75. Bankier AA, Janata K, Fleischmann D et al. Severity assessment of acute pulmonary embolism with spiral CT: evaluation of two modified angiographic scores and comparison with clinical data. J Thoracic Imaging 12:150–158.

76. Qanadli SD, El Hajjam M, Vieillard-Baron A et al. New CT index to quantify arterial obstruction in pulmonary embolism: comparison with angiographic index and echocardiography. AJR 2001; 176(6):1415–1420.

77. Wu AS, Pezzullo JA, Cronan JJ, Hou DD, Mayo-Smith WW. CT pulmonary angiography: quantification of pulmonary embolus as a predictor of patient outcome—initial experience. Radiology 2004; 230(3):831–835.

78. Garg K, Kemp JL, Russ PD, Baron AE. Thromboembolic disease: variability of interobserver agreement in the interpretation of CT venography with CT pulmonary angiography. AJR 2001; 176:1043–1047.

79. Richman PB, Wood J, Kasper DM et al. Contribution of indirect computed tomography venography of the chest for the diagnosis of thromboembolic disease in two United States emergency departments. J Thromb Haemost 2003: 1(4):652–657.

80. Bergin CJ, Sirlin C, Deutsch R, Fedullo P, Hauschildt J, Huynh T, Auger W, Brown M. Predictors of patient response to pulmonary thromboendarterectomy. AJR Am J Roentgenol 2000; 174(2):509–515.

81. Schwickert HC, Schweden FJ, Schild HH et al. Pulmonary arteries and lung parenchyma in chronic pulmonary embolism: preoperative and postoperative CT findings. Radiology 1994; 191:351–357.

82. Hasegawa I, Boiselle PM, Hatabu H. Bronchial artery dilatation on MDCT scans of patients with acute pulmonary embolism: comparison with chronic or recurrent pulmonary embolism. AJR 2004; 182(1):67–72.

83. Remy J, Remy-Jardin M, Wattinne L, Deffontaines C. Pulmonary arteriovenous malformations: evaluation with CT of the chest before and after treatment. Radiology 1992; 182(3):809–816.

84. Siegel MJ. Multiplanar and three-dimensional multi-detector row CT of thoracic vessels and airways in the pediatric population. Radiology 2003; 229(3):641–650.

85. Bozkurt AK, Oztunc F, Akman C, Kurugoglu S, Eroglu AG. Multiple pulmonary artery aneurysms due to infective endocarditis. Ann Thorac Surg 2003; 75(2): 593–596.

86. Akdag Kose A, Kayabali M, Sarica R, Saglik E, Azizlerli G. Pulmonary artery involvement in Behcet's disease. Adv Exp Med Biol. 2003; 528:419–422.

87. Park JH. Conventional and CT angiographic diagnosis of Takayasu arteritis. Int J Cardiol 1996; 54(Suppl):S165–S171.

88. Seo JB, Im JG, Chung JW, Song JW, Goo JM, Park JH, Yeon KM. Pulmonary vasculitis: the spectrum of radiological findings. Br J Radiol 2000; 73(875):1224–1231.

89. Tateishi U, Hasegawa T, Kusumoto M, Yamazaki N, Iinuma G, Muramatsu Y, Moriyama N. Metastatic angiosarcoma of the lung: spectrum of CT findings. AJR 2003; 180(6):1671–1674.

90. Yi CA, Lee KS, Choe YH, Han D, Kwon OJ, Kim S. Computed tomography in pulmonary artery sarcoma: distinguishing features from pulmonary embolic disease. J Comput Assist Tomogr 2004; 28(1):34–39.

Part III: Magnetic Resonance

6

Introduction to Magnetic Resonance Imaging

EDWIN J. R. VAN BEEK

University of Iowa,
Iowa City, Iowa, USA
University of Sheffield,
Sheffield, UK

STANISLAO FICHELE

University of Sheffield,
Sheffield, UK

DAVID A. LIPSON

University of Pennsylvania Medical Center,
Philadelphia, USA

I. Introduction

Magnetic resonance imaging (MRI) has made a tremendous impact on the way in which we use diagnostic tests. This was recently recognized, when the 2003 Nobel Prize for Medicine was awarded to two MRI pioneers (Paul Lauterbur and Sir Peter Mansfield). This was not the first (and probably not the last) Nobel Prize related to work in MRI, and it highlights the multidisciplinary nature of this area of medicine (Table 6.1). It is not surprising that it is not

Table 6.1 Nobel Prizes Related to Work Involving MRI

Year	Nobel Prize Area	Winner(s)
1952	Physics	Bloch and Purcell
1991	Chemistry	Ernst
2003	Medicine	Lauterbur and Mansfield

possible to describe all the potential applications of MRI in this short chapter. Furthermore, the authors of the following chapters have written the methods used in sufficient detail. However, for the uninitiated reader, it is important to have some basic information on the workings of MRI. If the interest should be awakened, there are many dedicated textbooks on the topic (ranging from basic to advanced).

MRI is a noninvasive imaging method capable of yielding information on the structure (and function) of the body without the need for ionizing radiation. Originally called "nuclear magnetic resonance" (NMR), the name was changed to MRI in the 1970s because of sensitivity to the word "nuclear." At present, the method appears entirely safe, albeit that some concerns have been raised with higher magnetic field strength systems (>3 T). Most clinical magnets work using a 1.5 T magnetic field. MRI works by applying radiofrequency (RF) radiation, while the body is positioned in a homogeneous magnetic field. Depending on the exact frequency used, it can portray the distribution and density of atoms—the most frequently employed method aims at hydrogen atoms, which are part of the water molecule. Thus, it becomes possible to distinguish water from fat due to different motion characteristics of the hydrogen nuclei within these environments. As 70% of the body is made up of water, there is sufficient signal to gain high-resolution images of virtually any part of the body.

As MRI became more established over the past few years, researchers quickly developed an increasing number of applications (initially mainly the central nervous system, but later all body systems became part of MRI investigations) for its use. Furthermore, improvements in spatial resolution (partly due to new sequences and partly due to better hardware) enhanced contrast methods (including the use of exogenous contrast agents, such as gadolinium and hyperpolarized helium-3 gas) and greater imaging speed (particularly, with the introduction of novel sequences and so-called parallel imaging methods) have made MRI the primary imaging technique for many diagnostic applications.

II. Basic Physics

MRI makes use of the behavior of nuclei that have an odd number of protons or neutrons, which will act as small magnetic dipoles within an external strong magnetic field. Thus, although proton (^{1}H) MRI has been used most extensively, other nuclei, such as ^{31}P and ^{133}Xe or ^{3}He, may also be studied using MRI. Within a strong magnetic field, the dipoles will align themselves along the direction of the field and will spin at a predetermined frequency, which is dependent on the field strength and the gyromagnetic ratio (Larmor frequency; Fig. 6.1).

A RF pulse may be directed into this system, which will cause a resonant effect to occur (magnetic resonance). The nuclei will be forced from their resting state by the application of the RF pulse by an angle α [the flip angle, Fig. 6.2(a) and (b)]. The flip angle is dependent on the duration and the strength of the RF pulse. The nuclei will subsequently return to the ground state, and during this return, the energy is released again as RF energy, which may be recorded using sensitive antennae [RF receiver coil, Fig. 6.2(c)]. This electrical signal is known as free induction decay (FID), and its magnitude and length are dependent on the longitudinal relaxation time (T1) and the transverse relaxation time (T2). The transverse relaxation time may be influenced by local magnetic field changes at molecular level, which will cause a decrease in T2, and this change is incorporated into the amended transverse relaxation time (T2*).

Applying the RF pulse will not allow any spatial resolution to take place. In order to achieve this, so-called gradient fields are applied in a different direction (x and y axes), which allow the returned signals to be pinpointed in location. This will result in complex FID signals, which can be analyzed using equally complex mathematics (Fourier analysis). Several methods may be employed, but it is sufficient to say that using combined gradient magnetic fields, it is possible to build a spatially encoded data array known as k-space. Subsequent Fourier analysis will transform this data into an image. A major difference with any other technique is that each element in k-space contains the information of the entire image

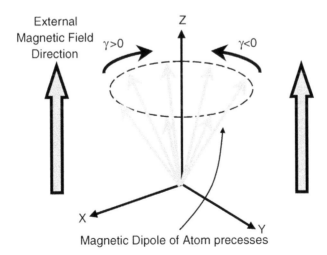

Figure 6.1 The magnetic dipoles associated with each atom precess about the external magnetic field direction. The frequency of this spin is determined by the strength of the magnetic field and the gyromagnetic ratio (γ).

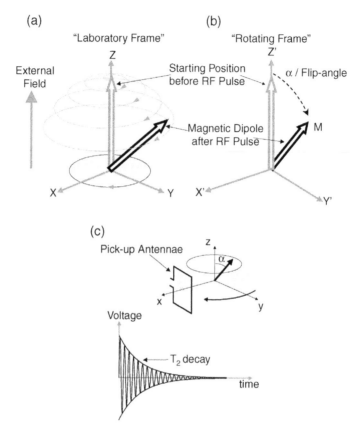

Figure 6.2 When the RF pulse is applied at the Larmour frequency, it excites the nucleus, causing the direction of spin to tip by an angle α (the flip angle). (a) The evolution of the spins is shown spiraling downward towards the *xy* plane. (b) The same evolution as in (a), but now seen from the position of the nucleus, thus demonstrating a rotating frame. (c) The excited nuclear spin can be detected using a RF antenna. The signal will change over time, as the spin direction returns to the resting state. This oscillating signal is what constitutes FID, which ultimately becomes zero over time (this equals the time constant, T2).

(Fig. 6.3). However, the amount of data generated in particular parts of the *k*-space will influence the signal-to-noise ratio and the spatial resolution of the image, and this forms an essential part of MR sequence design. Thus, sequences can be faster by filling *k*-space in a different manner (for instance, using spiral or radial techniques) or by only filling part of *k*-space during the imaging (for instance, single shot fast spine echo or fast low angle single shot half-Fourier techniques), although this will invariably affect the spatial resolution.

We will now briefly discuss the main sequence applications in chest MRI.

Image Space   K-Space

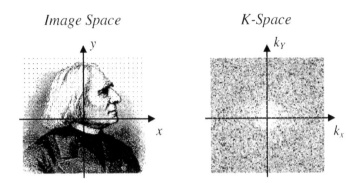

Figure 6.3 This figure shows an image as one perceives it in the "real world." The same image in *k*-space after the inverse mathematical Fourier geometry has been applied.

III. Proton Density MRI

This technique assesses the distribution of protons in any given area of the body. In the lungs, the airspaces are virtually devoid of protons, but the soft tissues of the chest wall, the mediastinum, and the interstitium of the lungs do contain protons. Furthermore, pathological conditions may change the number of (free moving) protons. For instance, edema, inflammation, tumors, and hemorrhage increase this number (and hence the signal at MRI), whereas fibrosis or calcification will decrease this number (and will lead to signal loss at MRI).

Proton density can be assessed using T1-weighted and T2-weighted sequences, which (at 1.5 T) will project water as low and high signal, respectively (Fig. 6.4). As fat has high signal using both sequences, a fat suppression technique may be used to detect the difference between fluid and water on T2-weighted images (Fig. 6.4b). One of the problems using proton density MRI is the time it takes to acquire the images. This is, generally, longer than a single breath-hold, and the reason why faster techniques were developed.

IV. Half-Fourier Techniques

The major difference with spin density MRI is that the technique only fills a part of *k*-space, which is typically just over >50%. The remaining *k*-space is filled in through extrapolation by the computer. Thus, the time required to fill *k*-space (and obtain an image) is significantly reduced. This allows for imaging during single breath-hold, even if the quality of the image will be slightly degraded (Fig. 6.5).

V. Arterial Spin Labeling

Arterial spin labeling (ASL), also known as arterial spin tagging (AST), was initially described by Detre et al. in 1991 (1,2). This technique involves

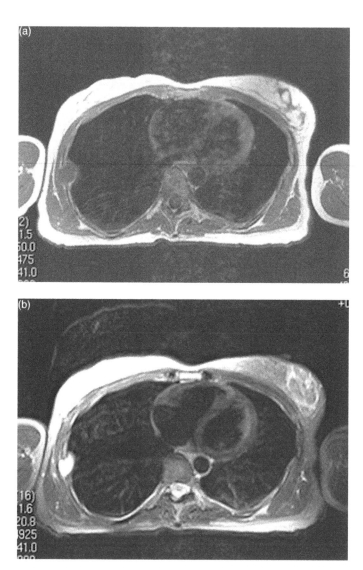

Figure 6.4   (a) Intercostal neuroma, demonstrating low signal on T1-weighted image. Notice that the lungs are virtually devoid of signal. (b) Intercostal neuroma, demonstrating high signal on T2-fat saturated image. Notice that the lungs remain virtually devoid of signal.

magnetically labeling arterial water (noninvasively) and using it as an endogenous contrast agent (3). The method is based on the fact that tissue magnetization of an organ changes according to its perfusion status. As an entirely noninvasive method, ASL avoids the risks and expenses of exogenous contrast agents such as

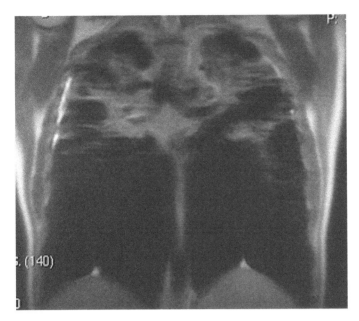

Figure 6.5 Single shot fast spin echo of a patient with cystic fibrosis, obtained during a single breath-hold. Notice high signal in the blood vessels and increased signal particularly in the upper lung zones, compatible with chronic infection.

gadolinium. The ASL method also offers the possibility of quantification and may therefore be used to follow patients during therapy (4). Finally, ASL methods may be used repeatedly in time to study dynamic processes (5,6), because there is no degradation in the perfusion image as is seen with gadolinium-enhanced imaging methods (7,8).

VI. MR Angiography

Although flow effects can be detected using noncontrast-enhanced techniques, the use of gadolinium-based agents has allowed a revolution in vascular imaging. Contrast agents work by significant shortening of the T1, allowing a massive increase in signal. This in turn allows a shorter imaging time, and, combined with novel sequences, has enabled the introduction of very fast techniques within a single breath-hold. The technique is explained in detail in Chapter 10.

VII. Hyperpolarized Noble Gas MRI

An alternative to endogenous contrast is the administration of external contrast agents. Hyperpolarized noble gases, such as 3-He, effectively lead to a massive increase in available signal. Furthermore, by exploiting intrinsic characteristics of the gas, one may obtain images in various physiologic situations. The method is extensively discussed in subsequent chapters.

References

1. Detre JA, Leigh JS, Williams DS, Koretsky AP. Perfusion imaging. Magn Reson Med 1991; 22:1–9.
2. Williams DS, Detre JA, Leigh JS, Koretsky AP. Magnetic resonance imaging of perfusion using spin inversion of arterial water. Proc Natl Acad Sci USA 1992; 89:212–216.
3. Rizi RR, Lipson DA, Dimitrov IE, Ishii M, Roberts DA. Operating characteristics of hyperpolarized 3He and arterial spin tagging in MR imaging of ventilation and perfusion in healthy subjects. Acad Radiol 2003; 10(5):502–508.
4. Lipson DA, Roberts DA, Hansen-Flaschen J, Gentile TR, Jones G, Thompson A, Dimitrov IE, Palevsky HI, Leigh JS, Schnall M, Rizi RR. Pulmonary ventilation and perfusion scanning using hyperpolarized helium-3 MRI and arterial spin tagging in healthy normal subjects, and in pulmonary embolism, and orthotopic lung transplant patients. Magn Reson Med 2002; 47:1073–1076.
5. Roberts DA, Gefter WB, Hirsch JA et al. Pulmonary perfusion: respiratory-triggered three-dimensional MR imaging with arterial spin tagging—preliminary results in healthy volunteers. Radiology 1999; 212(3):890–895.
6. Roberts DA, Rizi RR, Lipson DA et al. Dynamic observation of pulmonary perfusion using continuous arterial spin-labeling in a pig model. J Magn Reson Imag 2001; 14(2):175–180.
7. Williams DS, Detre JA, Zhang W, Koretsky AP. Fast serial MRI of perfusion in the rat brain during bicuculline induced seizures using spin inversion of arterial water. In: Proceedings of the Society of Magnetic Resonance in Medicine, 11th Annual Scientific Meeting, 1992, Berlin, SMRM, Berkeley, 1992, p. 711.
8. Roberts DA, Mai VM, Salerno M, Lipson DA, Rizi RR. Functional magnetic resonance imaging of the lung. Appl Radiol 2003; 32:4–48.

7

Noble Gas Ventilation Imaging Using ^{3}He and ^{129}Xe: An Introduction

EDWIN J. R. VAN BEEK

University of Iowa, Iowa City,
Iowa, USA

University of Sheffield,
Sheffield, UK

DAVID A. LIPSON

University of Pennsylvania Medical Center,
Philadelphia, Pennsylvania, USA

I. Introduction

Magnetic resonance imaging (MRI) using hyperpolarized noble gases, such as helium-3 (^{3}He) and xenon-129 (^{129}Xe), has been a novel addition to the arsenal of pulmonary diagnostic tests. It has enabled the development of MRI in the chest, which was traditionally hampered by the low number of protons and magnetic field inhomogeneities that exist at the boundaries of air/soft-tissues of the lung parenchyma. Hyperpolarized noble gas MRI makes use of the inherent properties of these nonradioactive isotopes, which have a nuclear spin of 1/2. This makes them sensitive to nuclear magnetic resonance (NMR) methodology, albeit that this would only be marginally detectable at normal thermal equilibrium. In a strong magnetic field, the atoms can exist in two ground states which are parallel or antiparallel to the magnetic field. It is the introduction of large quantities of energy using laser light in a process termed "optical pumping," which will allow one population of the ground states to grow (1–3). This imbalance of the normal distribution of ground states is called hyperpolarization, and the percentage of the population is what is generally described as the level of polarization. Thus, at 50–80% polarization, the signal that is introduced into the lungs by breathing in a small amount of gas is in the order of $>100,000\times$ at thermal equilibrium, and more than sufficient to allow for detailed images of the lungs to be obtained.

Hyperpolarized gas is produced through the transfer of angular momentum from circularly polarized laser light to the electron and nuclear spins of atoms, so-called optical pumping (1,4). Two methods are currently available at near-commercial levels of development. The "spin exchange optical pumping" method uses an alkali vapor (rubidium) as an intermediary for spin polarization transfer (3,5). This method was commercially developed and is presently undergoing testing to allow FDA approval (Fig. 7.1). This system can be adapted for production of either hyperpolarized ^{3}He or ^{129}Xe (6). This method uses circularly polarized laser at the wavelength of rubidium (794.8 nm), which is focused on a rubidium coated glass cell with a mixture of ^{3}He with a small amount of N_2 at high pressure (3 bar) within a homogeneous low magnetic field. The rubidium valence electron will become excited, and during collisions of these excited atoms with ^{3}He atoms, the angular momentum of the rubidium electrons is transferred to the nucleus of the ^{3}He atom. The costs of these individual systems are

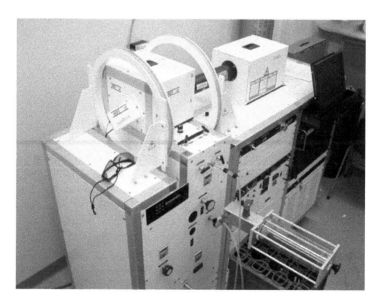

Figure 7.1 Prototype commercial polarizer (Amersham Health, Princeton, NJ), which is capable of performing either ^{3}He or ^{129}Xe polarization using the rubidium exchange method.

not negligible (in the order of 200–250,000 US$), and can produce ~1 L of gas polarized to 35–40%/24 h. The system is relatively easy to operate, and can be performed by an adequately trained technician.

The second method is known as "metastability exchange optical pumping," which takes place entirely between ^{3}He atoms without the need for an intermediary alkali metal atom (2,4). This system operates at low pressure with a weak radiofrequency (RF) discharge, which causes some valence electrons to become excited to a metastable state. Subsequently, laser light at the helium wavelength of 1083 nm is applied, ultimately leading to hyperpolarization of ^{3}He atoms. Following compression, the gas can be "harvested" and applied to humans. This methodology has been upscaled (Fig. 7.2), leading to the potential to produce many liters of highly polarized (>60%) gas every 24 h (7). Nevertheless, this technique may also be used for smaller tabletop systems using either a peristaltic (8) or a diaphragmatic (9) pump for compression of smaller quantities of gas.

There are advantages and disadvantages of the different technologies. Smaller systems allow flexibility for local use, but will require space, manpower, and compliance with pharmaceutical production requirements. This could hamper introduction in smaller thoracic imaging centers. The large-scale system offers a central production facility, which has to be complemented by a distribution network, allowing for purchase as required options. Recent work within the European project Polarized Helium Imaging of the Lung (Framework 5 program, European Community) has demonstrated that it is feasible to use a central production facility for a clinical trial in three centers (10). The time between

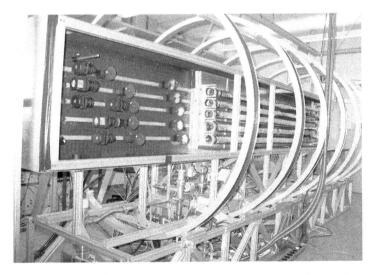

Figure 7.2 Large-scale ^{3}He polarizer of metastability exchange principle (Institute of Physics, University of Mainz, Germany).

gas production and use of gas for imaging was in the order of 18 h, and polarization levels were >30% at the time of imaging.

II. Hardware Requirements

Before one is able to perform hyperpolarized noble gas MRI, several hardware requirements need to be met. First, the MRI system will need to be tuned to the proper frequency (48 MHz at 1.5 T for ^{3}He, 17.6 MHz at 1.5 T for ^{129}Xe). This requires an upgradation in the RF amplifier of the system (or alternatively multinuclear capability) and also a dedicated RF coil that operates at the appropriate frequency. Bird-cage RF coils have been used in most clinical studies.

The delivery of the noble gas is another essential part of any working system. This can be achieved through the simple use of a Tedlar bag (which preserves polarization) and inhalation through a short length of tubing (Fig. 7.3). Alternatively, one may wish to introduce a more robust method, allowing for quantification and precise timing of bolus delivery through a respirator driven, computer-controlled delivery system (Fig. 7.4). The first method has the advantage of simplicity and low costs, whereas the second method may be able to yield additional information on gas flow patterns.

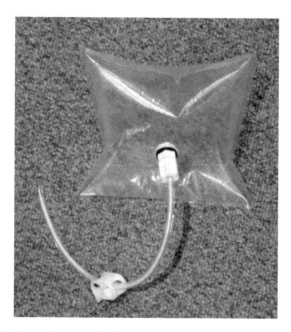

Figure 7.3 Delivery through a Tedlar bag method.

(a)

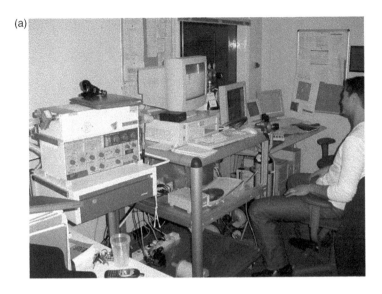

(b)

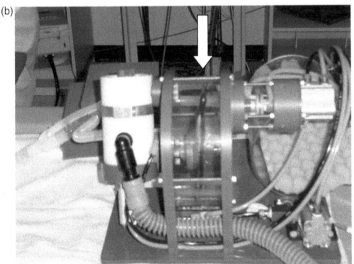

Figure 7.4 (a) Delivery through a respirator/computer-controlled system, which is located in the MRI control room. (b) Delivery system, demonstrating gas delivery chamber (arrow) and multiple valves to allow gas delivery, which is located on the end of the MRI table.

III. ³He MR Imaging

The use of ^{3}He was tested after initial success using ^{129}Xe, when *ex vivo* and *in vivo* experiments in animals (11,12) were followed by initial applications in humans (Fig. 7.5) (13–15). The technique is now nearly 10 years old, and has

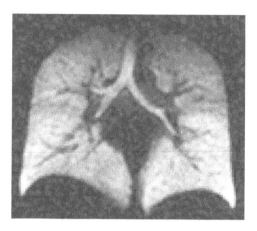

Figure 7.5   Coronal hyperpolarized ³He gas MR Image.

undergone a huge development as demonstrated in some of the following chapters. In fact, the use of ³He has largely taken over the potential use of ¹²⁹Xe, which is partly due to its complete inertness (¹²⁹Xe has anesthetic properties at high concentrations) and its ease of use. Nevertheless, there are issues such as availability and costs that will require attention if the technique is to survive into the future. ³He is a limited resource (produced as a by-product of tritium decay in the nuclear arms industry) and usually involves an active recycling program.

Several methods have been explored using hyperpolarized ³He MRI. These will be discussed in more detail in the chapters that follow. As an introduction, it suffices to briefly describe the methods and their potential implications regarding information concerning lung function.

The ventilation distribution method tends to make use of a single breath-hold fast sequence, whereby the actual helium gas distribution is imaged. This technique allows the demonstration of ventilation defects, which is analogous to that demonstrated by nuclear ventilation scintigraphic methods. However, the MRI technique has the added advantage of greater spatial resolution and newer sequences that are capable of allowing full three-dimensional analysis of the lungs, including reformatting in different slice directions.

The apparent diffusion coefficient method also makes use of a single breath-hold, and incorporates a time interval within the sequence to assess the diffusion distance of the ³He atoms (see Chapter 15). This method is capable of probing the microstructure of the lung, and can depict maps of airspace size throughout the lungs. This method is of particular interest in the assessment of patients with small airway diseases, and is a main competitor for high-resolution computed tomography.

Oxygen sensitive imaging uses a breath-hold technique, where two sequences are run with different flip angles and different interscan delays (see Chapter 16).

The technique has huge potential for spatial resolution of oxygen uptake within the lungs, which could have an impact on treatment effect assessment and preoperative planning of patients. In this method, analysis of helium signal decay provides information regarding regional alveolar oxygen partial pressures. While this in itself is very important information, solving mass balance equations using this regional oxygen data also yields information regarding regional ventilation/perfusion relationships.

Finally, dynamic ventilation imaging has allowed time-resolved inflow and outflow of ^{3}He during a single respiratory cycle (see Chapter 8). The technique has become faster with novel sequences, such as spiral and radial techniques, and the reconstruction has allowed a smoothing of data with sliding-window reconstruction. It has allowed, for the first time, the spatial resolution of spirometry data within the lungs and lung regions. This could allow more precise targeting of therapy and also increase the knowledge of pathophysiology.

IV. ^{129}Xe MR Imaging

The use of laser-polarized ^{129}Xe gas in human lung imaging dates to the past decade (16,17). Interestingly, despite its wide availability and increased natural abundance in the atmosphere, pulmonary MRI using ^{129}Xe has not achieved the same success as has ^{3}He. There are several reasons for this observation. Although pure ^{129}Xe is slightly easier to produce than ^{3}He (albeit at considerable cost), the main disadvantages of ^{129}Xe are its anesthetic properties stemming from its lipophilic nature, its rapid uptake into the blood through the lung membrane-capillary barrier, and its relatively inferior polarization levels. Polarization of ^{129}Xe is also more technically complex, the polarization levels that can be achieved are lower as a result of the smaller spin exchange cross-sections and the T1 relaxation times are shorter than for ^{3}He, meaning the polarization has a shorter half-life. Freezing and then sublimating the gas prior to inhalation does prolong the polarization half-life. Finally, the gyromagnetic ratio of ^{129}Xe is smaller than ^{3}He, so its inherent sensitivity to NMR is lower.

^{129}Xe dissolves in lipophilic compounds almost 10 times more readily than does ^{3}He. Although this is a disadvantage for formal airspace imaging, the fact that ^{129}Xe has a large dissolved/gas partition coefficient allows for study of the alveolar/capillary membrane, and provides information regarding the diffusion capacity of the lung. This holds promise in the early detection of lung pathology, disease monitoring, or potentially as a surrogate endpoint in drug intervention trials.

Compared with hyperpolarized ^{3}He, the spectral analysis of ^{129}Xe is chemically shifted by a significant amount depending on whether it is in a gaseous or soluble state. This property is important as it allows surveillance and examination of ^{129}Xe in either phase. In fact, it is this asset that may allow determination of diseased or healthy tissue, simply on the scrutiny of polarized ^{129}Xe NMR spectra. Further analysis of ^{129}Xe spectra promises to provide even more information regarding lung structure and function.

V. Conclusions

The use of hyperpolarized noble gases for lung imaging is still in its infancy, despite the fact that a tremendous amount of research has occurred that has allowed the field to progress to its present state. The following chapters will provide a state-of-the-art overview of the field of magnetic resonance lung imaging using hyperpolarized noble gases. The field promises to provide knowledge about pulmonary structure and function that would have been unthinkable just a decade ago.

References

1. Kastler A. Quelques suggestions concernant la production optique et la detection optique d'une inégalité de population des niveaux de quantification spatiale des atomes. Application à l'expérience de Stern et Gerlach et à la resonance magnétique. J Phys Radium 1950; 11:255–265.
2. Colegrove FD, Schearer LD, Walters GK. Polarisation of ^{3}He gas by optical pumping. Phys Rev 1963; 132:2561–2572.
3. Miron E, Schaefer S, Schreiber D, Van Wijngaarden WA, Zeng X, Happer W. Polarisation of the nuclear spins of noble-gas atoms by spin exchange with optically pumped alkali-metal atoms. Phys Rev 1984; A29:3092–3110.
4. Goodson BM. Nuclear magnetic resonance of laser-polarized noble gases in molecules, materials, and organisms. J Magn Reson 2002; 155:157–216.
5. Walker TG, Happer W. Spin-exchange optical pumping of noble-gas nuclei. Rev Mod Phys 1997; 69:629–642.
6. Driehuys B, Cates GD, Miron E, Sauer K, Walter DK, Happer W. High-volume production of laser-polarized ^{129}Xe. Appl Phys Lett 1996; 69:1668–1670.
7. Becker J, Heil W, Krug B et al. Study of mechanical compression of spin-polarized ^{3}He gas. Nucl Instrum Meth A 1994; 346:45–51.
8. Nacher PJ, Tastevin G, Maître X, Dollat X, Lemaire B, Olejnik J. A peristaltic compressor for hyperpolarized helium. Eur Radiol 1999; 9:B18.
9. Gentile TR, Jones GL, Thompson AK et al. Demonstration of a compact compressor for application of metastability-exchange optical pumping of ^{3}He to human lung imaging. Magn Reson Med 2000; 43:290–294.
10. Wild JM, Schmiedeskamp J, Paley MNJ et al. MR imaging of the lungs with hyperpolarized 3-helium transported by air. Phys Med Biol 2002; 47:N185–N190.
11. Middleton H, Black RD, Saam B et al. MR imaging with hyperpolarized ^{3}He gas. Magn Reson Med 1995; 33:271–275.
12. Black RD, Middleton HD, Cates GD et al. *In vivo* He-3 MR images of guinea pig lungs. Radiology 1996; 199:867–870.
13. Ebert M, Großmann T, Heil W et al. Nuclear magnetic resonance imaging on humans using hyperpolarised ^{3}He. Lancet 1996; 347:1297–1299.

14. MacFall JR, Charles HC, Black RD et al. Human lung air spaces: potential for MR imaging with hyperpolarized ^{3}He. Radiology 1996; 200:553–558.
15. Kauczor HU, Hofmann D, Kreitner KF et al. Normal and abnormal pulmonary ventilation: visualization at hyperpolarized ^{3}He MR imaging. Radiology 1996; 201:564–568.
16. Mugler JP III, Driehuys B, Brookeman JR et al. MR imaging and spectroscopy using hyperpolarized ^{129}Xe gas: preliminary human results. Magn Reson Med 1997; 37:809–815.
17. Albert MS, Cates GD, Driehuys B et al. Biological magnetic resonance imaging using laser-polarized ^{129}Xe. Nature 1994; 370:199–201.

8

Dynamic Imaging of Lung Ventilation with Hyperpolarized Gas MRI

JIM M. WILD

University of Sheffield,
Sheffield, UK

EDWIN J. R. VAN BEEK

University of Iowa, Iowa City,
Iowa, USA

University of Sheffield,
Sheffield, UK

I. Introduction

Hyperpolarized (HP) gas magnetic resonance imaging (MRI) has shown to be effective at visualizing breath-hold images of ventilation in humans (1). Optical pumping techniques permit high nuclear spin polarization levels of the noble gas nuclei, irrespective of the strength of the MRI scanner static field (B_0). As the polarization is not constrained by the processes of saturation recovery, but more so by radio-frequency (RF) depletion, imaging with very fast repetition times at high signal-to-noise ratio (SNR) is a realistic prospect *in vivo*. This has enabled the dynamic study of gas inhalation and visualization of the respiratory cycle with fast imaging techniques. Aside from providing visually striking cinematic movies of ventilation in the lungs, the study of ventilation dynamics may give insights into lung pathophysiology such as obstruction and air trapping.

In this chapter, a methodological review of the MRI pulse sequences used to date is given in the context of a discussion of their relative performance and ease of implementation. Some of the physical and physiological factors are then considered, which influence the appearance of the images of the lungs. To conclude, an overview of some of the clinical applications of dynamic HP gas MRI is provided and methods of quantification of the signal time course are reviewed.

II. MRI Methodology

Dynamic HP gas MR images are influenced by a set of physical properties of the gas and its surroundings. When choosing an MRI pulse sequence repetitively to sample k-space, these factors should be considered in conjunction with the MRI hardware and software limitations imposed by the system's performance. They are outlined in the following text.

A. Sequence Design and k-Space Sampling

A fast acquisition of a complete k-space data set is conducive to dynamic imaging. The inspiratory phase in human ventilation typically lasts between 1 and 3 s, as such there is much to be said for either ultrafast multishot sequences that have very short repetition times between RF pulses or single shot sequences, such as EPI, that convert all of the longitudinal magnetization into transverse magnetization in one go.

Multishot Sequences

In the first case, a short TE offers a short TR and such gradient echo based multishot sequences have been adopted as the first choice for dynamic tracking of gas flow. MacFall et al. (2) were the first to demonstrate dynamic images in humans using a fast gradient echo spin-warp (FLASH) technique with thick slices in a coronal orientation, at a temporal resolution of 1800 ms. The TR of a FLASH sequence was subsequently reduced by Schreiber et al. (3) by using an asymmetric echo with a nonselective RF pulse, giving a frame time of 130 ms for a 65-view FLASH image (Fig. 8.1). With this temporal resolution, it is just possible to observe the rapid inspiratory phase in the upper airways. However, the early phase images suffer from ghosting and motion related artifacts owing to the discontinuity in signal intensity experienced between high and low *k*-space (Fig. 8.1). A drawback of the rectilinear Cartesian sampling used is that the center of *k*-space is only sampled once per frame, meaning that without keyhole type undersampling strategies, the dynamic update rate of contrast in the image is limited by the overall frame rate (4).

An alternative means of sampling *k*-space in multiple views is offered by non-Cartesian strategies of radial projection and spiral imaging. These have the advantage that both central and outer parts of *k*-space are sampled per RF excitation (view) meaning that a fast refresh rate in the reconstructed image can be achieved by employing a "sliding window" reconstruction and sampling *k*-space in a continuously revolving manner (5). The oversampling of the low spatial frequencies also makes both sequences self-compensating to phase shifts relating to motion and flow. Viallon et al. presented both radial projection

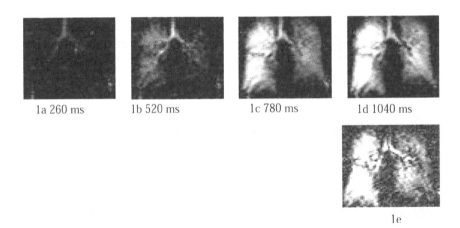

| 1a 260 ms | 1b 520 ms | 1c 780 ms | 1d 1040 ms |

1e

Figure 8.1   Dynamic time series (1a–d) obtained from a healthy normal with a spin-warp. FLASH sequence; TR 4 ms 65 phase encodes matrix; frame rate 3.8 s^{-1}. The temporal resolution is just about fast enough to resolve signal in the airways before the alveolar airspace is ventilated. Schreiber et al. (19) used an ultrafast version of this sequence and achieved an almost 2-fold increase in temporal resolution with a TR of 2 ms. One means of increasing temporal resolution is to use half-Fourier phase encodings. (e) An image acquired with 40 views as opposed to 65 views from the same part of the inspiratory phase as 1 d. The SNR is worse than the full-Fourier image.

(6) and interleaved spiral cine sequences (7) of inhaled ^{3}He gas in animal experiments. When combined with sliding window reconstruction, these experiments gave high quality images with a fast pseudo-temporal image contrast refresh rate.

Several studies have been performed in humans using interleaved spiral pulse sequences, the design of which offers a compromise between spin-warp gradient echo and EPI in terms of number of RF pulses, effectively a trade-off between consumption of polarization and spatial resolution (8,9). The effects of the short T_2^* for ^{3}He in the lung (discussed subsequently) are accounted for by the shorter echo time that can be achieved with spiral imaging when compared with single shot EPI.

More recently, Wild et al. (10) demonstrated radial projection imaging in humans with sliding window reconstruction. The simplicity of sequence design of a radial sequence means that TR can be minimized to as low as 2 ms without slice selection and 5.4 ms with slice selection leading to very fast refreshment rates. Oversampling in the radial direction combined with angular undersampling allows the time taken to acquire a complete image data set to be further reduced without much compromise to spatial resolution, but with a loss in SNR and increased radial streaking artifacts. Thus, undersampled radial imaging offers an accurate means of tracking gas flow in the upper airways, where SNR is typically high (Fig. 8.2).

There has been some discussion as to which of these three multishot sampling strategies offers the highest SNR/unit time and most accurate tracking of fast gas flow for dynamic HP gas imaging and a rigorous comparative theoretical analysis awaits. The drawback of all of these multishot sequences is that each trajectory in k-space requires an RF pulse, and each time an RF pulse is applied, the polarization of the ^{3}He is reduced, introducing a complicated magnetization time course, which weights the image appearance.

Single Shot Sequences

For efficient use of the non-equilibrium magnetization, single shot sequences, such as EPI, offer an advantage over multishot methods, because only one RF pulse is required per image, meaning that the TR is the limiting factor on the temporal resolution. In addition, changes in image appearance can be more directly equated to freshly inhaled polarized gas without having to consider the temporal variation of signal from view to view, which can weight a multiple shot acquisition from both depolarization and fresh influx of gas. The drawback is that the spatial resolution is limited by the high diffusion coefficient of ^{3}He and its short T_2^* in the lungs (discussed subsequently). Gierada et al. (11) used EPI with a temporal resolution of 40 ms in healthy and emphysematous lungs; however, the technique was limited by its spatial resolution. An EPI sequence has a longer frequency readout, it is prone to off-resonance effects owing to field inhomogeneity; Gierada et al. (11) noticed marked signal loss around vessels and Saam et al. (12) observed a limited success with the sequence in planes other than axial (Fig. 8.3).

The use of an interleaved EPI sequence can lessen the diffusion and susceptibility limitations of EPI; however, the fact that the *k*-space becomes

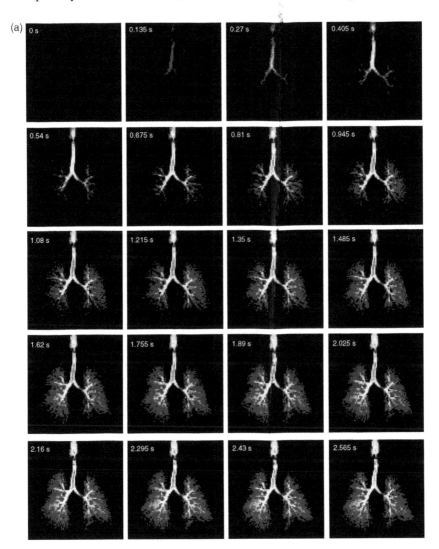

Figure 8.2 Dynamic images collected using a sliding window radial sequence. (a) Images from a healthy normal (128 views per frame) selected at intervals from the first part of an inhalation of 300 mL of ^{3}He polarized to 40%. The temporal passage of gas, down the trachea, into the bronchi and peripheral lung is clearly resolved. (b) Dynamic time series from a COPD patient showing regions of ventilation obstruction in both lungs particularly in the upper lobes and a delayed emptying/depolarization of gas in the lower left lobe which could be indicative of air trapping.

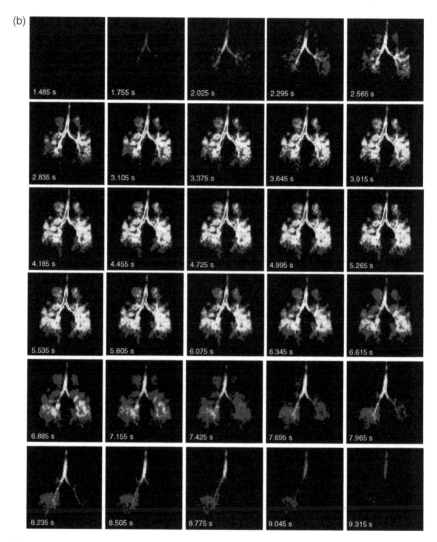

Figure 8.2 *Continued.*

segmented means that interleaved EPI is more prone to motion artifacts due to lung wall motion (13). Ruppert et al. (8) observed homogeneous and steady influx of gas into the peripheral airspaces, using axial slices, and confirmed a substantial gravity dependent inflow into the posterior lung zones in the supine position. Several of the pros and cons of the pulse sequences mentioned earlier are described in Table 8.1 in terms of their ease of implementation and performance.

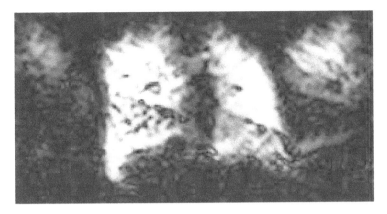

Figure 8.3 Coronal EPI image acquired from a healthy normal from a whole lung projection with 64 readouts. Note the substantial blurring, ghosting artifacts and distortion of the image around the diaphragm.

B. Spin Polarization

How can one best use the available finite spin polarization in terms of the number of RF pulses used to build up the image. The effects of size of flip angle and rate of influx of fresh polarized gas (see Section II.C) will also have a bearing on the image appearance. In short-duration breath-hold studies of ventilation, the longitudinal magnetization (M) can be approximated by a monotonic decay from view to view due to the RF flip angle θ: $M = M_0(\cos \theta)^{n-1}$. This imposes a smooth k-space filter on the data. In dynamic studies of gas flow, a more complicated filtering of the data will arise due to this effect as the RF depletion decay is convolved with a "bolus passage" time envelope as fresh gas is inhaled into the lungs [Fig. 8.2(b)] (14). Studies in guinea pigs (15) and in humans show that a larger flip angle introduces a higher degree of contrast between the airways and the lung periphery (16,17). This is because the earlier generation major airways are higher up the respiratory tree and receive a higher volume flow rate of fresh gas.

Figure 8.4 shows the time course of signal measured in ROI's in the trachea and apex of the left lung from a time series from a healthy normal at different

Table 8.1 Pros (Check or Double Checks) and Cons ($\times$ or $\times\times$) of Various MR Sequences

	EPI	Spin-warp FLASH	Spiral	Radial
Single shot	✓	✗	✗	✗
Sliding window	✗	✗	✓	✓
Difficult to implement	✓	✓✓	✗✗	✗
Susceptibility to diffusion attenuation	✗	✗	✓	✓
Eddy current/B_0 sensitive	✗✗	✓	✗	✓

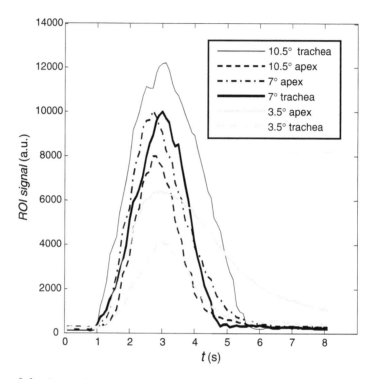

Figure 8.4 Graph of signal vs. time as a function of the flip angle.

flip angles. A high flip angle weights the dynamic contrast towards the major airways, a low flip angle depletes gas less quickly allowing the passage of polarized gas to the periphery. Furthermore, the time course of a dynamic imaging study is typically longer (3–10 s) than the time taken to acquire a single 2D slice (subsecond) and as such longitudinal relaxation due to paramagnetic oxygen may contribute more to signal change especially in the late stages of inspiration. B_1 homogeneity could influence the persistence of ^{3}He polarization, especially at the extreme periphery, where B_1 is likely to be smaller due to the smaller flip angles than at the center of the coil. This could cause the appearance of air trapping in the extreme peripheries of the lung.

C. Breathing Factors

The breathing factors related closely to the above, the appearance of the time course is strongly influenced by the subjects posture, rate of inhalation, and replenishment of the polarization in the region of interest. Ruppert et al. (8) showed homogeneous and steady influx of gas into the peripheral airspaces, using axial slices, and confirmed a substantial gravity dependent inflow into the posterior lung zones in supine position. The mode of delivery of the HP gas and its repeatability will also have an influence. Most dynamic studies in humans have used either inhalation from a 1 L Tedlar bag (9,10,18) or an automated ventilator device (19,20). The first method is simple to operate but is less repeatable, relying entirely on the subject's rate of inhalation. A slow breath of highly polarized gas can provide striking images of the lungs, but may be less reliable and indicative of the true inspiratory phase than a quick breath. The second route offers a higher degree of certainty in the timing of the dose but is more invasive. We have performed studies with both methods and have observed different transit times of gas from trachea to lung periphery when imaging with the same sequence using the two modes of delivery. Tooker et al. (21) chose to build up very high spatial resolution, low temporal resolution images of the airways by imaging following sequentially delivered doses of helium. Any residual polarization contributes to the subsequent images and with careful choice of flip angle, this technique results in excellent delineation of the major airways beyond the fifth generation.

To date, all clinical studies have focused on the inspiratory phase. However, further information on particular clinical conditions, such as air trapping, may well be better suited to imaging in the expiratory phase. In this case, gas can penetrate into the deep alveolar air space before polarization starts to be depleted. This could mean that there is a greater chance of detecting the prolonged signal of a residual gas volume in these regions where SNR is typically much lower than in the large airways. Figure 8.4 shows a high and low flip angle time series from a healthy normal subject.

D. Local Static Magnetic Field Homogeneity

The localized magnetic susceptibility gradients that exist between the parenchyma and the air in the lungs create an inhomogeneous magnetic field. This is exacerbated at higher field strengths and leads to very short transverse relaxation times of the FID of ^{3}He in the alveolar airspace at the typical clinical field strength of 1.5 T ($T_2^* \approx 5$–20 ms). The short T_2^* imposes a limit on the time duration of a readout sampling period for imaging due to k-space filtering effects and can limit the spatial resolution attainable with fast imaging sequences, such as EPI, which rely on the sampling of multiple gradient echoes per RF excitation (12). Furthermore, localized susceptibility gradients are a significant source of localized signal dephasing in gradient echo imaging, which could be misdiagnosed as ventilation defects (16). These artifacts can be minimized by using a very short TE, which is possible with a spin-warp gradient echo sequence that uses a very asymmetric echo (3). Radial and spiral sequences (9,10) can offer even shorter TEs over spin-warp as there is no need for a blipped phase encode gradient prior to the frequency encoding.

E. Localized Diffusion

[3]He has a very high apparent diffusion coefficient in free air (0.9×10^{-4} cm^2/s), but this becomes restricted in the alveolar space leading to lower values (typically measured $\sim 0.2 \times 10^{-4}$ cm^2/s). Nevertheless, the diffusion is high enough that the imaging gradients can cause significant dephasing of the FID. So care should be taken to minimize the associated diffusion attenuation *b*-values of the imaging gradients themselves. As fast temporal resolution demands rapid sampling and associated high readout bandwidths, there is a tendency for such sequences to have strong readout gradients, which will attenuate the signal. The effect of the read gradient can be mitigated by using an asymmetric readout in the case of spin-warp or alternatively a spiral or radial gradient—all of these sample the center of *k*-space early and thus minimize the loss in SNR. For the same reason, the spatial resolution attainable with multiple echo sequences such as EPI and single shot fast spin echo is severely restricted by the *b*-value that accrues as the echo train develops (12).

III. Quantitative Evaluation

The sequences described earlier have been shown to provide striking cine movies of lung ventilation. However, with the dynamic images being affected by the physical factors related to the lung environment, the breathing maneuver and the pulse sequence design, there are questions as to the inference of meaningful functional information from the data.

A. Spatio-Temporal Parametric Analysis

The obvious procedure is to generate signal time curves (Fig. 8.4) in defined lung regions or on a pixel by pixel basis. Figure 8.5 shows transit time maps in healthy subjects and in patients with chronic obstructive pulmonary disease (COPD) with ROI graphs.

From such parametric maps, we may be able to identify abnormalities such as delayed ventilation, opening up the possibility that the technique can detect delayed expiratory time constants in patients with COPD (11). A recent paper by Gast et al. (20) evaluated the possibility to derive quantifiable parameters of airflow using HP [3]He-MRI. A FLASH sequence with an image refreshment rate of 128 ms was used, and signal characteristics were observed and plotted. A simple motion correction algorithm involving a one-dimensional translation or stretching of the lung projections was applied to try and maintain a constant region of interest. An accurate image registration would require complicated algorithms for dealing with the motion of nonrigid structures. The following parameters were proposed and reference ranges obtained: tracheal transit time (0.11–1.21 s), tracheo–alveolar interval (0.0–0.02 s), alveolar rise time (0.22–0.62 s), and alveolar amplitude (0–76.6 arbitrary units). This latter measure will be difficult to normalize, as the signal will depend on many external factors such as level of polarization, amount of gas inhaled, and dilution volume.

In more recent work in animals, Dupuich et al. (22) addressed the issue of gas depolarization during influx (Sections II.C and II.D). They normalized the signal based on knowledge of the RF flip angle and the fact that a radial sliding window method constantly updates the SNR in the image. With these factors accounted for, parametric maps of transit times, total inhaled volume and rate of flow (slope of the transit time curve in the airways) were produced. The technique was called SPIRO as it shows good correlation with spirometric tests of lung function in these animal models. In recent work, we have applied these algorithms to our human *in vivo* data acquired with a radial projection sequence and the results look promising (Fig. 8.5).

IV. Clinical Applications

With most of the reported dynamic imaging of ^{3}He in humans coming from research studies in a handful of sites worldwide, comprehensive clinical

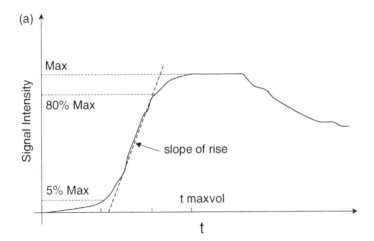

Figure 8.5 **(See color insert)** Schematic showing some of the temporal parameters that can be derived from (a) the signal time course. (b) Maps from a healthy normal. The rise time to maximum in the healthy normal shows a definite grading from the major airways outwards indicating quite isotropic progression of the flow front. Furthermore, the slope of the flow front is highest in the airways. The corrected signal represents the flip angle corrected integral of the signal passing through the pixel over the whole breath. Summation over all pixels in the lungs gives an estimate of total inhaled volume of gas. (c) The parametric maps from the COPD patient [time series shown in Fig. 8.2(b)] show less grading with distance away from the major airways in the rise time to maximum. This might be expected in a patient where obstruction is significant. The map of the slope of the rise shows some hyperintensity in areas other than the major airways which may reflect co-lateral flow routes of lower resistance than those found in the peripheral airways in healthy subjects.

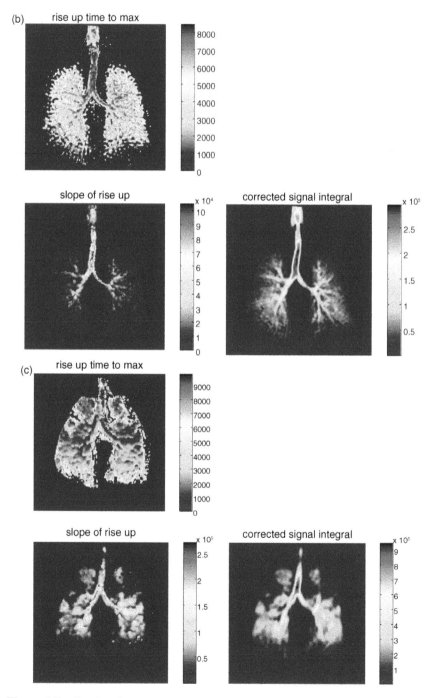

Figure 8.5   *Continued.*

information is yet to filter into the published domain. We can, however, report on some early clinical results from the literature and from our own preliminary studies on patients with asthma, COPD, and cystic fibrosis.

A. Cystic Fibrosis

By the very nature of the technique, the dynamic imaging procedure is only sensitive to long regions which are ventilated. We, therefore, feel that the technique will have limited use in diseases, which cause permanent obstruction, such as advanced stages of CF in adults. In a group of four adult CF patients, the two patients with the most homogeneous inflow had the best $FEV_1 > 50\%$ predicted. The two patients with significant inflow impairment both had $FEV_1 < 30\%$ predicted. Furthermore, these latter two patients both demonstrated delayed emptying of >1 s in the lower right lobe. This corresponded with significantly worse peak flow in these patients ($<50\%$ vs. $>60\%$ in those with normal gas emptying) and a higher residual volume ($>230\%$ predicted vs. $<170\%$ predicted) (23).

In children with CF, the disease tends to be less advanced and, therefore, the lungs are generally more homogeneously ventilated and a systematic analysis of dynamic ventilation may be more useful. In a study of eight children aged 6–15 years (mean age 11.4 years), we focused on the slope of the time course as it may shed some light on levels of obstruction as a measure of the rate of flow in the different regions. Figure 8.6(a) shows a dynamic time series from a child of 11 years, obtained during inspiration and Fig. 8.6(b) shows some images from the same subject when imaging commenced from a point of full inspiration during the expiratory phase. By first calculating the rate of signal influx in the trachea, we have a means of normalizing the signal in the periphery as all gas enter via the trachea. Thus, we used the relative slope of the curve defined as a linear fit to the curve in the region between 5% and 80% of the maximum signal intensity. We observed a trend of a smaller gradient in the upper lobes,

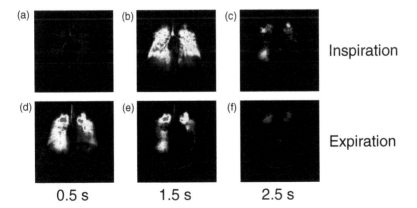

Figure 8.6 (See color insert) Imaging in CF.

indicating a more severe involvement of the upper zones, a typical feature of cystic fibrosis [Fig. 8.6(c)]. Furthermore, when we plot the mean relative slope observed in the peripheral lung zones against the FEV_1 predicted from spirometry we see evidence of correlation in Fig. 8.6(d).

B. Asthma

Asthma is an obstructive disease that has been shown to change with time. Spirometry is used routinely in the clinic as a means of diagnosing the severity of asthma and assessing response of patients to therapy. With the ability to rapidly monitor changes in ventilation dynamic ³He-MRI may well prove to be a powerful tool in the diagnosis and treatment of the disease. Our experience with asthmatics is limited to a group of six patients pre- and post-bronchodilator therapy; however, some interesting observations have arisen. For instance, we have observed delayed inflow of gas that was reversible by bronchodilator therapy (as illustrated in Fig. 8.7).

C. Chronic Obstructive Pulmonary Disease

COPD is currently the fourth leading cause of death in the world and is increasing in prevalence. In the condition, airflow obstruction gives rise to prolonged expiration of affected lung units with incomplete expiration, known as air trapping. Prolonged activity of the respiratory muscles in expiration occurs, this is associated with acute bronchospasm and so contributes to the air trapping. Surgeons are also becoming involved in COPD, performing operations such as lung volume reduction surgery. Patients with upper lobe predominant emphysema seem to

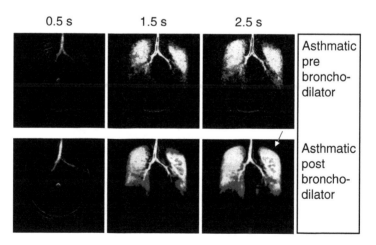

Figure 8.7 (**See color insert**) Asthma before and after bronchodilator therapy. Images of an asthmatic pre- and post-bronchodilator therapy. Note the increased SNR indicating better ventilation in particular in the upper left lobe (arrow) where a defect is seen to resolve.

yet benefit most from the procedure (24). Perfusion scintigraphy, has been shown to help predict which patients are likely to benefit from the surgery, as apical hypoperfusion likely indicates good target regions for surgical resection (25). Ventilation scintigraphy with 133-xenon has been proposed as a means of measuring air trapping in patients with smoking related emphysema who typically shows a relative lack of upper lobe ventilation on the first breath. This is followed by a longer period of rebreathing during which time the initially underventilated regions accumulate radioactive gas, then retain it for a prolonged period during a washout phase of several minutes (26,27).

With dynamic ^{3}He-MRI we can potentially diagnose obstruction and air trapping. We have preliminary experience with a group of three COPD patients who showed large ventilation defects, particularly in the upper lobes where smoking-related, centrilobular emphysema tends to be most severe. All three subjects were judged to have regions of delayed expiration. This is most likely due to bronchiolar obstruction, where the regions distal to the obstruction are ventilated by collateral air passages through alveolar pores; however, on expiration the alveolar pores are smaller and hence the air is trapped [see later images in the time series of the COPD patient in Fig. 8.2(b)]. B_1 inhomogeneity could cause the appearance of air trapping in the extreme peripheries of the lung; however, from our study the persistence of signal intensity in the COPD patients is localized to specific lung regions, which is not indicative of this effect. Furthermore, we do not see delayed depolarization of signal in the healthy normals indicating that there is some collateral flow mechanism at work. Gast et al. (28) performed dynamic ^{3}He-MRI on a group of 11 single and six double lung transplant recipients who had undergone surgery for treatment of COPD. Results from grafts and native lungs were compared with a different median alveolar rise time, of 0.28 s for the graft and 0.48 s for the native lung.

D. Hemidiaphragm

Dynamic ^{3}He-MRI may well supply complementary information to dynamic proton MRI of the lung walls and diaphragm in patients who suffer from mechanical problems associated with the diaphragm and ribs (Refer Section V). Figure 8.8 shows sagittal ventilation images acquired from a patient with paralysis of the right hemidiaphragm.

V. Dynamic Imaging Using Proton MRI

The dynamics of respiration has already been discussed in Chapter 4. However, this chapter has mainly focused on CT technology in this respect and only hinted at the fact that MRI is also extremely capable of visualization of chest wall and diaphragm motion. For completeness, we will discuss the most salient publications in this area.

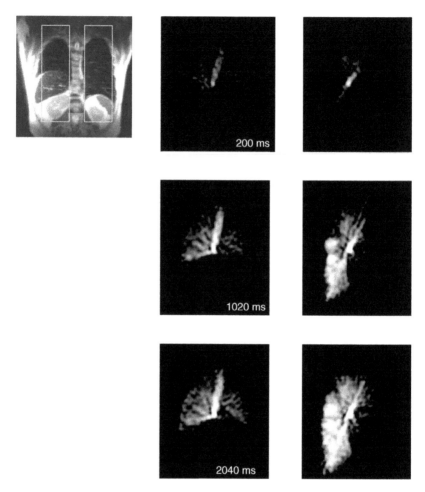

Figure 8.8   Dynamic dual sagittal slice images acquired from 13 cm thick slices centered on the left and right lungs of a patient with hemi-paralysis of the left diaphragm. The image refresh rate per slice in this dual slice acquisition was 10.8 ms. Note the motion of the base of the right lung whilst the left remains static, and also how the right lung becomes better ventilated.

MRI has the major advantage of gaining information on movement of the thoracic cage without the need for ionizing radiation and has the capability of ultrafast imaging to allow good temporal resolution of movements. Gierada et al. (29) applied fast MRI to demonstrate the feasibility of diaphragmatic movement assessment in healthy volunteers for the first time. Cluzel et al. (30) demonstrated the exquisite detail of diaphragm movement and volume calculations using high resolution MRI in comparison with spirometry in five healthy subjects. It was shown that the shape of the diaphragm changes significantly with inspiratory volumes of the lungs. In patients with COPD, several authors have assessed changes in diaphragmatic motion and demonstrated impaired respiratory mechanics compared to controls (31). The technique has even been employed to assess the changes in patients with emphysema before and after lung volume reduction surgery (32).

However, one of the limitations of all this work was the supine position of subjects in the MRI environment, which makes it difficult to compare the findings with the standard lung function assessment in the sitting position. A more recent study has addressed the change in diaphragm motion between supine and vertical positioning of 10 healthy subjects (33). Measurement of diaphragmatic excursion was performed at six preset points, which demonstrated that diaphragmatic excursion was greatest with subjects in the supine position, and that the posterior part of the diaphragm moves over a greater distance. This finding probably reflects the greater intra-abdominal pressure in the supine position, leading to more compression of the diaphragm at end-expiration. However, other explanations such as lung volume changes and gravity induces changes on the lungs themselves could also have a role to play.

In conclusion, dynamic proton imaging is probably capable of addressing respiratory dynamics both in healthy and in diseased states. Ultrafast imaging is capable of MR fluoroscopy, which will further enhance the potential of probing respiratory mechanics. The introduction of vertical MR systems may also be of interest in this respect.

References

1. Moller HE, Chen XJ, Saam B, Hagspiel KD, Johnson GA, Altes TA, de Lange EE, Kauczor HU. MRI of the lungs using hyperpolarized noble gases. Magn Reson Med 2002; 47:1029–1051.
2. MacFall JR, Charles HC, Black RD, Middleton H, Swartz JC, Saam B, Driehuys B, Erickson C, Happer W, Cates GD, Johnson GA, Ravin CE. Human lung air spaces: potential for MR imaging with hyperpolarized helium-3. Radiology 1996; 200(2):553–558.
3. Schreiber WG, Weiler N, Kauczor HU, Markstaller K, Eberle B, Hast J, Surkau R, Grossmann T, Deninger A, Hanisch G, Otten EW, Thelen M. Ultrafast MRI of lung ventilation using hyperpolarized helium-3. Rofo Fortschr Geb Rontgenstr Neuen Bildgeb Verfahr 2000; 172(2):129–133.
4. van Vaals JJ, Brummer ME, Dixon WT, Tuithof HH, Engels H, Nelson RC, Gerety BM, Chezmar JL, den Boer JA. "Keyhole" method for accelerating imaging of contrast agent uptake. J Magn Reson Imaging 1993; 3:671–675.
5. Riederer SJ, Tasciyan T, Farzaneh F, Lee JN, Wright RC, Herfkens RJ. MR fluoroscopy: technical feasibility. Magn Reson Med 1998; 8:1–15.
6. Viallon M, Cofer GP, Suddarth SA, Moller HE, Chen XJ, Chawla MS et al. Functional MR microscopy of the lung using hyperpolarized ^{3}He. Magn Reson Med 1999; 41:787–792.

7. Viallon M, Berthezene Y, Callot V, Bourgeois M, Humblot H, Briguet A et al. Dynamic imaging of hyper-polarised ³He distribution in rat lungs using interleaved-spiral scans. NMR Biomed 2000; 13:207–213.
8. Ruppert K, Brookeman JR, Mugler JP. Real-time MR imaging of pulmonary gas-flow dynamics with hyperpolarized ³He. 1998 Proceedings of the ISMRM, 1909.
9. Salerno M, Altes TA, Brookeman JR, de Lange EE, Mugler JP III. Dynamic spiral MR imaging of pulmonary gas flow using hyperpolarized ³He: Preliminary studies in healthy and diseased lungs. Magn Reson Med 2001; 46:667–677.
10. Wild JM, Paley MNJ, Kasuboski L, Swift A, Fichele S, Woodhouse N, van Beek EJR. Dynamic radial projection MRI of inhaled hyperpolarised ³He. Magn Reson Med 2003; 49(6):991–997.
11. Gierada DS, Saam B, Yablonskiy D, Cooper JD, Lefrak SS, Conradi MS. Dynamic echo planar MR imaging of lung ventilation with hyperpolarized ³He in normal subjects and patients with severe emphysema. NMR Biomed 2000; 13:176–181.
12. Saam B, Yablonskiy DA, Gierada DS, Conradi MS. Rapid imaging of hyper-polarized gas using EPI. Magn Reson Med 1999; 42:507–514.
13. Mugler JP, Brookeman JR, Knight-Scott J, Maier T, de Lange EE, Bogorad PL. Interleaved echo-planar imaging of the lungs with hyperpolarized ³He. Proceedings of the ISMRM, 1998, 448.
14. Johnson GA, Cates G, Chen XJ et al. Dynamics of magnetization in hyperpolarized gas MRI of the lung. Magn Reson Med 1997; 38:66–71.
15. Chen BT, Brau AC, Johnson GA. Measurement of regional lung function in rats using hyperpolarized ³He dynamic MRI. Magn Reson Med 2003; 49(1):78–88.
16. Wild JM, Fichele S, Woodhouse N, Paley MNJ, Swift A, Kasuboski L, Griffiths PD, van Beek EJR. Assessment and compensation of susceptibility artifacts in gradient echo MRI of hyperpolarised ³He gas. Magn Reson Med 2003; 50:417–422.
17. Wild JM, Paley MNH, Viallon M, Schreiber WG, van Beek EJR, Griffiths PD. *k*-Space filtering in 2D gradient echo breath-hold hyperpolarized ³He MRI: spatial resolution and signal to noise considerations. Magn Res Med 2002; 47:687–695.
18. Roberts DA, Rizi RR, Lipson DA, Aranda M, Baumgardner J, Bearn L et al. Detection and localization of pulmonary air leaks using laser-polarized ³He MRI. Magn Reson Med 2000; 44:379–382.
19. Schreiber WG, Markstaller K, Kauczor HU, Eberle B, Surkau R, Hanisch G et al. Ultrafast imaging of the lungs ventilation using hyperpolarized helium-3. Proceedings of the ISMRM, 1999, 2096.
20. Gast KK, Puderback MU, Rodriguez I, Eberle B, Markstaller K, Hanke AT et al. Dynamic ventilation ³He-magnetic resonance imaging with lung motion correction: gas flow distribution analysis. Invest Radiol 2002; 37:126–134.
21. Tooker AC, Hong KS, McKinstry EL, Costello P, Jolesz FA, Albert MS. Distal airways in humans: dynamic hyperpolarized ³He MR imaging-feasibility. Radiology 2003; 227(2):575–579.
22. Dupuich D, Berthezene Y, Clouet PL, Stupar V, Canet E, Cremillieux Y. Dynamic ³He imaging for quantification of regional lung ventilation parameters. Magn Reson Med 2003; 50(4):777–783.
23. van Beek EJR, McMahon CJ, Dodd JD, Hill C, Woodhouse N, Fichele S, Gallagher SG, Skehan SJ, Masterson JB, Wild JM. Hyperpolarized ³He MRI in

adults with cystic fibrosis: comparison with HRCT (Bhalla score) and body plethysmography. Proc UKRC 2004, 55.

24. National Emphysema Treatment Trial Research Group. A randomized trial comparing lung-volume—reduction surgery with medical therapy for severe emphysema. N Engl J Med 2003; 348:2059–2073.

25. Kotloff RM, Hansen-Flaschen J, Lipson DA, Tino G, Arcasoy SM, Kaiser LR et al. Apical perfusion fraction as a predictor of short term functional outcome following bilateral lung volume reduction surgery. Chest 2001; 120(5):1609–1615.

26. Suga K, Tsukuda T, Awaya H, Matsunaga N, Sugi K, Esato K. Interactions of regional respiratory mechanics and pulmonary ventilatory impairment in pulmonary emphysema: assessment with dynamic MRI and xenon-133 single-photon emission CT. Chest 2000; 117(6):1646–1655.

27. Suga K, Kume N, Matsunaga N, Ogasawara N, Motoyama K, Hara A, Matsumoto T. Relative preservation of peripheral lung function in smoking-related pulmonary emphysema: assessment with 99mTc-MAA perfusion and dynamic ^{133}Xe SPET. Eur J Nucl Med 2000; 27(7):800–806.

28. Gast KK, Zaporozhan J, Ley S, Biedermann A, Knitz F, Eberle B, Schmiedeskamp J, Heussel CP, Mayer E, Schreiber WG, Thelen M, Kauczor HU. [3]He-MRI in follow-up of lung transplant recipients. Eur Radiol 2004; 14(1):78–85.

29. Gierada DS, Curtin JJ, Erickson SJ, Prost RW, Strandt JA, Goodman LR. Diaphragmatic motion: fast gradient-recalled-echo MR imaging in healthy subjects. Radiology 1995; 194:879–884.

30. Cluzel P, Similowski T, Chartrand-Lefebvre C, Zelter M, Derenne J-P, Grenier PA. Diaphragm and chest wall: assessment of the inspiratory pump with MR imaging—preliminary observations. Radiology 2000; 215:574–583.

31. Suga K, Tsukuda T, Awaya H et al. Impaired respiratory mechanics in pulmonary emphysema: evaluation with dynamic breathing. J Magn Reson Imaging 1999; 10:510–520.

32. Iwasawa T, Kagei S, Gotoh T et al. Magnetic resonance analysis of abnormal diaphragmatic motion in patients with emphysema. Eur Respir J 2002; 19:225–231.

33. Takazakura R, Takahashi M, Nitta N, Murata K. Diaphragmatic motion in the sitting and supine positions: healthy subject study using a vertically open magnetic resonance system. J Magn Reson Imaging 2004; 19:605–609.

9

Oxygen-Enhanced Ventilation Imaging

VU M. MAI

Evanston Northwestern Healthcare,
Evanston, Illinois

Feinberg School of Medicine at
  Northwestern University,
Chicago, Illinois, USA

QUN CHEN

New York University School of Medicine,
New York, New York, USA

181

I. Introduction

Assessment of ventilation is crucial in the evaluation of a host of pulmonary disorders because sufficient ventilation of the lung tissue is a major determinant of efficient gas exchange in the lung. There are several imaging methods available to evaluate lung ventilation such as radionuclide scintigraphy and the recently developed hyperpolarized gas magnetic resonance imaging (MRI). Radionuclide scintigraphy encounters limitations such as poor spatial resolution and the need for a radioactive tracer (1). Hyperpolarized ^{3}He and ^{129}Xe MR imaging have provided detailed images of the lung, but the high cost of the laser polarizer, the expenses for the ^{3}He and ^{129}Xe gases, and the need for nonproton imaging apparatus currently limit its wide spread application (2–4).

An alternative approach to hyperpolarized gas MRI is oxygen-enhanced ventilation imaging, which exploits the paramagnetic T_1-shortening property of inhaled oxygen (5,6). When compared with hyperpolarized gas imaging, oxygen-enhanced imaging offers several advantages: (1) oxygen is readily available as part of emergency equipment in most MR suites, (2) oxygen-enhanced imaging does not impose the burden of the high cost of the laser-polarizing unit, noble gases, and the need for nonproton imaging apparatus, and (3) most importantly, the oxygen ventilation imaging technique potentially provides a means to directly study oxygen diffusivity (oxygen uptake) from the air space to the pulmonary vasculature.

In this chapter, we will discuss the current advances and all the issues regarding the oxygen-enhanced ventilation imaging technique. These include the effect of paramagnetic properties of dissolved oxygen to the longitudinal relaxation time (T_1), general procedures of the image acquisition schemes and image post-processing, and the potential applications of oxygen-enhanced imaging. The goal of this chapter is to provide interested readers with the detailed technical and logistical backgrounds necessary to implement oxygen-enhanced ventilation imaging.

II. Paramagnetic Properties of Oxygen

The weakly paramagnetic property of molecular oxygen caused by the presence of two unpaired electrons is the underlying principle of oxygen-enhanced ventilation imaging. Each electron has a magnetic moment that is 1000 times that of a nucleus, and the resulting fluctuating magnetic field can produce a greater dipole–dipole interaction than that of the neighboring nuclei, thus causing a faster rate of spin–lattice relaxation (R_1). Chiarotti et al. (7) first reported that an increase in dissolved oxygen in water shortens its T_1 ($1/R_1$). They also concluded that a linear relationship exists between R_1 and the concentration of dissolved oxygen in water, and the results in Fig. 9.1 confirm this observation. Figure 9.2 shows a change in T_1 would thus translate into a change in MR

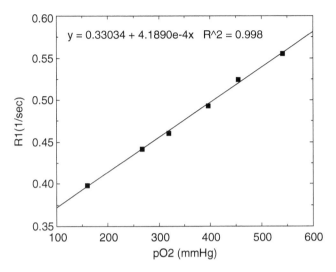

Figure 9.1 The linear relation between R_1 and partial oxygen pressure in the saline solution. An excellent correlation between the R_1 and the partial oxygen pressure can be observed between the different data points and the fitted straight line ($r^2 = 0.998$).

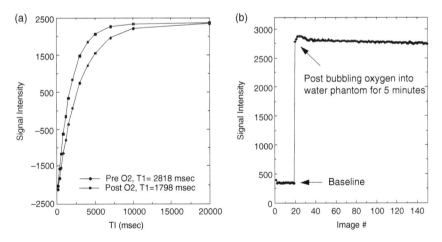

Figure 9.2 Change in signal intensity after bubbling of oxygen into saline solution. (a) Signal intensities measured at different TI between pre- and post-oxygen, which can be fitted to calculate for T_1 of the saline solution. Clearly, there is a shortening of T_1 in post-oxygen ($T_1 = 1798$ ms) relative to preoxygen ($T_1 = 2818$ ms). (b) Noticeable signal change from the baseline can be observed after 5 min of bubbling of oxygen into the saline solution.

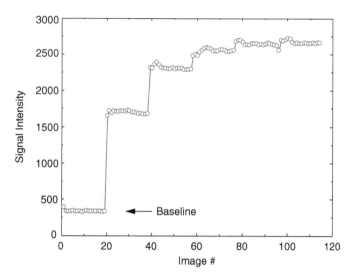

Figure 9.3 Graded MR signal changes corresponding to repeated oxygen bubbling periods of 30 s at a flow rate of 3L/min. Signal intensity increase develops a plateau toward the end, indicating a saturation of concentration of oxygen in the solution.

signal intensity, whereas Fig. 9.3 illustrates the graded signal changes of the saline solution corresponding to different degrees of 100% oxygen bubbling into the solution (8). The signal plateau in both Figs. 9.2(b) and 9.3 suggests a saturation of dissolved oxygen in the saline solution.

Young et al. (9) extended Chiarotti's study and reported the shortening of T_1 and an increase in signal intensity of blood in the left ventricle after the volunteers inhale 100% oxygen in their investigation of the potential use of oxygen as a paramagnetic contrast agent. Expanding on these results, Edelman et al. (5) first proposed the use of oxygen for ventilation imaging in the lung. Though oxygen is weakly paramagnetic, its overall effect on the lung is considerable, given the large surface area of the lung and the large difference in partial pressures between room air and 100% oxygen. These two factors facilitate an environment that allows more oxygen to diffuse across the parenchyma and dissolve in blood.

III. Prerequisites for Oxygen-Enhanced Imaging

The ability to detect MR signal of the lung is a requisite because oxygen-enhanced imaging is essentially a subtraction technique. Generally, oxygen-enhanced imaging involves the acquisition of series of images as the subject alternately inhales room air (21% oxygen) and 100% oxygen (5,6). The signal difference between the two reflects the change in the oxygen level dissolved in blood and/or lung tissues. The acquired images are then averaged and subtracted to produce the oxygen ventilation image. However, detection of MR signal of the lung, until recently, has been particularly difficult owing to the inherent architecture of the lung. The lung, designed for efficient gas exchange, contains a large number of alveoli, which produce large air-to-tissue interfaces. These large air–tissue interfaces in turn generate an inhospitable environment for MRI of the lung (10,11). First, the numerous alveoli result in low-proton density, which produces an inherently weak signal for detection relative to other organs in the body. Secondly, the air–tissue interfaces create large local magnetic field gradients that rapidly dephase the already weak MR signal and significantly reduce the apparent transverse relaxation time (T_2^*), which has been measured at 1.5 ms (12). This makes MRI of the lung difficult using conventional sequences. Lastly, involuntary respiratory and cardiac motion potentially introduce artifacts in the image that may significantly degrade image quality.

Despite these challenges, numerous efforts have been attempted to demonstrate the feasibility of MRI of the lung. Early attempts have focused on shortening the TE of gradient echo sequences in an effort to overcome the ultra-short T_2^* of the lung. Bergin et al. (13) proposed a back projection reconstruction imaging method, whereas Alsop et al. (12) exploited the advance of gradient hardware technology and designed a submillisecond TE sequence. Though they have demonstrated the visualization of the lung, these gradient echo sequences are quite sensitive to magnetic field susceptibility. The measured signal-to-noise ratio (SNR) remains poor, and as a result, gradient echo sequences are not quite suitable for oxygen-enhanced imaging. Spin echo sequences, on the other hand, are more immune to magnetic field susceptibility. Its signal is dictated by the transverse relaxation time (T_2), which tends to be longer than that of T_2^*, thus making more time available for signal detection. Consequently, spin echo sequences are more suitable for MRI of the lung. However, the acquisition time of a conventional spin echo sequence is generally long and this makes it more susceptible to motion artifact. Single-shot fast spin echo (SSFSE) sequences with an acquisition time in the order of hundreds of milliseconds are relatively immune to motion artifacts, and are, therefore, often used.

Mayo et al. (14) were one of the first to explore the use of a spin echo sequence for MRI of the lung, but the visualization of the lung remained poor owing to the bright signals from the surrounding tissues such as fat and muscle. To enhance the visualization of the lung, preparatory inversion recovery (IR) and multiple IR (MIR) along with a half-Fourier SSFSE (such as HASTE) sequences have been proposed to specifically suppress signal contributions from the thoracic muscle and fat based on the T_1 of these tissues (15–17). For the IR sequence, it has been determined that a time of inversion (TI) of 600 ms, which is the null point of muscle, is optimal for the visualization of the lung (15). To suppress the MR signal of fat, a frequency selective saturation pulse is used. On the other hand, two preparatory inversion radiofrequency pulses in the MIR sequence are used to simultaneously suppress MR signals from

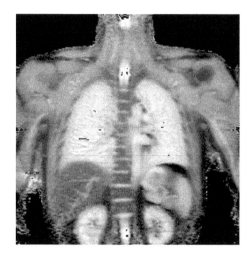

Figure 9.4 T_1 map from a healthy volunteer calculated from a series of nonselective IR-HASTE images of the lung at different TIs of 100, 500, 1000, 1400, and 3000 ms. The average T_1 of the lung parenchyma is 1371 ± 90 ms. The average T_1s of the liver, cerebrospinal fluid, renal cortex, renal medulla, and spleen are 618.2 ± 43.2 ms, 2173.5 ± 280.5 ms, 1103.5 ± 118.7 ms, 830.4 ± 105.0 ms, 1018.0 ± 39.8 ms, respectively.

fat and muscle by setting the appropriate time delays (TDs). Assuming the T_1 of 250 ms for fat and 1400 ms for the lung, the TI_1 of 800 ms and TI_2 of 150 ms have been used in the MIR sequence (16). This assumption of T_1 of the lung has been validated experimentally (Fig. 9.4). As shown in Figs. 9.5 and 9.6, the IR-HASTE and MIR-HASTE images clearly depict the lung, even at an effective TE of 38 ms. This is because preliminary measurement of the T_2 of the lung has been reported to be between 60 and 100 ms depending on the phase of the cardiac cycle (18). In addition, motion artifacts are negligible in these images. These results suggest that there is more than adequate detectable signal to measure the change in oxygen-enhanced imaging.

IV. Implementation

A. Image Acquisition

Image acquisition of oxygen-enhanced studies involves two aspects: the MR sequence and the experimental protocol. To date, a cardiac triggered IR or MIR SSFSE sequence has often been used in oxygen-enhanced ventilation imaging due to their inherent advantages (5,6,19). Basically, cardiac triggering ensures that data acquisition would occur in the late diastole, assuming that the heart rate of the subject is relatively stable over time (19). The TI in the IR

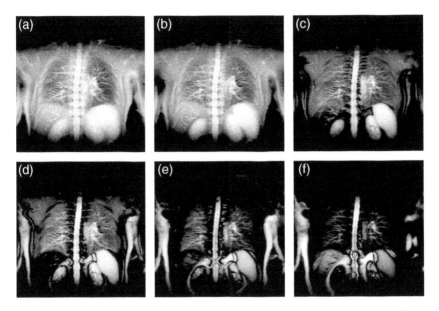

Figure 9.5 IR-HASTE lung images from a normal male volunteer at different TIs of (a) 100, (b) 150, (c) 300, (d) 400, (e) 500, and (f) 600 ms. Different contrast is observed between the lung and the background tissues such as muscle and fat. At short TIs of 100 and 150 ms, the pulmonary vessels are clearly distinguished, but visualization of the lung is poor (a and b). As TI increases, improved visualization of the lung parenchyma is observed, even though the signal intensities of muscle and/or fat are not completely suppressed (c–f). Optimized visualization of the lung appears in (f).

sequence is normally set to ~1200–1300 ms to optimize for signal change (6,20). As described earlier, the two TIs in the MRI sequence are set at TI_1 of 800 ms and TI_2 of 150 ms to concurrently suppress the signal from muscle and fat because the longitudinal magnetization of these issues would simultaneously approach their null points (Fig. 9.7). As a result, a MIR scheme would improve the subtraction of the background tissues because its source images have less starting signal, but would sacrifice some signal loss (16,19). The SSFSE sequences used are either centric reordered or half-Fourier *k*-space sampling with a short echo spacing of 3.6–4.5 ms. Subsequently, a time delay (TD) of 2–4 s is set to allow for the magnetization recovery.

The fundamental protocol of an oxygen-enhanced experimentation is the alternating inhalation of room air and 100% oxygen by the subjects, who are asked to remain still and perform normal, quiet breathing for the duration of the imaging session (5,6). The 100% oxygen flow is delivered at a rate of 15 L/min through a nonrebreathing ventilatory mask and a series of 20–30 images are acquired. Each data acquisition period lasts ~3 min and may be repeated if necessary. Image acquisition during the oxygen inhaling period can

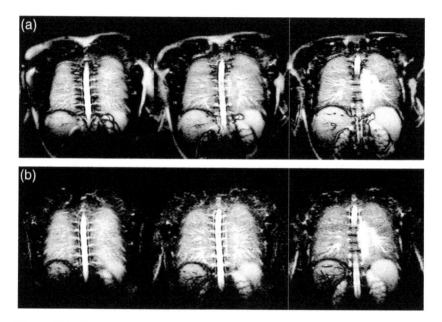

Figure 9.6 Comparison between IR-HASTE and MIR-HASTE images of the lung. Shown are three contiguous slices acquired with (a) IR-HASTE with fatsat and (b) MIR-HASTE sequences. MIR-HASTE images show excellent suppression of both fat and muscular signal. Similar pulmonary features are observed in both IR- and MIR-HASTE images. The average SNR of 37.2 ± 5.8 for IR-HASTE and 26.6 ± 8.4 for MIR-HASTE are measured.

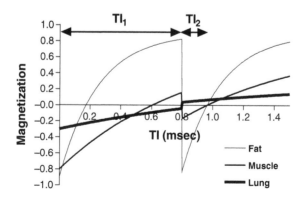

Figure 9.7 Longitudinal magnetization of different tissues in a MIR sequence for a TI_1 of 800 ms and TI_2 of 150 ms. Both magnetizations of muscle and fat are nulled at TI ($TI_1 + TI_2$) of 950 ms but not that of the lung.

be obtained in either dynamic or steady-state schemes. In the steady-state scheme, at the end of the period of inhalation of room air, oxygen flow is initiated for ~1–2 min before the start of image acquisition. This allows for the oxygen level in the lung to reach steady-state. Similarly, a delay of 1–2 min is applied at the end of 100% oxygen period before the next image acquisition during room air to allow return of the arterial oxygen level to room air. On the other hand, image acquisition in the dynamic scheme continues from the period of inhalation of room air into the period of inhalation of 100% oxygen as the oxygen flow is initiated or ceased. The steady-state scheme results in an immediate and abrupt transition in signal intensity between the periods of inhalation of room air and 100% oxygen, whereas the dynamic scheme shows a progressive rise in signal intensity from the room air to 100% oxygen period until it reaches a steady-state. Similar observations would also occur following cessation of 100% oxygen and the return to room air levels. The average signal intensities are measured from the regions of interest (ROI) drawn in the upper right or left lung, where the lung is minimally affected by respiratory motion.

B. Image Post-processing

Oxygen-enhanced ventilation images can be reconstructed by calculating the difference, percentage, or correlation on a pixel-by-pixel basis (5,6,19–22). For the difference and the percentage images, the average images of the room air and 100% oxygen are first determined. To minimize misregistration artifact, a reference image, usually at maximal expiration, is first selected and only images from the steady-state segment of the series that match within a few pixels of the right lung–liver interface as reference will be selected and averaged. The difference image is then calculated by subtracting the average images obtained during room air and oxygen images. The percentage image is obtained by dividing the difference to the average image of either room air or 100% oxygen.

The qualitative correlation map is reconstructed by recognizing that the modulation of signal intensity between room air and 100% oxygen periods approximates the box-car pattern (Fig. 9.8). This pattern can be exploited to determine the correlation map using statistical analysis, which has been previously applied in brain activation studies to confidently localize regions of brain activation (23,24). Pixel-by-pixel correlation maps of oxygen-enhanced ventilation are generated by computing the cross-correlation between the time response function of each pixel and the ideal box-car waveform that describes the expected time response. If the time response of each given pixel was denoted by the vector $\mathbf{A} = \{A_i\}$, where $i = 1-N$, the number of images, and the expected time response was represented by the vector $\mathbf{B} = \{B_i\}$, the correlation coefficient, r, was computed using the following equation (23,24):

$$r = \frac{\sum_{n=1}^{N} (A_i - \bar{A})(B_i - \bar{B})}{\sqrt{\sum_{n=1}^{N} (A_i - \bar{A})^2} \sqrt{\sum_{n=1}^{N} (B_i - \bar{B})^2}} \tag{9.1}$$

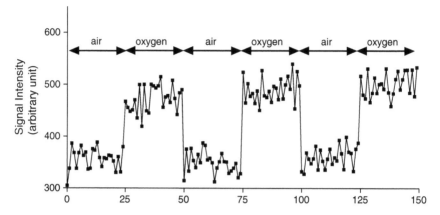

Figure 9.8   Time course of signal intensities of the lung during periods of inhalation of room air and 100% oxygen in a steady-state image acquisition. The average signal intensities were measured from a region-of-interest drawn in the upper right lung. Modulation of signal intensity between room air and 100% oxygen approximates the box-car pattern.

where $\bar{A}$ is the average value of vector **A**, and $\bar{B}$ is the average value of the vector **B**. The correlation coefficient reflects the degree to which the shapes of **A** and **B** are similar but does not reflect their relative amplitudes.

V. Healthy Volunteer Studies and Experimental Optimizations

The signal difference in oxygen-enhanced ventilation imaging has been reported in studies of healthy volunteers using IR or MIR sequences (5,6,19–22). Figure 9.9 shows the IR oxygen-enhanced difference and percentage images along with the correlation map and Fig. 9.10 shows the MIR images along with their oxygen-enhanced difference images from three contiguous slices. The signal distribution in the difference image is consistent with previous reports (5,7,8). Signal difference of pulmonary veins in Figs. 9.9 and 9.10 reflects the exchange of molecular oxygen from the air space to pulmonary veins following inhalation of 100% oxygen. Similarly, the signal of the descending aorta, spleen, subclavian arteries, or the kidneys is indicative of the substantial increased concentration of oxygen in blood. The minimal change in the pulmonary arteries, however, results from the tissue and systemic venous uptake of oxygen in blood before it returns to pulmonary arteries. Consequently, oxygen concentration in blood plasma in the pulmonary arteries only increases slightly, which contributes to the poor signal change.

Signal difference in the lung parenchyma between the inhalation of room air (21% oxygen) and 100% oxygen is on the order of ~10–20% (6,19,20).

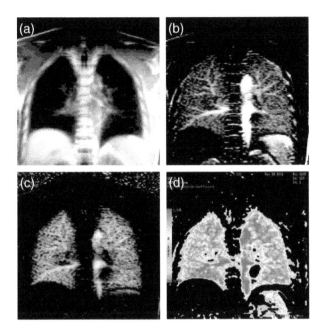

Figure 9.9 (**See color insert**) Oxygen-enhanced ventilation images of a healthy volunteer obtained through different calculations. Shown are the (a) anatomical image, (b) difference image, (c) percentage image, and (d) correlation map. Normal ventilation and similar pulmonary anatomy is observed among the images.

The observed signal change results mainly from the effect of increased concentration of oxygen dissolved in blood. It has been hypothesized that the paramagnetic effect of oxygen on T_1 is the dominant mechanism that induces decrease in signal intensity, and the results in Fig. 9.11 experimentally show the shortening of T_1 after the inhalation of 100% oxygen. A difference of 100–200 ms in T_1 of the lung parenchyma between breathing room air and 100% oxygen has been reported (6,20,25–27). However, T_1 shortening is not the only mechanism that can cause change in signal intensity. Increase in concentration of oxygen also affects T_2^* by decreasing the susceptibility of blood through its binding with hemoglobin. This increase of MR signal intensity, parallel to a decrease of paramagnetic deoxyhemoglobin, has been referred to as blood oxygen level dependent (BOLD) effect (28,29). The potential signal changes due to BOLD should be minimal in the oxygen-enhanced ventilation imaging because a fast spin echo sequence with short echo spacing time is quite insensitive to susceptibility effect (T_2^*). These results have proven the feasibility of oxygen-enhanced ventilation imaging using 100% oxygen and the outlined technical and experimental parameters. On the basis of the theoretical equation of the magnetization recovery for the IR sequence, there should be different degrees of signal enhancement

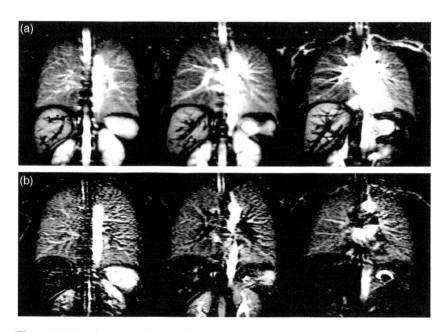

Figure 9.10 Shown are three contiguous coronal MIR anatomical image and their corresponding oxygen-enhanced difference images. Note the high signal difference occurs mainly in the lung parenchyma, pulmonary veins, the descending aorta, the spleen and the kidneys, but not in pulmonary arteries. Excellent subtraction of the background tissues and a minimal presence of motion or spatial misregistration artifacts are observed.

for different TI. In addition, as oxygen solubility in blood is poor, there may be different degrees of signal enhancement for different oxygen flow rates. Therefore, there should exist an optimal signal enhancement for these parameters. Previous studies have determined that the optimal TI is $\sim$1200 ms and the optimal oxygen flow rate through a nonrebreathing ventilatory mask, as shown in Fig. 9.12, is 15 L/min (6,20,30).

VI. Potential Clinical Applications

The described oxygen-enhanced ventilation imaging technique offers a potential tool in the diagnosis of pulmonary diseases. It may be directly used to reliably evaluate healthy and diseased lung tissues in airway obstructive pulmonary pathologies such as emphysema and cystic fibrosis. It may also be used in conjunction with Gd-DTPA or arterial spin labeling (ASL) perfusion imaging to constitute a MR ventilation–perfusion (V/Q) scan to assess pulmonary diseases such as acute pulmonary embolism (5,31–34). The use of combined MR V/Q imaging is discussed elsewhere (Chapter 14).

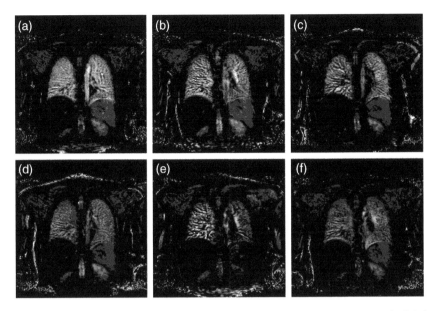

Figure 9.11 T_1 maps of the lung at different oxygen flow rates of (a) room air (0 L/min), (b) 5 L/min, (c) 10 L/min, (d) 15 L/min, (e) 20 L/min, and (f) 25 L/min. A shortening of T_1 of the lung can be observed between that measured during inhalation of room air and 100% oxygen.

A. Oxygen-Enhanced Ventilation Imaging of Pulmonary Diseases

Despite the fact that oxygen-enhanced imaging has been developed only recently, it has been successfully used to detect regional ventilation defects in various pulmonary diseases (5,32,33). Edelman et al. (5) showed ventilation defects in a patient with bullous emphysema. Figure 9.13 shows an oxygen-enhanced ventilation image from a patient with emphysema, where a ventilatory defect can easily be distinguished in the lower left lung (arrow). Nakagawa et al. (32) concluded that V/Q using oxygen-enhanced and bolus gadolinium contrast-enhanced techniques can be used to comprehensively assess pulmonary V/Q abnormalities in patients with lung diseases. Ohno et al. (35) studied 18 patients with lung cancer who also may or may not have emphysema. Among many findings, they found that the mean slope of the signal enhancement was significantly lower in patients with lung cancer than in healthy volunteers and also significantly lower in lung cancer patients with emphysema than in those without emphysema. They also reported a strong correlation between the mean slope of relative enhancement and forced expiratory volume in 1 s and a good correlation between the maximum mean relative enhancement and the high-resolution CT emphysema score. Another preliminary study also shows promising results in

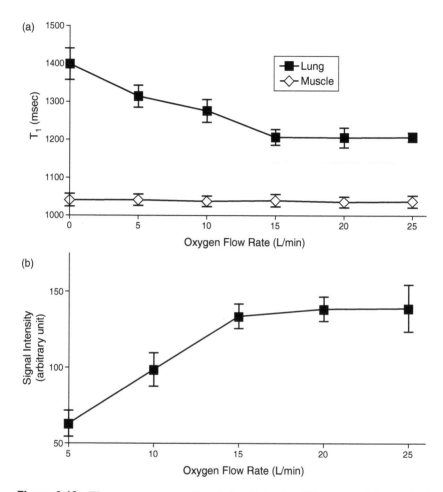

Figure 9.12 The average measure T_1 and signal intensity differences and the standard error of the mean of the lung and muscle of six volunteers at different oxygen flow rates. Both (a) the plot of the average T_1 and (b) the average signal differences reach a plateau at the flow rate of ~15 L/min, suggesting an optimal oxygen flow rate for oxygen-enhanced ventilation imaging.

differentiating between normal and abnormal lung tissues in patients with cystic fibrosis. In this study, T_1 maps are acquired during the inhalation of oxygen at five different concentrations and the measured average R_1 were then plotted in Fig. 9.14. The average R_1 of the lung progressively increases, that is, T_1 shortening, in normal tissues (ROI2) as the concentration of the inhaled oxygen increases, but remains practically unchanged in a region cystic lung disease (ROI1).

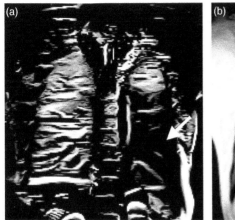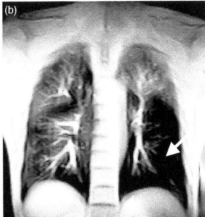

Figure 9.13 Oxygen-enhanced ventilation and gadolinium contrast-enhanced perfusion images from a patient with emphysema. Matched ventilation and perfusion defects can be observed in the lower left lung (arrows).

B. V/Q Imaging

The matching of ventilation to pulmonary perfusion determines the efficiency of gas exchange in the lung. Ventilation and perfusion mismatching causes hypoxemia and impairs the gas exchange of both oxygen and carbon dioxide (36–40). A thorough understanding of the distribution of V/Q ratio is, therefore, essential to elucidate the pathophysiologic mechanisms leading to impaired gas exchange (40). Pulmonary perfusion is an important physiological indicator in the evaluation of different lung diseases such as pulmonary embolism (PE). However, an abnormal perfusion lung scan by itself is nonspecific as a variety of cardiorespiratory disorders, for example chronic obstructive pulmonary disease (COPD), can also result in pulmonary perfusion disturbances. Consequently, a complementary ventilation scan is concurrently evaluated to ascertain V/Q patterns that reflect probabilities of PE and obstructive lung disease. Generally, a mismatch between V/Q scan (normal ventilation and abnormal perfusion) indicates a high probability of PE, whereas a matched V/Q (abnormal ventilation and perfusion) reduces this probability and increases the likelihood for obstructive lung disease.

One of the widely used screening modalities for PE is radionuclide V/Q scanning. However, this technique uses radioactive tracer, has limited resolution, and is nonspecific in about two-third of clinically suspected PE cases (41,42). Several V/Q imaging methods using magnetic resonance have been proposed combining aerosolized gadolinium and hyperpolarized gas for ventilation and gadolinium contrast-enhanced (43–47). Oxygen-enhanced ventilation imaging can also be combined with either gadolinium contrast-enhanced or ASL perfusion imaging technique to form a MR V/Q scan as shown in Figs. 9.15 and 9.16 (5,6,31–34). Contrast-enhanced perfusion imaging uses exogenous

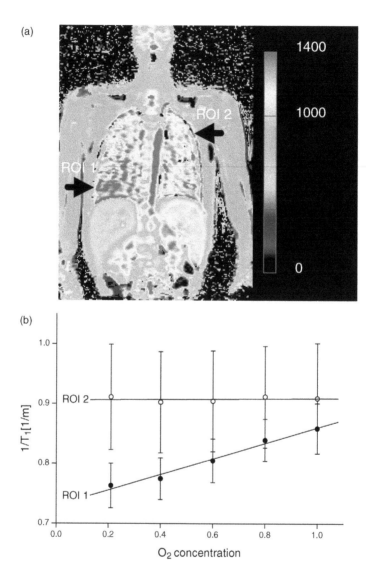

Figure 9.14 (**See color insert**) Shown are (a) a T_1 map acquired with a preparatory inversion recovery fast gradient echo sequence during inhalation of room air (21% oxygen) and (b) a graph of the average regional R_1 of the ROI1 and ROI2 as a function of different concentration of inhaled oxygen. A bar indicates the scale of the T_1 values in ms. ROI1 denotes a region of normal lung tissue, whereas ROI2 points to a region of lung destruction in a patient with cystic fibrosis. The R_1 of the normal lung increases progressively as the concentration of inhaled oxygen increases, but the region of cystic destruction remains constant. (Courtesy of Peter Jakob, Ph.D. of the University of Wuerzburg.)

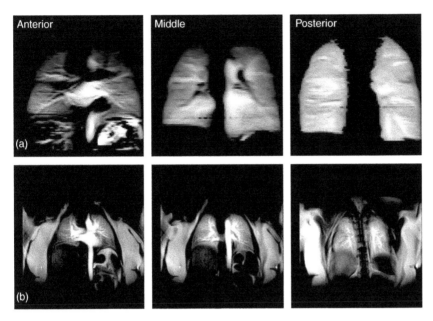

Figure 9.15 Three coronal V/Q images using oxygen-enhanced and gadolinium contrast-enhanced perfusion from a healthy volunteer. Normal ventilation and perfusion in both lungs are observed.

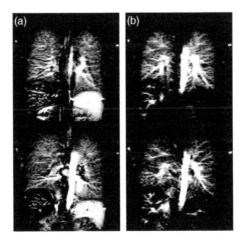

Figure 9.16 V/Q imaging using oxygen-enhanced ventilation and ASL perfusion imaging techniques. (a) MIR-HASTE oxygen ventilation images at two different anatomical positions and (b) corresponding FAIRER perfusion images at the same slice positions of the oxygen-enhanced MIR ventilation images. Normal ventilation and perfusion in both lungs are observed.

tracer such as gadolinium chelates, whereas ASL, originally proposed to measure cerebral blood flow, uses blood water as an endogenous, freely diffusible tracer, and has been successfully demonstrated to image pulmonary perfusion (48–57).

V/Q Imaging in Animal Models

V/Q scanning has been successfully demonstrated in animal models of airway obstruction and pulmonary embolism. Chen et al. (31) used oxygen-enhanced ventilation and gadolinium contrast-enhanced perfusion imaging to investigate the feasibility of the technique in seven Yorkshire pigs and showed matched ventilation and perfusion defects in a porcine model of airway obstruction and mismatched ventilation and perfusion defects in PE as shown in Figs. 9.17 and 9.18, respectively. Preliminary V/Q results, depicted in Fig. 9.19, have also shown promises in using oxygen-enhanced ventilation and ASL techniques called flow-sensitive alternating IR with an extra radiofrequency pulse (FAIRER) to

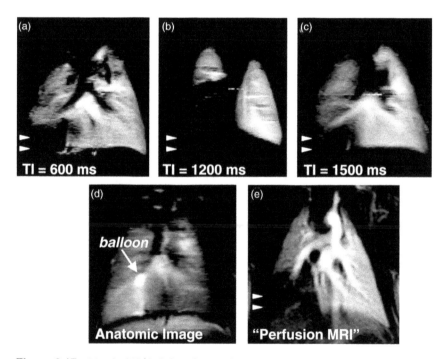

Figure 9.17   Matched V/Q defects in an animal model of airway obstruction. Oxygen-enhanced ventilation images at three different TI of (a) 600 ms, (b) 1200 ms, and (c) 1500 ms show regional ventilation defects in the lower right lung. (d) Anatomical image shows the location of the inflated balloon catheter, and (e) contrast-enhanced perfusion image also shows regional perfusion defect in the lower right lung.

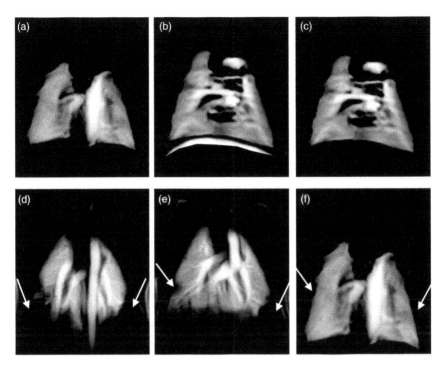

Figure 9.18 Mismatched V/Q defects in an animal model of pulmonary embolism. (a–c) Oxygen-enhanced ventilation images at three different anatomical positions show normal ventilation in both lungs. (d and e) Contrast-enhanced perfusion images at two different slices corresponding to (a) and (b), respectively, show peripheral wedge-shaped perfusion defects in the lower left and right lungs (arrows). (f) Composite of the oxygen-enhanced ventilation images (a–c).

detect matched ventilation and perfusion defects in a porcine model of airway obstruction (33).

V/Q Imaging in Patients

To date, the full clinical potential of V/Q scanning using oxygen-enhanced and contrast-enhanced or ASL perfusion MR has not been studied sufficiently. However, there have been preliminary studies on a limited patient population. Edelman et al. (5) have shown matched ventilation and perfusion defects in patients with emphysema and matched ventilation and perfusion defects in patients diagnosed with PE using oxygen-enhanced and gadolinium contrast-enhanced techniques. V/Q images using oxygen-enhanced and ASL show a matched ventilation and perfusion defect in a patient with Swyer–James syndrome and a mismatched ventilation and perfusion defect in a patient with suspected PE in Fig. 9.20, respectively. The perfusion defects in the ASL images

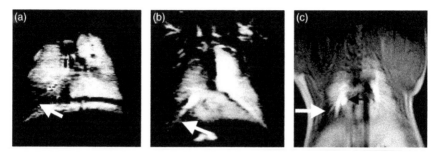

Figure 9.19 V/Q imaging using oxygen-enhanced ventilation and an ASL technique called FAIRER in a porcine model of airway obstruction. As regional pulmonary airway obstruction occurs, blood flow to such area is responsively reduced due to hypoxic vasoconstriction. Consequently, it is expected that both ventilation and perfusion images will exhibit corresponding abnormalities. The balloon catheter is positioned in a bronchiole of the right lung. (a) Ventilation, (b) FAIRER perfusion, and (c) gadolinium perfusion images are shown. Regional matched ventilation and perfusion deficits distal to the balloon catheter are observed between oxygen-enhanced and FAIRER images (arrows). The result in gadolinium perfusion image confirms the finding of regional perfusion defect in FAIRER image.

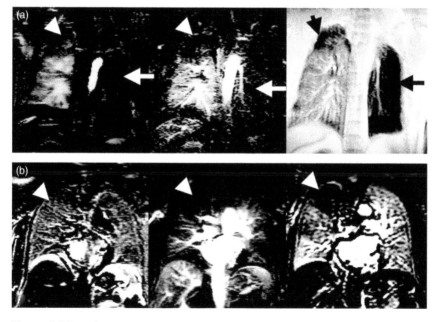

Figure 9.20 V/Q images from patients diagnosed with (a) Swyer–James syndrome and (b) pulmonary embolism. Shown are oxygen-enhanced ventilation (left), ASL (middle), and gadolinium perfusion (right) images. Matched V/Q defects (arrows and arrowheads) are observed in (a) whereas mismatched V/Q defects are detected in (b).

are confirmed by gadolinium contrast-enhanced perfusion images (arrows and arrowheads in Fig. 9.20).

V/Q Ratio of Signal Intensity

The established method to measure the V/Q distribution in the lung is the multiple inert gas elimination technique (MIGET), and the V/Q distribution has a characteristic unimodal logarithmic normal distribution in healthy volunteers, and a matching distribution of ventilation and perfusion over a range of V/Q ratios with the average at ~0.8 (58–60). Another technique, using fluorescent microspheres, can provide high-resolution V/Q scan but is currently limited to experimental studies (61,62).

Assuming that the signal difference in oxygen-enhanced and an ASL techniques called flow-sensitive alternating IR (FAIR) reflects that of ventilation and perfusion, respectively, V/Q ratios of signal intensity on a pixel-by-pixel basis can be determined (Fig. 9.21) and its distribution also shows a unimodal logarithmic normal distribution in healthy volunteers (Fig. 9.22) (63). The V/Q method of oxygen-enhanced ventilation and FAIR perfusion imaging differs from other methods in several ways. The established MIGET technique characterizes the matching of pulmonary ventilation and perfusion, but it does not provide the heterogeneous anatomical distribution of ventilation and perfusion within the lung. Furthermore, its data analysis is complex and time consuming. The fluorescent microsphere technique can provide high-resolution V/Q mapping, but it requires the removal of the lung after the injection of the fluorescent dyes for data measurement. Other V/Q imaging schemes have been proposed using MR imaging but none have determined or mapped V/Q ratios (43–47). Furthermore, hyperpolarized Helium-3 MR imaging may provide information on oxygen uptake by the lungs, as discussed in Chapter 7. Our V/Q imaging technique provides good spatial resolution without the use of radioactive materials. However, it should be emphasized that the V/Q ratios reported here are those of the signal intensity of the oxygen-enhanced ventilation and FAIR perfusion images and not the ratios of the ventilation and perfusion rates as measured in the MIGET technique. To accurately compare our method and MIGET, quantitative measurement of perfusion and ventilation rates should be performed using oxygen-enhanced and FAIR techniques. ASL methods can theoretically quantify pulmonary perfusion rates (53,54,64). Regarding the quantification of ventilation rate, to date, no studies have been proposed to measure ventilation rate with the subjects inhaling 100% oxygen. Therefore, quantitative measurement of V/Q ratios using oxygen-enhanced and ASL techniques requires further studies and development.

C. Dynamic Oxygen-Enhanced Imaging

The progressive increase in signal intensity in the dynamic data acquisition of oxygen-enhanced studies may provide potentially useful information regarding

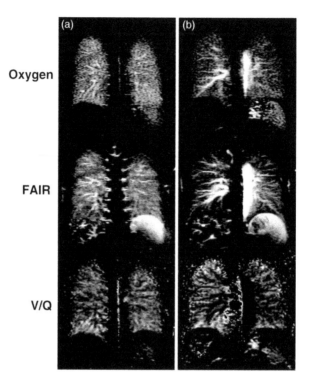

Figure 9.21 Shown are oxygen-enhanced ventilation and FAIR perfusion images at TI of 1200 ms along with the V/Q signal intensity ratio maps from two anatomically different coronal slices (a and b) from the same volunteer. Normal ventilation and perfusion are observed. Good subtraction of the background tissues such as fat and muscle indicates the observed signal enhancement is due to increased oxygen in blood in ventilation and inflowing blood in FAIR perfusion. The V/Q signal intensity ratio maps exhibit heterogeneous distributions in the lung.

the ventilation, diffusion, and perfusion, as the signal changes are the net result of these three factors. Ventilation determines the amount of oxygen being delivered to the lung, diffusion indicates the rate of oxygen crossing from the alveolar air space into blood, and perfusion is the rate of blood flow that carries the oxygenated blood away from the imaging slice. Muller et al. (65) have shown that the mean slopes of the signal intensity are different between healthy volunteers and patients with pulmonary diseases and the slopes correlate with the diffusion capacity of the lung for carbon monoxide (DLco). Ohno et al. (66) have also shown that mean relative enhancement ratios correlate with DLco.

Additional parameters such as time shift and time to peak may be extracted from fitting the dynamic time course of the signal intensities using a mathematical function such as hyperbolic tangent, linear, sine, and so on as shown in

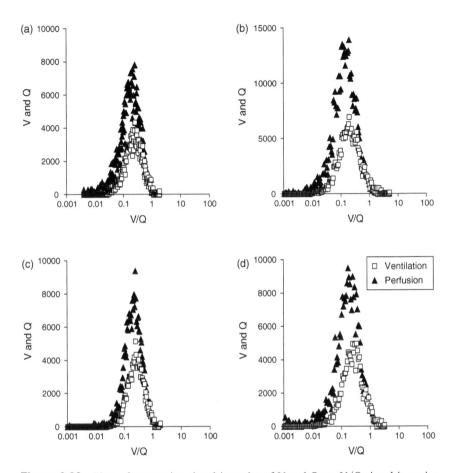

Figure 9.22 Plots of summative signal intensity of V and Q vs. V/Q signal intensity ratio of (a) the left lung that includes large pulmonary vessels, (b) the right lung that includes large pulmonary vessels, (c) the left lung that excludes large pulmonary vessels, and (d) the right lung that excludes large pulmonary vessels. All show characteristic unimodal, logarithmic normal distributions, and matching of ventilation and perfusion over a range of V/Q signal intensity ratios.

Fig. 9.23. The time courses along with the hyperbolic tangent and sine fitting and the resulting pixel-by-pixel maps of these parameters are shown in Fig. 9.24. Together, these may provide complementary and comprehensive regional information that may help in improving the specificity of the diagnosis of pulmonary diseases. While the values of the maps of the difference and the slope have been shown (65,66), the maps of the time shift and time to peak may potentially differentiate between a complete and a partial airway occlusion. However, there has not been any extensive study to evaluate the clinical use of this technique.

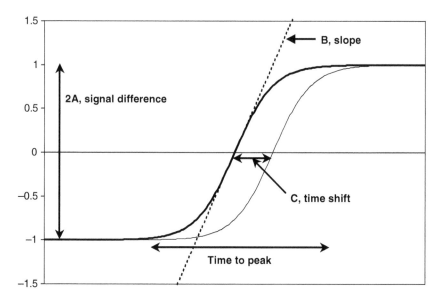

Figure 9.23 A graphic representation of the potentially extracted parameters from a fitted hyperbolic tangent of a time course of signal intensity of a dynamic data acquisition scheme.

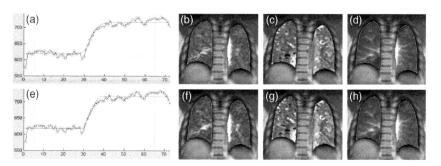

Figure 9.24 (**See color insert**) The dynamic time course of oxygen-enhanced signal intensities of the up-slope ramp. Signal intensity during the period of inhalation of room air progressively increases when oxygen flow was initiated and subsequently reaches steady-state. Shown are (a) the time course of signal intensities with the fitted hyperbolic secant line, (b) the slope map, (c) time shift map, and (d) the difference map. Also shown are (e) the time course of signal intensities with the fitted linear line, (f) the slope map, (g) time shift map, and (h) the difference map. Similar maps between the two different mathematical fits can be observed.

D. Mapping Partial Pressure of Oxygen in the Lung

Oxygen-enhanced imaging offers a promising tool to map regional tissue oxygenation in the lung on the basis of excellent correlation between R_1 of the lung and partial oxygen pressure in water, saline solution (Fig. 9.1), and blood (7–9). However, additional information is needed, such as the hematocrit level, as it has been shown that the T_1 changes are dependent on the hematocrit (67).

VII. Oxygen-Enhanced Imaging at 3.0 T

MRI of the lung at 3.0 T systems poses additional problems, but at the same time offers attractive advantages. As it has already been mentioned, the lung presents a challenging environment for MRI in that its magnetic susceptibility is quite severe due to its large air–tissue interfaces. This magnetic susceptibility worsens as the static magnetic field increases from 1.5 to 3.0 T. However, at higher field, the T_1 of the lung lengthens and the signal-to-noise ratio improves. These would be particularly helpful in oxygen-enhanced imaging. Preliminary experimental results show that oxygen-enhanced ventilation imaging is feasible (Fig. 9.25). Additional work such as shortening of the effective echo time and echo spacing is required to optimize oxygen-enhanced imaging at 3.0 T.

In conclusion, oxygen-enhanced imaging of the lung is a relatively new and exciting means to study gas exchange in the lung and a promising clinical tool for the diagnosis of various pulmonary diseases. It should be noted that MR oxygen-enhanced ventilation imaging is different from hyperpolarized gas imaging in several aspects. The signal of hyperpolarized ^{3}He or ^{129}Xe gas imaging directly reflects the air spaces of the lung, whereas the signal of oxygen ventilation imaging technique arises mainly from the pulmonary tissue water or blood. As a result, oxygen-enhanced MRI is an indirect method of imaging ventilation. In addition, as oxygen plays a major role in functional gas exchange, the technique may provide a means to directly study oxygen transfer from the air

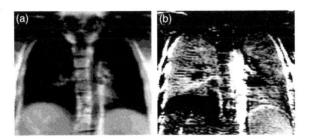

Figure 9.25 (a) A cropped anatomical image of the lung acquired on a 3.0 T MR system using a SSFSE sequence and (b) the corresponding oxygen-enhanced ventilation image are shown. This preliminary result proves that oxygen-enhanced ventilation imaging at 3.0 T is feasible.

space to the pulmonary vasculature. Additionally, oxygen is readily available as part of emergency equipment in most MR suites and is safe and inexpensive. The only limitation, however, is the longer examination time compared with noble gas imaging. Finally, oxygen-enhanced imaging is not limited to studying the lung but also other organs such as the eyes, heart, and kidney (68–72). The oxygen-enhanced MRI technique has the potential to open new therapeutic and diagnostic possibilities and offers itself a powerful tool to study oxygenation in the lung and other organs.

Acknowlegdment

VMM is supported by a grant from the American Heart Association. We sincerely thank Peter Jakob, Ph.D. of the Department of Physics, University of Wuerzburg, Wuerzburg, Germany for his contribution.

References

1. Hayes M, Taplin GV. Lung imaging with radioaerosols for the assessment of airway disease. Semin Nucl Med 1980; 10:243–251.
2. Middleton H, Black RD, Saam B, Cates GD, Cofer GP, Guenther R, Happer W, Hedlund LW, Johnson GA, Juvan K, Swartz J. MR imaging with hyperpolarized ^{3}He gas. Magn Reson Med 1995; 33:271–275.
3. Bachert P, Schad LR, Bock M, Knopp MV, Ebert M, Grobman T, Heil W, Hofmann D, Surkau R, Otten EW. Nuclear magnetic resonance imaging of airways in humans with use of hyperpolarized ^{3}He. Magn Reson Med 1996; 36:192–196.
4. Mugler JP, Driehuys B, Brookeman J, Gates G, Berr SS, Bryant R, Daniel T, de Lange E, Downs J, Eikson C, Harper W, Hinton D, Kassel N, Maier T, Phillips C, Saam B, Sauer K, Wagshul M. MR imaging and spectroscopy using hyperpolarized ^{129}Xe gas: preliminary human results. Magn Reson Med 1997; 38:809–812.
5. Edelman RR, Hatabu H, Tadamura E, Li W, Prasad PV. Noninvasive assessment of regional ventilation in the human lung using oxygen-enhanced magnetic resonance imaging. Nat Med 1996; 2:1236–1239.
6. Chen Q, Jakob PM, Griswold MA, Levin DL, Hatabu H, Edelman RR. Oxygen enhanced MR ventilation imaging of the lung. MAGMA 1998; 7:153–161.
7. Chiarotti G, Cristiani G, Bliulotto L. Proton relaxation in pure liquids and in liquids containing paramagnetic gases in solution. Nuovo Cimento 1955; 1:863–873.
8. Chen Q, Levin D, Mai V, Edelman R, Hatabu H. Magnetic resonance imaging using oxygen as a T1 contrast agent. International Society of Magnetic Resonance in Medicine 7th Annual Meeting, Philadelphia, PA, 1999; p. 2104.
9. Young IR, Clarke GJ, Bailes DR, Pennock JM, Doyle FH, Bydder GM. Enhancement of relaxation rate with paramagnetic contrast agents in NMR imaging. J Comput Tomogr 1981; 5:543–546.
10. Case TA, Durney CH, Ailion DC, Cutillo AG, Morris AH. A mathematical model of diamagnetic line broadening in lung tissue and similar heterogeneous systems: calculations and measurements. J Magn Reson 1987; 73:304–314.

11. Durney CH, Bertolina J, Ailion DC et al. Calculation and interpretation of inhomogeneous line broadening in models of lungs and other heterogeneous structures. J Magn Reson 1989; 85:554–570.

12. Alsop DC, Hatabu H, Bonnet M, Listerud J, Gefter W. Multislice, breathhold imaging of the lung with submillisecond echo times. Magn Reson Med 1995, 33:678–682.

13. Bergin CJ, Pauly JM, Macovski A. Lung parenchyma: projection reconstruction MR imaging. Radiology 1991; 179:777–781.

14. Mayo JR, MacKay A, Muller NL. MR imaging of the lungs: value of short TE spin echo pulse sequences. Am J Roentgenol 1992; 159:951–956.

15. Mai VM, Knight-Scott J, Edelman RR, Chen Q, Keilholz-George S, Berr SS. ^{1}H magnetic resonance imaging of human lung using inversion recovery turbo spin echo. J Magn Reson Imaging 2000; 11:616–21.

16. Mai VM, Knight-Scott J, Berr SS. Improved visualization of the human lung in ^{1}H MRI using multiple inversion recovery to simultaneously suppress signal contributions from fat and muscle. Magn Reson Med 1999; 41:866–870.

17. Mai VM, Chen Q, Li W, Hatabu H, Edelman RR. Effect of respiratory phases on MR lung signal intensity and lung conspicuity using segmented multiple inversion recovery turbo spin echo (MIR-TSE). Magn Reson Med 2000; 43:760–763.

18. Hatabu H, Gaa J, Tadamura E, Edinburgh KJ, Stock KW, Garpestad E, Edelman RR. MR imaging of pulmonary parenchyma with a half-Fourier single shot turbo spin echo (HASTE) sequence. Eur J Radiol 1999; 29:152–159.

19. Mai VM, Chen Q, Bankier AA, Edelman RR. Multiple inversion recovery MR subtraction imaging of human ventilation from inhalation of room air and pure oxygen. Magn Reson Med 2000; 43:913–916.

20. Loffler R, Muller CJ, Peller M, Penzkofer H, Deimling M, Schwaiblmair M, Scheidler J, Reiser M. Optimization and evaluation of the signal intensity change in multisection oxygen-enhanced MR lung imaging. Magn Reson Med 2000; 43:860–866.

21. Muller CJ, Loffler R, Deimling M, Peller M, Reiser M. MR lung imaging at 0.2 T with T_1-weighted true FISP: native and oxygen-enhanced. J Magn Reson Imaging 2001; 14:164–168.

22. Mai VM, Chen Q, Li W, Liu B, Prasad PV, Chen C, Polzin PA, Kurucay S, Tutton S, Edelman RR. Computing correlation maps of the lung in oxygen-enhanced ventilation imaging. Magn Reson Med 2003; 49:591–594.

23. Bandettini PA, Wong EC, Hinks RS, Tikofsky RS, Hyde JS. Time course EPI of human brain function during task activation. Magn Reson Med 1992; 25:390–397.

24. Bandettini PA, Jesmanowicz A, Wong EC, Hyde JS. Processing strategies for time-course data sets in functional MRI of the human brain. Magn Reson Med 1993; 30:161–173.

25. Stock KW, Chen Q, Morrin M, Hatabu H, Edelman RR. Oxygen-enhanced magnetic resonance ventilation imaging of the human lung at 0.2 T and 1.5 T. J Magn Reson Imaging 1999; 9:838–841.

26. Mai VM, Chen Q, Bankier AA, Hatabu H, Edelman RR. Mapping T_1 changes in oxygen-enhanced ventilation imaging in the human lung using MIR. Proceedings of the International Society for Magnetic Resonance in Medicine 8th Annual Meeting, Denver, CO, 2000; p. 2178.

27. Jakob PM, Hillenbrand CM, Wang T, Schultz G, Hahn D, Haase A. Rapid quantitative lung ^{1}H T_1 mapping. J Magn Reson Imaging 2001; 14:795–799.

28. Ogawa S, Lee TM, Kay AR, Tank DW. Brain magnetic resonance imaging with contrast dependent of blood oxygenation. PNAS 1990; 87:9868–9872.

29. Ogawa S, Menon RS, Tank DW, Kim SG, Merkle H, Ellermann JM, Ugurbil K. Functional brain mapping by blood oxygenation level-dependent contrast magnetic resonance imaging. A comparison of signal characteristics with a biophysical model. Biophys J 1993; 64:803–812.

30. Mai VM, Liu B, Li W, Polzin JA, Kurucay S, Chen Q, Edelman RR. Influence of oxygen flow rate on signal and T_1 changes in oxygen-enhanced ventilation imaging. J Magn Reson Imaging 2002; 16:37–41.

31. Chen Q, Levin DL, Kim D et al. Pulmonary disorders: ventilation–perfusion MR imaging with animal models. Radiology 1999; 213:871–879.

32. Nakagawa T, Sakuma H, Murashima S, Ishida N, Matsumura K, Takeda K. Pulmonary ventilation–perfusion MR imaging in clinical patients. J Magn Reson Imaging 2001; 14:419–424.

33. Mai VM, Chen Q, Gladstone S, Li W, Hatabu H, Edelman RR. Noninvasive ventilation–perfusion MR imaging using oxygen and FAIRER in humans and in a porcine model of airway obstruction (abstr). Proceedings of the ISMRM, 7th Annual Meeting, Philadelphia, PA, 1999; p. 137.

34. Mai VM, Bankier AA, Prasad PV et al. MR ventilation–perfusion imaging of human lung using oxygen-enhanced and arterial spin labeling techniques. J Magn Reson Imaging 2001; 14:574–579.

35. Ohno Y, Hatabu H, Takenaka D, Adachi S, Van Cauteren M, Sugimura K. Oxygen-enhanced MR ventilation imaging of the lung: preliminary clinical experience in 25 subjects. Am J Roentgenol 2001; 177:185–194.

36. Krogh A, Lindhard J. The volume of the dead space in breathing and the mixing of gases in the lungs of man. J Physiol 1917; 51:59–90.

37. Haldane JS. Respiration. New Haven, CT: Yale University Press, 1922.

38. Fenn WO, Rahn H, Otis AB. A theoretical study of the composition of alveolar air at altitude. AM J Physiol 1946; 146:637–653.

39. Riley RL, Cournand A. "Ideal" alveolar air and the analysis of ventilation–perfusion relationships in the lungs. J Appl Physiol 1949; 1:825–847.

40. West JB, Wagner PD. Ventilation–perfusion relationships. In: Crystal RG, West JB, Barnes PJ, Cherniack NS, Weibel ER, eds. The Lung: Scientific Foundations. New York: Raven Press, 1991:1289–1305.

41. Amis TC, Crawford ABH, Davison A, Engel LA. Distribution of inhaled ^{99m}technetium-labelled ultrafine carbon particle aerosol (Technegas) in human lungs. Eur Respir J 1990; 3:679–685.

42. Glenny RG, Polissar NL, McKinney S, Robertson HT. Temporal heterogeneity of regional pulmonary perfusion is spatially clustered. J Appl Physiol 1995; 79:986–1001.

43. Berthezene Y, Vexler V, Clement O, Muhler A, Moseley ME, Brasch RC. Contrast-enhanced MR imaging of the lung: assessments of ventilation and perfusion. Radiology 1992; 183:667–672.

44. Cremillieux Y, Berthezene Y, Humblot H, Viallon M, Canet E, Bourgeois M, Albert T, Heil W, Briguet A. A combined ^{1}H perfusion/^{3}He ventilation NMR study in rat lungs. Magn Reson Med 1999; 41:645–648.

45. Viallon M, Berthezene Y, Decorps M, Wiart M, Callot V, Bourgeois M, Humblot H, Briguet A, Cremillieux Y. Laser-polarized ³He as a probe for dynamic regional measurements of lung perfusion and ventilation using magnetic resonance imaging. Magn Reson Med 2000; 44:1–4.

46. Callot V, Canet E, Brochot J et al. Vascular and perfusion imaging using encapsulated laser-polarized helium. MAGMA 2001; 12:16–22.

47. Rizi RR, Roberts DA, Dimitrov IE, Schnall MD, Leigh JS. MRI of pulmonary ventilation/perfusion using hyperpolarized ³He gas and arterial spin-tagging: preliminary results in healthy subjects. Proceedings of the ISMRM, 6th Annual Meeting, Sydney, Australia, 1998; p. 447.

48. Meaney JF, Weg JG, Chenevert TL, Stafford-Johnson D, Hamilton BH, Prince MR. Diagnosis of pulmonary embolism with magnetic resonance. N Engl J Med 1997; 336:1422–1427.

49. Hatabu H, Gaa J, Kim D, Li W, Prassad PV, Edelman RR. Pulmonary perfusion: qualitative assessment with dynamic contrast-enhanced MRI using ultra-short TE and inversion recovery turbo FLASH. Magn Reson Med 1996; 36:503–508.

50. Amundsen T, Kvaerness J, Jones RA, Waage A, Bjermer L, Odegard A, Haraldseth O. Pulmonary embolism: detection with MR perfusion imaging of lung–a feasibility study. Radiology 1997; 203:181–185.

51. Detre JA, Leigh JS, Williams DS, Koretsky AP. Perfusion imaging. Magn Reson Med 1992; 23:37–45.

52. Edelman RR, Siewert B, Darby DG et al. Quantitative mapping of cerebral blood flow and functional localization with echo-planar MR imaging and signal targeting with alternating radio frequency. Radiology 1994; 192:513–520.

53. Kwong KK, Chesler DA, Weisskoff RM et al. MR perfusion studies with T1-weighted echo planar imaging. Magn Reson Med 1995; 34:878–887.

54. Kim SG. Quantification of relative cerebral blood flow change by flow-sensitive alternating inversion recovery (FAIR) technique: application to functional mapping. Magn Reson Med 1995; 34:293–301.

55. Mai VM, Hagspiel KD, Christopher JM et al. Noninvasive MR perfusion imaging of pulmonary parenchyma using flow-sensitive alternating inversion recovery with an extra radiofrequency pulse (FAIRER). Magn Reson Imaging 1999; 17:355–361.

56. Mai VM, Berr SS. MR perfusion imaging of pulmonary parenchyma using pulsed arterial spin labeling techniques: FAIRER and FAIR. J Magn Reson Imaging 1999; 9:483–487.

57. Roberts DA, Gefter WB, Hirsch JA, Rizi RR, Dougherty L, Lenkinski RE, Leigh JS Jr, Schnall MD. Pulmonary perfusion: respiratory-triggered three-dimensional MR imaging with arterial spin tagging—preliminary results in healthy volunteers. Radiology 1999; 212:890–895.

58. Wagner PD, Saltzman HA, West JB. Measurement of continuous distributions of ventilation–perfusion ratios: theory. J Appl Physiol 1974; 36:588–599.

59. Evans JW, Wagner PD. Limits on V_A/Q_A distributions from analysis of experimental inert gas elimination. J Appl Physiol 1977; 42:889–898.

60. Berne RM, Levy MN. Physiology. St. Louis, MO: Mosby Year Book, 1993.

61. Robertson HT, Glenny RB, Stanford D, McInnes LM, Luchtel DL, Covert D. High-resolution maps of regional ventilation utilizing inhaled fluorescent microspheres. J Appl Physiol 1997; 82:943–953.

62. Altemeier WA, Robertson HT, Glenny RB. Pulmonary gas-exchange analysis by using simultaneous deposition of aerosolized and injected microspheres. J Appl Physiol 1998; 85:2344–2351.

63. Mai VM, Liu B, Polzin PA, Li W, Kurucay S, Bankier AA, Knight-Scott J, Madhav P, Edelman RR, Chen Q. Ventilation–perfusion ratio of signal intensity in human lung using oxygen-enhanced and arterial spin labeling techniques. Magn Reson Med 2002; 48:341–350.

64. Mai VM, Chen Q, Edelman RR. Absolute quantification of pulmonary perfusion rates using flow sensitive alternating inversion recovery with an extra radiofrequency pulse (FAIRER). Proceedings of the International Society of Magnetic Resonance in Medicine, 8th Annual Meeting, Denver, CO, 2000; p. 171.

65. Muller CJ, Schwaiblmair M, Scheidler J, Deimling M, Weber J, Loffler RB, Reiser MF. Pulmonary diffusing capacity: assessment with oxygen-enhanced lung MR imaging preliminary findings. Radiology 2002; 222:499–506.

66. Ohno Y, Hatabu H, Takenaka D, Van Cauteren M, Fujii M, Sugimura K. Dynamic oxygen-enhanced MRI reflects diffusing capacity of the lung. Magn Reson Med 2002; 47:1139–1144.

67. Silvennoinen MJ, Kettunen MI, Kauppinen RA. Effects of hematocrit and oxygen saturation level on blood spin–lattice relaxation. Magn Reson Med 2003; 49:568–571.

68. Ito Y, Berkowitz BA. MR studies of retinal oxygenation. Vision Res 2001; 41:1307–1311.

69. Berkowitz BA. Role of dissolved plasma oxygen in hyperoxia-induced contrast. Magn Reson Imaging 1997; 15:123–126.

70. Berkowitz BA, Wilson CA. Quantitative mapping of ocular oxygenation using magnetic resonance imaging. Magn Reson Med 1995; 33:579–581.

71. Fidler F, Hirn S, Wacker CM, Bauer WR, Jakob PM, Haase A. Quantitative assessment of myocardial perfusion in human heart under rest and adenosine induced stress breathing room air and oxygen at 2 Tesla. Proceedings of the International Society of Magnetic Resonance in Medicine, 10th Annual Meeting, Honolulu, HI, 2002; p. 514.

72. Jones RA, Ries M, Moonen C, Grenier N. Functional imaging of the kidneys using inhalation of pure O_2: a feasibility study. Proceedings of the International Society of Magnetic Resonance in Medicine, 9th Annual Meeting, Glasgow, Scotland, 2002; p. 523.

10

MR Angiography and Direct Thrombus Imaging for Diagnosis of Pulmonary Embolism

EDWIN J. R. VAN BEEK

University of Iowa,
Iowa City, Iowa, USA
University of Sheffield,
Sheffield, UK

MATTHIJS OUDKERK

State University Hospital,
Groningen, The Netherlands

I. Introduction

Pulmonary embolism (PE) is proved in approximately 0.5 per 1000 population annually, with an estimated 600,000 cases in the United States alone (1,2). Of these, 90% of patients will reach hospital to allow a diagnosis to be made. Recently, it has been proposed to classify PE as massive, submassive, or non-massive PE, according to clinical severity at the time of presentation (3). Less than 5% of patients will suffer from massive PE and these patients benefit from rapid (thrombolytic) intervention using echocardiography as (bed-side) diagnostic test (3). A small subgroup of patients will present with submassive PE, that is, those with echocardiographic signs of right ventricular dysfunction.

There is some evidence that more aggressive therapy may be indicated in these patients (4–6), but further studies are required. However, the vast majority of cases will have nonmassive (hemodynamically stable) PE and can undergo standard diagnostic tests.

Overall, only ~20–40% of patients who were initially suspected of PE will have their diagnosis confirmed (7–10). Thus, the group without disease is much larger than those with disease. The reference method, pulmonary angiography, is invasive and carries a (small) complication risk (11) and is not likely to be performed in up to 20% of patients in many institutions (12). Traditionally, the diagnostic management of PE was largely concentrated around lung scintigraphy. A normal perfusion lung scan result effectively rules out PE, whereas a high-probability lung scan carries a positive predictive value of 90% (7–11,13). In the large remaining group of patients (40–60%), the lung scan does not give a conclusive, diagnostic result. Novel, noninvasive tests have been developed to try and avoid angiography, including plasma D-dimer (10,14,15), ultrasonography of the leg veins (15,16), and most importantly helical/spiral computed tomography (hCT) with CT-pulmonary angiography with or without extended CT venography of the pelvis and leg veins (17,18). These tests have been tried in several diagnostic strategies, and satisfactory results are reported, but these strategies are based on local availability, local expertise, and circumstances (7–10,15–22). More details of the diagnostic strategies can be found in the chapter on PE later in this book (Chapter 23). Although these strategies may work well, their main concerns are complexity, invasive nature, use of nephrotoxic contrast agents, and almost universal need for ionizing radiation.

Magnetic resonance imaging (MRI) of the chest is a relatively new development, which needed to overcome technical challenges such as motion of heart and lungs, lack of protons for signal, and magnetic susceptibility or air–soft tissue interfaces. Contrast-enhanced MR has solved many of these issues for imaging of pulmonary arteries using relatively safe contrast agents, whereas direct thrombus MRI involves no contrast injection at all. Advances in computing, gradient strengths, and magnetic resonance hardware have enabled the use of these techniques even in breathless patients.

II. Magnetic Resonance Angiography

A. Techniques

Several methods may be employed to perform magnetic resonance angiography (MRA), ranging from time-of-flight angiography to Gadolinium-enhanced 3D MRA. Initially, time-of-flight MRA was applied with some success for imaging of the central pulmonary arteries, but the spatial resolution was insufficient, there was inherent insensitivity to slow flow, respiratory and pulsation artifacts were difficult to correct, and field distortion artifacts were further degrading the image quality (23–26). Although another noncontrast-enhanced sequence used variable angle uniform signal excitation during free breathing (3D-VUSE), this was not developed into a population of patients with PE (27).

Single breath-hold 3D contrast-enhanced MRA was developed after the introduction of improved gradient strength systems (>30 mT/m) and the development of short repetition time 3D gradient echo sequences (Fig. 10.1) (28–30). Another innovation that is currently under investigation is the application of parallel imaging techniques which greatly improve the speed of data acquisition (31–33). Recently, these techniques have become available for imaging of the pulmonary vasculature (34,35).

With improvements in technique, hardware, and image sequence, breath-hold times were gradually reduced from 30 s to <10 s (29,30,34–41). Thus, the potential role of MRA in breathless patients has increased, as the image quality has improved because of the decreased reliance on a prolonged breath-hold.

B. Hardware and Software Requirements

High-performance gradient systems with amplitudes >20 mT/m and slew rates >120 mT/m per ms have enabled the development of ultrafast, short breath-hold MRA. Table 10.1 describes some of the recently documented image sequences employed (41,42). The introduction of high gradient strength systems (40 mT/m) and increased slew rates, that can now be obtained (200 mT/m per ms), has resulted in a significant reduction of breath-hold time. It has become

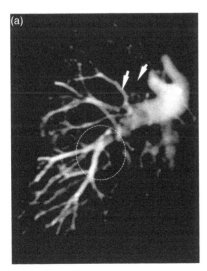 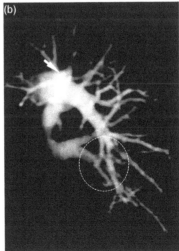

Figure 10.1 Corresponding conventional pulmonary angiogram and gadolinium-enhanced 3D MRA in a patient with PE.

Table 10.1 Contrast-Enhanced 3D MR Pulmonary Angiography Techniques as Described in the Literature (40,41)

Scan parameter	1.5 T unit with enhanced gradients (40)	1.5 T unit with high-performance 3-axial gradients (41)
Field-of-view (minimum)	200×320 mm	360×360 mm
Matrix	90–106×512	140×256
Flow compensation	No	No
Breath-hold	Yes, 2×15 s	Yes, 5×4 s (19 s total)
Slab thickness	125 mm Sagital	110 mm
Encoded partitions	44	40
Reconstructed images	100	100
Slice thickness	1.25 mm	2.75 mm
Coil	Phased array body	Phased array body
Scan mode	3D	3D
Scan technique	Fast low angle single shot	
TE (ms)	1.6	0.6
TR (ms)	3.65	1.64
Flip angle (degrees)	25	15
Bandwidth readout	390 Hz/pixel	1295 Hz/pixel
Encoding	Center of data at half scan time	
Test bolus	4 mL	No
Contrast total volume	20 mL For each lung	20 mL
Contrast injection	2 mL/s, 10 s Each lung	3 mL/s, Saline flush
Mode of injection	Biphasic: 1 mL/s 5 s, 2 ml/s remainder	
Scan duration	40 s	3.74 s per dataset (×5)

feasible to image both lungs in a single breath-hold and following a single contrast bolus.

Gadolinium is the most commonly used exogenous MR contrast agent. Gadolinium should be injected using a power injector and is generally followed by a saline flush (41). A dose range of 0.1–0.3 mmol/kg has been attempted, but general consensus is that a dose of 0.2 mmol/kg is optimal and that increasing this dose does not enhance image quality (42,43). Gadolinium concentration should be optimal at the time of central k-space acquisition, as this will determine the vascular signal intensity. In standard sequences, the center of k-space will be sampled in the second half of the imaging time, whereas spiral sequences will sample the center of k-space during the first one-third of the imaging time (44). In sequences that require prolonged second breath-holding, a trial bolus is advocated to optimize the delay between contrast injection and imaging (40). However, in ultrafast imaging sequences this is no longer required in the majority of patients and a routine delay time of 5 s following the initiation of contrast injection will result in excellent quality images in patients with suspected acute PE (45).

An alternative method, which is less reliant on (ultra)short imaging and/or breath-holding, is the use of contrast agents which remain in circulation for prolonged periods of time (Fig. 10.2) (46,47). These blood pool agents allow repeated data acquisition and also open the possibility of extending the imaging protocol to the deep venous system of the pelvis and lower extremities (47). Although several agents are under development and undergoing initial clinical tests, the results are not sufficient to suggest their clinical usefulness at present.

Image analysis should be performed on a workstation. This allows maximal use of post-processing techniques such as volume rendering, maximum intensity projections, and multiplanar reformatting (48). Although these techniques allow for a 3D evaluation, one should also evaluate the source data to ensure that post-processing has not altered essential data (such as small filling defects).

C. Clinical Applications

Only a limited number of clinical studies have evaluated the role of 3D gadolinium-enhanced MRA for the diagnosis of PE in reasonable patient samples. The first study to compare MRA with pulmonary angiography was performed by Loubeyre et al. (28), who obtained a sensitivity of 70% and a

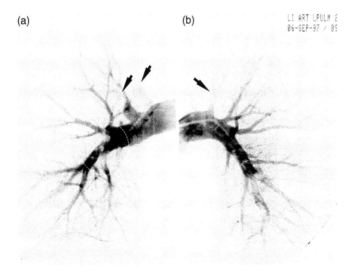

(a)   (b)   LI ART LPULM   06-SEP-97 / 09

Figure 10.2 Selective pulmonary angiogram of same subject as Fig. 10.1, demonstrating corresponding pulmonary emboli. (Images courtesy of Prof. A.R. Moody, Toronto, Canada.)

specificity of 100% in a group of 23 patients with PE. A study by Isoda et al. (36) evaluated 3D gadolinium-enhanced MRA in 13 patients, but these patients suffered from a variety of lung disorders other than PE.

A ground-breaking study was performed by Meaney et al. (39), who investigated the performance of a coronal gadolinium-enhanced 3D time-of-flight sequence during a single breath-hold in 30 patients with suspected PE. A total of eight patients had pulmonary emboli demonstrated by angiography. The study design included independent assessment of MRA by three radiologists and the use of pulmonary angiography as reference standard. In 10% of patients, the images were of insufficient quality to be diagnostic. The interobserver correlation was good to excellent (kappa values of 0.57–0.83), while sensitivity and specificity of MRA for PE for the remaining 27 patients varied between 75–100% and 95–100%, respectively (39). Some of the criticisms of this study were possible selection bias (no subsegmental emboli were diagnosed) and the fact that many patients with suspected PE would not be able to hold their breath for 27 s.

An alternative approach is to use MRA in conjunction with other diagnostic tests. Thus, using perfusion lung scintigraphy to safely exclude PE seems a cost-effective and sensible approach in terms of availability of diagnostic tests. One study took place in 36 consecutive patients with intermediate or low probability lung scan result and high clinical suspicion (49). Patients underwent pulmonary angiography and MRA, and assessment of these investigations was independent. A total of 19 emboli was demonstrated in 13 patients by angiography, and MRA diagnosed 12 patients as PE (one false positive; specificity 96%) and missed two cases (sensitivity 85%). Both missed pulmonary emboli were isolated and subsegmental in location.

A more recent study performed contrast-enhanced 3D MR pulmonary angiography in 141 consecutive patients with an abnormal perfusion lung scintigram and compared the findings with pulmonary angiography (40). A double contrast injection was employed with a 20 s breath-hold for each lung. MRA was contraindicated in 13 patients (9%), whereas images were not interpretable in eight patients (6%). MRA could be performed in two patients in whom conventional pulmonary angiography was contraindicated. Thus, both MRA and pulmonary angiography were available in 118 patients (84%). The prevalence of PE was 30%, partially as a result of exclusion by normal scintigraphy as initial test. Images were read independently in 115 patients, and agreement was obtained in 105 cases (91%), with a kappa value of 0.75. MRA demonstrated 27 of 35 patients with confirmed emboli for an overall sensitivity of 77%. The sensitivity for isolated subsegmental, segmental, and central/lobar PE was 40%, 84%, and 100%, respectively. MRA demonstrated emboli in two patients with a normal angiogram for a specificity of 98%. These latter two studies demonstrate the difficulty of diagnosing isolated subsegmental pulmonary emboli, while the sensitivity for segmental or larger emboli is high (40,49). Isolated subsegmental emboli are relatively uncommon, occurring between 6% and

15% of cases (7,40,49,50). These results are comparable with the early (single detector spiral) CT data in the literature (13,17).

Most recently, the use of a very fast imaging technique with the use of the newest gradient systems (1.5 T, amplitude 40 mT/m, slew rate 200 mT/m per ms) has resulted in a gadolinium-enhanced 3D MRA sequence that can be performed in <4 s per image dataset, with five datasets acquired within a 19 s breath-hold (41). The sequence has been tested in three healthy volunteers and eight patients with dyspnea and demonstrated emboli in all four subsequently confirmed cases, whereas those without emboli were also adequately identified. A problem was that only two of the eight patients could hold their breath for 19 s, whereas all patients could hold their breath for 8 s, during which time two datasets were acquired.

It is concluded that 3D gadolinium-enhanced MRA may offer a fast, reliable test for the diagnosis of PE, but further studies will be required to confirm this. In particular, management studies will need to demonstrate the additional value of MRA, especially in terms of cost-effectiveness. The use of blood pool agents to image the entire venous system may be useful in the future.

III. Direct Thrombus Imaging

Direct thrombus imaging is based on the principle that $T1$ changes over time are predictable (51,52). Thus, it is possible to perform a subtraction image leaving only the signal of clot, without the need for gadolinium-based contrast agents, which can be applied in PE and deep vein thrombosis (Figs. 10.3 and 10.4) (53,54). One of the potential pitfalls is that the $T1$ value will eventually equal that of normal (flowing) blood, rendering the technique susceptible to the aging process of blood clots.

Initial pilot studies employed an MRI sequence consisting of a $T1$-weighted magnetization-prepared 3D gradient echo sequence. A water-only excitation radiofrequency pulse was administered, and the effective inversion time was chosen to nullify the blood signal. Using a body coil, two imaging blocks resulted in coverage from ankle to inferior vena cava, with each block requiring 3.5 min acquisition time (55). Subsequently, a study applied this technique in 101 patients with suspected deep vein thrombosis and compared with contrast venography (56). Although the cohort was not a consecutive group of patients, the authors prevented selection bias by including all patients with a positive venogram and randomly selecting 25% of patients who had a normal venogram result. Images were reviewed independently, and sensitivity and specificity were in the range of 94–96% and 90–92%, respectively. The interobserver agreement was formally assessed, and kappa values of greater than 0.8 were obtained. As could be expected, the diagnostic accuracy for isolated calf vein thrombosis was slightly lower than that for ileofemoral thrombosis, yielding a sensitivity range of 83–92%.

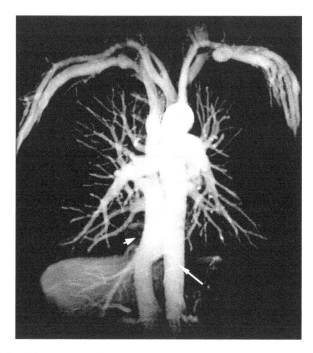

Figure 10.3 Pulmonary angiogram using an experimental blood pool agent (NC100150), demonstrating both arterial and venous systems in one image. This is the result of the prolonged imaging time and the recirculation of the contrast agent.

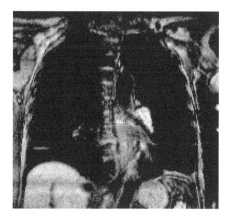

Figure 10.4 MR direct thrombus imaging, demonstrating central PE. (Images courtesy of Prof. A.R. Moody, Toronto, Canada.)

The same technique is currently applied in a randomized clinical management study, comparing direct thrombus MRI as single test with the following three management strategies: (1) lung scintigraphy followed by ultrasonography of the deep venous system of the leg, if the lung scan is nondiagnostic; (2) same as strategy 1, but with pulmonary angiography as final diagnostic test, if ultrasonography was normal; (3) helical CT pulmonary angiography (57).

Recently, interim results of the study were presented, with 157 patients randomized to undergo management solely based on MR direct thrombus imaging (57). A total of 33 patients (21%) did not undergo MR investigations because of various reasons such as having a pacemaker, claustrophobia, or for logistical reasons. This feasibility of 80% is similar to that shown for conventional pulmonary angiography (12). Eight patients died during the follow-up period, but none of these deaths were due to thromboembolism. Furthermore, no clinically overt episodes of recurrent disease were encountered in the negative group, nor were there incidences of bleeding in the positive group. PE was detected directly in the positive group in 19 patients (Fig. 10.5) and by the presence of deep vein thrombosis alone in 13 for a total incidence of venous thromboembolism of 32 patients (25%), which corresponds well with the literature. The outcome of the MR direct thrombus imaging management protocol was similar to that of the other management strategies. If these results can be reproduced, it would show that MR direct thrombus imaging could replace other technologies in the management of venous thromboembolic diseases and provide a comprehensive, essentially noninvasive, imaging technique.

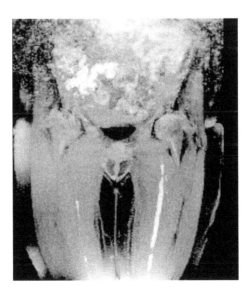

Figure 10.5 Concurrent left lower limb deep venous thrombosis. (Images courtesy of Prof. A.R. Moody, Toronto, Canada.)

IV. Conclusions

MRA and direct thrombus MRI are two techniques which offer potential for the evaluation of suspected PE in the future. Several demands will still need to be met, most notably an increase in the available MR table time. Although initial results have shown excellent diagnostic accuracy, the main competitor for this modality remains (multidetector) CT angiography. This latter technique offers better sensitivity and specificity at present, while the availability of CT is also better in almost every hospital. Nevertheless, further developments in this area of MRI technology need to be encouraged in order to prepare for the future. A diagnostic strategy including MRI can currently be advocated for pregnant patients, where ionizing radiation is a particular concern. Furthermore, patients who require regular follow-up, for instance, those with chronic thromboembolic pulmonary hypertension and those at increased risk of incomplete clot resolution (e.g., those with familial thrombophilia), could benefit from repeated MRA to evaluate vessel patency and clot resolution.

References

1. van Beek EJR, ten Cate JW. The diagnosis of venous thromboembolism: an overview. In: Hull RD, Raskob GE, Pineo GF, eds. Venous Thromboembolism: An Evidence-Based Atlas. Armonk: Futura Publishing Co., 1996:93–99.
2. Hirsh J, Hoak J. Management of deep vein thrombosis and pulmonary embolism. A statement for health professionals. Council on Thrombosis (In Consultation with the Council on Cardiovascular Radiology), American Heart Association. Circulation 1996; 93:2212–2245.
3. ESC Task Force on Pulmonary Embolism. Guidelines on management of acute pulmonary embolism. Eur Heart J 2000; 21:1301–1336.
4. Goldhaber SZ, Haire WD, Feldstein ML et al. Alteplase versus heparin in acute pulmonary embolism: randomised trial assessing right-ventricular function and pulmonary perfusion. Lancet 1993; 341:507–511.
5. Konstantinides S, Geibel A, Olschewski M et al. Association between thrombolytic treatment and the prognosis of hemodynamically stable patients with major pulmonary embolism. Circulation 1997; 96:882–888.
6. Konstantinides S, Geibel A, Heusel G, Heinrich F, Kasper W et al. Heparin plus alteplase compared with heparin alone in patients with submassive pulmonary embolism. N Engl J Med 2002; 347:1143–1150.
7. The PIOPED Investigators. Value of the ventilation-perfusion scan in acute pulmonary embolism. JAMA 1990; 263:2753–2759.
8. van Beek EJR, Kuijer PMM, Büller HR, Brandjes DPM, Bossuyt PMM, ten Cate JW. The clinical course of patients with suspected pulmonary embolism. Arch Intern Med 1997; 157:2593–2598.
9. Wells PS, Ginsberg JS, Anderson DR et al. Use of a clinical model for safe management of patients with suspected pulmonary embolism. Ann Intern Med 1998; 129:997–1005.

10. Perrier A, Desmarais S, Miron MJ et al. Noninvasive diagnosis of venous thromboembolism. Lancet 1999; 353:190–195.
11. van Beek EJR, Brouwers E, Song B, Stein PD, Oudkerk M. Clinical validity of a normal pulmonary angiogram in patients with suspected pulmonary embolism—a critical review. Clin Radiol 2001; 56:838–842.
12. van Beek EJR, Reekers JA, Batchelor D, Brandjes DPM, Peeters FLM, Büller HR. Feasibility, safety and clinical utility of angiography in patients with suspected pulmonary embolism and non-diagnostic lung scan findings. Eur Radiol 1996; 6:415–419.
13. van Beek EJR, Brouwers EMJ, Bongaerts AH, Oudkerk M. Lung scintigraphy and helical computed tomography in the diagnosis of pulmonary embolism: a meta-analysis. Clin Appl Thromb Hemost 2001; 7:87–92.
14. van Beek EJR, Schenk BE, Michel BC, van den Ende A, van der Heide YT, Brandjes DPM, Bossuyt PMM, Büller HR. The role of plasma D-dimer concentration in the exclusion of pulmonary embolism. Br J Hematology 1996; 92:725–732.
15. Perrier A, Bounameaux H, Morabia A et al. Diagnosis of pulmonary embolism by a decision analysis-based strategy including clinical probability, D-dimer levels, and ultrasonography: a management study. Arch Intern Med 1996; 156:531–536.
16. Turkstra F, Kuijer PMM, van Beek EJR, Brandjes DPM, Büller HR, ten Cate JW. Value of compression ultrasonography for the detection of deep venous thrombosis in patients suspected of having pulmonary embolism. Ann Intern Med 1997; 126:775–781.
17. Ghaye B, Remy J, Remy-Jardin M. Non-traumatic thoracic emergencies: CT diagnosis of acute pulmonary embolism: the first 10 years. Eur Radiol 2002; 12:1886–1905.
18. Ghaye B, Dondelinger RF. Non-traumatic thoracic emergencies: CT venography in an integrated diagnostic strategy of acute pulmonary embolism and venous thrombosis. Eur Radiol 2002; 12:1906–1921.
19. Oudkerk M, van Beek EJR, Van Putten WLJ, Büller HR. Cost-effectiveness analysis of various strategies in the diagnostic management of pulmonary embolism. Arch Intern Med 1993; 153:947–954.
20. Ginsberg JS. Management of venous thromboembolism. N Engl J Med 1998; 335:1816–1823.
21. Goodman LR, Lipchik RJ, Kuzo RS, Liu Y, McAuliffe RL, O'Brien DJ. Subsequent pulmonary embolism: risk after a negative helical CT pulmonary angiogram—prospective comparison with scintigraphy. Radiology 2000; 215:535–542.
22. Tillie-Leblond I, Mastora I, Radenne F et al. Risk of pulmonary embolism after a negative spiral CT angiogram in patients with pulmonary disease: 1-year clinical follow-up study. Radiology 2002; 223:461–467.
23. MacFall JR, Sostman HD, Foo TKF. Thick-section, single breath-hold magnetic resonance pulmonary angiography. Invest Radiol 1992; 27:318–322.
24. Kauczor HU, Gamroth AH, Tuengerthal S et al. MR angiography: clinical applications in thoracic surgery. Eur Radiol 1992; 2:214–222.
25. Wielopolski P, Haacke E, Adler L. Evaluation of the pulmonary vasculature with three-dimensional magnetic resonance imaging techniques. MAGMA 1993; 1:21–34.

26. Schiebler ML, Holland GA, Hatabu H et al. Suspected pulmonary embolism: prospective evaluation with pulmonary MR angiography. Radiology 1993; 189:125–131.

27. Friedli JL, Paschal CB, Loyd JE, Halliburton SS. Quantitative 3D VUSE pulmonary MRA. Magn Reson Imag 1999; 17:363–370.

28. Loubeyre P, Revel D, Douek P et al. Dynamic contrast enhanced MR angiography of pulmonary embolism: comparison with pulmonary angiography. Am J Roentgenol 1994; 162:1035–1039.

29. Leung D, McKinnon G, Davis C, Pfammatter T, Krestin G, Debatin J. Breath-hold, contrast-enhanced, three-dimensional MR angiography. Radiology 1996; 201:569–571.

30. Steiner P, McKinnon GC, Romanowski B, Goehde SC, Hany T, Debatin JF. Contrast-enhanced, ultrafast 3D pulmonary MR angiography in a single breath-hold: initial assessment of imaging performance. J Magn Reson Imaging 1997; 7:177–182.

31. Sodickson DK, Manning WJ. Simultaneous acquisition of spatial harmonics (SMASH): fast imaging with radiofrequency coil arrays. Magn Reson Med 1997; 38:591–603.

32. Pruessmann KP, Weiger M, Scheidegger MB, Boesiger P. SENSE: sensitivity encoding for fast MRI. Magn Reson Med 1999; 42:952–962.

33. Weiger M, Pruessmann KP, Kassner A, Roditi G, Lawton T, Reid A, Boesiger P. Contrast-enhanced 3D MRA using SENSE. J Magn Reson Imaging 2000; 12:671–677.

34. Fujii M, Ohno Y, Kawamitsu H et al. Multiphase 3D contrast-enhanced MRA of the lung using SENSE. Proc ISMRM 2002:1780.

35. Nikolaou K, Schoenberg SO, Nittka M et al. Magnetic resonance imaging in the diagnosis of pulmonary arterial hypertension: high resolution angiography and fast perfusion imaging using intelligent parallel acquisition techniques (iPAT). Radiology 2002; 225(P):473.

36. Isoda H, Ushimi T, Masui T et al. Clinical evaluation of pulmonary 3D time-of-flight MRA with breath-holding using contrast media. J Comput Assist Tomogr 1995; 19:911–919.

37. Wielopolski P, Hicks S, Obdeijn AIM, Oudkerk M. PE detection using contrast-enhanced breathhold 3D magnetic resonance angiography. Preliminary experience. Proc ISMRM 1996; 2:705.

38. Leung DA, Debatin JF. Three-dimensional contrast-enhanced magnetic resonance angiography of the thoracic vasculature. Eur Radiol 1997; 7:981–989.

39. Meaney JFM, Weg JG, Chenevert TL et al. Diagnosis of pulmonary embolism with magnetic resonance angiography. N Engl J Med 1997; 336:1422–1427.

40. Oudkerk M, van Beek EJR, Wielopolski P et al. Comparison of contrast-enhanced MRA and DSA for the diagnosis of pulmonary embolism: results of a prospective study in 141 consecutive patients with an abnormal perfusion lung scan. Lancet 2002; 359:1643–1647.

41. Goyen M, Laub G, Ladd ME et al. Dynamic 3D MR angiography of the pulmonary arteries in under four seconds. J Magn Reson Imaging 2001; 13:372–377.

42. Boos M, Lentschig M, Scheffler K, Bongartz GM, Steinbrich W. Contrast enhanced magnetic resonance angiography of peripheral vessels. Different contrast agent applications and sequence strategies: a review. Invest Radiol 1998; 33:538–546.

43. Hany TF, Schmidt M, Hilfiker PR, Steiner P, Bachmann U, Debatin JF. Optimization of contrast dosage for gadolinium enhanced 3D MRA of the pulmonary and renal arteries. Magn Reson Imaging 1998; 16:901–906.

44. Maki JH, Prince MR, Londy FJ, Chenevert TL. The effects of time varying intravascular signal intensity and k space acquisition order on three dimensional MR angiography image quality. J Magn Reson Imaging 1996; 6:642–651.

45. Kauczor HU. Contrast-enhanced magnetic resonance angiography of the pulmonary vasculature. A review. Invest Radiol 1998; 33:606–617.

46. Abolmaali ND, Hietschold V, Appold S, Ebert W, Vogl TJ. Gadomer-17-enhanced 3D navigator-echo MR angiography of the pulmonary arteries in pigs. Eur Radiol 2002; 12:692–697.

47. Hoffmann U, Loewe C, Bernhard C et al. MRA of the lower extremities in patients with pulmonary embolism using a blood pool contrast agent: initial experience. J Magn Reson Imaging 2002; 15:429–437.

48. Davis CP, Hany TF, Wildermuth S, Schmidt M, Debatin JF. Postprocessing techniques for gadolinium enhanced three-dimensional MR angiography. Radiographics 1997; 17:1061–1077.

49. Gupta A, Frazer CK, Ferguon JM et al. Acute pulmonary embolism: diagnosis with MR angiography. Radiology 1999; 210:353–359.

50. Oser RF, Zuckermann DA, Gutierrez FR, Brink JA. Anatomic distribution of pulmonary emboli at pulmonary angiography: implications for cross-sectional imaging. Radiology 1996; 199:31–35.

51. Cohen MD, McGuire W, Cory DA, Smith JA. MR appearance of blood and blood products: an in vitro study. Am J Roentgenol 1986; 146:1293–1297.

52. Sostman D, Pope CF, Smith GJW, Carbo P, Core JC. Proton relaxation in experimental clots varies with the method of preparation. Invest Radiol 1987; 22:509–512.

53. Moody AR, Liddicoat A, Krarup K. Magnetic resonance pulmonary angiography and direct imaging of embolus for the detection of pulmonary emboli. Invest Radiol 1997; 32:431–440.

54. Moody AR, Pollock JG, O'Connor AR, Bagnall M. Lower-limb deep venous thrombosis direct MR imaging of the thrombus. Radiology 1998; 209:349–355.

55. Moody AR. Direct imaging of deep vein thrombosis with magnetic resonance imaging. Lancet 1997; 350:1073.

56. Fraser DGW, Moody AR, Morgan PS, Martel AL, Davidson I. Diagnosis of lower-limb deep venous thrombosis: a prospective blinded study of magnetic resonance direct thrombus imaging. Ann Intern Med 2002; 136:89–98.

57. Moody AR, Crossley I, Moorby S, Delay G. Magnetic resonance direct thombus imaging (MRDTI) as a first line investigation for pulmonary embolism—the PDQ trial. In: Proceedings of the 11th Annual Scientific Meeting of ISMRM, Toronto, Canada, 2003.

11

Gadolinium-Enhanced MR Perfusion Imaging

YOSHIHARU OHNO

Kobe University Graduate
   School of Medicine,
Kobe, Japan

HIROTO HATABU

Beth Israel Deaconess Medical Center and
   Harvard Medical School,
Boston, Massachusetts, USA

I. Introduction

To be effective at gas exchange, the lung cannot act in isolation; the lung must interact with the central nervous system (which provides the rhythmic drive to breathe), the diaphragm, and muscular apparatus of the chest wall (which respond to signals from the central nervous system and act as a bellows for movement of air), and the circulatory system (which provides blood flow and, therefore, gas transport between the tissues and the lungs). The processes of oxygen uptake and carbon dioxide elimination by the lungs depend on the proper functioning of all affected systems, and a disturbance in any of them can result in clinically important abnormalities in gas transport and arterial blood gases.

Matched distribution of regional pulmonary blood flow (perfusion) and ventilation is required for this process to occur efficiently (1). The large amount of ventilation in lungs is matched by correspondingly high perfusion; 100% of the cardiac output from the right ventricle goes to the lungs. The balance between pulmonary perfusion and ventilation alters in various states. In pulmonary disease, the normal pattern of pulmonary blood flow is often changed, sometimes exacerbating the disturbance in gas exchange (2,3). Therefore, assessment of these changes in regional perfusion patterns is important to understand the physiology and the pathophysiology of the lung. Currently, multiple methods are available to quantitatively evaluate pulmonary perfusion.

Regional pulmonary perfusion has been evaluated in normal subjects and patients using nuclear medicine studies requiring radioactive macroaggregates (2–6). The scintigraphic method is an established clinical tool; however, it is limited by poor spatial and temporal resolution, artifacts from diaphragm and breast tissue, or overlap due to projection. In addition, clinical utility is hampered within the setting of pulmonary embolism due to a frequent occurrence of indeterminate studies (7). Moreover, absolute quantification of pulmonary perfusion by radionuclide scanning requires arterial sampling and correction for tissue attenuation of gamma radiation emitted by technetium-99m. Although positron emission tomography (PET) with O-15 water can measure the absolute pulmonary perfusion (4), it requires a cyclotron for production of tracer with an extremely short half-life (2 min).

MR imaging provides higher spatial and temporal resolution than any of the techniques described earlier. However, until recently, MR imaging of lung parenchyma has not been comprehensively pursued for several reasons. Although air-soft tissue interfaces of lung parenchyma facilitate gas exchange (8), these air-soft tissue interfaces produce extremely heterogeneous magnetic susceptibility in the lung, resulting in a reduction of the MR signal. Moreover, intrinsic low proton density, respiratory and cardiac motion, pulmonary perfusion, and molecular diffusion are other factors which decrease the signal from lung parenchyma (9). In recent years, an ultra-short echo time (TE) spin-echo (10), single-shot fast spin-echo (SE) sequence (11), and gradient-echo (12,13) has enabled MR imaging of the pulmonary parenchyma despite the short T_2^* of lung tissue. Projection reconstruction techniques, in which the data are acquired during the free induction decay, have also been introduced to lung imaging (14). These developments in MR imaging now provide a platform for MR perfusion imaging of the lung.

Thus far, two major techniques have been used for MR perfusion imaging. The more widely studied technique utilizes fast scanning of the lung parenchyma following an intravenous bolus injection of gadolinium (Gd). An alternative MR perfusion technique known as arterial spin labeling (ASL) or spin tagging, requires no exogenous contrast agent, an important advantage of this protocol.

In this chapter, we review Gd contrast-enhanced MR perfusion imaging of the lung, whereas ASL is described in Chapter 6.

II. First-Pass Contrast Agent Technique—Basics

As previously stated, MR imaging of lung parenchyma has been hampered by the extremely heterogeneous magnetic susceptibility of the lung, which derives from its unique architecture of multiple air-soft tissue interfaces (8). Although essential for gas exchange, these air-soft tissue interfaces produce large magnetic field gradients that dephase the MR signal. The T_2^* value of the lung parenchyma is very short, ranging from 0.9 to 2.2 ms (13). Moreover, intrinsic low proton density, respiratory and cardiac motion, pulmonary blood flow, and molecular diffusion are other factors which also reduce the signal from lung parenchyma (14). However, the accurate assessment of pulmonary perfusion is required to evaluate various diseases including pulmonary embolism, pulmonary arteriovenous malformation (AVM) and lung cancer.

The recent development in MR imaging of pulmonary parenchyma has proved feasible despite the short T_2^* of lung tissue by using contrast-enhanced dynamic MR imaging using gradient-echo (8–10). Two-dimensional (2D) T_1-weighted ultra-short repetition time (TR) and TE MR imaging with contrast agents has emerged as a platform for visualization of lung perfusion (15–17). Breath-hold three-dimensional (3D) contrast-enhanced MR imaging with short TR and TE has also been proven to be useful (18–22). After the bolus administration of a low dose gadopentetate dimeglumine (Gd-DTPA), the pulmonary arterial tree was visualized beyond the segmental branches, followed by a gradual diffuse increase in the signal intensity of the lung parenchyma by using both 2D and 3D contrast-enhanced MR imaging techniques (Fig. 11.1). Both the pulmonary perfusion and the pulmonary vasculature were depicted in a single breath-hold with this technique. To clearly demonstrate the difference between the pulmonary circulation and the systemic circulation of pulmonary parenchyma, a 5 mL/s injection rate is recommended for *in vivo* studies (21).

III. Basics of Quantitative Assessment of Pulmonary Perfusion Imaging

Using signal intensity–time course curves, quantitative assessment of regional pulmonary perfusion parameters have been reported by a few investigators using 2D dynamic contrast-enhanced MR imaging in pulmonary embolic pig models and humans (16,17,21). Quantitative analysis of dynamic contrast-enhanced MR imaging was attempted based on the indicatory dilution principle similar to that used in PET examinations. The quantitative indices [the inverse of apparent mean transit time ($1/\tau_{app}$), distribution volume (V), and V/τ_{app}] were obtained. In order to exact quantitative indices, the signal intensity time curves

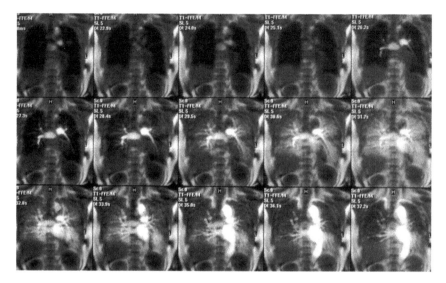

Figure 11.1 3D dynamic contrast-enhanced MR perfusion imaging (TR 2.7 ms/TE 0.7 ms/flip angle 30°, 120 mm slab thickness, 12 partition, 128 × 128 matrix, 45 cm FOV) in 32-year-old male normal volunteer. After bolus administration of low dose GD-DTPA followed by 20 mL saline, the pulmonary arterial tree was visualized beyond the segmental branches followed by a faint diffuse blush of lung parenchyma. Diffuse gradual increase in signal intensity of lung parenchyma was observed. Temporal resolution of dynamic contrast-enhanced MR perfusion imaging is every 1.1 s.

were fitted to a gamma variate function (23) described by the equation:

$$C_{\text{tissue}}(t) = \kappa(t)^{\alpha}e^{St/\beta} \tag{11.1}$$

where t is the time, $C_{\text{tissue}}(t)$ is the measured signal intensity as a function of time which is related to the concentration of the agent; κ is a constant scale factor, α and β are parameters that define the shape of the curve. From the fitted values for α and β one could deduce perfusion indices such as time to reach peak concentration [t_p] and apparent mean transit time (τ_{app}) as follows:

$$t_p = \alpha\beta \tag{11.2}$$
$$\tau_{\text{app}} = \beta(\alpha + 1) \tag{11.3}$$

Additionally, from measurements of the tissue concentration curve [$C_{\text{tissue}}(t)$], and arterial concentration curves [$C_{\text{arterial}}(t)$], the distribution volume of the agent was calculated directly as follows:

$$V = \frac{\oint_0^{\infty} C_{\text{tissue}}(t)\,\mathrm{d}t}{\oint_0^{\infty} C_{\text{arterial}}(t)\,\mathrm{d}t} \tag{11.4}$$

The central volume principle (24) relates the terms perfusion (f), blood tissue partition coefficient (ρ), and the mean transit time (τ):

$$f = \frac{\rho}{\tau} \tag{11.5}$$

The principle applies to any agent, whether it is extracted from the blood or not. We assumed that contrast media behaves as an intravascular agent during the first pass. Therefore, the mean transit time equals τ_{app} and the partition coefficient can be determined as V by MR.

$$f = \frac{\rho}{\tau} = \frac{V}{\tau_{app}} \tag{11.6}$$

Therefore, by using quantitative analysis of regional pulmonary perfusion, we are able to assess the physiology and pathophysiology of lung diseases more precisely than by using qualitative analysis of regional pulmonary perfusion.

IV. Animal Studies of Contrast-Enhanced MR Perfusion Imaging

From late 1990s to early 2000s, some investigators tried to demonstrate the utility of dynamic contrast-enhanced MR perfusion imaging for assessment of regional pulmonary perfusion and analysis of pulmonary perfusion abnormalities in animal models with pulmonary embolism (15,16,25–28).

Regarding qualitative assessment of pulmonary perfusion abnormalities, Chen et al. (25) examined MR ventilation and perfusion imaging using oxygen-enhanced MR imaging and dynamic contrast-enhanced MR perfusion imaging of pulmonary embolic and bronchial obstructed pig models. In this study, MR imaging was shown to clearly demonstrate ventilation–perfusion mismatch. Other investigators demonstrated dynamic MR perfusion imaging with and without contrast enhancement (26–28). Dynamic contrast-enhanced MR perfusion imaging can demonstrate higher signal-to-noise ratio (SNR), and visualize regional perfusion abnormalities with higher image quality than non-contrast-enhanced MR perfusion imaging.

Hatabu et al. (15,16) compared $f = V/\tau_{app}$ with the absolute perfusion obtained with the colored microsphere technique. In addition, V and $1/\tau_{app}$ were also correlated with the absolute values of perfusion. The f, V, and $1/\tau_{app}$ correlated well with the absolute lung perfusion (15) (Fig. 11.2). Recently, parametric mapping of lung perfusion was attempted (17). The τ_{app}, V, and f were calculated for each voxel. Quantitative measurements can be obtained to place ROIs on these parametric maps (17). This quantitative analysis demonstrated slightly faster τ_{app} in the lung apex compared with the lung base.

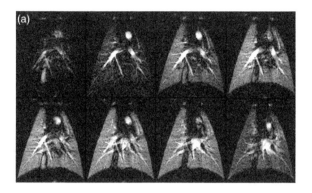

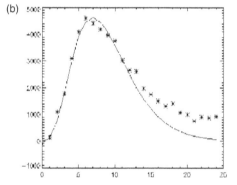

Figure 11.2   2D perfusion MR imaging (TR 6.3 ms/TE 1.3 ms/flip angle 45°, 10 mm section thickness, 128 × 128 matrix, 24 cm FOV) of lung in a pig model. (a) Five milliliter of Gd-DTPA is administered, followed by a 20 mL saline flush. Eight selected coronal images are shown from the total of 40 coronal images obtained every 0.8 s in the plane of the pulmonary hila. (b) Example of region of interest generated in lung field and gamma variate fit of signal intensity–time course curve. Graph shows change in MR imaging signal intensity (∗) following injection of contrast media and gamma variate fit (line) for first pass.

V.   *In Vivo* Study of Contrast-Enhanced MR Perfusion Imaging

Recently, qualitative assessment of pulmonary perfusion has been adapted for various pulmonary diseases (19–22,29–35). Some investigators adapted the 2D or 3D dynamic contrast-enhanced MR imaging technique to demonstrate feasibility and for characterization of pulmonary perfusion abnormalities in pneumonia, chronic obstructive pulmonary disease, and pulmonary embolism patients (29–35). However, these studies only demonstrated the capability of dynamic contrast-enhanced MR imaging to visualize pulmonary perfusion abnormalities, and did not show the clinical utility of this technique. Therefore, we have adapted 3D dynamic contrast-enhanced MR perfusion imaging technique for assessment of therapeutic effect of embolotherapy of pulmonary AVM, characterization of solitary pulmonary nodules (SPNs), and management of SPNs to demonstrate its clinical utility (19,20).

In pulmonary AVM patients, assessment of the nidus blood supply following embolotherapy can currently only be achieved by dynamic contrast-enhanced MR perfusion imaging due to its temporal and spatial resolution, although multidetector CT technology is increasing imaging speed (Fig. 11.3) (19). This information is very important for follow-up study of post-embolized pulmonary AVM, as the nidus represents the arterial-to-venous anastomosis, which is the

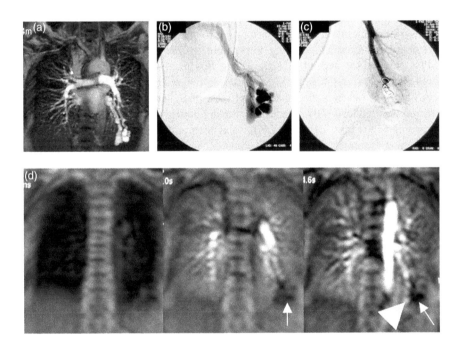

Figure 11.3 A 51-year-old female with pulmonary AVM in left lower lobe. (a) Pretherapeutic contrast-enhanced MR angiography clearly demonstrates simple-type pulmonary AVM. Diameter of aneurysmal sac is 15 mm. Diameters of feeding artery and draining vein are 7 and 10 mm, respectively. (b) Pretherapeutic pulmonary angiogram shows simple-type pulmonary AVM. Diameter of aneurysmal sac is 15 mm. Diameters of feeding artery and draining vein are 7 and 10 mm, respectively. (c) Follow-up angiogram shows successful embolotherapy. (d) Follow-up contrast-enhanced MR perfusion images (L to R; $t = 0$ s, $t = 5.5$ s, $t = 11.0$ s) demonstrates nonenhanced area in left lower lobe (arrow) which does not have pulmonary arterial blood supply. The post occluded pulmonary AVM (arrow head) is enhanced at 11.0 s. The post occluded pulmonary AVM has a blood supply from systemic circulation considered to be bronchial artery-to-pulmonary artery collateral flow.

main site of recurrence and rupture of pulmonary AVM. Therefore, when embolotherapy is performed, pulmonary AVM patients are advised to undergo dynamic contrast-enhanced MR perfusion imaging as a follow-up study (19).

Another promising result of qualitative assessment of dynamic contrast-enhanced MR perfusion imaging is its use in the characterization and management of SPNs (20). Considering the characterization and management of SPN, which is one of the most common findings on chest radiographs, many investigators have evaluated the radiological features, blood supply, and metabolism of SPNs to differentiate malignant SPN from benign SPN, and demonstrated promising results using computed tomography, MR imaging, and PET with 2-[fluorine-18]-fluoro-2-deoxy-D-glucose (FDG) (36–39). However, significant overlap between malignant SPNs and benign SPNs were observed in all studies. Recent advances in MR sequences can now demonstrate the pulmonary and systemic circulation in the entire lung by using 3D radio-frequency spoiled gradient-echo imaging, making it possible to analyze the hemodynamics of SPNs (Figs. 11.4 and 11.5) (20). Using this technique, the overlap between malignant SPN and benign SPNs, such as tuberculoma and hamartoma, was not observed, whereas the overlap between malignant SPN and active inflammation was reduced (20). In addition, the diagnostic capability of this technique is similar to that of FDG-PET, and can differentiate SPNs into two

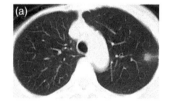

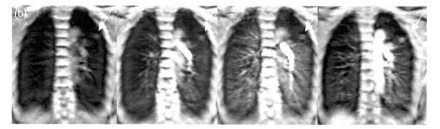

Figure 11.4 A 73-year-old female lung cancer patient with SPN in left upper lobe. (a) Chest routine computed tomograph (lung window setting) shows small nodule with pleural indentation in the left upper lobe. (b) Dynamic MR images (L to R; $t = 0$ s, $t = 5.5$ s, $t = 9.9$ s, $t = 11.0$ s) demonstrate enhancement in the left upper lobe. Maximum relative enhancement is 0.64 and slope of enhancement is 0.12 s^{-1}. Therefore, dynamic MR imaging can diagnose as a malignant SPN requiring further intervention and treatment according to Ohno et al. (20).

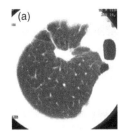

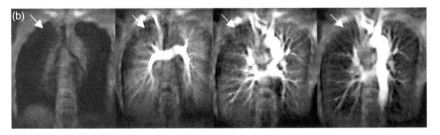

Figure 11.5 A 54-year-old male patient with tuberculoma in the right upper lobe. (a) Chest thin-section computed tomograph (lung window setting) shows nodule in the right upper lobe. (b) Dynamic MR images (L to R; $t = 0$ s, $t = 5.5$ s, $t = 9.9$ s, $t = 13.2$ s) demonstrate enhancement in the right upper lobe. Maximum relative enhancement is 0.2 and slope of enhancement is 0.02 s^{-1}. Therefore, dynamic MR imaging can diagnose a benign SPN requiring no further evaluation according to Ohno et al. (20).

categories: those requiring subsequent intervention or treatment and those requiring no treatment with high diagnostic precision (20). Thus, qualitative assessment of perfusion within the SPN by using dynamic contrast-enhanced MR pulmonary perfusion imaging technique may play an important role in the future management of SPNs.

A few investigators have reported the qualitative assessment of regional pulmonary perfusion parameters in humans (17,21,22). Levin et al. (17) adapted 2D dynamic contrast-enhanced MR perfusion imaging technique, the indicator dilution theory and the central volume principle for assessment of mean transit time, relative regional pulmonary perfusion and blood volume, and demonstrated preliminary experience in normal volunteers. Ohno et al. (22) adapted 3D dynamic contrast-enhanced MR perfusion imaging technique using the same theory and principle for comparison of regional pulmonary perfusion and capability of prediction of post-operative lung function with perfusion scintigraphy in 60 lung cancer patients. In our study, when compared with perfusion scintigraphy, a very high correlation of regional perfusion between 3D dynamic contrast-enhanced MR perfusion imaging and perfusion scintigraphy was obtained ($r = 0.84$, $p < 0.0001$), and the limits of agreement between the two methods were between -5.2% and 8.0%, and small enough for clinical purposes (22).

Moreover, the correlation between actual post-operative lung function and predicted post-operative lung function by 3D dynamic contrast-enhanced MR perfusion imaging was also excellent ($r = 0.93$, $p < 0.0001$), and slightly better than that between actual post-operative lung function and predicted post-operative lung function by perfusion scintigraphy ($r = 0.89$, $p < 0.0001$). In addition, the mean and limits of agreement between actual post-operative lung function and predicted post-operative lung function by 3D dynamic contrast-enhanced MR perfusion imaging were between -9.5% and 11.3%, smaller than those between actual post-operative lung function and predicted post-operative lung function by perfusion scintigraphy, and small enough for clinical purposes (22). Thus, 3D dynamic contrast-enhanced MR perfusion imaging may be able to substitute pulmonary perfusion scintigraphy in clinical situations, such as pretreatment assessment of lung cancer.

VI. Limitations of Dynamic Contrast-Enhanced MR Perfusion Imaging

When assessing regional pulmonary perfusion by using dynamic contrast-enhanced MR imaging, there are some limitations.

Concerning qualitative assessment, the spatial resolution of dynamic contrast-enhanced MR perfusion imaging has been limited. To overcome this limitation, a higher gradient system at 1.5 T permits dynamic acquisition of 3D MR data sets of the entire pulmonary tree in <4 s for qualitative assessment of pulmonary circulation, and in <1.2 s for semiquantitative and quantitative assessment of pulmonary circulation in the entire lung (18–22). Although the increased slew rate of this gradient system is limited in clinical situations, the newly developed parallel imaging techniques such as sensitivity encoding (22) have been introduced as a promising technique to improve temporal resolution for assessment of pulmonary circulation (22). SENSE has been introduced to reduce image acquisition time and increase spatial resolution for various MR imaging techniques such as diffusion weighted imaging, MR angiography, and conventional MR imaging (40–49). SENSE permits unfolding of reduced-field of view (FOV) images (i.e., images obtained by equal reduction in FOV and the number of phase-encoding steps) into a full FOV image with commensurate reductions in imaging time and maintenance of spatial resolution by using multiple surface coils, each with its own receiver circuit, and operating in a phased-array configuration. Therefore, SENSE makes it possible to enhance spatial resolution and time resolution of contrast-enhanced 3D pulmonary MR imaging without increasing acquisition time or the need for high-performance gradient systems, and also makes it convenient to use dynamic contrast-enhanced MR perfusion imaging in clinical settings (22).

On the other hand, the quantitative assessment of pulmonary perfusion parameters has been limited due to the need for adaptation of the indicator dilution theory and central volume principle similar to cerebral perfusion, soft tissue perfusion, and cardiac perfusion studies (50–57). First, direct application of these principles to contrast-enhanced, first-pass dynamic perfusion MR imaging experiments is difficult, although indicator dilution theories are frequently used to determine regional blood volume and regional blood flow by various perfusion MR imaging techniques. Regional blood volume can be determined by direct calculation of the area under the observed tissue concentration curve. However, the calculated regional blood flow and mean transit time is less straightforward. Wisskoff et al. (50,52) pointed out that the use of the central volume principle to calculate mean transit time for locations within a tissue volume is incorrect. This is because MRI signal intensity changes for specific tissue regions of interest reflect the tracer concentration remaining within the tissue rather than that leaving the tissue. Secondly, the method also assumes that the signal intensity observed is linearly related to the concentration of contrast within the blood. Theoretically, this relationship is not linear. However, over a limited range of contrast concentrations this appears to be sufficiently linear to be valid (56). Thirdly, the model used also assumes that the contrast agent remains within the intravascular space (55). To the extent that the contrast agent acts as a pure intravascular marker, the volume of distribution will reflect the blood volume. As mentioned, preliminary studies found a strong correlation between blood volume divided by apparent mean transit time, which is an MR imaging measure of regional flow, and regional perfusion as measured with microspheres (15). Similar results were obtained by Wilke et al. (51,53) who were able to obtain a quantitative assessment of myocardial perfusion using similar techniques. This suggests that indicator dilution techniques can provide measures of regional blood flow despite these limitations. Recently, several blood pool contrast agents have been introduced mainly for research purposes. The use of blood pool agents ensures the acquisition of consistent high spatial-resolution pulmonary angiography images with equal vascular contrast (58–61). A single injection of blood pool contrast agent demonstrated the potential for the acquisition of pulmonary perfusion and angiographic imaging with sufficient SNRs and without noticeable artifact (58–61). Although the application for routine clinical practice is still limited, blood pool contrast agents may have an important role in perfusion MR imaging of the lung.

VII. Conclusions

Dynamic contrast-enhanced MR perfusion imaging of the lung is increasingly useful in clinical settings. Although the first-pass contrast agent technique method is minimally invasive and associated with risks and expenses for contrast administration, this technique is simple and easily applied in the clinical setting. Moreover, dynamic contrast-enhanced MR perfusion imaging has the potential for quantitative assessment of regional pulmonary perfusion parameters and analysis of the physiology and pathophysiology of the lung.

References

1. Wagner HN Jr. The use of radioisotope techniques for the evaluation of patients with pulmonary disease. Am Rev Respir Dis 1976; 113:203–218
2. Schuster DP. ARDS: clinical lessons from the oleic acid model of acute lung injury. Am J Respir Crit Care Med 1994; 149:245–260.
3. Pistolesi M, Miniati M, Di Ricco G, Marini C, Giuntini C. Perfusion lung imaging in the adult respiratory distress syndrome. J Thorac Imaging 1986; 1:11–24.
4. Schuster DP, Kaplan JD, Gauvain K, Welch MJ, Markham J. Measurement of regional pulmonary blood flow with PET. J Nucl Med 1995; 36:371–377.
5. Nyren S, Mure M, Jacobsson H, Larsson SA, Lindahl SG. Pulmonary perfusion is more uniform in the prone than in the supine position: scintigraphy in healthy humans. J Appl Physiol 1999; 86:1135–1141.
6. Wilson JE III, Bynum LJ, Ramanathan M. Dynamic measurement of regional ventilation and perfusion of the lung with Xe-133. J Nucl Med 1977; 18:660–668.
7. The PIOPED Investigators. Value of the ventilation/perfusion scan in acute pulmonary embolism. Results of the prospective investigation of pulmonary embolism diagnosis (PIOPED). JAMA 1990; 263:2753–2759.
8. Hatabu H, Chen Q, Stock KW, Gefter WB, Itoh H. Fast magnetic resonance imaging of the lung. Eur J Radiol 1999; 29:114–132.
9. Bergin CJ, Glover GM, Pauly J. Magnetic resonance imaging of lung parenchyma. J Thorac Imaging 1993; 8:12–17.
10. Mayo JR, MacKay A, Muller NL. MR imaging of the lungs: value of short TE spin-echo pulse sequences. AJR Am J Roentgenol 1992; 159:951–956.
11. Hatabu H, Gaa J, Tadamura E et al. MR imaging of pulmonary parenchyma with a half-Fourier single-shot turbo spin-echo (HASTE) sequence. Eur J Radiol 1999; 29:152–159.
12. Alsop DC, Hatabu H, Bonnet M, Listerud J, Gefter W. Multi-slice, breathhold imaging of the lung with submillisecond echo times. Magn Reson Med 1995; 33:678–682.
13. Hatabu H, Alsop DC, Listerud J, Bonnet M, Gefter WB. T2* and proton density measurement of normal human lung parenchyma using submillisecond echo time gradient echo magnetic resonance imaging. Eur J Radiol 1999; 29:245–252.
14. Bergin CJ, Pauly JM, Macovski A. Lung parenchyma: projection reconstruction MR imaging. Radiology 1991; 179:777–781.
15. Hatabu H, Gaa J, Kim D, Li W, Prasad PV, Edelman RR. Pulmonary perfusion: qualitative assessment with dynamic contrast-enhanced MRI using ultra-short TE and inversion recovery turbo FLASH. Magn Reson Med 1996; 36:503–508.
16. Hatabu H, Tadamura E, Levin DL, Chen Q, Li W, Kim D, Prasad PV, Edelman RR. Quantitative assessment of pulmonary perfusion with dynamic contrast-enhanced MRI. Magn Reson Med 1999; 42:1033–1038.
17. Levin DL, Chen Q, Zhang M, Edelman RR, Hatabu H. Evaluation of regional pulmonary perfusion using ultrafast magnetic resonance imaging. Magn Reson Med 2001; 46:166–171.
18. Hatabu H, Gaa J, Kim D, Li W, Prasad PV, Edelman RR. Pulmonary perfusion and angiography: evaluation with breath-hold enhanced three-dimensional fast imaging

steady-state precession MR imaging with short TR and TE. AJR Am J Roentgenol 1996; 167:653–655.

19. Ohno Y, Hatabu H, Takenaka D, Adachi S, Hirota S, Sugimura K. Contrast-enhanced MR perfusion imaging and MR angiography: utility for management of pulmonary arteriovenous malformations for embolotherapy. Eur J Radiol 2002; 41:136–146.

20. Ohno Y, Hatabu H, Takenaka D, Adachi S, Kono M, Sugimura K. Solitary pulmonary nodules: potential role of dynamic MR imaging in management initial experience. Radiology 2002; 224:503–511.

21. Ohno Y, Kawamitsu H, Higashino T et al. Time-resolved contrast-enhanced pulmonary MR angiography using sensitivity encoding (SENSE). J Magn Reson Imaging 2003; 17:330–336.

22. Ohno Y, Hatabu H, Higashino T et al. Dynamic perfusion MRI versus perfusion scintigraphy: prediction of postoperative lung function in patients with lung cancer. Am J Roentgenol 2004; 182:73–78.

23. Thompson HK Jr, Starmer CF, Whalen RE, Mcintosh HD. Indicator transit time considered as a gamma variate. Circ Res 1964; 14:502–515.

24. Meier P, Zierler Kl. On the theory of the indicator-dilution method for measurement of blood flow and volume. J Appl Physiol 1954; 6:731–744.

25. Chen Q, Levin DL, Kim D et al. Pulmonary disorders: ventilation-perfusion MR imaging with animal models. Radiology 1999; 213:871–879.

26. Suga K, Ogasaware N, Matsunaga N, Sasai K. Perfusion characteristics of oleic acid—injured canine lung on Gd-DTPA—enhanced dynamic magnetic resonance imaging. Invest Radiol 2001; 36:386–400.

27. Suga K, Ogasawara N, Okada M, Matsunaga N, Arai M. Regional lung functional impairment in acute airway obstruction and pulmonary embolic dog models assessed with gadolinium-based aerosol ventilation and perfusion magnetic resonance imaging. Invest Radiol 2002; 37:281–291.

28. Ogasawara N, Suga K, Karino Y, Matsunaga N. Perfusion characteristics of radiation-injured lung on Gd-DTPA-enhanced dynamic magnetic resonance imaging. Invest Radiol 2002; 37:448–457.

29. Amundsen T, Torheim G, Waage A, Bjermer L, Steen PA, Haraldseth O. Perfusion magnetic resonance imaging of the lung: characterization of pneumonia and chronic obstructive pulmonary disease. A feasibility study. J Magn Reson Imaging 2000; 12:224–231.

30. Torheim G, Amundsen T, Rinck PA, Haraldseth O, Sebastiani G. Analysis of contrast-enhanced dynamic MR images of the lung. J Magn Reson Imaging 2001; 13:577–587.

31. Nakagawa T, Sakuma H, Murashima S, Ishida N, Matsumura K, Takeda K. Pulmonary ventilation-perfusion MR imaging in clinical patients. J Magn Reson Imaging 2001; 14:419–424.

32. Matsuoka S, Uchiyama K, Shima H et al. Detectability of pulmonary perfusion defect and influence of breath holding on contrast-enhanced thick-slice 2D and on 3D MR pulmonary perfusion images. J Magn Reson Imaging 2001; 14:580–585.

33. Amundsen T, Torheim G, Kvistad KA et al. Perfusion abnormalities in pulmonary embolism studied with perfusion MRI and ventilation-perfusion scintigraphy: an intra-modality and inter-modality agreement study. J Magn Reson Imaging 2002; 15:386–394.

34. Iwasawa T, Saito K, Ogawa N, Ishiwa N, Kurihara H. Prediction of postoperative pulmonary function using perfusion magnetic resonance imaging of the lung. J Magn Reson Imaging 2002; 15:685–692.

35. Seo JB, Im JG, Goo JM et al. Comparison of contrast-enhanced ct angiography and gadolinium-enhanced MR angiography in the detection of subsegmental-sized pulmonary embolism. An experimental study in a pig model. Acta Radiol 2003; 44:403–410.

36. Patz EF Jr, Lowe VJ, Hoffman JM et al. Focal pulmonary abnormalities: evaluation with F-18 fluorodeoxyglucose PET scanning. Radiology 1993; 188:487–490.

37. Gupta NC, Maloof J, Gunel E. Probability of malignancy in solitary pulmonary nodules using fluorine-18-FDG and PET. J Nucl Med 1996; 37:943–948.

38. Dewan NA, Shehan CJ, Reeb SD, Gobar LS, Scott WJ, Ryschon K. Likelihood of malignancy in a solitary pulmonary nodule: comparison of Bayesian analysis and results of FDG-PET scan. Chest 1997; 112:416–422.

39. Goo JM, Im JG, Do KH et al. Pulmonary tuberculoma evaluated by means of FDG PET: findings in 10 cases. Radiology 2000; 216:117–121.

40. Pruessmann KP, Weiger M, Scheidegger MB, Boesiger P. SENSE: sensitivity encoding for fast MRI. Magn Reson Med 1999; 42:952–962.

41. Weiger M, Pruessmann KP, Boesiger P. Cardiac real-time imaging using SENSE. Sensitivity Encoding scheme. Magn Reson Med 2000; 43:177–184.

42. Golay X, Pruessmann KP, Weiger M et al. PRESTO-SENSE: an ultrafast whole-brain fMRI technique. Magn Reson Med 2000; 43:779–786.

43. Weiger M, Pruessmann KP, Kassner A et al. Contrast-enhanced 3D MRA using SENSE. J Magn Reson Imaging 2000; 12:671–677.

44. Weiger M, Pruessmann KP, Leussler C, Roschmann P, Boesiger P. Specific coil design for SENSE: a six-element cardiac array. Magn Reson Med 2001; 45:495–504.

45. Golay X, Brown SJ, Itoh R, Melhem ER. Time-resolved contrast-enhanced carotid MR angiography using sensitivity encoding (SENSE). AJNR Am J Neuroradiol 2001; 22:1615–1619.

46. Bammer R, Keeling SL, Augustin M et al. Improved diffusion-weighted single-shot echo-planar imaging (EPI) in stroke using sensitivity encoding (SENSE). Magn Reson Med 2001; 46:548–554.

47. Sodickson DK, McKenzie CA. A generalized approach to parallel magnetic resonance imaging. Med Phys 2001; 28:1629–1643.

48. Pruessmann KP, Weiger M, Boesiger P. Sensitivity encoded cardiac MRI. J Cardiovasc Magn Reson 2001; 3:1–9.

49. Dydak U, Weiger M, Pruessmann KP, Meier D, Boesiger P. Sensitivity-encoded spectroscopic imaging. Magn Reson Med 2001; 46:713–722.

50. Weisskoff RM, Chesler D, Boxerman JL, Rosen BR. Pitfalls in MR measurement of tissue blood flow with intravascular tracers: which mean transit time? Magn Reson Med 1993; 29:553–558.

51. Wilke N, Simm C, Zhang J, Ellermann J, Ya X, Merkle H, Path G, Ludemann H, Bache RJ, Ugurbil K. Contrast-enhanced first pass myocardial perfusion imaging: correlation between myocardial blood flow in dogs at rest and during hyperemia. Magn Reson Med 1993; 29:485–497.

52. Weisskoff RM, Zuo CS, Boxerman JL, Rosen BR. Microscopic susceptibility variation and transverse relaxation: theory and experiment. Magn Reson Med 1994; 31:601–610.

53. Wilke N, Jerosch-Herold M, Stillman AE et al. Concepts of myocardial perfusion imaging in magnetic resonance imaging. Magn Reson Q 1994; 10:249–286.
54. Sinha S, Sinha U, Czernin J, Porenta G, Schelbert HR. Noninvasive assessment of myocardial perfusion and metabolism: feasibility of registering gated MR and PET images. AJR Am J Roentgenol 1995; 164:301–307.
55. Donahue KM, Weisskoff RM, Burstein D. Water diffusion and exchange as they influence contrast enhancement. J Magn Reson Imaging 1997; 7:102–110.
56. Jerosch-Herold M, Wilke N, Stillman AE. Magnetic resonance quantification of the myocardial perfusion reserve with a Fermi function model for constrained deconvolution. Med Phys 1998; 25:73–84.
57. Maeda M, Yuh WT, Ueda T et al. Severe occlusive carotid artery disease: hemodynamic assessment by MR perfusion imaging in symptomatic patients. AJNR Am J Neuroradiol 1999; 20:43–51.
58. Berthezene Y, Vexler V, Price DC et al. Magnetic resonance imaging detection of an experimental pulmonary perfusion deficit using a macromolecular contrast agent. Polylysine-gadolinium-DTPA40. Invest Radiol 1992; 27:346–351.
59. Ahlstrom KH, Johansson LO, Rodenburg JB, Ragnarsson AS, Akeson P, Borseth A. Pulmonary MR angiography with ultrasmall superparamagnetic iron oxide particles as a blood pool agent and a navigator echo for respiratory gating: pilot study. Radiology 1999; 211:865–869.
60. Weishaupt D, Hilfiker PR, Schmidt M, Debatin JF. Pulmonary hemorrhage: imaging with a new magnetic resonance blood pool agent in conjunction with breathheld three-dimensional magnetic resonance angiography. Cardiovasc Intervent Radiol 1999; 22:321–325.
61. Zheng J, Carr J, Harris K et al. Three-dimensional MR pulmonary perfusion imaging and angiography with an injection of a new blood pool contrast agent B-22956/1. J Magn Reson Imaging 2001; 14:425–432.

12

Proton Perfusion Imaging

TAE IWASAWA

Kanagawa Cardiovascular and Respiratory Center,
Yokohama, Japan

I. Introduction

This chapter is divided into four sections that focus on methodology: perfusion imaging with contrast material, perfusion imaging with arterial spin labeling (ASL), proton perfusion imaging, and gas imaging. The first three techniques use a signal from protons. In this chapter, proton perfusion imaging is strictly defined as a method that employs flow-related "signal change" mainly due to dephasing of protons. While no extrinsic contrast materials are used in proton perfusion imaging, the author will distinguish proton perfusion imaging from ASL, which uses magnetically labeled water in blood as an endogenous, freely diffusible contrast agent (1,2). Proton perfusion imaging of the lung parenchyma is divided into two groups, one uses intrinsic signal change only accompanied by cardiac contraction (3,4) while the other is based on signal change evoked by the addition of gradients (5).

   Proton perfusion imaging of the lung was given various names in the past in relation to the sequence used, and include the following: "cardiac-triggered half-Fourier single-shot turbo spin echo" (HASTE) (3), fresh-blood imaging (FBI) (6), "diffusion-weighted HASTE" (5), the intravoxel incoherent motions (IVIM) method (7), and the flow dephased/flow compensated approach (8). Thus,"proton perfusion imaging" denotes a comprehensive term comprising all previous work; although this might be replaced by a new term in the future with further technical advances.

   In this section, the basic principles and historical aspects of proton perfusion imaging will be introduced. Subsequently, the HASTE sequence (9), which is widely used for proton perfusion imaging of the lung, will be described and its applications and limitations will be discussed. Lastly, several representative cases and clinical applications will be demonstrated.

II. Blood Flow and MR Signal

A. Flow-Related Phenomena

Proton perfusion imaging is based on flow-related signal change. Since the early days of conventional spin echo, it has been well known that flow increases or decreases blood signal in MR images (Fig. 12.1) (10). This effect is due to several independent factors. The main factors that contribute to the decrease of blood signal are high velocity, turbulence, and dephasing. These factors collectively lead to the flow void, which is a comprehensive name for signal loss related to the flow. In contrast, the factors that increase the blood signal are even-echo rephasing, diastolic pseudo-gating, and flow-related enhancement (11,12).

   These phenomena are closely related to blood flow velocity and the diameter of blood vessels. For example, high-velocity signal loss occurs when protons do not remain for a long-enough period of time within the selected slice to

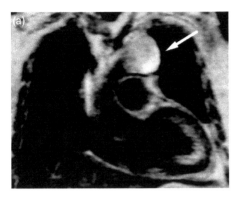 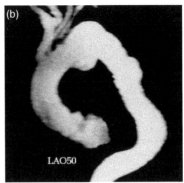

Figure 12.1 Flow-related phenomena in the thoracic aortic aneurysm. (a) Fast spin echo coronal section of a 67-year-old male demonstrates normal flow void in the pulmonary artery and lumen of the left ventricle. The aneurysm of aortic arch shows marked high signal intensity due to turbulent flow (arrow). Note that bilateral lungs show very low signal intensity. (b) Three-dimensional contrast-enhanced MR angiography shows fusiform dilatation of the aorta.

acquire the 90° and 180° pulses. The magnitude of the high-velocity signal loss is a linear function of velocity. Turbulence is present when randomly fluctuating velocity components are found in both axial and nonaxial directions. Turbulence occurs even in slow-flow vessels if they have large diameters (12).

Dephasing causes flaring of the magnetization because some proton processes are faster and some are slower than average because of the relatively stronger and weaker local magnetic field (11). In conventional spin echo, magnetization vectors begin to flare after 90° pulses. As 180° pulse is applied, flared magnetization vectors begin to rephase. At echo time (TE), rephasing is complete and coherent spin echo is emitted (Fig. 12.2). When blood flows, not all protons in the voxel move at the same velocity through the magnetic field gradient, rather, they process at different frequencies and exhibit a variety of phase shifts. This results in incomplete rephasing and total signal loss of that voxel (11).

B.   Velocity Measurement in Great Vessels Using Phase Shift

Because the phase shift can be directly related to the velocity of flowing spins, it has been applied for quantitative flow measurement since 1980s (13), and its potential has been known since the 1960s (14,15). When bipolar gradient pulses are applied to modulate the phase of proton spins, the velocity v can be determined by the phase difference acquired in the two interleaved measurements (16,17):

$$\Delta\Phi = \gamma\Delta mv$$

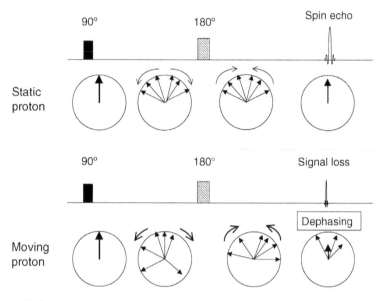

Figure 12.2 Dephasing.

where $\Delta\Phi$ is the phase shift, γ is the gyromagnetic ratio determined by static magnetic field strength, and Δm is the difference of the first moment of the gradient–time curve of velocity encoding gradients. For rectangular bipolar gradient pulses, m is simply defined as the product of the gradient area and the time. Flow volume can also be obtained by measurement of the area of the vessel (15,16,18). The imaging time remains unchanged, stronger gradient amplitudes are required to encode smaller velocities. Hence, this method was applied for velocity measurements of large vessels before the advancement of MR performance. Determination of cardiac output can be easily performed with this method based on measurement of velocity in the ascending aorta (18). It has been recently reported that the cardiac output based on velocity measurements agrees with that determined by right heart catheterization, overall difference in the measurements of blood velocity and cardiac output between the two methods is $\sim10\%$ (19,20).

In the same manner, it is possible to assess the stroke volume into both lungs and each lung, separately (21) (Fig. 12.3). In healthy adults, $\sim55\%$ of pulmonary blood flow passes though the right pulmonary artery and 45% into the left pulmonary artery (22). The regional pulmonary flow measured using phase shift on MR images agrees with the count ratios in perfusion scintigraphy using 99m-Tc MAA SPECT (23). Although lung perfusion scintigraphy is considered the gold standard for quantitative evaluation of pulmonary perfusion, in certain situations, MR measurement is superior to scintigraphy. For example, in patients with congenital heart disease such as Fontan-like circulation (i.e., atriopulmonary

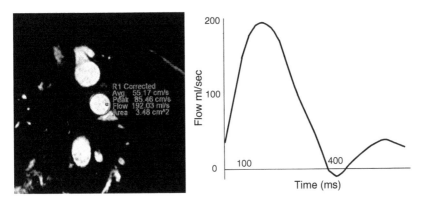

Figure 12.3 Magnitude image of the left pulmonary artery and time–velocity curve for phase-shift velocity measurement using gradient-echo technique (FLASH). The imaging plane is positioned orthogonal to the main direction of flow of the left pulmonary artery and through-plane flow encoding is used. Other imaging parameters are TR: 57 ms, TE: 3.7 ms, flip angle 15°.

anastomosis, total cavopulmonary connection, or partial cavopulmonary connection; i.e., caval blood into the right or left pulmonary arteries), lung perfusion scintigraphy does not optimally reflect the genuine perfusion ratio in this setting. Recent studies indicate that MR provides accurate assessment of pulmonary perfusion ratios in these patients (24). The phase-encoding velocity measurement of pulmonary artery is sometimes called "pulmonary perfusion" (25). However, it is stressed that this method cannot evaluate blood flow in pulmonary segmental or subsegmental regions.

C. Micromovement Evaluation by MRI

Ideal perfusion imaging would describe blood flow at a capillary level, or at least at the arteriole and/or venule level, which approaches 400–800 μm/s of velocity in the vessel (26). Dephasing is based on a change in the local strength of the magnetic field felt by each proton, and may occur not only due to high flow but also due to very small movement in a given voxel. Stejskal and Tanner (27) provided "mapping" methods to detect very small movement, IVIM, which means that protons in a voxel move at different velocities in different directions. The idea of Stejskal and Tanner has developed into diffusion and perfusion imaging; it allows the detection of diffusion of the proton as low as 10^{-6} mm/s (28).

Although dephasing was expected to detect perfusion, initially it could not be applied to lung perfusion imaging. Several reasons explain this limitation. First, in an actual voxel in the tissue, variable motions coexist. Le Bihan et al. (7) proposed a model in which IVIM composed of diffusion and perfusion

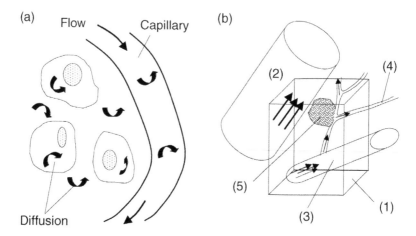

Figure 12.4 (a) Intravoxel incoherent motion (IVIM). A tissue can be divided into volume fractions: water flowing (arrow) and diffusing (curved arrow) in capillaries and water in the cells and interstitial tissues, which is involved in diffusion only (curved arrow). [Reprinted from Le Bihan et al. (7).] (b) Five-compartment model: (1) stationary component, (2) constant velocity, (3) anisotropic coherent component, (4) isotropic coherent component, and (5) isotropic incoherent component. [From Maki et al. (8).]

(Fig. 12.4a). Maki et al. (8) introduced the five-compartment model (Fig. 12.4b). Even the most vascular organs (brain, kidney, liver, and spleen) contain <2–3% volume fraction of capillaries. The majority of the signals come from static spin or dephasing due to diffusion in the cells and interstitial tissue. Thus, considering only the capillaries, the signal differences between organs with and without capillary flow would be <1–1.5% based on the IVIM method (7,29).

The second reason is the unique architecture of the lung tissue. With regard to blood volume, the lung has larger fraction of blood volume than extravascular tissue volume (30). A lot of blood flow, however, evokes marked washout effects and dephasing, leading to significant reductions of signal (31). The volume of air in normal lungs is as much as 80% of their volume, with a resultant high air–tissue interface, which increases local heterogeneity of the magnetic field and decreases the signal from lung tissue including blood (32). In the conventional spin echo sequence, it is difficult to obtain the signal of the lung parenchyma itself. Moreover, IVIM sequence requires large gradients to detect very slow flow (<1 mm/s), it makes the image extremely sensitive to bulk movement during the TE, such as respiration-related chest wall movements and cardiac contraction, resulting in degraded images. Thus, perfusion imaging based on IVIM method could not be utilized for pulmonary perfusion, although this method was applied to investigate the microcirculation of the brain and kidney in the 1980s and 1990s (33,34).

D. Development of Lung Parenchymal Perfusion Imaging

von Shulthess et al. (35) are credited with the first description of signal changes in the lung using MRI in 1985. Spin echo images of the lung were obtained with cardiac and respiratory gating using a MR unit of 0.35 T. They observed that the signal of the lung field changed with the cardiac cycle in normal volunteers and that such cyclic changes disappeared in patients with pulmonary hypertension caused by pulmonary arterial embolism. They considered that their method could be useful for evaluating pulmonary perfusion. It is evident that these changes were easier to observe using a low magnetic field system, which decreases magnetic heterogeneity and enhances the signal from the lung parenchyma.

During the 1990s, Hatabu et al. (36) reported that the HASTE sequence allows visualization of the lung parenchyma using 1.5 T MR systems. HASTE is one of the fastest sequences, which has certain advantages for lung imaging (9). First, it uses radiofrequency (RF) pulses to obtain the echo signal, which is solid to magnetic heterogeneity compared with the gradient-recalled sequence. Second, HASTE with short echo train spacing (ETS) reduces the time of recording signal, and allows one to obtain signal from the lung before it has significantly decreased due to dephasing. Lastly, and most importantly with regard to perfusion imaging, HASTE with short ETS is sensitive to dephasing of the proton. Hatabu et al. (36) reported that T2 values of the lung tissues changed with cardiac trigger delay time and speculated this signal change was related to the flow effects or blood volume. In 2001, Knight-Scott et al. (3) and Tadamura et al. (4) independently reported the use of HASTE to evaluate pulmonary perfusion. Recently, Miyazaki et al. (6) developed FBI, a new MR angiography sequence based on HASTE. This technique has also been applied to proton perfusion imaging (37–39). At present, most proton perfusion imaging of the lung is performed with HASTE-based sequences.

III. Perfusion Imaging with HASTE

A. Principle of HASTE

HASTE is one of the fastest spin echo sequences derived from rapid acquisition with relaxation enhancement (RARE) (9). Figure 12.5 shows the pulse-sequence diagram and the k-space trajectory of conventional spin echo and fast spin echo (40). The major difference between conventional spin echo and fast spin echo is that in the former, all echoes are preceded by a single value of the phase-encoding gradient, whereas in the latter, each echo is preceded by variable phase encoding gradients. Because each value of the phase encoding gradients corresponds to a separate line in the k-space, the k-space is filled faster in HASTE (see Chapter 6).

k-Space is a representation of how raw image data are acquired (40). When fully sampled, the k_x and k_y information of k-space is redundant, because positive

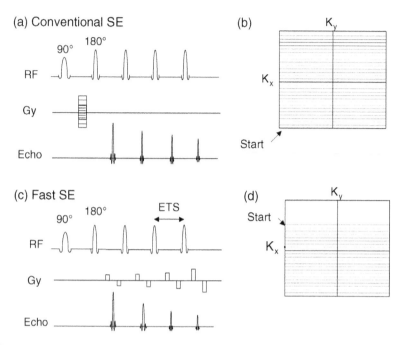

Figure 12.5 The pulse-sequence diagram and k-space trajectory of conventional four echo-train spin echo (a, b) and fast spin echo with four echo train length (ETL: number of 180° pulses and the number of echoes) (c, d). [Modified from Bradley et al. (40).] HASTE is a single-shot fast SE sequence, 72 echoes are acquired after single RF excitation for 128 × 256 matrixes. In conventional spin echo the phase encoding gradients apply after the 90° pulse. The echoes decrease in amplitude as a result of T2 decay. In fast spin echo, the amplitude of the echo is also determined by the magnitude of the phase encoding gradient preceding it. In this figure the center of k-space (smallest phase encode amplitude) is acquired on the first echo resulting in a short effective TE for the image.

and negative special frequencies are conjugate symmetrical (Fig. 12.5b). In HASTE, only half of the data along k_y is acquired to cut the imaging time (Fig. 12.5d). Neglecting half of the data requires a phase correction that is commonly derived from the 16 central, low spatial frequencies along k_y. For this reason, data are acquired sequentially, beginning with the eight lines above the center. Thus, the data of the center 16 lines are acquired first after 90° pulses, and these center 16 lines of k-space are used to calculate the phase correction for the entire data set in HASTE. The phase encoding gradient is weakest in the center of k-space. This leads to a minimum amount of dephasing along phase-encoding axis and thus the strongest echo signal. At the same time, the signal closest to the center of k-space is more resistant to respiratory and cardiac movements (3,4,36). Thus, HASTE with short ETS is sufficiently resistant to dephasing to obtain signal from the lung parenchyma, and at the same time, HASTE is sensitive to dephasing based on the flow.

B. Relationships Between Diffusion Imaging and HASTE with Cardiac Gating

Figure 12.6 provides a comparison of representative diffusion sequences, HASTE with cardiac gating, and diffusion-weighted HASTE. In single-echo sequence (Fig. 12.6a), which was the earliest developed sequence to detect micromovement, a constant gradient is applied during the TE, and dephasing evoked by this extrinsic continuous gradient induces signal loss when the protons move (28,41). This sequence could not be applied directly *in vivo* because this single-echo sequence requires strict homogeneity of the magnetic field. Moreover, the presence of a gradient during the recording of echo signal markedly reduces the signal-to-noise ratio.

In HASTE with cardiac gating (Fig. 12.6c), no extrinsic gradient exists. Instead, continuation of the blood flow during TE evokes dephasing. The magnitudes of these phase errors are proportional to blood velocity, and thus the image signal is dependent on the average velocity of the blood between the excitation pulse and acquisition of the center of k-space. It is well known that multiple-echoes reduce the signal change by dephasing compared with the single-echo

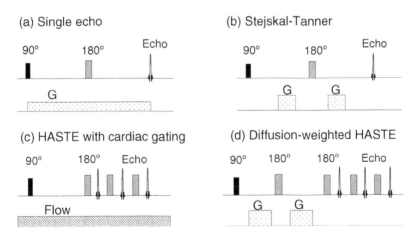

Figure 12.6 Comparison of (a) single echo sequence, (b) Stejskal–Tanner sequence, (c) HASTE with cardiac gating, and (d) diffusion-weighted HASTE. (a) In single echo sequence, the constant gradient pulse evokes a phase shift due to micromovement. (b) In Stejskal–Tanner sequence, very large and short gradient pulses are placed on each side of 180° pulse of spin echo sequence. These gradients are balanced and therefore transparent for static proton; accurate measurements of micromovement can be achieved. (c) In HASTE with cardiac gating the flow evokes the phase shift. (d) Diffusion-weighted HASTE uses the preparation pulse similar to the pattern of Stejskal–Tanner sequence.

approach (28,42). HASTE uses multiple echoes; however, the central k-space ordering and the use of RF pulses to obtain the signal minimize the influence from multiple echoes (28,42). Thus, the lung parenchyma shows high signal intensity (SI) in relatively slow and steady flow during cardiac diastole and low SI in high blood flow during systole (Fig. 12.7). The subtraction images

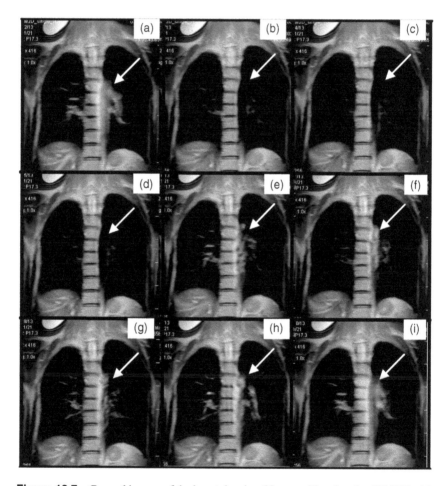

Figure 12.7 Coronal images of the lung taken in a 30-year-old male using HASTE with cardiac gating at 1.5 T MR system (Siemens medical systems, Erlangen, Germany) (acquisition parameters: TEeff, 35 ms; ETS, 4.52 ms; bandwidth, 349 Hz/pixel; slice thickness, 10 mm; and acquisition time, 260 ms). Images are taken at various points of the cardiac cycle: (a) 35 ms, (b) 135 ms, (c) 235 ms, (d) 335 ms, (e) 435 ms, (f) 535 ms, (g) 635 ms, (h) 735 ms, and (i) 835 ms. The true delay time is delay time (0–800 ms) added by TE (35 ms). R-R interval is ~750 ms. Note that the signal of aorta changes markedly during the cardiac cycle (arrows).

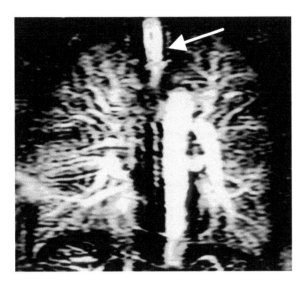

Figure 12.8 A subtraction image between coronal sections b and h shown in Fig. 12.7. The lung field shows high signal intensity. The cerebrospinal fluid in the spine also shows high signal intensity (arrow).

from the two images obtained at systolic and diastolic phases can provide a clear visualization of pulmonary perfusion (Fig. 12.8). Moreover, in the FBI sequence (6), image acquisition is segmented into several shots and k-space is filled with the data from each shot in an interleaved manner (Fig. 12.9). This reduces the

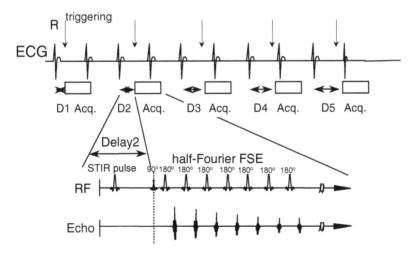

Figure 12.9 Sequence diagram of FBI (ECG-synchronized 3D half-Fourier FSE). The 3D half-Fourier FSE sequence is ECG synchronized for each slice encoding to have the same cardiac phase in every slice partition. [From Miyazaki et al. (6).]

number of echoes for each shot and increases the sensitivity to flow-related dephasing.

Figure 12.6d shows HASTE with extrinsic gradients (diffusion-weighted HASTE) proposed by Knight-Scott and Mai (5), and Fig. 12.10 shows the images obtained by diffusion-weighted HASTE. The diffusion preparation with Stejskal–Tanner type gradients (27,28) (Fig. 12.6b) is settled before signal acquisition using HASTE. During this preparation, diffusion attenuation is produced by pulsed gradients. The image is obtained with cardiac gating and the delay time after the QRS complex is fixed at diastole, which effectively cancels fast flow effects. The micromovement of the protons may then be detected by diffusion gradients on the subtraction image between two images with or without diffusion preparation gradients.

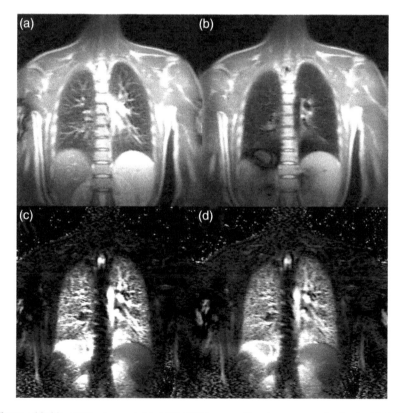

Figure 12.10 Diffusion-weighted HASTE images. Two images are obtained with 1.5 T magnet (Siemens medical systems, Erlangen, Germany) using phased array coil. Images were taken at end-expiration, 400–500 ms after QRS complex with b-factor = 0.015 s/mm^2 (a) and 1.5 s/mm^2 (b). (c) Corresponding calculated difference image [(a − b)/b]. (d) Dispersion image of the decay constant. [From Knight-Scott et al. (5).]

Diffusion-weighted HASTE is a promising method for quantitative evaluation of pulmonary perfusion. The signal obtained by HASTE with cardiac gating is influenced by T2 relaxation, and it includes random phase errors, which may have occurred during signal accumulation. This causes problems for the quantitative measurement of perfusion. On the other hand, in diffusion imaging such as the Stejskal–Tanner sequence, signal S depends on decay constant D and the factor b, which is a measure of degree of diffusion weighting that depends on the timing diagram and strength of the diffusion gradient pulses (28):

$$S = \exp(-bD)$$

If two different images with different b values are obtained using b values $b1$ and $b2$ respectively, then

$$D = \frac{\ln(S1/S2)}{b2 - b1}$$

D includes several factors, true T2 decay, flow-related dephasing, and diffusion. When the b value is very large, T2 relaxation and flow-related dephasing can be neglected (7). On the other hand, when b values are very small, signal attenuation is dominated by flow-related phase dispersion. Knight-Scott called D the dispersion constant Dp (5). The author expects that the Dp can be developed as a tool for quantitative measurement of perfusion.

IV. Signal Change in HASTE with Cardiac Gating

A. Signal Change and Cardiac Cycle

Although the diffusion-weighted HASTE sequence is a promising technique, it has not yet gained widespread acceptance in the MR community. Therefore, HASTE with cardiac gating will be described in more detail as an alternative method of imaging. Figure 12.11 shows the signal changes in the lung parenchyma, aorta, and muscle during the cardiac cycle and the HASTE images obtained with cardiac gating in a normal volunteer. The basic temporal pattern of the lung signal first demonstrates a large fall in the SI, followed by a recovery period, then a second and smaller reduction, and finally another recovery period (3,4,39). The initial drop corresponds to the high velocity in the aorta and pulmonary arteries (Fig. 12.11). Closure of the aortic and pulmonary valves signals the beginning of the ventricular diastole, followed by a sudden reduction in arterial and aorta blood velocities. The lung signal begins its recovery and reaches peak intensity only 60 ms after closure of the pulmonary valve. The lung signal is relatively stable over the next 80 ms before the second drop. The atrioventricular valves open, followed by a rapid flow of blood from the atria into the ventricles resulting in the second drop (Fig. 12.12). The recovery period of the second trough signifies the beginning of diastole.

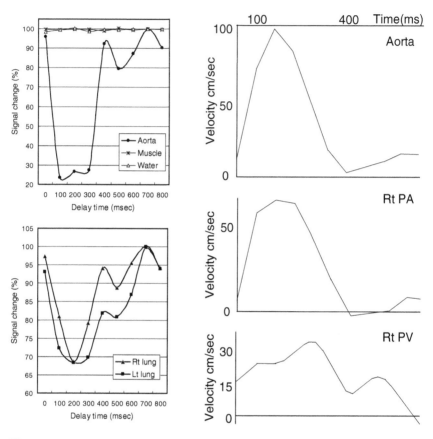

Figure 12.11 Left panel: Time intensity curve of both lungs, aorta, muscle, and water phantom (shown in left upper corner in Fig. 12.7a–i). Right side: time–velocity curves of the descending aorta (top), right pulmonary artery (middle), and right pulmonary vein (bottom), obtained using phase-shift velocity measurement in the same volunteer of Fig. 12.7. Signal changes were measured using the region of interests (ROIs) settled in Fig. 12.7. Velocity was measured in a manner similar to that shown in Fig. 12.4. The signal change in the lung field shows a biphasic pattern (left panel). The change in muscle signal is small. The aorta and lung signals show similar temporal dependencies, except the systolic signal change which is greater in the aorta. Compared with the velocity changes, the initial drop in the signal change of the lungs corresponds to the high velocities of the pulmonary artery and vein during systole. Note that the velocity of the pulmonary vein shows a biphasic pattern.

B. Velocity and Signal Change

The signal change in the aorta in HASTE imaging with cardiac gating and time–velocity curve in the aorta measured by phase-shift imaging (Fig. 12.11) indicate that the difference in the SI between the systolic and diastolic phases mainly

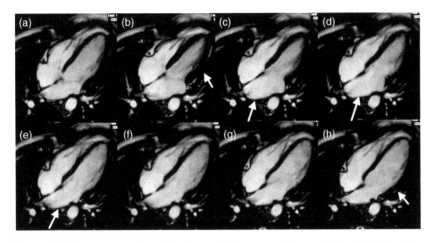

Figure 12.12   Cine imaging of the heart of the same volunteer of Fig. 12.8. The delay time after R-trigger is (a) 35.6 ms, (b) 106.9 ms, (c) 285.6 ms, (d) 392 ms, (e) 427 ms, (f) 499 ms, (g) 605 m, and (h) 712 ms. Compared with Fig. 12.11, shrinking of the left ventricle (b) corresponds to the timing of the initial drop of the signal change of the lungs. The second drop of the signal change of the lungs corresponds to the timing of (d) opening of the mitral valve and inflow of blood in the left ventricle, and (e, f) a rapid fall in left atrial volume.

reflects differences in velocities, (at least in large blood vessels such as aorta and the main pulmonary artery). Part of the signal change in the lung parenchyma may reflect the differences in velocities in small vessels, such as arteries and veins, and possibly the arterioles and venules (37). Several studies demonstrated that blood flow in microvessels is pulsatile. Laser Doppler velocimetry or particle image velocimetry revealed that, at least in arterioles, the velocity increases sharply toward peak systole and then decreases moderately toward late diastole, in synchronicity with the cardiac cycle (43,44).

However, the difference in velocity between systolic and diastolic phases is very small in microvessels. Suga et al. (37) showed that HASTE with cardiac gating could not detect velocity changes that are <10 cm/s in a flow phantom study (Fig. 12.13). Hence, signal change in the lung parenchyma cannot be explained only by the velocity change in images of HASTE with cardiac gating.

C.   Blood Volume and Signal Change

Another possible cause of signal change in the lung parenchyma could be blood volume (36–39). Topulos et al. (45) showed fractional changes in capillary blood volume and oxygen saturation during the cardiac cycle in the rabbit lung using dual-wavelength diffuse light-scattering technique. The finding of gravity dependence of pulmonary perfusion also supports the notion that blood volume influences the signal (Fig. 12.14) (37,38). The high pulmonary arterial pressure in the

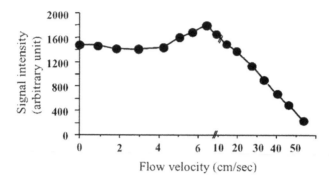

Figure 12.13 Relationship between water flow velocity and signal intensity of water stream measured on HASTE images. The SI of the water stream decreases linearly at high flow velocity (>7.2 cm/s) as a result of flow void effect. The increase in SI in velocities raging from 4.3 to 7.2 cm/s is due to the inflow effect. The SI is almost steadily high and unchanged at low flow velocity (<4.3 cm/s). [From Kawanami et al. (39).]

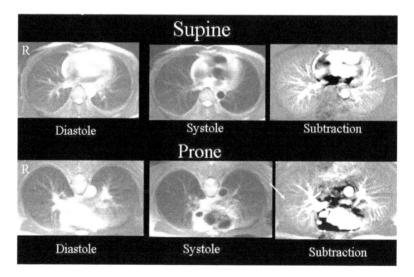

Figure 12.14 Proton perfusion imaging with FBI sequence from a 30-year-old male, using 1.5 T magnet (Toshiba, Tokyo, Japan), with the following imaging parameters: $TE_{eff} = 80$ ms, echo train spacing (ETS) = 4 ms, slice thickness = 30 mm, using eight shots with 12 number of excitation (NEX) without breath-holding. The signal change between systolic and diastolic phases is greater in the dorsal portion of the lung than in the ventral part in the supine position. In the prone position, the difference in signal is greater in the ventral part. The lesser signal area in the left lung is the fissure. The fissure is commonly seen in normal subject. (Courtesy of Dr. Kazuyoshi Suga.)

dorsal lung normally increases the transmural pressure in the dorsal vascular networks, which distends the capillary and lowers vascular resistance to blood flow, resulting in greater pulmonary arterial blood flow and volume (46–48). Changes in blood volume directly correlate with changes in total proton density in an imaging voxel on MRI, because the component of blood is large in the lung tissues compared with other organs (30,49), and the change in blood volume in the imaging voxel would directly relate to the signal.

It is well known that the pulmonary microcirculation is a complex network containing a distribution of vascular path lengths and resistance, and the blood volume is one of the important factors in some physiological and pathological states of pulmonary perfusion. For example, capillary distension and new capillary recruitment occurs during exercise. When cardiac output increases during exercise, capillary transit time decreases. The latter, however, is partially offset by an increase in capillary volume that occurs though recruitment of new capillaries and distension of existing capillaries. This capillary recruitment increase the cross-sectional area of the microvascular bed and the surface area available for gas exchange (50–53).

On the other hand, in patients with pulmonary thromboembolism (PTE), the occluded vessels show abrupt tapering and diminished pulsation. High-resolution computed tomography (HRCT) can clearly demonstrate low attenuation caused by oligemia in the affected lung (54–56). It has been reported that proton perfusion images can detect perfusion defects caused by PTE in an animal model (Fig. 12.15) (4,37) and in clinical cases (Fig. 12.16). It was suggested that low signal in the affected area on proton perfusion images reflects a marked decrease in not only pulsatile signal change, but also in total signal from the lung parenchyma.

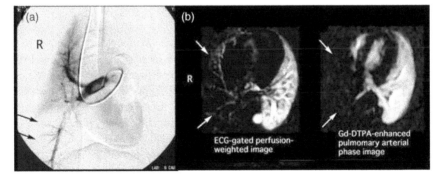

Figure 12.15 MR studies performed soon after embolization (right) and in a pulmonary embolic model with relatively large embolized area in the right lung (left). Proton perfusion imaging (obtained using the same sequence described in Fig. 12.14) demonstrates a perfusion defect, which corresponds with the perfusion image of Gd-DTPA. [Modified Fig. 12.5 from Kawanami et al. (39) with permission.]

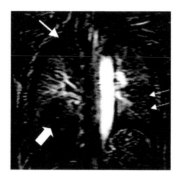

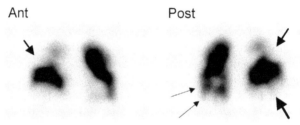

Figure 12.16 Proton perfusion image (top) and perfusion scintigraphy (bottom) of a 64-year-old female with acute thromboembolism of the pulmonary artery. The proton perfusion image (obtained with a sequence similar to that reported in Fig. 12.9) demonstrates perfusion defects in both lungs, similar to the corresponding images of perfusion scintigraphy.

V. Clinical Applications

A. Potential Applications

Because proton perfusion imaging of the lung was only developed over the past few years, clinical trials or comparative studies in a large population have not yet been performed. As described earlier, animal experiments have demonstrated that proton perfusion imaging could identify perfusion abnormalities in a pig model of pulmonary embolism (4), similar to the perfusion imaging using Gd-DTPA (Fig. 12.14) (36). Hence, the most promising clinical application of proton perfusion imaging is PTE.

For assessment of the perfusion defects in patients with PTE, the readers should be reminded that the normal fissure is commonly seen as a low signal area in proton perfusion images (Fig. 12.15). The reason for this finding is likely the ability of proton perfusion imaging to detect hypoperfusion in the subpleural region (Dr. Kazuyoshi Suga, personal communication, 2003). This argument is supported by previous anatomical and physiological studies, for example, the subpleural capillary networks have a coarser mesh and thus occupy a smaller fraction of alveolar wall than do interior capillary networks (48,57). The number of red blood cells in the subpleural alveolar wall is also smaller than those in interior regions, especially with low alveolar pressure (58).

Proton perfusion imaging could also be applied to several other diseases with perfusion abnormalities. Figure 12.17 shows images taken in a child with unilateral absence of the right pulmonary artery. Unilateral absence of a pulmonary artery (UAPA) is a rare congenital disorder of the pulmonary circulation, and the term isolated UAPA is used when it is not associated with various cardiac and other vascular malformation (59). With the FBI technique (6), proton perfusion imaging can be obtained without breath-holding, and can thus be applied to children under sedation rather than under general anesthesia.

Figure 12.18 shows a patient with Takayasu arteritis. Takayasu arteritis is an uncommon vasculitis principally affecting the aorta and its major branches. Pulmonary artery involvement is found in an appreciable number of cases (60). It has been reported that MR clearly demonstrates various vascular regions such as wall thickening of the involved vessels (61). MR angiography with Gd-DTPA can also depict vascular narrowing and occlusion, similar to conventional angiography (62). Proton perfusion imaging, which uses no contrast materials, is potentially of value in the assessment of the pulmonary circulation in these patients.

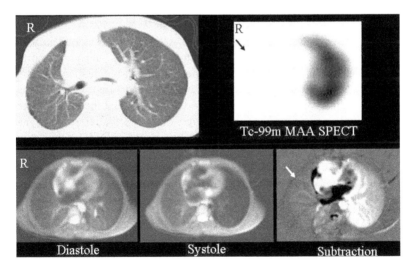

Figure 12.17 A 9-year-old girl with congenital right pulmonary artery atresia, a rare anomaly of the pulmonary artery. CT image (top, left) shows the volume loss and oligemia of the right lung. Perfusion scintigraphy shows complete perfusion defect of the right lung (arrow, top right). Proton perfusion images (bottom) also demonstrate the perfusion defect (white arrow) corresponding to scintigraphy. The proton perfusion image is obtained using the same sequence described in Fig. 12.14. (Courtesy of Dr. Kazuyoshi Suga.)

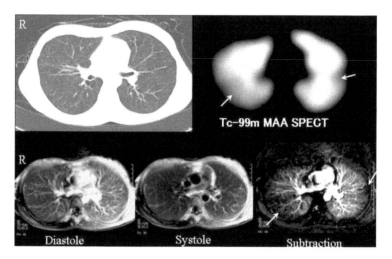

Figure 12.18 Takayasu arteritis in a 32-year-old female patient. Perfusion defects are evident in both lungs by both perfusion scintigraphy and proton perfusion imaging (obtained using the same sequence described in Fig. 12.14). (Courtesy of Dr. Kazuyoshi Suga.)

Another remarkable characteristic of proton perfusion is its repeatability. Suga et al. (37) observed a gradual reduction of the pulmonary signal on proton perfusion images after bronchial occlusion (Fig. 12.19). Regional hypoxemia after airway obstruction has a direct action on the smooth muscles of pulmonary arteries measuring 200–300 μm in diameter, and partly on small veins, and elicits hypoxic vasoconstriction leading to regional hypoperfusion (63–65). Suga et al. (37) indicated that the signal reduction reflected a gradual decrease in pulmonary arterial blood flow due to a gradual increase in hypoxic vasoconstriction in the hypoventilated lungs. Such observation of the dynamic change in pulmonary perfusion is not possible using Gd-DTPA-enhanced perfusion imaging or perfusion scintigraphy. Thus, the author predicts that proton perfusion imaging, which can be safely repeated, will be beneficial for monitoring perfusion changes after anticoagulation or thrombolysis in patients with pulmonary embolism.

B. Guidelines for Clinical Applications

Proton perfusion imaging using HASTE with cardiac gating requires a system with a large slew rate (i.e., a large phase-encoding gradient evoked within short time), which allows shorter ETS. Minimizing ETS to <4.5 ms is required for this technique. The phase shift during an acquisition window (ETS multiplied by number of echoes) reduces total signal, resulting in a decrease in the fraction of the signal change due to flow. Hence, a long ETS will decrease the difference

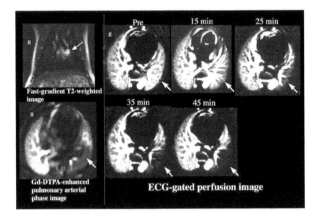

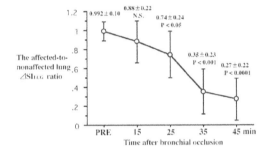

Figure 12.19 (a) MR studies of an airway obstruction dog model. The right main bronchus was occluded with a balloon catheter. Mid-coronal localized fast-gradient T2 weighted images show the site of the inflated balloon (top left, arrow). After balloon inflation, the cardiac-gated perfusion-weighted images show a gradual decrease of SI, corresponding to the hypoventilated lung areas. The location of this low perfusion is nearly consistent with that on the subtracted, Gd-DTPA- enhanced pulmonary arterial perfusion image (left bottom). The proton perfusion images were obtained using the same sequence described in Fig. 12.14. (b) Serial changes in signal intensity ΔSI_{ECG} ratio of affected-to-nonaffected contralateral lung after bronchial occlusion with a balloon catheter. $\Delta SI_{ECG} = [(\text{maximal SI} - \text{background noise SI}) - (\text{minimal SI} - \text{background noise SI})]$. Data are mean $\pm$ SD of 8 dogs. [From Kawanami et al. (39).]

in the signal change between systole and diastole. To obtain the maximal signal change, the delay time after R-trigger should be settled for each case by monitoring the signal change in the lung field (6,37).

The imaging time of HASTE with cardiac gating requires a few seconds to allow for single breath-hold imaging (3,4). The expiratory phase is preferable for perfusion imaging due to the smaller amount of air in the lung during this phase, which increases the signal from the lung parenchyma (3). Moreover, deep inspiration reduces pulmonary blood flow, compared with measurements during spontaneous breathing (66). SENSE (sensitivity encoding), a recently developed technique used with proton perfusion imaging should allow for further decreases in acquisition times (67).

There is a heated debate on the importance of other imaging parameters. Knight-Scott et al. used short TE (3,5), while Suga et al. used long TE (37). Short TE sequences increase the signal from lung parenchyma and minimize T2 effect. Longer TE increases the phase shift due to flow, but the influence of T2 relaxation is also larger. It also decreases the signal-to-noise ratio. Suga et al. increased the number of excitations to increase the signal-to-noise ratio, for example, 12 excitation episodes were used in their animal experiments.

VI. Conclusion

Proton perfusion imaging is based on signal changes due to blood flow in the pulmonary vessels and is one of the most physiological methods of imaging. In images taken by HASTE with cardiac gating, the signal is influenced by both perfusion (including blood velocity and blood volume) and T2 relaxation; hence, quantitative evaluation of perfusion using HASTE has not yet been established. Diffusion-weighted HASTE is expected to provide a quantitative assessment of pulmonary perfusion.

Proton perfusion imaging does not use radiation or contrast material. It can be repeated within a short period without any adverse effects. This method could be applied to patients with perfusion abnormalities such as pulmonary embolism. As the technique does not require long breath-holds it may be particularly useful in children.

Acknowledgments

The author gratefully acknowledges the help of all colleagues at the Department of Radiology, Yokohama City University School of Medicine. The author also gratefully acknowledges the help and advice of Drs. Tommie Inoue, Kazuyoshi Suga, Yasuyuki Kurihara, Mitue Miyazaki, and Jack Knight-Scott.

References

1. Edelman RR, Siewert B, Darby DG, Thangaraj V, Nobre AC, Mesulam MM, Warach S. Qualitative mapping of cerebral blood flow and functional localization with echo-planar MR imaging and signal targeting with alternating radio frequency. Radiology 1994; 192:513–520.
2. Mai VM, Hagspiel KD, Christopher JM, Do HM, Altes T, Knight-Scott J, Stith AL, Maier T, Berr SS. Perfusion imaging of the lung using flow-sensitive alternating inversion recovery with an extra radio-frequency pulse (FAIRER). Magn Reson Imaging 1999; 17:355–361.

3. Knight-Scott J, Keilholz-George SD, Mai VM, Christopher JM. Temporal dynamics of blood flow effects in half-Fourier fast spin echo ^{1}H magnetic resonance imaging of the human lungs. J Magn Reson Imaging 2001; 14:411–418.

4. Tadamura E, Hatabu H. Assessment of pulmonary perfusion using a subtracted HASTE image between diastole and systole. Eur J Radiol 2001; 37:179–183.

5. Knight-Scott J, Mai VM. Diffusion-weighting as a contrast enhancement mechanism for ^{1}H MR lung imaging. Proc Int Soc Mag Reson Med 2002; 10:410.

6. Miyazaki M, Sugiura S, Fumiaki T, Hirofumi A, Kassai Y, Abe H. Non-contrast-enhanced MR angiography using 3D ECG-synchronized half-Fourier fast spin echo. J Magn Reson Imaging 2000; 12:776–783.

7. Le Bihan D, Breton E, Lallemand D, Aubin ML, Vignaud J, Laval-Jantet M. Separation of diffusion and perfusion in intravoxel incoherent motion MR imaging. Radiology1988; 168:497–505.

8. Maki JH, Mac Fall JR, Johnson GA. The use of gradient flow compensation to separate diffusion and microcirculatory flow in MRI. 1991 Magn Reson Med 1991; 17:95–107.

9. Nitz W. Fast and ultrafast non-echo-planar MR imaging techniques (Review). Eur Radiol 2002; 12:2866–2882.

10. Fisher MR, Higgins CB. Central thrombi in pulmonary arterial hypertension detected by MR imaging. Radiology 1986; 158:223–226.

11. Bradley WG Jr, Waluch V. Blood flow: magnetic resonance imaging. Radiology 1985; 154:443–450.

12. Bradley WG Jr, Waluch V, Lai KS, Fernandez EJ, Spalter C. The appearance of rapidly flowing blood on magnetic resonance images. Am J Roentgenol 1984; 143:1167–1174.

13. Maier SE, Meier D, Boesiger P, Moser UT, Vieli A. Human abdominal aorta: comparative measurements of blood flow with MR imaging and multigated Doppler US. Radiology 1989; 171:487–492.

14. Singer JR. Blood flow rates by nuclear magnetic resonance measurements. Science 1959; 130:1652–1653.

15. Singer JR, Crooks LE. Nuclear magnetic resonance blood flow measurements in the human brain. Science 1983; 221:654–665.

16. Lotz J, Meier C, Leppert A, Galanski M. Cardiovascular flow measurement with phase-contrast MR imaging: basic facts and implementation. Radiographics 2002; 22:651–671.

17. Moran PR, Moran RA, Karstaedt N. Verification and evaluation of internal flow and motion. True magnetic resonance imaging by the phase gradient modulation method. Radiology 1985; 154(2):433–441.

18. Kondo C, Caputo GR, Semelka R, Foster E, Shimakawa A, Higgins CB. Right and left ventricular stroke volume measurements with velocity-encoded cine MR imaging: *in vitro* and *in vivo* validation. AJR Am J Roentgenol 1991; 157:9–16.

19. Hoeper MM, Tongers J, Leppert A, Baus S, Maier R, Lotz J. Evaluation of right ventricular performance with a right ventricular ejection fraction thermodilution catheter and MRI in patients with pulmonary hypertension. Chest 2001; 120:502–507.

20. Laffon E, Laurent F, Bernard V, De Boucaud L, Ducassou D, Marthan R. Noninvasive assessment of pulmonary arterial hypertension by MR phase-mapping method. J Appl Physiol 2001; 90:2197–2202.

21. Marcus JT, Vonk Noordegraaf A, De Vries PM, Van Rossum AC, Roseboom B, Heethaar RM, Postmus PE. MRI evaluation of right ventricular pressure overload in chronic obstructive pulmonary disease. J Magn Reson Imaging 1998; 8:999–1005.

22. Henk CB, Schlechta B, Grampp S, Gomischek G, Klepetko W, Mostbeck GH. Pulmonary and aortic blood flow measurements in normal subjects and patients after single lung transplantation at 0.5 T using velocity encoded cine MRI. Chest 1998; 114:771–779.

23. Osada H, Machida K, Honda N. Quantification of regional pulmonary flow with ^{99m}Tc-MAA SPECT and cine phase contrast MR imaging. Ann Nucl Med 2002; 16:423–429.

24. Fratz S, Hess J, Schwaiger M, Martinoff S, Stern HC. More accurate quantification of pulmonary blood flow by magnetic resonance imaging than by lung perfusion scintigraphy in patients with fontan circulation. Circulation 2002; 106:1510–1513.

25. Silverman JM, Julien PJ, Herfkens RJ, Pelc NJ. Quantitative differential pulmonary perfusion: MR imaging versus radionuclide lung scanning. Radiology 1993; 189:699–701.

26. Kuhnle GE, Reichenspurner H, Lange T, Wagner F, Groh J, Messmer K, Goetz AE. Microhemodynamics and leukocyte sequestration after pulmonary ischemia and reperfusion in rabbits. J Thorac Cardiovasc Surg 1998; 115:937–944.

27. Stejskal EO, Tanner JE. Spin diffusion measurements: spin echoes in presence of a time-dependent field gradient. J Chem Phys 1965; 42:288–292.

28. Basser PJ. Diffusion and diffusion tensor MR imaging. In: Atlas SW, ed. Magnetic Resonance Imaging of the Brain and Spine. 3rd ed. Philadelphia: Lippincott Williams & Wilkins, 2002:197–214.

29. Patel MR, Siewert B, Warach S, Edelman RR. Diffusion and perfusion imaging techniques. Magn Reson Imaging Clin N Am 1995; 3:425–438.

30. Brudin LH, Rhodes CG, Valind SO, Jones T, Jonson B, Hughes JM. Relationships between regional ventilation and vascular and extravascular volume in supine humans. J Appl Physiol 1994; 76:1195–1204.

31. Stock KW, Chen Q, Hatabu H, Edelman RR. Magnetic resonance T2* measurements of the normal human lung *in vivo* with ultra-short echo times. Magn Reson Imaging 1999; 17:997–1000.

32. Hatabu H, Alsop DC, Listerud J, Bonnet M, Gefter WB. T2* and proton density measurement of normal human lung parenchyma using submillisecond echo time gradient echo magnetic resonance imaging. Eur J Radiol 1999; 29:245–252.

33. Young IR, Hall AS, Bryant DJ, Thomas DG, Gill SS, Dubowitz LM, Cowan F, Pennock JM, Bydder GM. Assessment of brain perfusion with MR imaging. J Comput Assist Tomogr 1988; 12:721–727.

34. Turner R, Le Bihan D, Maier J, Vavrek R, Hedges LK, Pekar J. Echo-planar imaging of intravoxel incoherent motion. Radiology1990; 177:407–414.

35. von Shulthess GK, Fisher MR, Higgins C. Pathologic blood flow in pulmonary vascular disease as shown by gated magnetic resonance imaging. Ann Int Med 1985; 103:317–323.

36. Hatabu H, Gaa J, Tadamura E, Edinburgh KJ, Stock KW, Garpestad E, Edelman RR. MR imaging of pulmonary parenchyma with a half-Fourier single-shot turbo spin-echo (HASTE) sequence. Eur J Radiol 1999; 29:152–159.

37. Suga K, Ogasawara N, Okada M, Tsukuda T, Matsunaga N, Miyazaki M. Lung perfusion impairments in pulmonary embolic and airway obstruction with noncontrast MR imaging. J Appl Physiol 2002; 92:2439–2451.
38. Kurihara Y, Yakushiji Y, Arakawa H, Tani I, Niimi H, Matsumoto J, Nakajima Y, Hirose K, Higashi M, Miyazaki M. A new perfusion weighted image of the lung without contrast material: difference of parenchymal signal intensity between systolic and diastolic phases. Proc Intl Soc Magn Reson Med 2001; 9:1991.
39. Kawanami S, Nakamura K, Miyazaki M, Sugiura S, Yamamoto A, Nakata H. Flow-weighted MRI of the lungs with the ECG-gated Half-Fourier FSE technique: evaluation of the effect of cardiac cycle. Magn Reson Medical Sciences 2002; 1:137–147.
40. Bradley WG Jr, Chen DY, Atkinson DJ, Edelman RE. Fast spine-echo and echo-planar imaging. In: Stark DD, Bradley JR, eds. Magnetic Resonance Imaging. 3rd ed. New York: Mosby, 1999:125–157.
41. Carr HY, Purcell EM. Effects of diffusion on free precession in nuclear magnetic resonance experiments. Phys Rev 1954; 94:630–638.
42. Hinks RS, Constable RT. Gradient moment nulling in fast spin echo. Magn Reson Med 1994; 32:698–706.
43. Singh SS, Singh M. Detection of pulsatile blood flow cycle in frog microvessels by image velocimetry. Med Biol Eng Comput 2002; 40:269–272.
44. Sugii Y, Nishio S, Okamoto K. Measurement of a velocity field in microvessels using a high resolution PIV technique. Ann NY Acad Sci 2002; 972:331–336.
45. Topulos GP, Lipsky NR, Lehr JL, Rogers RA, Butler JP. Fractional changes in lung capillary blood volume and oxygen saturation during the cardiac cycle in rabbits. J Appl Physiol 1997; 82:1668–1676.
46. Glenny RW, Bernard S, Robertson HT, Hlastala MP. Gravity is an important but secondary determinant of regional pulmonary blood flow in upright primates. J Appl Physiol 1999; 86:623–632.
47. Brudin LH, Rhodes CG, Valind SO, Jones T, Jonson B, Hughes JM. Interrelationships between regional blood flow, blood volume, and ventilation in supine humans. J Appl Physiol 1994; 76:1205–1210.
48. Stock KW, Chen Q, Levin D, Hatabu H, Edelman RR. Demonstration of gravity-dependent lung perfusion with contrast-enhanced magnetic resonance imaging. J Magn Reson Imaging 1999; 9:557–561.
49. Treppo S, Mijailovich SM, Venegas JG. Contributions of pulmonary perfusion and ventilation to heterogeneity in V(A)/Q measured by PET. J Appl Physiol 1997; 82:1163–1176.
50. Sackner MA, Greeneltch D, Heiman MS, Epstein S, Atkins N. Diffusing capacity, membrane diffusing capacity, capillary blood volume, pulmonary tissue volume, and cardiac output measured by a rebreathing technique. Am Rev Respir Dis 1975; 111:157–165.
51. Capen RL, Hanson WL, Latham LP, Dawson CA, Wagner WW Jr. Distribution of pulmonary capillary transit times in recruited networks. J Appl Physiol 1990; 69:473–478.
52. Presson RG Jr, Hanger CC, Godbey PS, Graham JA, Lloyd TC Jr, Wagner WW Jr. Effect of increasing flow on distribution of pulmonary capillary transit times. J Appl Physiol 1994; 76:1701–1711.
53. Presson RG Jr, Baumgartner WA Jr, Peterson AJ, Glenny RW, Wagner WW Jr. Pulmonary capillaries are recruited during pulsatile flow. J Appl Physiol 2002; 92:1183–1190.

54. Greaves SM, Hart EM, Brown K, Young DA, Batra P, Aberle DR. Pulmonary thromboembolism: spectrum of findings on CT. AJR Am J Roentgenol 1995; 165:1359–1363.

55. Bergin CJ, Sirlin CB, Hauschildt JP, Huynh TV, Auger WR, Fedullo PF, Kapelanski DP. Chronic thromboembolism: diagnosis with helical CT and MR imaging with angiographic and surgical correlation. Radiology 1997; 204:695–702.

56. Sherrick AD, Swenson SJ, Hartman TE. Mosaic pattern of lung attenuation on CT scans: frequency among patients with pulmonary artery hypertension of different causes. AJR Am J Roentgenol 1997; 169:79–82.

57. Shraufnagel DE, Mehta D, Harshbarger R, Treviranus K, Wang N. Capillary remodeling in bleomycin-induced pulmonary fibrosis. Am J Pathol 1986; 125:97–106.

58. Short AC, Montoya ML, Gebb SA, Presson RG, Wagner WW, Capen RL. Pulmonary capillary diameters and recruitment characteristics in subpleural and interior networks. J Appl Physiol 1996; 80:1568–1573.

59. Maeda S, Suzuki S, Moriya T, Suzuki T, Chida M, Suda H, Sakuma H, Kondo T, Sasano H. Isolated unilateral absence of a pulmonary artery: influence of systemic circulation on alveolar capillary vessels. Pathol Int 2001; 51:649–653.

60. Yamato M, Lecky J, Hiramatu K, Kohda E. Takayasu arteritis: radiographic and angiographic findings in 59 patients. Radiology 1986; 161:329–334.

61. Matsunaga N, Hayashi K, Sakamoto I, Matsuoka Y, Ogawa Y, Honjo K, Takano K. Takayasu arteritis: MR manifestations and diagnosis of acute and chronic phase. J Magn Reson Imaging 1998; 8:406–414.

62. Yamada I, Nakagawa T, Himeno Y, Kobayashi Y, Numano F, Shibuya H. Takayasu arteritis: diagnosis with breath-hold contrast-enhanced three-dimensional MR angiography. J Magn Reson Imaging 2000; 11:481–487.

63. Chen Q, Levin DL, Kim D, David V, McNicholas M, Chen V, Jakob PM, Griswold MA, Goldfarb JW, Hatabu H, Edelman RR. Pulmonary disorders: ventilation–perfusion MR imaging with animal models. Radiology 1999; 213:871–879.

64. Suga K, Nishigauchi K, Kume N, Uchisako H, Yoshimizu T, Nakanishi T. Delayed restoration of lung perfusion after removal of aspirated foreign body. Clin Nucl Med 1995; 20:1032–1033.

65. Morrell NW, Nijran KS, Biggs T, Seed WA. Changes in regional pulmonary blood flow during lobar bronchial occlusion in man. Clin Sci (Lond) 1994; 86:639–644.

66. Sakuma H, Kawada N, Kubo H, Nishide Y, Takano K, Kato N, Takeda K. Effect of breath holding on blood flow measurement using fast velocity encoded cine MRI. Magn Reson Med 2001; 45:346–348.

67. Pruessmann KP, Weiger M, Scheidegger MB, Boesiger P. SENSE: sensitivity encoding for fast MRI. Magn Reson Med 1999; 42:952–962.

13

Intravascular Imaging Using Hyperpolarized Nuclei

YANNICK CRÉMILLIEUX

Laboratoire de Résonance Magnétique Nucléaire,
Domaine Scientifique de la Doua, Villeurbanne, France

I. Introduction

Since the first demonstration of the magnetic resonance imaging (MRI) potential of laser-polarized nuclei by Albert et al. (1), polarized nuclei ventilation imaging studies have demonstrated the greatest advancements in terms of clinical application and research. Numerous studies in animal models, volunteers, and patients have been reported (2–6) and a large spectrum of applications, from partial alveolar oxygen pressure assessments (7) to diffusion measurements (8), has been demonstrated.

Besides these well-known ventilation imaging techniques, several research teams have investigated the development of new intravascular contrast agents using hyperpolarized nuclei. The prime objective of this research area is to obtain images or localized spectra of the distribution of these exogenous contrast agents in the body. The applications envisioned for these intravascular polarized contrast agents are the assessment of tissue perfusion, the acquisition of angiographic images, and improved characterization of biological tissues.

In order to perform such intravascular experiments, several problems need to be addressed first. First of all, one must develop a safe and efficient way for delivery of the polarized nuclei to the blood and the tissues. At the same time, the delivery process and the contrast agent media used must preserve the polarization level of the nuclei on a time scale compatible with NMR experiments. Finally, new dedicated MRI protocols and sequences have to be developed to use these contrast agents.

The answers to these problems depend greatly on the various polarized nuclei used in the experiments, as they have different solubilities, chemical affinities, and relaxation values. As a result, specific imaging strategies have to be defined depending on the polarized nuclei investigated. The scope of biomedical applications that may be obtained is dictated by the properties of the individual polarized nuclei. This chapter is divided into three sections dedicated, respectively, to xenon-129, helium-3, and carbon-13 studies. The conclusion will summarize the relative advantages and limitations of these polarized intravascular contrast agents, compare these agents to traditional MRI contrast agents, and discuss their potential clinical applications.

II. Intravascular Xenon-129 Imaging

Xenon-129, represents a stable isotope of xenon and has a natural abundance of 26.4%. Its gyromagnetic ratio, equal to 11.7 MHz/T, is about one-fourth of the proton gyromagnetic ratio, and one-third of helium-3. As a consequence, magnetic field gradient amplitudes four times larger than traditional proton imaging are required to obtain an image with equivalent acquisition parameters [such as the field-of-view (FOV) and the acquisition bandwidth]. The polarization of xenon-129 is obtained using the spin-exchange optical pumping technique. This method provides typical polarization on the order of 15%.

Two features of xenon are of great interest regarding its use as an intravascular contrast agent. First of all, it possesses a relatively high solubility (especially in lipid-based media) and it exhibits a large chemical shift spectrum, making it very sensitive to its environment and to chemical binding sites.

A. Xenon Delivery to Tissues

Although xenon is not able to participate in covalent chemical bonds, its large electronic polarizability results in a high solubility in polar solvents. This polarizability also accounts for its high affinity for lipids and hydrophobic sites in proteins. Its Ostwald coefficient (mL of dissolved gas/mL of solution) in blood is about 0.17 ($>10\times$ larger than that of helium). In lipid solutions, its Ostwald coefficient is more than 100 times larger than that of helium-3, which means that xenon is much more likely to become dissolved in lipid solutions.

Two different techniques have been developed to deliver polarized xenon to blood and tissues. Xenon can be delivered directly in the form of inhaled gas, or alternatively, it can be incorporated in an appropriate carrier agent and injected in a venous or an arterial blood vessel. Obviously, the simplest approach for xenon delivery to tissues is through the respiratory system (9). Because of its high solubility in tissues and blood, xenon can easily diffuse from the alveolar space to the intravascular compartment where it can be transported to organs and tissues of interest. This delivery method is, however, limited by the relatively small longitudinal relaxation times (T_1) of xenon in blood that ultimately limit the available xenon polarization (and, therefore, imaging ability) in tissues. These values also depend on the oxygenation level of blood. At 1.5 T and for a temperature of 37°C, T_1 values of 6.4 and 4 s in arterial and venous blood, respectively, have been reported (10). These differences between arterial and venous blood have been attributed to conformational changes of hemoglobin induced by oxygen binding (11) affecting the accessibility of xenon to binding sites and/or the xenon binding dynamics to those sites.

The second approach for xenon delivery to tissues relies on venous or arterial injection of a biocompatible carrier agent containing the polarized xenon. The most investigated carrier agents for xenon (12) are Intralipid suspensions, perfluorocarbon emulsions, xenon-filled liposomes, and saline solution. In lipid emulsion such as Intralipid, xenon's affinity for lipids allows the dissolution of large quantities of polarized xenon in a biocompatible injectable solution. Ostwald solubility values of xenon in 20% Intralipid and 30% Intralipid are equal to 0.4 and 0.6, respectively. The T_1 values of dissolved xenon were measured to be in the order of 25 and 30 s at magnetic field of 2 (13) and 2.35 T, respectively (14). At 2 T, the dissolved xenon resonance line was measured 197 ppm shifted relative to the xenon gas resonance.

Perflurocarbon emulsions represent interesting candidates for the transportation and the delivery of polarized xenon. These emulsions are chemically and biologically inert and they offer a high solubility for xenon. The xenon Ostwald coefficient in pure perfluorooctyl bromide (PFOB) emulsion is equal to 1.2. In 90% PFOB emulsion, the Ostwald coefficient is estimated to be in the order of 0.6.

The xenon spectrum shape in PFOB emulsion has been shown to depend on the PFOB droplet size distribution (15). This effect on the xenon NMR line has been attributed to xenon exchange between PFOB droplets and the aqueous environment. Larger droplet size results in reduced xenon exchange and narrower xenon resonance lines that can be more easily exploited in NMR experiments. In order to reach a compromise between biocompatible droplet size and narrow spectral lines, one may control the droplet size distribution by varying the emulsifier content, such as egg yolk phospholipid in the solution. In appropriate conditions, the chemical shift of xenon dissolved in PFOB droplets has been measured 111 ppm shifted relative to xenon gas phase. Xenon T_1 value in 20% PFOB emulsion was found equal to 83 s (16). Xenon has been shown to be also possibly encapsulated in liposomes of 8 ± 2 μm diameter (16). The T_1 of xenon in these liposomes has been measured to be 118 s.

Several groups have proposed compartmental models in order to predict the concentration of polarized xenon in tissues and blood following xenon delivery. Martin et al. (17) focused on xenon delivery through gas inhalation and have estimated the concentration of polarized xenon in the cerebral blood compartment and in brain tissues. In this model, the maximum breathed xenon concentration was set to 80% with a polarization level of 50%. The authors found that the estimated signal-to-noise ratio (SNR) of hyperpolarized xenon obtainable in the brain gray matter was 50 times less than the proton SNR at 2 T. The concentration in arterial blood was found to be 10 times greater than the concentration in gray matter.

Using a similar compartmental model, Lavini et al. (18) compared the expected polarized xenon concentration in brain tissues using either inhaled xenon or an intravenous injection of a xenon carrier agent. The authors studied the dependence of the tissue signal on the T_1, the xenon solubility in the compartments, and the injection rate. At first glance, the use of a xenon carrier agent represented an interesting alternative to the inhalation delivery technique because an appropriate solvent (with a large Ostwald coefficient and long xenon T_1) allowed for the dissolution of large quantities of xenon while preserving xenon polarization. However, the authors' experiments demonstrated that this approach suffered from large polarized xenon concentration losses due to xenon passage in the lung air spaces, solvent dilution with blood, and concomitant T_1 losses in mixed blood. These effects could be minimized by using solvents with larger xenon Ostwald coefficients. Lower tissue uptake would then be compensated by the reduced polarization losses. In experiments where xenon is encapsulated in structures such as liposomes, xenon polarization losses in lungs and blood could be further decreased, but the xenon gas would remain purely intravascular. Overall, predicted xenon signal in gray and white matter of the brain is comparable using inhalation or injection techniques, although, injection techniques require less polarized xenon.

The use of dissolved intraarterial xenon solutions represents one approach for the optimization of xenon tissues concentrations (14). Although this method is invasive and restricted to animal studies, it has been shown to provide interesting information regarding regional measurement of absolute cerebral perfusion values.

B. Polarized Xenon NMR in Tissues

The main interest of *in vivo* xenon NMR lies in its large chemical shift and its sensitivity to different biological environments. The assignment of xenon NMR lines to different biological environments has been investigated by several groups. Although there are still some controversies about the precise assignment of the *in vivo* xenon resonances, general trends emerge from the most recent *in vivo* studies (Fig. 13.1). Following xenon inhalation, Swanson et al. (19) observed *in vivo* resonance lines in rat body (brain, heart, and kidney) that have been attributed to blood (210 ppm shift relative to gas phase), tissues (199 ppm shift), and fat (192 ppm) compartments. In human studies, Kilian et al. (20) attributed the resonance lines to xenon in blood, gray matter (197 ppm), and white matter (193 ppm). In animal studies, using Intralipid injection with dissolved xenon, Duhamel et al. (14) observed resonance lines

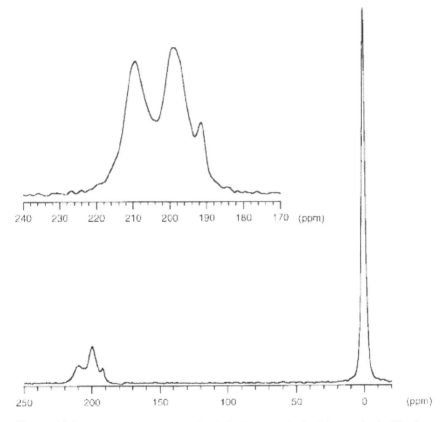

Figure 13.1 *In vivo* NMR spectra of polarized xenon obtained in a rat body. The four lines from left to right are attributed to xenon dissolved in blood, tissue, fat, and xenon gas in the lungs, respectively. The inset spectrum was acquired with a larger flip angle. [From Swanson et al. (19).]

attributed to xenon in brain tissue (199 ppm) and in Intralipid solution (194.5 ppm). One may note that the use of lipid-based solution for xenon delivery may not be compatible with the detection of xenon resonances in fat tissue or in white matter because of the resonance lines overlapping.

Wolber et al. (21) investigated the sensitivity of xenon longitudinal relaxation times and chemical shift depending upon the oxygenation state of blood. As mentioned previously, these effects have been attributed to conformational changes of hemoglobin induced by oxygen binding affecting the accessibility of xenon to the binding sites or the xenon binding dynamics to those sites. As suggested by the authors, these effects could be exploited for the assessment of blood oxygenation in tissues.

The same group has performed *in vivo* polarized xenon spectroscopy in animal tumors (22). They reported that xenon longitudinal relaxation times and spectrum shape depended on the investigated tumor types. These tumor specific xenon characteristics have been attributed to changes in xenon exchange dynamics between the xenon-dissolved medium and the biological compartments.

C. Polarized Xenon Imaging in Tissues

In order to take advantage of the xenon chemical shift in tissues and to avoid chemical shift artifacts, the chemical-shift imaging (CSI) technique has been widely used for *in vivo* xenon imaging. Using this technique, Swanson et al. (9) obtained the first *in vivo* image of the distribution of polarized xenon in a rat brain following xenon inhalation. The total acquisition time was 73 s for a $256 \times 16 \times 16$ data acquisition matrix and a voxel volume of 98 µL. In a more recent study, Swanson et al. (19) demonstrated the ability to obtain 2D CSI images of xenon at the level of a rat thorax corresponding to xenon in blood, tissue, and the alveolar space (Fig. 13.2). One-dimensional CSI acquisition in brain and kidney was also demonstrated.

Using the xenon inhalation technique, Kilian et al. (20) obtained the first two-dimensional CSI xenon images in human brain. These localized spectra were acquired at a 3 T magnetic field using a total volume of 1 L of xenon polarized at 15%. The phase gradient encoding matrix was 16×16 for a FOV equal to 32×32 cm.

Using an invasive approach restricted to animal studies, Duhamel et al. (23) demonstrated the feasibility of regional cerebral blood flow measurements using polarized xenon. In these studies, the authors used an injection of xenon dissolved in Intralipid solution into a rat carotid artery. A two-dimensional radial imaging sequence without slice selection was used to image the distribution of xenon in brain. The absolute quantification of perfusion and rCBF maps was obtained using the Kety–Schmidt formula (Fig. 13.3).

Angiographic imaging using xenon dissolved in Intralipid emulsion (Fig. 13.4) was also demonstrated by Möller et al. (13). These studies were performed in rats using intravenous injection of this lipid emulsion. The authors

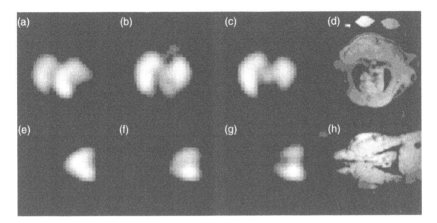

Figure 13.2 Two-dimensional CSI images of *in vivo* polarized xenon in rat thorax. Images A and E, xenon in blood; images B and F, xenon in tissue; images C and G, xenon gas in lungs; images D and H, axial and coronal proton images. [From Swanson et al. (19).]

obtained images of the pelvic and abdominal vasculature and demonstrated the possibility of measuring the mean blood flow velocity based on the dissolved xenon signal evolution.

A very interesting imaging application of xenon dissolved in tissue was proposed by Ruppert et al. (24). The technique, named xenon polarization

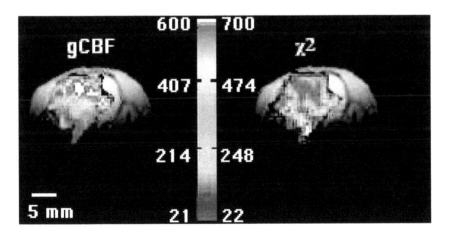

Figure 13.3 (**See color insert**) (Left) Perfusion maps (color) obtained in the rat brain using xenon washout analysis. (Right) The χ^2 map of the washout curve fitting procedure. The greyscale images correspond to the proton image at the same location. (Courtesy of Dr. Guillaume Duhamel and Dr. Anne Ziegler, Laboratoire Neuroimagerie Fonctionnelle et Métabolique, Inserm U594, Grenoble, France.)

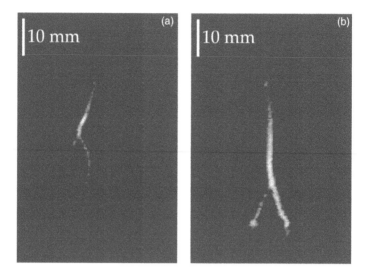

Figure 13.4 Coronal images of the rat vasculature following intravenous injection of an Intralipid solution with dissolved polarized xenon. (Left) The hypogastric and caudal veins, the right common iliac vein and the inferior vena cava. (Right) The right and left common iliac veins and the inferior vena cava. [From Möller et al. (13) reprinted with permission.]

transfer contrast (XTC), aims to probe the exchange of xenon between the alveolar space and blood/tissue compartments. The method is based on the selective destruction of xenon polarization in lung parenchyma. Because of the rapid exchange of xenon between the gas and the tissue phase, the depolarization of xenon dissolved in tissue affects the xenon signal from the gaseous phase. Using an appropriate pixel-based signal analysis of this effect, the authors obtained XTC lung images with a contrast related to the tissue and alveolar xenon exchange. According to the authors, this new type of contrast may lead to clinically useful information regarding the pathophysiologic state of the lungs.

III. Intravascular Helium-3 Imaging

A. Helium Delivery to Tissues

The nucleus of the helium-3 atom has a gyromagnetic ratio equal to about three-fourth of a proton. It can be hyperpolarized by two different optical pumping techniques: the spin-exchange technique and the metastability technique, with typical polarization levels equal to 30% and 60%, respectively.

In contrast to xenon, helium is characterized by a low solubility in fluids (~0.01 mL of dissolved gas per milliliter of fluid in blood and water). This precludes an efficient delivery of helium to the intravascular system via inhalation of polarized helium. Additionally, major difficulties are encountered in the prep-aration of an injectable solution of dissolved helium.

The first *in vivo* intravascular helium images have been obtained using helium microbubble suspensions. Chawla et al. (25) investigated several biocom-patible fluids for the production of a suspension of helium-3 microbubbles. The suspensions were formed after rapid and repeated flushing of the suspending fluid through a syringe containing the polarized helium. From all the tested fluids, the authors found that Hexabrix, a commercial radiographic contrast agent, enabled the best SNR. This suspension medium was used for *in vivo* imaging exper-iments. The longitudinal relaxation time of the helium suspension in this fluid was measured to be on the order of 40 s. The authors obtained arterial and venous angiographic images of the helium suspension in rats and obtained maximum SNR values equal to 55 (Fig. 13.5). However, the large mean bubble diameter of these suspensions (on the order of 30 μm) represented a major limitation for safe *in vivo* use of these solutions.

The problem of the low dissolution coefficient of helium can be overcome using appropriate carrier agents similar to the contrast agents designed for gas encapsulation in ultrasound contrast agent imaging. Chawla et al. (26) reported *in vivo* vascular images in rats using encapsulated helium-3 in microspheres.

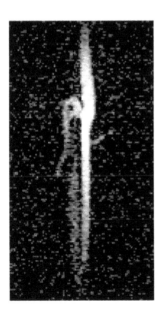 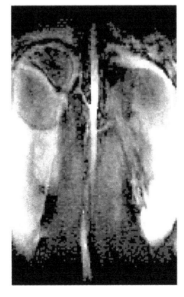

Figure 13.5 Coronal images of the rat vasculature using an injection of helium-3 microbubbles suspension. The abdominal aorta, the superior mesenteric artery, the right and left renal arteries and the vena cava are visible. The image on the right corresponds to proton image acquired at the same location. [From Chawla et al. (25) with permission. Copyright (1998) National Academy of Sciences, USA.]

These dual-walled microspheres (Point Biomedical, San Carlos, CA, USA) are composed of a bioabsorbable polymer inner wall and a cross-linked human serum albumin outer wall. The authors obtained two size distributions of polarized helium microspheres of 5.3 ± 1.3 and 10.9 ± 3.0 μm mean diameter. The gas concentration by volume in microsphere suspension varied between 0.9% and 7%. The T_1 longitudinal value of encapsulated helium was measured equal to ~64 s. Using these suspension of helium microspheres, the authors obtained MR images of a rat pelvic veins with SNR value of 15.

Using a similar approach, Callot et al. (27,28) demonstrated *in vivo* angiographic and perfusion images in rats and isolated reperfused pig heart (29). Lyophilized substrates for helium encapsulation were provided by Bracco-Research (Geneva, Switzerland). The encapsulating powder was made up of a combination of phospholipids and pharmaceutical grade polyethyleneglycol. This type of substrate and the encapsulation technique were similar to those used to generate microbubble ultrasound vascular contrast agent (30).

Using 300 mg of lyophilized substrate, the mean microbubble diameter was found equal to 3.0 ± 0.2 μm. The number of microbubbles per milliliter of solution and the total encapsulated volume of gas increased quasilinearly with the amount of lyophilisate used. Typically, a solution prepared with 300 mg of substrate and 4 mL of saline contained 8.1×10^8 microbubbles per milliliter, corresponding to 45 μL of encapsulated gas per milliliter of solution. Transverse and longitudinal relaxation values of encapsulated helium were measured *in vitro* in the syringe used to prepare the solution. Linewidths obtained after spectrum quantification yielded apparent transverse relaxation times T_2^* of 4.5 ± 0.1 ms. Transverse relaxation times T_2 were measured in the order of 300 ± 40 ms and a T_1 longitudinal relaxation time of 140 s was obtained (29).

B. Polarized Helium Imaging in Tissues

As described previously, angiographic images may be obtained using an injection of polarized helium microspheres or microbubbles. Another application of intravascular helium concerns the visualization of tissue perfusion. Callot et al. (27,28) demonstrated that obtaining images of helium microbubbles in lung vasculature is feasible (Fig. 13.6). The SNR values of these lung perfusion images were reasonable, on order of 30, and allowed good visualization of lung parenchymal perfusion. The potential of this technique for lung perfusion assessment was validated through an experimental pulmonary embolism model with visualization of perfusion defects. In recent experiments, the same group demonstrated the possibility of obtaining dynamic images of lung perfusion (Fig. 13.7).

Callot et al. (29) investigated the potential of helium microbubbles in coronary imaging. In a reperfused and beating pig heart model, they obtained dynamic coronary and myocardium perfusion images (Fig. 13.8). For this purpose, the authors used a combination of radial imaging and "sliding-window" technique. Coronary branches down to the third generation were visualized with vessel

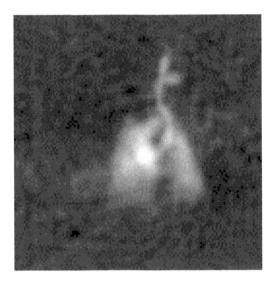

Figure 13.6 Rat lung perfusion image following a jugular venous injection of 1 mL solution of helium-3 microbubbles.

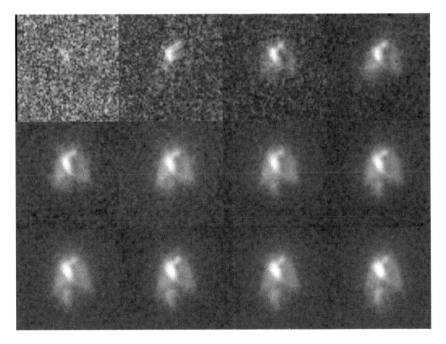

Figure 13.7 Dynamic rat lung perfusion images series following an intravenous injection of a solution of helium-3 microbubbles. The temporal image series resolution is 200 ms.

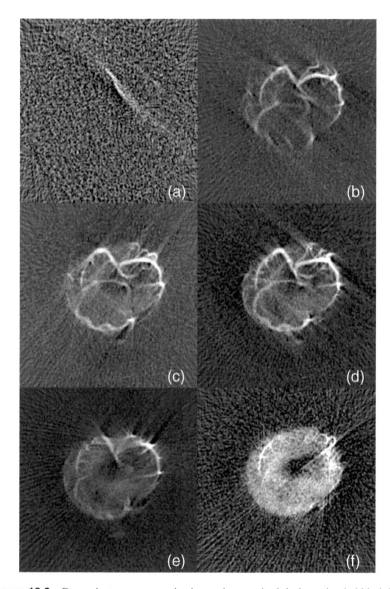

Figure 13.8 Dynamic transverse projection series acquired during microbubble injection in the coronaries of an isolated perfused beating heart. The different images correspond to (a) $t = 1.13$ s (preliminary arrival of the microbubbles in the coronaries), (b) $t = 2.48$ s (intermediate image), (c) $t = 3.37$ s (angiographic image: arteries are clearly outlined), (d) $t = 4.13$ s (myocardial tissue highlighting due to the presence of microbubbles in the capillaries), (e) $t = 4.88$ s (myocardial perfusion phase), (f) $t = 6.22$ s (total myocardial perfusion before the washout phase; left and right ventricles, free of microbubbles, are visible). The size of the major vessels varies between 1.6 and 2.8 mm, the SNR in the corresponding region of interest are 19 and 27.

diameter of 1 mm. An enhancement of the myocardium corresponding to the distribution of the microbubbles in the capillaries was also observed. The SNR was measured between 10 (myocardium) and 30 (coronary vessels).

IV. Intravascular Carbon-13 Imaging

A. Carbon-13 Polarization Techniques

Carbon-13 has a natural abundance of 1.1%. The polarization of carbon-13 for MR imaging applications has been demonstrated with two different techniques, parahydrogen-induced polarization (PHIP) (31) and dynamic nuclear polarization (32).

The parahydrogen-induced polarization method is based on the hydrogenation of ^{13}C-enriched molecules with parahydrogen. Parahydrogen is an isomeric form of molecular hydrogen where the two proton spins are aligned in antiparallel fashion. At thermal equilibrium, molecular hydrogen contains 25% of the parahydrogen state. In the first step of the PHIP method, the dihydrogen is enriched in parahydrogen by lowering the temperature at liquid nitrogen temperature (77 K) in the presence of paramagnetic compounds. Golman et al. (31) investigated the hydrogenation of a molecule of acetylene di-carboxylic acid dimethyl ester yielding maleic acid dimethyl ester. Following hydrogenation by parahydrogen, the second step of the method as proposed by the authors consists of the conversion of the spin order introduced in the molecule into longitudinal magnetization, leading to a high polarization level. For this purpose, the authors proposed a method using magnetic field cycling resulting in the final carbon-13 polarization level of 4%. The authors took advantage of the long longitudinal relaxation time (75 s) of carbon-13 to perform *in vivo* images in animal. They demonstrated carbon-13 angiographic images in a rat using a single-shot RARE imaging sequence.

Another approach based on the DNP technique has been proposed and demonstrated for the acquisition of *in vivo* images of polarized carbon (32). The principle of the DNP technique relies on a polarization transfer from the electron to the nuclear spin. The technique requires the presence of a paramagnetic agent, typically a free radical, whose electron spin is highly polarized using a large magnetic field and low temperatures. The irradiation and saturation of the electron spin resonance results in the transfer of the electron polarization to the nuclear spin.

In their experimental set-up, the authors cooled the imaging agent, (1-hydroxymethyl-1-^{13}C-cyclopropyl)-methanol, to a temperature of 1.3 K. The sample was doped with paramagnetic agent and placed into a magnetic field of 3.35 T. With these experimental parameters, the electron polarization was equal to 94%. The sample is saturated for 1 h using microwaves at a frequency of 93.925 GHz. Using this technique, the authors obtained a carbon-13 polarization level of 20%. Following this polarization procedure, the sample is warmed up, and a solution containing 200 mM of polarized imaging agent is prepared prior to injection.

B. Polarized Carbon-13 Imaging in Tissues

Using the PHIP technique, Golman et al. (31) demonstrated that subsecond angiographic images in rat could be obtained using molecules with polarized carbon-13. The authors took advantage of the long transverse relaxation time of the carbon nucleus ($T_2 > 2$ s) by using a RARE imaging sequence with multiple transverse magnetization refocusing pulses. The matrix size was equal to 128×64, and the total acquisition time was equal to 0.9 s.

The same group demonstrated the high efficiency of the trueFISP imaging sequence (33,34) for the optimization of the image SNR using intravascular imaging agents with polarized carbon-13. In the case of nonhyperpolarized spins, this gradient echo imaging sequence with short repetition times is based on the acquisition of the steady-state magnetization with zero gradient dephasing during the repetition time. In the case of hyperpolarized spins, this imaging sequence takes advantage of the very long relaxation times of the carbon-13 spins to complete the image acquisition before the magnetization decays towards the thermally polarized steady-state magnetization. Hence, the relaxation times of the (1-hydroxymethyl-1-^{13}C-cyclopropyl)-methanol *in vivo* were 40 and 2 s, respectively, for longitudinal and transverse magnetization. When compared with fast gradient echo imaging sequence with small flip angles, the gain in image SNR can be significantly improved up to one order of magnitude.

Using this trueFISP imaging sequence (33), angiograms with high SNR have been obtained in thoracic, abdominal, and head regions. In the cardiac and pulmonary regions, SNR's equal to 500 were measured (Fig. 13.9). Dynamic angiographic and perfusion images in rats were demonstrated in the heart, lung, and brain (34). On the basis of contrast agent first pass imaging techniques, perfusion maps of cerebral blood volume, blood flow, and mean transit times were also obtained (34).

V. Applications of Intravascular Polarized Imaging Agents

A. Compared Properties

The hyperpolarized spin species (xenon, helium, and carbon) and the proton spin can be compared with each other in terms of the available SNR per unit volume. In the case of polarized spins, the signal amplitude per unit volume is proportional to the magnetization per unit volume M multiplied by the nucleus Larmor frequency ω_0. The magnetization per unit volume is equal to the product of the following terms: the nucleus gyromagnetic ratio γ, the polarization level P, the spin density N, and the spin value I. For human imaging studies in standard magnetic field >1.5 T, the sample represents the predominant source

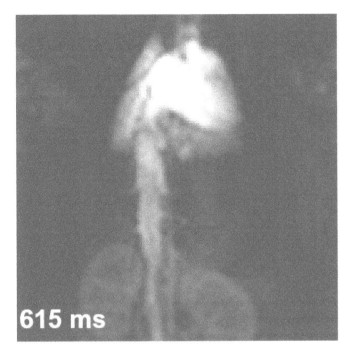

615 ms

Figure 13.9 Angiographic image in a rat thorax and abdomen following intravenous injection of 3 mL of a polarized carbon-13 imaging agent solution highlighting the lung and the kidney vasculature. [From Svensson et al. (33).]

of noise and is proportional to the squared Larmor frequency. With identical I spin value ($I = 1/2$) and at a fixed magnetic field, the SNR value per unit volume is then proportional to the product γPN. The typical values of the achievable SNR for intravascular polarized imaging applications are summarized in Table 13.1.

In the case of peripheral injection, dilution of the contrast agent with venous blood significantly reduces the blood concentration of the polarized imaging agent. This dilution coefficient has been estimated by Lavini et al. (18) and depends on the cardiac output and the contrast agent injection rate. For helium-3 and carbon-13 polarized imaging agents, the typical expected dilution factor is in the order of 12. For a polarized xenon suspension, Lavini et al. pointed out that an additional dilution coefficient corresponding to the xenon passage from the pulmonary capillary bed to the alveolar space has to be taken into account, yielding a total dilution coefficient equal to 60.

The imaging sequence represents an important parameter for the optimization of the image SNR. As shown by Svensson et al. (33), the use of magnetization refocusing imaging sequences (trueFISP or RARE) should be performed whenever possible for optimizing the image SNR. In this instance, the long

Table 13.1 Summary of NMR Parameters of Hyperpolarized Imaging Agents

	Proton	Xenon-129	Helium-3	Carbon-13
Gyromagnetic ratio γ (MHz/T)	42.6	11.7	32.5	10.7
Polarization (P)	5×10^{-6} (at 1.5 T and 310 K)	0.15	0.50 (metastable technique)	0.15 (32)
Concentration (M)	80 (in blood)	0.01 (natural abundance Ostwald coefficient of 1)	0.002 (27,28)	0.2 (32)
Relative SNR (imaging agent solution)	1	1	1.9	18.8
Dilution factor (18)	1	60	12	12
Relative SNR (peripheral injection)	1	0.017	0.16	1.6
Longitudinal relaxation times	1–3 s	80 s in PFOB (16)	140 s (29)	40 s (32)

Note: Numbers within parentheses indicate references.

relaxation times of polarized nuclei represent a substantial advantage, although not easily quantifiable, over conventional proton fast imaging acquisitions.

Several conclusions can be derived from the numerical values of Table 13.1. First of all, polarized xenon offers the lowest SNR values of all hyperpolarized nuclei, meaning that the use of polarized xenon should be probably restricted to applications where its large chemical shift can be exploited. Because of its larger concentration achievable in imaging agents, polarized carbon-13 solutions provide a larger available SNR than a polarized helium-3 microbubble suspension. In this sense, polarized carbon-13 imaging agents appear as the polarized nuclei of choice for intravascular imaging applications such as angiographic or perfusion studies. On the other hand, helium-3 microbubbles suspensions exhibit larger longitudinal relaxation times and benefit from the important expertise developed and accumulated in the ultrasound microbubbles-based contrast agent field.

B. Imaging Applications

The very large nonequilibrium magnetizations of polarized nuclei represent the first motivation for the use of polarized imaging agents. The signal increase resulting from the polarization process represents an indubitable competitive advantage of the void space of the pulmonary airways. However, this advantage is drastically reduced in the case of intravascular *in vivo* applications because of the much larger proton spin density in biological tissues. Furthermore, angiographic and perfusion imaging using conventional contrast agents such as gadolinium chelates or iron oxides nanoparticles represent very well established MR imaging techniques. Hence, the future of intravascular polarized imaging agents in the MRI field will depend strongly on their ability to allow new *in vivo* applications according to their specific properties.

The intrinsic high contrast to noise ratio (CNR) obtained with exogenous polarized spins represents one important feature of these imaging agents. The absence of disturbing background signal coming from surrounding tissues (i.e., fat, blood) has several important implications regarding the precise evaluation of the imaging agent distribution, signal quantification, and the reduction of image artifacts from motion and chemical shift.

The potential of the high CNR offered by polarized imaging agents is illustrated by the work of Callot et al. (29) on the isolated and perfused beating heart using helium-3 microbubbles injection in coronary vessels (Fig. 13.8). The visualization of the coronary vessels and the myocardium perfusion is greatly facilitated by the absence of background signal arising from fat, heart parenchyma, and blood in the heart cavities. As a consequence, projection images of the coronary vessels, similar to those obtained in X-ray coronary angiography, were acquired. Furthermore, because of the absence of signal from moving tissues or flowing blood, the fluoroscopic images obtained on the beating heart exhibited very few motion artifacts. This type of study allowing simultaneous coronary imaging and myocardium perfusion evaluation could have future applications in interventional MR imaging.

For hemodynamic measurements such as tissue perfusion, polarized imaging agents, in contrast to conventional contrast agents, demonstrate a direct relationship between the NMR signal amplitude and the polarized imaging agents concentration. Furthermore, the contrast agent re-circulation can be easily controlled using radio-frequency pulses for the suppression of the hyperpolarized magnetization.

Lung perfusion imaging using helium-3 or carbon-13 imaging agents (27,28,34) represents a promising application for intravascular polarized nuclei. MR proton imaging of the lungs is still a difficult matter because of the low proton density and the magnetic susceptibility heterogeneity of the lung. In this instance, polarized imaging agents represent a competitive alternative to proton lung imaging for the assessment of lung perfusion.

Besides the use of polarized imaging agents such as pure blood pool contrast agents, important applications lie in their potential for obtaining information about their biological environment through their chemical shift or their affinity for specific biological tissues. In the case of hyperpolarized xenon, these applications are, however, confronted with the problem of low SNR in xenon studies. For this reason, technical (polarization levels) or methodological (imaging sequences, xenon delivery) improvements will be certainly necessary to extend the application fields of this polarized spin. With respect to hyperpolarized carbon-13, the possible incorporation of polarized carbon-13 in organic molecules of biological interest could clearly open a large spectrum of imaging or spectroscopic applications for this nucleus. However, potential applications still rely on the successful demonstration of production of polarized ^{13}C-enriched organic molecules associated with long longitudinal relaxation times.

References

1. Albert MS, Cates GD, Driehuys B, Happer W, Saam B, Springer CS Jr, Wishnia A. Biological magnetic resonance imaging using laser-polarized ^{129}Xe. Nature 1994; 370:199–201.
2. Middleton H, Black RD, Saam B, Cates GD, Cofer GP, Guenther R, Happer W, Hedlund LW, Johnson GA, Juvan K, Swartz J. MR imaging with hyperpolarized ^{3}He gas. Magn Reson Med 1995; 33:271–275.
3. Black RD, Middleton HL, Cates GD, Cofer GP, Driehuys B, Happer W, Hedlund LW, Johnson GA, Shattuck MD, Swartz JC. In vivo ^{3}He MR images of guinea pig lungs. Radiology 1996; 199:867–870.
4. MacFall JR, Charles HC, Black RD, Middleton H, Swartz JC, Saam B, Driehuys B, Erickson C, Happer W, Cates GD, Johnson GA, Ravin CE. Human lung air spaces: potential for MR imaging with hyperpolarized helium-3. Radiology 1996; 200:553–558.
5. Bachert P, Schad LR, Bock M, Knopp MV, Ebert M, Grossmann T, Heil W, Hofmann D, Surkau R, Otten EW. Nuclear MRI of airways in humans with use of hyperpolarized helium-3. Magn Reson Med 1996; 36:192–196.
6. Viallon M, Berthezène Y, Décorps M, Wiart M, Callot V, Bourgeois M, Humblot H, Briguet A, Crémillieux Y. Laser-polarized ^{3}He as a probe for dynamic regional measurements of lung perfusion and ventilation using magnetic resonance imaging. Magn Reson Med 2000; 44(1):1–4.
7. Deninger AJ, Mansson S, Petersson JS, Pettersson G, Magnusson P, Svensson J, Fridlund B, Hansson G, Erjefeldt I, Wollmer P, Golman K. Quantitative measurement of regional lung ventilation using ^{3}He MRI. Magn Reson Med 2002; 48(2):223–232.
8. Saam BT, Yablonskiy DA, Kodibagkar VD, Leawoods JC, Gierada DS, Cooper JD, Lefrak SS, Conradi MS. MR imaging of diffusion of ^{3}He gas in healthy and diseased lungs. Magn Reson Med 2000; 44(2):174–179.
9. Swanson SD, Rosen MS, Agranoff BW, Coulter KP, Welsh RC, Chupp TE. Brain MRI with laser-polarized ^{129}Xe. Magn Reson Med 1997; 38(5):695–698.
10. Wolber J, Cherubini A, Dzik-Jurasz AS, Leach MO, Bifone Angelo. Spin-lattice relaxation of laser-polarized xenon in human blood. Proc Natl Acad Sci 1999; 96(7):3664–3669.
11. Wolber J, Cherubini A, Leach MO, Bifone A. On the oxygenation-dependent ^{129}Xe T1 in blood. NMR Biomed 2000; 13(4):234–237.
12. Goodson BM. Using injectable carriers of laser-polarized noble gases for enhancing NMR and MRI. Concepts in Magnetic Resonance 1999; 11(4):203–223.

13. Möller HE, Chawla MS, Chen XJ, Driehuys B, Hedlung LW, Wheeler CT, Johnson GA. Magnetic resonance angiography with hyperpolarized [129]Xe dissolved in a lipid emulsion. Magn Reson Med 1999; 41:1058–1064.
14. Duhamel G, Choquet P, Grillon E, Lamalle L, Leviel JL, Ziegler A, Constantinesco A. Xenon-129 MR imaging and spectroscopy of rat brain using arterial delivery of hyperpolarized xenon in a lipid emulsion. Magn Reson Med 2001; 46(2):208–212.
15. Wolber J, Rowland IJ, Leach MO, Bifone A. Perfluorocarbon emulsions as intravenous delivery media for hyperpolarized xenon. Magn Reson Med 1999; 41(3):442–449.
16. Venkatesh AK, Zhao L, Balamore D, Jolesz FA, Albert MS. Evaluation of carrier agents for hyperpolarized xenon MRI. NMR Biomed 2000; 13(4):245–252.
17. Martin CC, Williams RF, Gao JH, Nickerson LD, Nickerson LDH, Xiong J, Fox PT. The pharmacokinetics of hyperpolarized xenon: implications for cerebral MRI. J Magn Reson Imaging 1997; 7(5):848–854.
18. Lavini C, Payne GS, Leach MO, Bifone A. Intravenous delivery of hyperpolarized [129]Xe: a compartmental model. NMR Biomed 2000; 13(4):238–244.
19. Swanson SD, Rosen MS, Coulter KP, Welsh RC, Chupp TE. Distribution and dynamics of laser-polarized [129]Xe magnetization in vivo. Magn Reson Med 1999; 42(6):1137–1145.
20. Kilian W, Seifert F, Rinneberg H. MRI of human lung and brain using hyperpolarized [129]Xe. Helion 02, International Workshop on Polarized [3]He Beams and Gas Targets and Their Applications, Oppenheim, Germany, Sept 8–13, 2002.
21. Wolber J, Cherubini A, Leach MO, Bifone A. Hyperpolarized [129]Xe NMR as a probe for blood oxygenation. Magn Reson Med 2000; 43(4):491–496.
22. Wolber J, McIntyre DJ, Rodrigues LM, Carnochan P, Griffiths JR, Leach MO, Bifone A. In vivo hyperpolarized [129]Xe NMR spectroscopy in tumors. Magn Reson Med 2001; 46(3):586–591.
23. Duhamel G, Choquet P, Grillon E, Leviel JL, Décorps M, Ziegler A, Constantinesco A. Global and regional cerebral blood flow measurements using NMR of injected hyperpolarized xenon-129. Acad Radiol 2002; 9(suppl 2):S498–S500.
24. Ruppert K, Brookeman JR, Hagspiel KD, Mugler JP III. Probing lung physiology with xenon polarization transfer contrast (XTC). Magn Reson Med 2000; 44(3):349–357.
25. Chawla MS, Chen XJ, Möller HE, Cofer GP, Wheeler CT, Hedlung LW, Johnson GA. *In vivo* magnetic resonance vascular imaging using laser-polarized [3]He microbubbles. Proc Natl Acad Sci USA 1998; 95:10832–10835.
26. Chawla MS, Chen XJ, Cofer GP, Hedlung LW, Kerby MB, Ottoboni TB, Johnson GA. Hyperpolarized [3]He microspheres as a novel vascular signal source for MRI. Magn Reson Med 2000; 43:440–445.
27. Callot V, Canet E, Brochot J, Viallon M, Humblot H, Briguet A, Tournier H, Crémillieux Y. MR perfusion imaging using encapsulated laser-polarized 3He. Magn Reson Med 2001; 46(3):535–540.
28. Callot V, Canet E, Brochot J, Berthezene Y, Viallon M, Humblot H, Briguet A, Tournier H, Crémillieux Y. Vascular and perfusion imaging using encapsulated laser-polarized helium. MAGMA 2001; 12(1):16–22.

29. Callot V, Canet E, Brochot J, Humblot H, Briguet A, Tournier H, Crémillieux Y. Hyperpolarized helium-3 encapsulated in microbubbles: a new class of blood pool MRI contrast agent. Acad Radiol 2002; 9(suppl 2):S501–503.
30. Schneider   M.   Characteristics   of   SonoVue[TM].   Echocardiography   1999; 16(7):743–746.
31. Golman K, Axelsson O, Johannesson H, Mansson S, Olofsson C, Petersson JS. Parahydrogen-induced polarization in imaging: subsecond ^{13}C angiography. Magn Reson Med 2001; 46(1):1–5.
32. Golman K, Ardenkjaer-Larsen JH, Svensson J, Axelsson O, Hansson G, Hansson L, Johannesson H, Leunbach I, Mansson S, Petersson JS, Pettersson G, Servin R, Wistrand LG. ^{13}C-angiography. Acad Radiol 2002; 9(suppl 2):S507–510.
33. Svensson J, Mansson S, Johansson E, Petersson JS, Olsson LE. Hyperpolarized ^{13}C MR angiography using trueFISP. Magn Reson Med 2003; 50(2):256–262.
34. Golman K, Ardenkjaer-Larsen JH, Axelsson O, Petersson JS, Mansson S. Hyperpolarisation of ^{13}C, ^{15}N and ^{1}H for MR applications. Helion 02, International Workshop on Polarized ^{3}He Beams and Gas Targets and Their Applications, Oppenheim, Germany, Sept 8–13, 2002.

14

Combined MR Ventilation/Perfusion Imaging

YVES BERTHEZÈNE

Hôpital de la Croix Rousse,
Service de Radiologie,
Lyon, France

YANNICK CRÉMILLIEUX

Laboratoire de Résonance
  Magnétique Nucléaire,
Domaine Scientifique de la Doua,
Villeurbanne, France

I. Introduction

The major function of the lung is to permit gas exchange between the airways and the blood. Integral to this task is the matching of local alveolar ventilation and pulmonary blood flow. Both lungs together receive a total of ~4 L/min alveolar ventilation and 5 L/min of blood flow, for an overall ventilation/perfusion ratio of 0.8. However, even in the normal individual, ventilation and blood flow are not equally distributed among all alveoli. Some alveoli have more ventilation than perfusion (increased ventilation/perfusion ratio), whereas others have more perfusion than ventilation (decreased ventilation/perfusion ratio). The changes in ventilation/perfusion ratios are small in the healthy person and are in part due to the effects of gravity on the distribution of pulmonary blood flow and ventilation between the base and the apex of the lung. The reason there is a regional difference in ventilation is due to the normal gradient in pleural surface pressure caused by gravity and interactions with the chest wall. In addition, more gravity-dependent regions of the lung receive more blood flow per unit volume. The intravascular pressure in the lower regions of the lung is greater because of hydrostatic effects in blood flow. Blood vessels in the more dependent portions of the lung are, therefore, more distended leading to greater perfusion. It is important to recognize that in many types of lung disease there are alterations in ventilation, perfusion, and the ventilation/perfusion ratio, which can become significant.

In clinical practice, ventilation and perfusion testing is used for two major reasons: detection of pulmonary emboli and assessment of regional lung function. Ventilation and perfusion lung scanning to assess regional lung function is often performed before surgery involving resection of a part of the lung, usually one or more lobes. By visualizing which areas of the lung receive ventilation and perfusion, the physician can determine how much the area to be resected is contributing to the overall lung function. It is also possible to predict postoperative pulmonary function, which is a guide to postoperative respiratory problems and impairment. Ventilation and perfusion to broncho-pulmonary segments is matched in a healthy individual. In pulmonary embolic disease, segmental reduction in perfusion occurs with maintenance of normal ventilation. This leads to the mismatch of perfusion and ventilation in the broncho-pulmonary segment. In parenchymal lung disease, matched ventilation and perfusion defects are usually observed.

The techniques used to assess regional pulmonary ventilation and perfusion are limited. The only method that is routinely used in a clinical setting is radionuclide ventilation–perfusion scintigraphy. Although this technique is noninvasive and widely available, it is limited by poor spatial and temporal resolution and by the use of radioactive materials.

Traditional pulmonary function tests, such as spirometry or the determination of pulmonary diffusion capacity, evaluate the lung as a whole. These tests are incapable of identifying the magnitude and distribution of the abnormalities on a regional basis. Although computed tomography is an accurate method for the detection of regional morphologic lesions, it usually does not provide a direct functional assessment of the lung.

The composition of lung tissue makes the lung an intrinsically difficult organ to examine with magnetic resonance imaging. Little or no signal may be detected with conventional sequences because of both low proton density and local magnetic field gradient perturbance at the air–tissue interface which rapidly dephase the transverse magnetization. Cardiac and respiratory motion also create artifacts with conventional MR imaging techniques.

Different MR approaches for ventilation/perfusion have been implemented using magnetic resonance imaging. Paramagnetic contrast media have the potential to increase the MR signal from the lungs when using very short TE, which reduce the susceptibility effect arising from tissue–air interfaces. Extra-cellular or strictly intravascular contrast agents administered intravenously (Gd-chelates) have been used to evaluate lung perfusion. To image ventilation, Gd-chelates have been applied as an aerosol. As oxygen has paramagnetic properties, it can also be used as an inhaled contrast agent for direct imaging of pulmonary ventilation.

Beside proton MRI, other nuclei can be used for MRI. They include ^{3}He, ^{129}Xe, and ^{19}Fl. ^{3}He and ^{129}Xe are inert gases and they can be applied easily by inhalation. This chapter will give an overview of the various methods to perform combined perfusion–ventilation MR imaging. Many of these methods are still in infancy, but some are approaching clinical application.

II. Proton MR Imaging

A. Venous Injection of Gd-Chelates and Inhalation of Aerosolized Gadolinium

The classical method requires the administration of intravenous contrast agent (Gd-chelates) to evaluate lung perfusion. Gd-chelates will reduce the longitudinal relaxation (T_1) of blood resulting in an increase in signal intensity. Usually, imaging is performed during the first pass of the contrast agent through the lung using a fast imaging sequence with a short TE to reduce susceptibility artifacts.

In the early 1990s, Berthezène et al. (1) demonstrated the feasibility of MR ventilation imaging in a rat model with aerosolized gadopentetate-dimeglumine as a contrast agent. Combined with gadopentetate-dimeglumine perfusion imaging, it is possible to demonstrate regional pulmonary ventilation and perfusion (Fig. 14.1). Because of the relatively low lung enhancement after inhalation of aerosolized gadolinium, it is necessary to start with the ventilation techniques before the acquisition of the perfusion images. More recently, Suga et al. (2) demonstrated that Gd-based aerosol and perfusion MR imaging have the ability to assess regionally impaired lung function associated with acute airway obstruction and pulmonary embolism with matched perfusion–ventilation deficits in airway obstruction dog models and the regionally mismatched perfusion–ventilation in pulmonary embolism dog models. However, Gd-chelates are not yet approved in the form of an inhaled aerosol; thus, this approach is not available in clinical settings. Furthermore, the relatively long

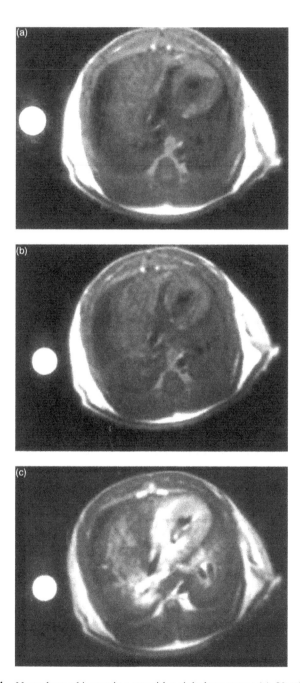

Figure 14.1 Nonenhanced image in a rat with a right lung tumor (a). Ventilation image obtained after inhalation of aerosolized gadolinium (b). Perfusion image obtained after venous injection of gadolinium chelates (c).

aerosol inhalation time (20 min) to obtain sufficient enhancement is also a drawback.

B. Venous Injection of Gd-Chelates and Oxygen Inhalation

Oxygen is safe and is readily available as part of emergency equipment in most MR suites. Oxygen ventilation imaging, therefore, does not induce additional costs. This imaging method does not require additional hardware and can be acquired with conventional MR imagers. The observed lung enhancement results from the shortening of the proton spin–lattice relaxation time in the lung tissue and blood, owing to paramagnetic effect of molecular oxygen. Oxygen is used as a T1 contrast agent to assess pulmonary ventilation and a bolus of Gd-chelates is used to assess lung perfusion (Fig. 14.2). In an animal model of airway occlusion, Chen et al. (3) demonstrated a mean 11-fold increase in ventilation enhancement in the normal lung compared with that in the obstructed lung. In the same experiment, MR perfusion imaging showed an associated decrease in lung perfusion, which probably reflects hypoxic vaso-constriction. In a model of pulmonary embolism, mismatched ventilation and perfusion patterns were observed in all animals.

More recently Nakagawa et al. (4) evaluated oxygen-enhanced MRI and contrast-enhanced perfusion MRI in patients with various lung diseases, includ-ing pulmonary embolism, lung malignancy, and bulla. Ventilation–perfusion mismatch was observed in all patients with pulmonary embolism and ventilation defects were observed in patients with bronchial stenosis.

However, in clinical practice, the enhancement with oxygen is relatively low and is influenced by the large and fast oxygen transfer into the blood stream. Misregistration can also occur between images obtained within the inter-vals of breathing room air and 100% oxygen. A more detailed description of this technique is available in Chapter 9.

C. Spin Labeling MR Perfusion and Oxygen Inhalation

This technique is completely noninvasive and does not require exogenous con-trast administration (5). First pass Gd imaging is somewhat invasive and cannot immediately be repeated, because time is required for washout of the tracer. This makes contrast-enhanced imaging unsuitable for studying perfusion changes over short time periods. This does not apply to spin labeling images, which can be acquired repeatedly without the need for contrast injection. In addition, depending on the gradient strength of the scanner, it might not be pos-sible to cover the whole lung with sufficient temporal and spatial resolution using contrast-enhanced imaging.

The arterial spin labeling method uses blood water as an endogenous con-trast agent and requires the acquisition of two images. Tagging pulses are applied so that the magnetization inside the slice is the same for both images, whereas the magnetization of the inflowing blood outside the slice is different. A delay

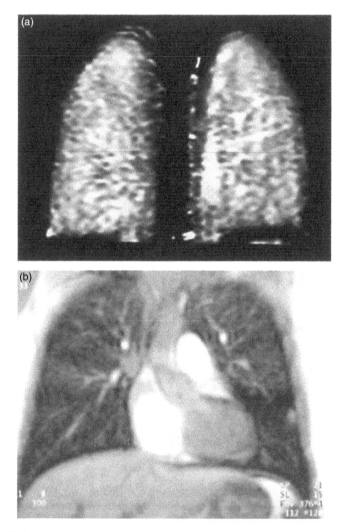

Figure 14.2 Oxygen coronal ventilation image in a patient with suspected pulmonary embolism demonstrates a homogeneous lung enhancement (a). Gadolinium perfusion image demonstrates a perfusion defect in the left lower lobe (b).

between the application of the tagging pulses and the acquisition of the image allows spins that were originally outside the imaging plane to perfuse in. Subtraction of these two images suppresses the signal from stationary tissue and yields a perfusion-weighted image. The lower signal-to-noise ratio of this method may render it unreliable for detecting very small defects but it is adequate for imaging moderate to large defects. According to Keilholz et al. (6), first pass contrast-enhanced perfusion imaging is more sensitive to defects than spin labeling technique, but spin labeling achieves acceptable image quality and may be used when repeated measurements are desirable.

Mai et al. (5) have successfully obtained combined V/Q images with this technique in 10 volunteers. Both lungs show normal ventilation and perfusion (with no ventilation or perfusion defects) in the oxygen-enhanced and perfusion images. In a patient in whom the left upper lobe was removed, matched ventilation and perfusion defects were observed (Fig. 14.3).

III. Hyperpolarized Gas Imaging

Hyperpolarized ^{3}He MRI is a new technology that provides a detailed image of lung ventilation with an excellent spatial and temporal resolution. Although MR imaging with hyperpolarized gas is an excellent and promising method, it will not be readily available for clinical hospitals, because laser polarizing equipment and nonproton MR imaging are required. A more detailed description of its applications can also be found in Chapters 7, 13, and 15.

A. Perfusion Imaging Using Encapsulated Polarized Helium and Inhalation of ^{3}He

Compared with xenon, helium is characterized by a much lower solubility (0.01 mL of dissolved gas per mL of fluid in blood and water vs. 0.1 for xenon). This precludes an efficient delivery of helium to the intravascular system from inhaled polarized helium. The first *in vivo* intravascular helium images were obtained using helium microbubble suspensions (Fig. 14.4). However, the large mean bubble diameter of these suspensions (on the order of 30 μm) represented a major limitation for the safe *in vivo* use of these solutions. Recently, Callot et al. (7) proposed an approach based on the encapsulation of ^{3}He in lipid-based carrier agents. The mean diameter of the resulting microbubbles and the corresponding NMR parameters of encapsulated ^{3}He are compatible with intravascular injection and *in vivo* MRI. Particularly, their structure and the helium polarization survive the passage through the heart cavities and pulmonary capillaries (Fig. 14.5). In a rat pulmonary embolism model, the ventilation image during inhalation of ^{3}He demonstrated normal ventilation, whereas the perfusion image demonstrated a defect in the embolized lung.

B. Venous Injection of Superparamagnetic Contrast Agent During ^{3}He Inhalation

Dynamic imaging acquisition during inhalation of ^{3}He during intravenous injection of a superparamagnetic contrast agent allows combined ventilation/perfusion imaging in a single breath of laser-polarized ^{3}He (8). Superparamagnetic iron oxide nanoparticles were injected as a bolus into the rat blood stream. During its first pass in the rat pulmonary vasculature, the magnetic susceptibility difference between the alveoli spaces and tissue increased, resulting in an enhanced

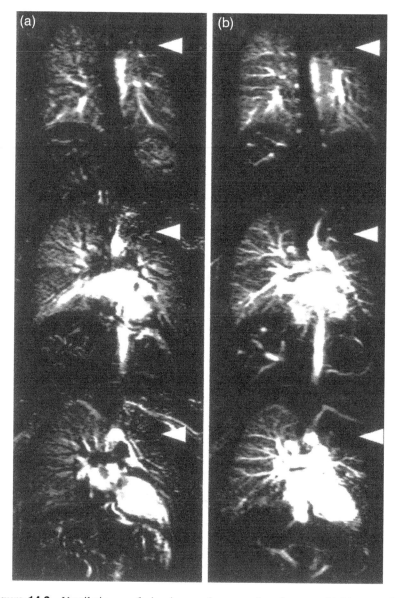

Figure 14.3 Ventilation–perfusion images from a male volunteer with his upper left lung partially removed. (a) MIR-HASTE oxygen ventilation images at three different anatomical positions. (b) The corresponding FAIRER perfusion images are shown. Ventilation and perfusion appear normal in the right lung. Relative to the contralateral upper right lung, matched ventilation and perfusion defects are observed in the upper left lung (arrowheads). This is in agreement with the fact that the volunteer had the upper left part of his lung partially removed when he was young. [Reproduced from Mai et al. (5) with permission.]

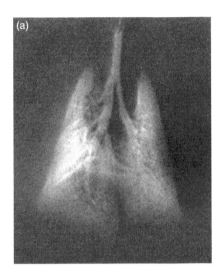 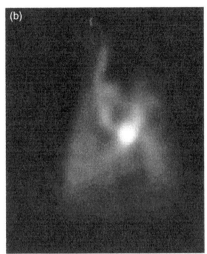

Figure 14.4 Coronal ^{3}He ventilation (a) and perfusion following the injection of micro-bubbles through the right jugular vein (b) in a normal rat.

dephasing of the ^{3}He nuclear spins in close proximity to the vessels. NMR signal variation can be analyzed using an approach similar to that in the standard blood volume and blood flow measurements based on dynamic proton signal variations during the first pass of a contrast agent (Fig. 14.6). According to the Stewart–Hamilton model, relative blood volume can be estimated by integrating the concentration of contrast agent in tissue. In NMR studies, the contrast agent tissues concentration is obtained from NMR signal variations, assuming that the apparent transverse relaxation rate is proportional to the contrast agent concentration. This technique was also validated in an animal model of pulmonary embolism (8). A blood volume map could be generated showing evidence of abnormal perfusion in the embolized region of the lung, while normal ventilation was demonstrated on the ventilation image.

The major advantage of this method is the simultaneous acquisition and the absence of misregistration between the perfusion and ventilation data. However, rapid bolus injection of superparamagnetic contrast agent is not yet approved in humans. Further studies using gadolinium chelates are needed.

IV. Proton Perfusion MR Imaging (Spin Labeling or Gd Injection) and ^{3}He Ventilation Imaging

Cremillieux et al. (9) demonstrates the feasibility of combined magnetic resonance imaging of ^{3}He lung ventilation and proton perfusion in rat lungs. Lung ventilation was assessed using hyperpolarized ^{3}He and lung perfusion proton imaging was demonstrated using Gd-chelates injection (Fig. 14.7). 3D proton

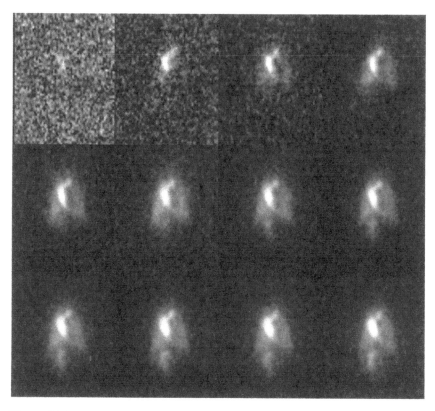

Figure 14.5 Dynamic perfusion images (temporal resolution: 200 ms) following intra-venous injection of ^{3}He microbubbles.

perfusion/helium ventilation imaging was demonstrated on an experimental rat model of pulmonary embolism showing normal lung ventilation associated with lung perfusion defect.

Lipson et al. (10) described the combined sequential use of a hyperpol-arized noble gas for ventilation images and arterial spin tagging for perfusion imaging in patients (Fig. 14.8). Using this technique in normal subjects, the V/Q signal was homogeneous throughout the lung field. In pulmonary emphy-sema, gas distribution and perfusion signal were heterogeneous similar to nuclear V/Q scan abnormalities.

V.   Indirect Measure of Ventilation/Perfusion Ratio by the Assessment of Alveolar Oxygen

Multiple MR approaches have been used for ventilation/perfusion MRI with their advantages and limitations. The matching of ventilation and perfusion

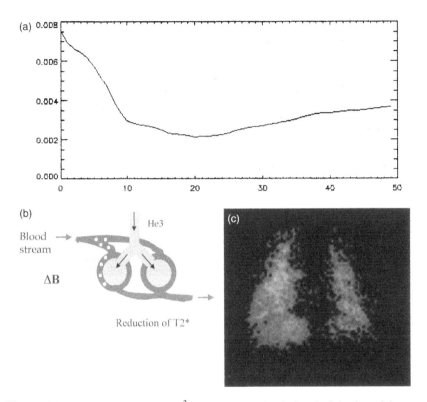

Figure 14.6 Evolution of the total ^{3}He signal intensity during the injection of the contrast injection. Note the large signal depletion corresponding to the contrast agent bolus pass in the capillary bed (a). This large signal decrease can presumably be attributed to the magnetic susceptibility difference between the alveoli and the iron oxide particles flowing through the surrounding capillaries (b). Relative pulmonary blood volume map obtained by integrating the concentration of contrast agent in the tissue (c).

provides important insights into the mechanisms of lung pathology and determines the effectiveness of gas exchange in the lung (Fig. 14.9). Recently, Mai et al. (11) investigated the distribution of ventilation–perfusion signal intensity ratio using oxygen-enhanced ventilation imaging and arterial spin labeling in volunteers. Excluding large pulmonary vessels, the average signal intensity V/P ratios were 0.355 ± 0.073 for the left lung and 0.371 ± 0.093 for the right lung. However, the real evaluation of V/P ratio will necessitate quantitative measurements of the ventilation and perfusion. Spin labeling methods can theoretically quantify pulmonary perfusion rates, whereas dynamic ventilation helium imaging is a promising tool for the assessment and quantification of local ventilation parameters (12). In addition to quantitative measurements, co-registration between ventilation and perfusion images in order to achieve spatially matched

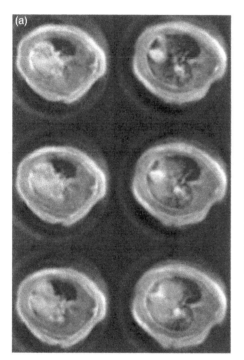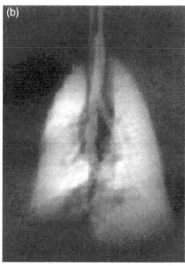

Figure 14.7 Axial proton images in a rat with pulmonary embolism in the upper lung after intravenous contrast injection (a). Coronal ³He image (b). Helium gas is homogeneously distributed in both lungs with a perfusion deficit in the upper lung.

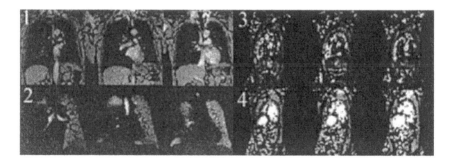

Figure 14.8 Corresponding (1) proton and (2) ³He coronal images of a patient with a history of emphysema. The patient had a left lung transplant. The ³He ventilation images show large defects in ³He distribution in the right (native) lung. The ³He distribution in the transplanted left lung allograft is uniform. Corresponding AST sagittal images perfusion images from (3) the right native lung show large defects in signal. In contrast, the images of (4) the left lung allograft show bright signal from normal blood perfusion. [Reproduced from Lipson et al. (10) with permission.]

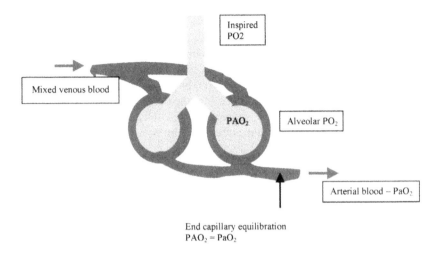

Figure 14.9 The rate at which oxygen reaches the alveolus is determined by its ventilation and the inspired PO_2. The rate at which oxygen leaves the alveolus is determined by its perfusion. Therefore, the alveolar PO_2 is determined by the ventilation–perfusion ratio. In an ideal lung, flip ventilation–perfusion ratio is equal to 1 but regional differences in the ventilation/perfusion ratio are observed with a vertical gradient (higher ventilation–perfusion ratio in the nondependent portion of the lung).

measures of regional ventilation and perfusion is necessary and is being evaluated by several research groups (13).

Given the difficulties in obtaining true spatially matched measures of ventilation and perfusion, the estimation of the alveolar oxygen concentration, which is an indirect measure of the ventilation/perfusion ratio might be an alternative to quantitative measurements. The $T1$ of ^{3}He in the lung is $\sim$20 s. In lung parenchyma, $T1$ is reduced primarily by radiofrequency pulses and the interaction with paramagnetic molecular oxygen, which leads to a linear relation between the relaxation rate and the oxygen partial pressure. By measuring the relaxation times of the hyperpolarized ^{3}He gas in the lungs during two different series, it is possible to compute the intrapulmonary oxygen concentration *in vivo* from ^{3}He images. As the intrapulmonary PO_2 distribution is governed by local ventilation, perfusion, and O_2 uptake, this represents a new approach to evaluate lung function. The rate at which oxygen reaches the alveolus is determined by its ventilation and the inspired PO_2. The rate at which oxygen leaves the alveolus is determined by its perfusion. Consequently, the determination of alveolar PO_2 is an indirect measure of the ventilation/perfusion ratio. Recently, the potential of ^{3}He imaging for detecting perfusion abnormalities due to their effect on alveolar PO_2 was demonstrated in an experimental pig model (13). After isolated pulmonary arterial occlusion using a balloon catheter a focal $T1$ reduction corresponding to an abnormally high PO_2 (because of the absence of perfusion) was observed, which normalized upon deflation of the balloon. Further explanation of this technique is given in Chapter 16.

In conclusion, the application of combined ventilation and perfusion MR imaging is a promising new tool. Various techniques are able to demonstrate V/Q mismatch and quantification is currently a main aim. It is expected that this technology will bring novel insights into the pathophysiology of major conditions, such as pulmonary embolism, while it will enhance our understanding of the gas exchange mechanism and the effects of illness on it. This could ultimately lead to better treatment for patients with pulmonary parenchymal and vascular disorders.

References

1. Berthezène Y, Vexler V, Clement O, Muhler A, Moseley ME, Brasch RC. Contrast-enhanced MR imaging of the lung: assessments of ventilation and perfusion. Radiology 1992; 183:667–672.
2. Suga K, Ogasawara N, Okada M, Matsunaga N, Arai M. Regional lung functional impairment in acute airway obstruction and pulmonary embolic dog models assessed with gadolinium-based aerosol ventilation and perfusion magnetic resonance imaging. Invest Radiol 2002; 37:281–291.
3. Chen Q, Levin DL, Kim D, David V, McNicholas M, Chen V, Jakob PM, Griswold MA, Goldfarb JW, Hatabu H, Edelman RR. Pulmonary disorders: ventilation–perfusion MR imaging with animal models. Radiology 1999; 213:871–879.
4. Nakagawa T, Sakuma H, Murashima S, Ishida N, Matsumura K, Takeda K. Pulmonary ventilation–perfusion MR imaging in clinical patients. J Magn Reson Imaging 2001; 14(4):419–424.
5. Mai VM, Bankier AA, Prasad PV, Li W, Storey P, Edelman RR, Chen Q. MR ventilation–perfusion imaging of human lung using oxygen-enhanced and arterial spin labeling techniques. J Magn Reson Imaging 2001; 14:574–579.
6. Keilholz SD, Mai VM, Berr SS, Fujiwara N, Hagspiel KD. Comparison of first-pass Gd-DOTA and FAIRER MR perfusion imaging in a rabbit model of pulmonary embolism. J Magn Reson Imaging 2002; 16:168–171.
7. Callot V, Canet E, Brochot J, Viallon M, Humblot H, Briguet A, Tournier H, Cremillieux Y. MR perfusion imaging using encapsulated laser-polarized ^{3}He. Magn Reson Med 2001; 46:535–540.
8. Viallon M, Berthezene Y, Decorps M, Wiart M, Callot V, Bourgeois M, Humblot H, Briguet A, Cremillieux Y. Laser-polarized ^{3}He as a probe for dynamic regional measurements of lung perfusion and ventilation using magnetic resonance imaging. Magn Reson Med 2000; 44:1–4.
9. Cremillieux Y, Berthezene Y, Humblot H, Viallon M, Canet E, Bourgeois M, Albert T, Heil W, Briguet A. A combined 1H perfusion/^{3}He ventilation NMR study in rat lungs. Magn Reson Med 1999; 41:645–648.
10. Lipson DA, Roberts DA, Hansen-Flaschen J, Gentile TR, Jones G, Thompson A, Dimitrov IE, Palevsky HI, Leigh JS, Schnall M, Rizi RR. Pulmonary ventilation and perfusion scanning using hyperpolarized helium-3 MRI and arterial spin

tagging in healthy normal subjects and in pulmonary embolism and orthotopic lung transplant patients. Magn Reson Med 2002; 47:1073–1076.

11. Mai VM, Liu B, Polzin JA, Li W, Kurucay S, Bankier AA, KnightScott J, Madhav P, Edelman RR, Chen Q. Ventilation–perfusion ratio of signal intensity in human lung using oxygen-enhanced and arterial spin labeling techniques. Magn Reson Med 2002; 48:341–350.

12. Dupuich D, Berthezene Y, Clouet PL, Stupar V, Canet E, Cremillieux Y. Dynamic ^{3}He imaging for quantification of regional lung ventilation parameters. Magn Reson Med 2003; 50:777–783.

13. Rizi RR, Saha PK, Wang B, Ferrante MA, Lipson D, Baumgardner J, Roberts DA. Co-registration of acquired MR ventilation and perfusion images–validation in a porcine model. Magn Reson Med 2003; 49(1):13–18.

14. Roberts D, Rizi R, Lipson DA, Hansen-Flaschen J, Yamomoto A, Gefter WB, Leigh JS, Schnall MS. Functional nonspecificity of T1-weighted MRI of laser-polarized helium-3 gas. In: Proceedings 9th ISMRM Scientific Meeting, Glasgow, 2001, p 946.

15

Assessment of Human Lung Microstructure with Hyperpolarized ^{3}He Diffusion MRI

MICHAEL SALERNO and **JOHN P. MUGLER**

University of Virginia School of Medicine,
Charlottesville, Virginia, USA

I. Introduction

Since the emergence of hyperpolarized ^{3}He gas as a novel contrast agent for MRI, there has been substantial interest in exploiting the unique properties of this gas for evaluating lung structure and function. Of particular relevance for assessing the microstructure of the lung, ^{3}He has a very high self-diffusion coefficient (2 cm^2/s at body temperature and a pressure of 760 Torr) which, in an unrestricted environment, results in relatively large diffusion-driven displacements of ^{3}He atoms during time periods of relevance for MRI, such as during the echo time of a gradient-echo (GRE) pulse sequence, as routinely used for hyperpolarized ^{3}He imaging. For example, within air in an unrestricted space, the root mean squared displacement of a ^{3}He atom is ~2 mm during 5 ms.

A second important characteristic of ^{3}He is its low tissue solubility, which effectively confines inhaled ^{3}He gas to the airspaces of the lung. When ^{3}He is confined to relatively small spaces such as the distal airway structures, which have characteristic lengths on the order of 0.1 mm, its motion is restricted resulting in reduced displacements and a decrease in the apparent diffusion coefficient (ADC) as measured by MRI (1–4). Depending on the parameters of the pulse sequence, these ADC values may exhibit a complex dependence on a variety of morphological features of the lung microstructure including the surface-to-volume ratio, the length scales of the distal airways, the anisotropy of airway orientation, and the tortuosity of airway connectivity. Application of diffusion MRI methods to hyperpolarized ^{3}He thus presents the opportunity to create image contrast on the basis of differences in the morphology of the microstructural environment between each voxel in the image, yielding a powerful tool to quantitatively evaluate disease processes that alter the underlying structure of the lung.

II. Background

A. Overview of Lung Structure

To provide the context for our discussion of measuring the diffusion properties of ^{3}He, we first briefly review the diffusion environment—the complex branching structure of airways that comprise the human lung. Air enters and leaves the lung through the conducting airways, which consist of the generations of airways from the trachea to the terminal bronchioles, the smallest airways without alveoli. These airways, which do not contribute to respiration, make up what is known as the anatomical dead space with a volume of ~150 mL (5). The generations of airways beyond the terminal bronchioles make up the pulmonary acini, which account for the majority of the total lung volume (5). In the healthy human lung there are approximately 30,000 pulmonary acini (6), each of which has a volume of ~0.2 mL (7). The average path-length from the terminal bronchioles to the alveolar sac is ~8 mm (6). The respiratory bronchioles, which typically branch for nine generations from the terminal bronchioles, contain a small portion of the alveoli. The internal airway dimensions of the respiratory bronchioles drop from 500 μm to ~270 μm from the proximal to the most distal branches (6). The respiratory bronchioles terminate in alveolar ducts, which are tubes with out-pouching alveoli, and alveolar sacs, which are blind-ending alveolar ducts. The size and number of alveoli increase toward the periphery of the acinus. On average, there are 10 alveoli per duct and approximately 7000 alveoli per acinus (7). The alveoli are polygonal in shape with an opening to the alveolar duct that is smaller than the alveolar diameter of 250 μm. The structure of the pulmonary acinus is similar in all lobes of the lung.

B. Techniques for Measuring the Diffusion of ^{3}He

Although the diffusion properties of water in various environments have been investigated extensively by using proton MRI methods, the high diffusion coefficient of ^{3}He (approximately 10^5 times larger than that for water in biological tissues) and the nonequilibrium nature of hyperpolarized magnetization require modification of established MRI diffusion measurement techniques for use with ^{3}He. The majority of ^{3}He ADC studies have used a GRE pulse sequence, modified by the addition of a bipolar pair of diffusion-sensitizing gradient pulses between the excitation radio frequency (RF) pulse and data acquisition (1–4,8). By collecting two or more images at each section position with different diffusion weightings, parametric images of the ADC values can be calculated. Other methods for ^{3}He diffusion imaging have also been explored, including spin-echo train pulse sequences (9,10) and magnetic tag dissolution (11,12). In the remainder of this section we review the theoretical basis for each of these techniques.

GRE Pulse Sequences with Bipolar Gradients

Diffusion sensitization using a bipolar pair of gradient pulses is a straightforward modification of the classic pulsed-gradient spin-echo method developed by Stejskal and Tanner (13). The effect of diffusion on the NMR signal can be understood by analyzing how a simple bipolar pair of magnetic field gradient pulses (Fig. 15.1) affects the phase of the magnetization in the presence of diffusion. The first gradient pulse of the bipolar pair imparts a position-dependent *phase tag* on the transverse magnetization in the direction of the gradient. The phase φ_1 accumulated by a spin during the application of this gradient pulse is

$$\varphi_1(x) = \gamma \int_0^\delta G_d(t)x(t)\,dt \tag{15.1}$$

where γ is the gyromagnetic ratio, $G_d(t)$ is the diffusion-gradient waveform, $x(t)$ is the position of the spin, and δ is the duration of the gradient pulse. A time period is then allowed to elapse, which is termed the mixing time, prior to the application of a gradient pulse with an identical shape but opposite polarity.

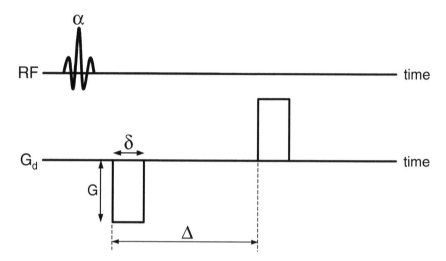

Figure 15.1 Diagram of a bipolar pair of diffusion-sensitizing gradient pulses applied just after an RF pulse with flip angle α. This configuration is commonly used in diffusion-sensitized GRE pulse sequences. Each gradient pulse has amplitude G and duration δ. The diffusion time for this bipolar-pulse pair is Δ. The diffusion gradient waveform G_d may be applied along the section-select, frequency-encoding or phase-encoding axis, or along an axis that has an arbitrary orientation.

This second gradient pulse results in a phase accumulation φ_2 given by:

$$\varphi_2(x) = \gamma \int_{\Delta}^{\Delta+\delta} G_d(t)x(t)\,dt \tag{15.2}$$

where Δ is as shown in Fig. 15.1.

The total phase φ accumulated by a given spin due to the application of the bipolar gradient-pulse pair is the sum of φ_1 and φ_2. In the absence of diffusion (or other motion), the second gradient pulse completely unwinds the phase tag imparted by the first gradient pulse, resulting in a value of zero for φ. The attenuation of the NMR signal due to the loss of phase coherence that results from diffusion in the presence of the bipolar gradient-pulse pair is found by integrating over all spins of interest (e.g., all spins within a voxel). For an isotropic, unbounded medium (e.g., ^{3}He in the central portion of a large container), this signal integral evaluates to an exponential decay:

$$S = S_0 e^{-bD} \quad \text{and} \quad b = (\gamma G \delta)^2(\Delta - \delta/3) \tag{15.3}$$

where S is the measured signal, S_0 is the signal that would be measured in the absence of diffusion, b describes the gradient-induced attenuation that results from the application of the bipolar gradient-pulse pair, D is the diffusion coefficient, and G is the amplitude of each gradient pulse in the bipolar pair. It should be noted that by increasing the diffusion-gradient amplitude (G), duration of application (δ), or the time between the diffusion gradients (Δ), we can control the amount of attenuation that will occur for a given diffusivity. The concept of the b value can be extended to arbitrary gradient waveforms by expressing the b value as a function of the k-space trajectory (14):

$$b(t) = \int_0^t |k(t')|^2 dt' \quad \text{and} \quad k(t) = \gamma \int_0^t G(t') dt' \tag{15.4}$$

The b-value expression corresponding to a bipolar gradient waveform composed of two trapezoidal segments is given in Ref. (8).

For hyperpolarized gas diffusion measurements using the bipolar-GRE technique, the phase-encoding lines corresponding to different b values, diffusion times, or diffusion directions are collected in an interleaved fashion to minimize the confounding signal-attenuation effects of T_1 decay and the application of RF pulses. Specifically, during the acquisition for each section, all phase-encoding data corresponding to a given line in k-space are collected before proceeding to the next line in k-space. Typically, between two and four diffusion-weighted images are obtained for each section, and parametric images of the ADC values corresponding to each section are calculated by fitting the signals as a function of b value corresponding to each pixel to the first of Eq. (15.3), wherein the ADC (which is termed *apparent* because it depends on the structure of the lung as well as the true diffusivity of the gas) replaces D. Other data-sampling schemes can be combined with bipolar diffusion-sensitization gradients. For example, an interleaved-spiral diffusion pulse sequence has been used to generate contiguous 15 mm thick ADC images of the whole lung in 5 s (15).

The bipolar-GRE pulse sequence is straightforward to implement, and the interleaved-acquisition approach minimizes bias of the ADC values due both to T_1 decay and flip angle effects. On state-of-the-art MR systems, the data required to calculate ADC images covering the whole human lung can be acquired within a single breath-hold period. As the diffusion-sensitization gradients are separate from the spatial-encoding gradients, different diffusion times or directions can be easily implemented. These advantages of the bipolar-GRE pulse sequence have made it the current method of choice for determining ADC values in the human lung (3,4).

There are some disadvantages of the bipolar-GRE approach. As the diffusion weightings of interest are acquired in interleaved, but separate, repetitions of the pulse sequence, the fundamental signal levels corresponding to different diffusion weightings are slightly different, which introduces a bias in the calculated ADC values. For example, the flip angle-dependent biases for two and four b-value ADC images obtained by using a flip angle of $10°$ are 0.01 and

0.03 cm^2/s, respectively (16). These biases are not easy to eliminate without accurate flip angle calibration and a map of the spatial dependence of the B1 field. Further, bias increases substantially if large flip angles are used or if a large number of diffusion-weighted images are obtained, effectively limiting the technique to small flip angles and a small number of diffusion weightings. Another disadvantage at high field strengths is that the short T_2^* of ^{3}He in the lung places an upper limit on the length scales that can be probed. Performing diffusion measurements at lower field strengths can mitigate this problem.

Spin-Echo Train Pulse Sequences

For an ideal, symmetric frequency-encoding gradient pulse of duration T_s (Fig. 15.2), the diffusion-induced attenuation of transverse magnetization during a Carr–Purcell–Meiboom–Gill (CPMG) spin-echo train with m echoes can be calculated by using:

$$b = \frac{m}{4}(\gamma G T_s)^2 \left(ESP - \frac{2}{3}T_s \right) \tag{15.5}$$

where ESP is the echo spacing. This b value is just m times that given in the second of Eq. (15.3) with the substitutions $\delta = T_s/2$ and $\Delta = ESP - T_s/2$. Thus, the CPMG echo train has an effective diffusion time of $ESP - T_s/2$

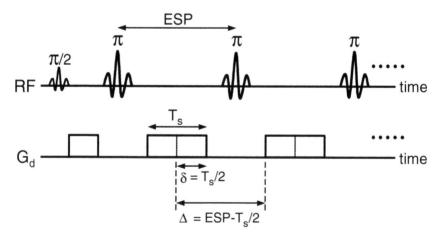

Figure 15.2 Diagram of a CPMG spin-echo-train pulse sequence wherein the frequency-encoding gradient waveform is interpreted as a diffusion-sensitization gradient. The other encoding gradients are omitted for clarity. In analogy to the bipolar-pulse pair shown in Fig. 15.1, the variable δ is equal to half of the data-sampling period per echo (T_s) and the diffusion time Δ is equal to the echo spacing (ESP) minus δ.

independent of the number of echoes, since for each echo the magnetization is refocused.

In contrast to the bipolar-GRE technique, which has been widely used, only a small number of experiments have been performed using CPMG-based methods at 0.1 Tesla (9,10). These methods include: (i) using a diffusion-sensitized CPMG echo train as a magnetization preparation for a GRE image acquisition; (ii) measuring the global signal decay during a diffusion-sensitized CPMG echo train; and (iii) acquiring multiple diffusion-weighted images by using a single CPMG echo train in which the acquisition of 10 images are linked together. With these techniques, Durand et al. (9,10) measured mean ADC values in the healthy human lung that ranged between 0.11 to 0.23 cm^2/s at 0.1 Tesla and that depended on the details of the measurement technique. In comparison, mean ADC values obtained by using the bipolar-GRE technique at 1.5 Tesla have typically ranged between 0.2 and 0.3 cm^2/s (1,3,4). The disparity between these values may be due to differences in the magnitude of susceptibility-induced gradients in the lung at 0.1 vs. 1.5 Tesla or in the effective diffusion times for the CPMG vs. bipolar-GRE techniques.

Because spin echoes, as opposed to gradients echoes, are acquired in CPMG-based techniques, they permit longer diffusion times to be probed when T_2^* values are relatively short, such as in the lung at 1.5 Tesla. On the other hand, substantial bias in the estimated ADC values can be introduced if the flip angle for the refocusing RF pulses is not 180° due to inaccurate calibration, B1-field inhomogeneity, or a poorly defined section profile.

Magnetic Tag Dissolution

The ADC can be calculated by measuring the rate of dissolution, or decay, of a magnetic *tag* applied by using a SPAMM (spatial modulation of magnetization) tagging pulse (17). Such tagging pulses are commonly used in cardiac MRI to evaluate heart function. Whereas the techniques discussed in the previous two sections are based on the effect of diffusion on *phase-tagged* transverse magnetization; tag-dissolution techniques measure the effect of diffusion on the *amplitude-tagged* longitudinal magnetization.

If T_1 relaxation is neglected, which is reasonable in the lung for time scales of a few seconds, the spatial and temporal dependence of the SPAMM-tagged hyperpolarized longitudinal magnetization, M, is:

$$M(x,t) = M_0 \cos(kx) e^{-k^2 Dt} \tag{15.6}$$

where $k = 2\pi/\lambda$ and λ is the wavelength of the tag pattern. The diffusion sensitivity and the spatial length scales that can be probed are determined by k, the spatial frequency of the tagging pulse. Equation (15.6) shows that the tag pattern will remain sinusoidal in space and decay exponentially with a rate that is proportional to the square of k. As shown in Fig. 15.3, the diffusion time, Δ,

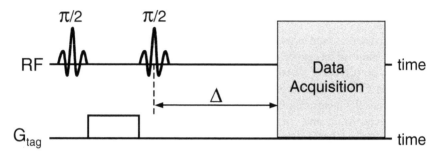

Figure 15.3 Diagram illustrating the general scheme for the tag-dissolution technique of measuring the ADC. A tagging pulse, which is a combination of RF pulses and a gradient pulse, is followed by a time delay, which is the diffusion time Δ. The data acquisition block is comprised of a pulse sequence that is used to monitor the decay of the tagged longitudinal magnetization.

for the tag-dissolution method is the time period from the end of the SPAMM tagging pulse to the application of the imaging pulse sequence that is used to monitor the decay of the tag pattern. This pulse sequence should be designed to avoid biases from T_1 decay, the effect of the RF pulses and B1 inhomogeneity.

Using the tag-dissolution method, Owers-Bradley et al. (11,12) measured ADC values for the healthy human lung. The decay of the tag patterns was monitored by a nonphase-encoded RARE pulse sequence that used a low excitation flip angle. A mean ADC value of $0.02 \ cm^2/s$ was found; ADC values were not a function of the tag wavelength, although these wavelengths were relatively large (several centimeters) compared with the characteristics lengths of the distal airways in the lung.

The measured ADC for restricted diffusion should decrease as the diffusion time, and hence the length scales that are probed, increase. The length scales probed by a tag-dissolution technique with tag wavelengths on the order of centimeters are at least a factor of 10 longer than those that can be probed by bipolar-GRE or CPMG pulse sequences, thus potentially allowing tortuosity or other long-time-scale parameters to be determined. On the other hand, a disadvantage of the tag-dissolution technique is that only very long length scales can be interrogated because the minimum tag wavelength is limited by the spatial resolution of the image.

C. Quantitative Models of Diffusion in the Lung

It is important to note that the equations discussed earlier for the signal attenuation are strictly true only for isotropic diffusion in an unbounded medium. When confining boundaries restrict atomic or molecular motion, and the associated displacements are on the order of the separation between these boundaries, the measured diffusion coefficient will be a function of the size and geometry of the confining space. As ³He gas in the lung is in the restricted regime, the term *apparent* diffusion coefficient is used for the parameter that is measured by MRI diffusion experiments. Calculating the diffusion coefficient for a restricting environment is typically quite difficult, and thus there are no general analytical expressions. The actual signal attenuation can be obtained only by experiment or, in sufficiently simple cases, by numerical simulation or modeling. Solutions for the signal attenuation due to diffusion have been developed for simple restricted environments such as within spherical shells and between planes (18–20).

Spherical Shells

A straightforward and simple model for the diffusion environment of the lung is a collection of spherical shells that have an average radius equal to that for a typical alveolus. However, using established solutions for restricted diffusion within a spherical shell, we find that the estimated ADC for this model is several orders of magnitude smaller than the values that have been measured by using a bipolar-GRE pulse sequence. This large discrepancy between predicted and measured ADC values supports that ³He atoms visit multiple alveoli and the associated connecting airways during the diffusion-sensitization period of the pulse sequence, which is several milliseconds for the bipolar-GRE technique. Thus, any model that is likely to yield results that are consistent with experimental measurements must, at a minimum, account for the diffusion of ³He atoms among groups of alveoli and their connecting airways.

Isotropically Distributed Cylinders

A more sophisticated approach was recently proposed by Yablonskiy et al. (21), who modeled the lung structure as a collection of isotropically distributed cylinders. In this model, the fundamental structure that is probed by diffusing ³He atoms during the pulse sequence is a cylindrical acinar airway that is embedded in an *alveolar sleeve*. The ADC is separated into D_L, the diffusion along the acinar airway, and D_T, the diffusion perpendicular to the acinar airway. Each voxel in the image is assumed to contain a large number of randomly oriented cylindrical airways. The signal equation for this model is (21):

$$S = S_0 \exp\left(-b\bar{D}\right)\sqrt{\frac{\pi}{4bD_{AN}}}\exp\left(\frac{bD_{AN}}{3}\right)\Phi\left[\sqrt{bD_{AN}}\right] \tag{15.7}$$

where

$$\bar{D} = \frac{D_L}{3} + \frac{2D_T}{3} \quad \text{and} \quad D_{AN} = D_L - D_T$$

In the first of Eq. (15.7), $\Phi()$ is the error function. The mean airway outer radius can be estimated from the D_T values, providing the potential to quantitatively evaluate the changes in microstructural dimensions that occur with disease progression.

This model represents a significant advance toward understanding how measured ADCs reflect the underlying architecture of the lung. Nonetheless, it does not account for the range of airway dimensions that are present in the acini, and does not address potential contributions that depend on the nature of the connectivity between various acinar airway segments, although such contributions may be negligible for relatively short diffusions times.

The Lung as a Porous Medium

Another potentially fruitful approach is to model the lung as a complex porous medium with a large number of dead-end pores and a high tortuosity. Porous media consist of a system of interconnected spaces within which atoms or molecules are free to diffuse. The effects of restricted diffusion in porous media have been the subject of many investigations in the field of petrophysics (22–25). Recently, diffusion measurements using xenon gas have been made in packed glass-bead phantoms and sedimentary rocks (26,27).

By analyzing the lung as a complex porous structure, we can utilize some of the established mathematical framework to understand the underlying parameters that affect the ADCs that are measured by using hyperpolarized-gas MRI. The measured diffusion coefficient, $D(t)$, in a porous medium will decrease compared to the free diffusion coefficient as the diffusion time is increased because more of the particles encounter boundaries owing to their random diffusive motion. For short diffusion times, only a small fraction of the particles are restricted by the boundaries of the pores. In the short-time limit, Mitra et al. (22) have shown that the time-dependent diffusion coefficient is proportional to the surface-to-volume ratio. For long diffusion times, $D(t)$ approaches an asymptotic limit, which is the inverse of the tortuosity of the porous medium (28).

The tortuosity is a parameter that describes the connectivity between pores within the medium and is independent of the length scales of the system. As these length scales increase, it takes longer to reach the tortuosity limit. For intermediate diffusion times, such as those that can be probed in the lung by using a bipolar-GRE pulse sequence, the dependence on the diffusion time is not well described but can be estimated by the two-point Pade approximation, which extrapolates between the short- and the long-time behavior (29).

An advantage of the porous media model is that structural changes in lung diseases such as emphysema, and their effects on ADC values, can be framed in terms of changes in length scales and connectivity of airways. This approach could be useful if measurement techniques are developed that are able to probe a larger range of diffusion length scales than those that can be probed currently by using bipolar-GRE or CPMG techniques. One disadvantage of this model is that the measured diffusion coefficient has a complex dependence both on the parameters of the pulse sequence and on those of the network such as the pore surface-to-volume ratio, the relevant length scales, and the tortuosity. On the time scales that can be probed *in vivo* by using ^{3}He gas, the ADC is likely to be affected primarily by changes in tortuosity and length scale rather than by changes in the surface-to-volume ratio.

III. ADC Measurements in Human Subjects

The vast majority of ^{3}He ADC measurements in humans have used a bipolar diffusion-sensitization gradient waveform in combination with a GRE pulse sequence. The results from these studies are summarized in this section. First, we review investigations performed in healthy and diseased subjects which, by using a measurement protocol that acquires diffusion-weighted images for two to four *b* values and a fixed diffusion time, determined ADC values on the basis of the assumption of a simple mono-exponential decay in signal strength with increasing *b* value as described by the first of Eq. (15.3). This is the measurement protocol that has been used most frequently for ADC studies in humans. Next, we discuss some of the more subtle issues involved with ^{3}He diffusion measurements—the dependence of ADC values on the duration and direction of the diffusion sensitization and on the level of lung inflation. Finally, we review results on the basis of the model of Yablonskiy et al. (21) in Eq. (15.7), wherein the assumption of a more complex dependence of the signal decay on *b* value is used to estimate the longitudinal and transverse diffusion coefficients for a cylindrical acinar airway as well as the mean airway radius.

A. Studies in Healthy and Diseased Subjects

A number of investigators have measured the ADC of ^{3}He in healthy or diseased human lungs using some variation of the bipolar-GRE technique (1,3,4). Mugler et al. (1) performed the first ADC study in humans. By using a bipolar diffusion-sensitization gradient waveform that was integrated into the frequency-encoding gradient waveform, and *b* values of 0.4, 0.8, 1.2, and 1.6 s/cm^2, an overall (i.e., averaged over all subjects) mean ADC value of 0.25 cm^2/s (range among subjects: 0.21–0.33 cm^2/s) was measured in the lungs of three healthy volunteers. In a study of 11 healthy volunteers, Saam et al. (3) found an overall mean ADC of 0.20 cm^2/s (range among subjects: 0.17–0.25 cm^2/s) by using a pair of bipolar gradient waveforms (to achieve first-order flow compensation) with a total duration of 7.5 ms and *b* values of 0 and 2.75 s/cm^2. In a study of 16 healthy subjects, Salerno et al. (4) measured an overall mean ADC of 0.23 cm^2/s (range among subjects: 0.18–0.34 cm^2/s) by using the same pulse sequence configuration as that used by Mugler et al. and either two or four *b* values. In another study that included 16 healthy subjects, Salerno et al. found an overall mean ADC of 0.25 cm^2/s by using a bipolar gradient waveform with a total duration of 2.9 ms and *b* values of 0 and 1.6 s/cm^2 (unpublished data). In summary, despite somewhat different diffusion-sensitization schemes, similar ADC values in the healthy human lung were measured in multiple investigations. These studies indicate that the ADC of ^{3}He in the healthy lung is restricted by about a factor of four compared to the diffusion coefficient for unrestricted ^{3}He in air at body temperature.

Figure 15.4 shows a ^{3}He ventilation image, a parametric ADC image, and a histogram of the corresponding ADC values from a representative healthy volunteer. The ventilation image appears homogeneous without any poorly ventilated regions, and the ADC image appears homogeneous without any focal regions of increased ADC values. The ADC values for this subject were typically between 0.16 and 0.30 cm^2/s, with a mean value of 0.21 cm^2/s. The distribution of ADC values is narrow, having a standard deviation of 0.06 cm^2/s.

The majority of the studies involving subjects with lung disease have focused on the microstructural changes that occur in emphysema (3,4). In a study of five patients with severe emphysema, Saam et al. (3) found that the

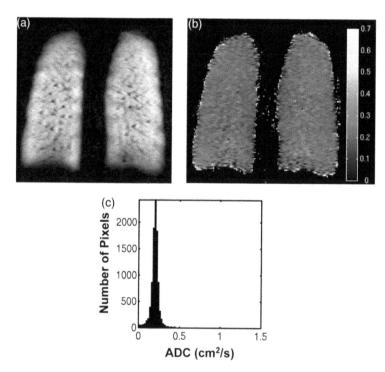

Figure 15.4 (**See color insert**) Coronal (a) ventilation and (b) ADC ^{3}He MR images and (c) the corresponding ADC histogram from a representative healthy volunteer. The signal intensities in (a) and (b) are homogeneous, and (c) depicts the low values for the mean ADC (0.21 cm^2/s) and standard deviation (0.06 cm^2/s) in this image section. The color bar for the ADC image is in units of cm^2/s. [From Ref. (4).]

mean ADC was increased by a factor of 2.5 as compared with the value for healthy volunteers, indicating that the diffusion of ^{3}He is less restricted in the emphysematous lung. In a study by Salerno et al. (4) including 11 patients with emphysema of varying severity, the mean ADC was increased by a factor of 2.0 compared with that for healthy volunteers. This study also demonstrated a statistically significant correlation in patients with emphysema between the decrease in the FEV$_1$/FVC ratio as determined by spirometry and the increase in the mean ADC. In subjects with emphysema, both of these studies showed that the variance of the ADC values increases substantially compared with that for healthy volunteers, consistent with regional variations in ADC values that are evident from visual inspection of the corresponding ADC images. More recently, Yablonskiy et al. (30) found that ADC values correlate with CT linear attenuation coefficients. Similar results in emphysema patients have been found by Salerno et al. (unpublished data).

Figure 15.5 shows ^{3}He ventilation images, parametric ADC images, and histograms of the corresponding ADC values from three subjects with emphysema. In the first subject, the ventilation image appears uniform in the upper right lung; however, on the ADC image, this area corresponds to the region with the highest ADC values. This region was hypodense on CT, indicating emphysema. The second subject shows a more diffuse pattern of emphysema. It should be noted that there is no one-to-one correlation between the ADC image and the ventilation image—the contrast in the images is created by different mechanisms. In the third subject, who had emphysema secondary to the genetic disease α-1 antitrypsin deficiency, ADC values are highest in the lower lung zones, which is consistent with the most common distribution of emphysema in this disease.

ADC changes in smokers have also been investigated. In a study of five healthy smokers, Leawoods et al. (31) found no increase in the mean ADC as compared with that for healthy volunteers. As emphysema develops only in a subset of smokers, it is possible that this negative finding may be due to the small number of subjects or an insufficient smoking history. Salerno et al. (32) demonstrated an increase in the mean ADC for smokers with a history of more than 20 pack years. Furthermore, ADC defects were found to correlate with hypodense regions on CT. Figure 15.6 shows high-resolution CT and ADC images from a healthy smoker with a 45-pack year history. Good correlation is seen between hypodense regions on CT and regions of elevated ADC values. In addition, there are regions of increased ADC values that are not apparent on the CT image, potentially indicating early emphysematous changes.

B. Time Dependence

Since the diffusion of ^{3}He is restricted in the human lung, we expect that ADC values will decrease toward an asymptotic long-time limit as the diffusion time is increased. Salerno et al. (16,33) studied the time dependence of ADC values

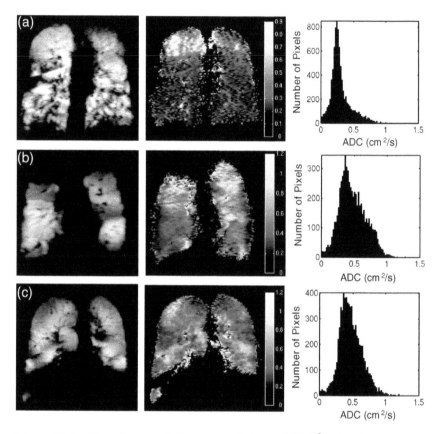

Figure 15.5 (See color insert) Coronal ventilation and ADC ^{3}He MR images and the corresponding histograms from three patients with differences in the regional distribution of ADC values. (a) The ADC values were increased primarily in the apices (mean, 0.31 cm^2/s; standard deviation, 0.17 cm^2/s). (b) A patient with more severe emphysema showed a multifocal pattern of increased ADC values (mean, 0.49 cm^2/s; standard deviation, 0.20 cm^2/s). (c) In a patient with α-1 antitrypsin deficiency, the ADC values in the lower regions of the lung were generally higher than those in upper regions (mean, 0.48 cm^2/s; standard deviation, 0.18 cm^2/s). The means and standard deviations correspond to the individual sections shown. The color bars for the ADC images are in units of cm^2/s. [From Ref. (4).]

in six healthy subjects and four emphysema patients for diffusion times of 1.8, 3.8, and 5.8 ms. Within this range of diffusion times, measured ADC values showed a significant decrease with increasing diffusion times.

For the healthy subjects, there was a statistically significant difference in mean ADC values between each of the diffusion times and a 21% drop between the shortest and longest diffusion times. ADC histograms from a representative healthy subject for the three diffusion times are shown in Fig. 15.7(a). The ADC histogram shifts toward lower values with increasing diffusion time.

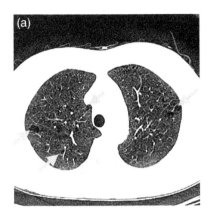 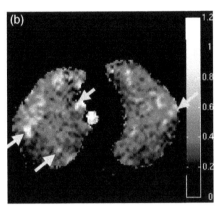

Figure 15.6 **(See color insert)** Axial (a) CT and (b) ADC images at the same anatomic level in a heavy smoker (45 pack-years) with no clinical evidence of emphysema. There is excellent concordance between emphysematous regions on CT (low density) and regions of elevated ADC (yellow) as indicated by the arrows. The color bar for the ADC image is in units of cm^2/s.

This trend is consistent with the results obtained by Maier et al. (34) in a healthy subject; in this study, bipolar diffusion-sensitization gradients were used in a simple pulse-acquire spectroscopic acquisition to measure global ADC values for diffusion times between 1 and 6 ms.

For the emphysema patients, the mean ADC dropped by only 12% between the shortest and longest diffusion times. Nonetheless, the diffusion coefficients measured at each time point were statistically different. Figure 15.7(b) shows ADC histograms from an emphysema patient for the three diffusion times. Again, the ADC histogram shifts to lower values as the diffusion time increases. When the ADC values between the healthy and emphysema groups were compared, there were a statistically significant differences at all diffusion times, and the greatest difference occurred for the shortest diffusion time suggesting, for this measurement protocol, that shorter diffusion times may be preferred to detect the structural changes that occur in emphysema. The ideal diffusion time has yet to be elucidated.

C. Directional Dependence

If the lung architecture with its single, centrally located inlet (the trachea) is considered, it is reasonable to expect some degree of preferential orientation of the lung airways. Depending on the extent of the airways that is sampled by a diffusing ^3He atom, it therefore also seems reasonable to expect that measured ADC values may exhibit dependence on the direction of diffusion-sensitization. To investigate this possibility, Salerno (16) measured ADC values in six healthy subjects and four emphysema patients by performing three sequential diffusion

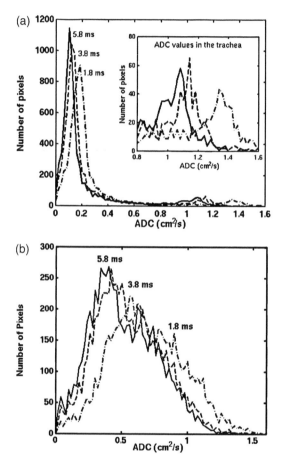

Figure 15.7 ADC histograms from (a) a representative healthy volunteer and (b) a patient with severe emphysema for diffusion times of 1.8, 3.8, and 5.8 ms. For both subjects, the histograms shifted to lower ADC values as the diffusion time was increased.

measurements with diffusion-sensitization in the anterior–posterior (A–P), head–foot (H–F), and left–right (L–R) directions.

Directional dependence was evaluated by calculating the percent difference between each of the three ADC images corresponding to a given diffusion-sensitization direction and the mean of these three images. Although in general the results indicated that the lung parenchyma of the healthy subjects was not far from being isotropic on the basis of this measure, there were some differences among the sensitization directions. The mean percent differences in ADC values for the A–P, H–F, and L–R directions were −5.28%, 3.30%, and 1.99%, respectively. The percent difference in the A–P direction was always negative and was statistically less than that for either the H–F or L–R directions. The

H–F direction always had a value that was higher than those for the other directions, but this value was not statistically greater than that in the L–R direction. The differences as a function of the diffusion-sensitization direction may be related to preferential orientation of the airways. Although one might expect that at the alveolar level the structure should be isotropic, smaller conductive airways may still have a preferred orientation.

In emphysema patients the values showed a similar trend, with mean percent differences of -2.78%, 3.13%, and 0.3% for the A–P, H–F, and L–R directions, respectively. When percent-difference values between the healthy and emphysema groups were compared, those in the A–P direction were significantly different. In addition, for the emphysema patients, the magnitude of the percent-difference values, averaged over the three directions of diffusion sensitization, was significantly lower than that for healthy subjects. Thus, it appears that the directional dependence of ADC values may be decreased in emphysematous regions of the lung.

Destruction of parenchyma and coalescence of distal airway structures may make the lung parenchyma more isotropic in emphysema, thus decreasing measures of anisotropy. Diffusion tensor imaging could be used to better assess such changes. Furthermore, it may be fruitful to extend the distributed-cylinder model discussed earlier to include an anisotropic distribution of cylinders.

D. Dependence on Lung Inflation

If ^{3}He diffusion measurements indeed convey information about the microstructural dimensions of the lung, one may expect to find a difference between ADC values that are measured at various states of lung inflation. Salerno et al. (16,35) evaluated the dependence of ADC values on lung inflation in seven healthy subjects by performing measurements at inspiration and expiration in the sagittal or axial orientation. There was a statistically significant decrease in the mean ADC values in the exhalation images compared with those in the inhalation images; the differences in mean ADC values ranged between 0.02 and $0.04 \, \mathrm{cm}^2/\mathrm{s}$. In the sagittal orientation, there was also a statistically significant difference between the mean ADC values in the anterior portion of the lung compared with those in the posterior portion at both inhalation and exhalation. In the axial orientation, the same phenomenon was observed, but the difference was statistically significant only at exhalation.

Figure 15.8 shows a set of sagittal ADC images from a 60-year-old male subject at inspiration and expiration. In this subject, the A–P gradient of ADC values was particularly pronounced at exhalation.

The decrease in ADC values between inhalation and exhalation results from structural changes that occur in the lung. The average size of the airways decreases which, without any other structural change, should in turn decrease the measured ADC. In addition, there may be a decrease in the sizes of the

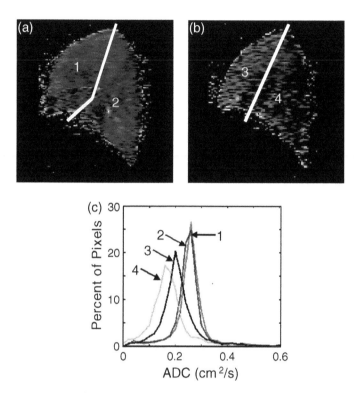

Figure 15.8 Sagittal ³He ADC MR images measured at (a) inhalation and (b) exhalation. (c) ADC histograms for the four regions that are labeled in the ADC images. The exhalation image had a lower mean ADC value. There was an A–P gradient of ADC values at inhalation that increased markedly at exhalation.

openings between different respiratory units. This would result in an increase in the tortuosity and potentially a decrease in the ADC for a given diffusion time.

E. Model-Based Diffusion Results

On the basis of the model of isotropically distributed cylinders, Yablonskiy et al. (21) calculated transverse (D_T) and longitudinal (D_L) components of the ADC for two healthy volunteers and four patients with severe emphysema by using a six b-value bipolar-GRE pulse sequence. In both subject groups, ³He diffusion was anisotropic, that is, the mean D_L values were 2–4 times larger than the mean D_T values. Parametric maps of the orientationally averaged diffusivity, the longitudinal and transverse diffusion coefficients, and the mean airway radius are shown in Fig. 15.9 for one of the healthy volunteers and two of the emphysema patients.

In the healthy volunteers, the mean D_L and D_T values were 0.35 and 0.11 cm²/s, respectively. The mean airway radius, calculated from D_T, was

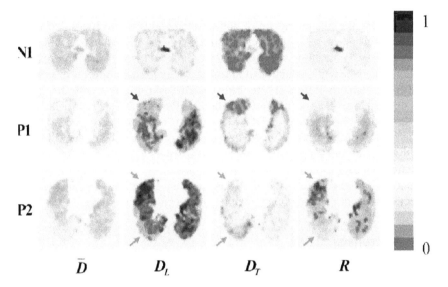

Figure 15.9 (**See color insert**) Representative ^{3}He parametric MR images of diffusivity from a normal subject (N1) and two patients with severe emphysema (P1 and P2). From left to right, the columns display the orientationally averaged diffusivity $\bar{D}$, the longitudinal ADC value D_L, the transverse ADC value D_T, and the mean airway radius R. The color scale on the right represents diffusivity coefficients in cm^2/s and airway radii in millimeters. Each color corresponds to 0.05 unit. Brown arrows point to an area of emphysematous lung with minor airway destruction, pink arrows point to an area of emphysematous lung with moderate airway destruction, and green arrows point to a lung area with severe emphysema. The small high-diffusivity regions in N1 are the two major bronchi just below their branching from the trachea. [From Ref. (21).]

0.36 mm, which is in agreement with previous *in vitro* morphometric measurements of 0.35 mm (6). In emphysema patients, both D_L and D_T increased markedly, with D_L approaching the free diffusion coefficient of ^{3}He in air for highly emphysematous regions. The mean D_L and D_T values were 0.72 and 0.25 cm^2/s, respectively. In regions of severe emphysema, the ratio of D_L to D_T decreased, possibly indicating a decrease in anisotropy owing to tissue destruction.

Studies will need to be performed in larger numbers of patients with a range of disease severity to assess the usefulness of this model in sensitively detecting emphysematous changes in the lung.

IV. Conclusion

The high diffusion coefficient and low tissue solubility of ^{3}He enable hyperpolarized diffusion MRI to be used as a novel probe of lung microstructure.

This technique has already demonstrated substantial potential for noninvasively characterizing the microstructure of both healthy and diseased lungs. Diffusion measurements have been performed using a variety of techniques, most of which are based on measuring the attenuation of phase-tagged transverse magnetization due to the random motion of diffusing ^{3}He gas. Measurements in subjects with emphysema indicate that ^{3}He diffusion MRI is a sensitive indicator of the structural changes that occur with this disease. Preliminary studies of the time and directional dependence of ADC values, as well as studies performed at inspiration and expiration, have yielded useful information about the diffusion environment of the lung. This complex diffusion environment makes simple analytical models difficult to develop. The model of isotropically distributed cylinders is an important first step toward understanding how measured ADCs reflect changes in the underlying complex architecture of the lung.

References

1. Mugler JP III, Brookeman JR, Knight-Scott J, Maier T, de Lange EE, Bogorad PL. Regional measurement of the ^{3}He diffusion coefficient in the human lung. In: Proceedings of the International Society for Magnetic Resonance in Medicine, 6th Meeting, 1998; 1906.
2. Chen XJ, Möller HE, Chawla MS et al. Spatially resolved measurements of hyperpolarized gas properties in the lung in vivo. Part I: diffusion coefficient. Magn Reson Med 1999; 42:721–728.
3. Saam BT, Yablonskiy DA, Kodibagkar VD et al. MR imaging of diffusion of ^{3}He gas in healthy and diseased lungs. Magn Reson Med 2000; 44:174–179.
4. Salerno M, de Lange EE, Altes TA, Truwit JD, Brookeman JR, Mugler JP III. Emphysema: hyperpolarized helium-3 diffusion MR imaging of the lungs compared with spirometric indexes—initial experience. Radiology 2002; 222:252–260.
5. West JB. Respiratory Physiology—the Essentials. 6th ed. Baltimore, Maryland, USA: Lippincott Williams and Wilkins, 2000: 1–19.
6. Haefeli-Bleuer B, Weibel ER. Morphometry of the human pulmonary acinus. Anat Rec 1988; 220:401–414.
7. Schreider JP, Raabe OG. Structure of the human respiratory acinus. Am J Anat 1981; 162:221–232.
8. Bock M. Simultaneous T2* and diffusion measurements with ^{3}He. Magn Reson Med 1997; 38:890–895.
9. Durand E, Guillot G, Darrasse L, Tastevin G, Nacher PJ. Diffusion imaging of hyperpolarized helium-3 in the human lung, with CPMG sequences at 0.1 T. In: Proceedings of the International Society for Magnetic Resonance in Medicine, 8th Meeting, 2000; 2184.
10. Durand E, Guillot G, Darrasse L et al. CPMG measurements and ultrafast imaging in human lungs with hyperpolarized helium-3 at low field (0.1 T). Magn Reson Med 2002; 47:75–81.
11. Owers-Bradley JR, Bennattayalah A, Fichele S et al. Diffusion and tagging of hyperpolarised ^{3}He in the lungs. In: Proceedings of the International Society for Magnetic Resonance in Medicine, 10th Meeting, 2002; 2016.

12. Owers-Bradley JR, Fichele MS, Bennattayalah A et al. MR tagging of human lungs using hyperpolarized ^{3}He gas. J Magn Reson Imaging 2003; 17:142–146.
13. Stejskal EO, Tanner JE. Spin diffusion measurements: spin echoes in the presence of a time-dependent field gradient. J Chem Phys 1965; 42:288–292.
14. Turner R, Le Bihan D, Maier J, Vavrek R, Hedges LK, Pekar J. Echo-planar imaging of intravoxel incoherent motion. Radiology 1990; 177:407–414.
15. Salerno M, Altes TA, Brookeman JR, de Lange EE, Mugler JP III. Rapid hyperpolarized ^{3}He diffusion MRI of healthy and emphysematous human lungs using an optimized interleaved-spiral pulse sequence. J Magn Reson Imaging 2003; 17:581–588.
16. Salerno M. Hyperpolarized ^{3}He Diffusion MRI for Characterizing the Human Lung. Ph.D. dissertation, University of Virginia, 2002.
17. Axel L, Dougherty L. MR imaging of motion with spatial modulation of magnetization. Radiology 1989; 171:841–845.
18. Neuman CH. Spin echo of spins diffusing in a bounded medium. J Chem Phys 1974; 60:4508–4511.
19. Kuchel PW, Lennon AJ, Durrant C. Analytical solutions and simulations for spin-echo measurements of diffusion of spins in a sphere with surface and bulk relaxation. J Magn Reson B 1996; 112:1–17.
20. Balinov B, Jonsson B, Linse P, Soderman O. The NMR self-diffusion method applied to restricted diffusion. Simulation of echo attenuation from molecules in spheres and between planes. J Magn Reson A 1993; 104:17–25.
21. Yablonskiy DA, Sukstanskii AL, Leawoods JC et al. Quantitative in vivo assessment of lung microstructure at the alveolar level with hyperpolarized ^{3}He diffusion MRI. Proc Natl Acad Sci USA 2002; 99:3111–3116.
22. Mitra PP, Sen PN, Schwartz LM. Short-time behavior of the diffusion coefficient as a geometrical probe of porous media. Phys Rev B—Condens Matter 1993; 47:8565–8574.
23. Sen PN, Schwartz LM, Mitra PP, Halperin BI. Surface relaxation and the long-time diffusion coefficient in porous media: periodic geometries. Phys Rev B—Condens Matter 1994; 49:215–225.
24. Latour LL, Kleinberg RL, Mitra PP, Sotak CH. Pore-size distributions and tortuosity in heterogenous porous media. J Magn Reson A 1995; 112:83–91.
25. Latour LL, Li LM, Sotak CH. Improved PFG stimulated-echo method for the measurement of diffusion in inhomogenous fields. J Magn Reson B 1993; 101:72–77.
26. Mair RW, Wong GP, Hoffmann D et al. Probing porous media with gas diffusion NMR. Phys Rev Let 1999; 83:3324–3327.
27. Mair RW, Hürlimann MD, Sen PN, Schwartz LM, Patz S, Walsworth RL. Tortuosity measurement and the effects of finite pulse widths on xenon gas diffusion NMR studies of porous media. Magn Reson Imaging 2001; 19:345–351.
28. de Swiet TM, Sen PN. Time dependent diffusion coefficient in a disordered medium. J Chem Phys 1996; 104:206–209.
29. Latour LL, Mitra PP, Kleinberg RL, Sotak CH. Time-dependent diffusion coefficient of fluids in porous media as a probe of surface-to-volume ratio. J Magn Reson A 1993; 101:342–346.
30. Yablonskiy DA, Lee M, Leewoods JC, Cooper JD, Gierada DS, Conradi MS. ^{3}He diffusional MRI provides quantitative information on lung tissue structure in patients with emphysema [abstr]. Radiology 2001; 221(P):631.

31. Leawoods J, Yablonskiy DA, Gierada D, Conradi MS. Ventilation abnormalities and diffusion coefficients in the lungs of asymptomatic smokers. In: Proceedings of the International Society for Magnetic Resonance in Medicine, 9th Meeting, 2001; 185.
32. Salerno M, Mugler JP III, Cooley B, Brookeman JR, de Lange EE, Altes TA. Hyperpolarized [3]He diffusion imaging in smokers: comparison with computed tomography and spirometry. In: Proceedings of the International Society of Magnetic Resonance Medicine, 10th Meeting, 2002; 760.
33. Salerno M, Brookeman JR, Mugler JP III. Time-dependent hyperpolarized [3]He diffusion MR imaging: initial experience in healthy and emphysematous lungs. In: Proceeding of the International Society for Magnetic Resonance in Medicine, 9th Meeting, 2001; 950.
34. Maier T, Knight-Scott J, Mai VM, Mugler JP III, Brookeman JR. Restricted diffusion of hyperpolarized 3He in the human lung. In: Proceedings of the International Society for Magnetic Resonance in Medicine, 6th Meeting, 1998; 1913.
35. Salerno M, Brookeman JR, de Lange EE, Knight-Scott J, Mugler JP III. Demonstration of an alveolar-size gradient in the healthy human lung: A study of the reproducibility of hyperpolarized [3]He diffusion MRI. In: Proceedings of the International Society for Magnetic Resonance in Medicine, 8th Meeting, 2000; 2195.

16

Regional Oxygen Balance

BALTHASAR EBERLE

University of Berne,
Berne, Switzerland

WOLFGANG G. SCHREIBER

Johannes Gutenberg University
Medical School,
Mainz, Germany

I. Introduction

The local ratio between ventilation ($\dot{V}_A$) and perfusion ($\dot{Q}$) and its distribution throughout the lung is one of the most important defining factors of alveolar gas composition (1). Until recently, direct and simultaneous regional measurement of alveolar and capillary gas concentrations has not been possible. Information about the regional pO_2 distribution within the pulmonary biocompartments would (i) add to the understanding of $\dot{V}_A/\dot{Q}$ distribution and heterogeneity in the normal lung, for example, with regard to species differences, maturation, structural, gravitational, exertional, and many other effects; (ii) contribute to diagnosis and monitoring of obstructive, interstitial, inflammatory, and embolic pulmonary diseases; and (iii) help to monitor the effects of drugs upon the pulmonary vasculature or the airways.

Conventionally, the clinical assessment of gas exchange in the lung is performed using global measurements and simple models of lung function. Partial pressures of O_2 (pO_2) and CO_2 (pCO_2) are measured in inspired, end-expiratory, and mixed expiratory gas. Mass spectrometry, polarographic, or paramagnetic principles are used for pO_2 measurements in respiratory gas. Expired pCO_2 is conveniently detected, for example, by its infrared absorption. Blood gas analysis and oximetry in mixed venous and arterial blood use electrochemical detection and multiwavelength spectrometry.

Using such data, gas exchange is conventionally modeled to occur in a single "ideal" alveolar compartment of the whole lung. A ventilated but nonperfused compartment (dead space, $\dot{V}_A/\dot{Q} = \infty$) and a nonventilated but perfused compartment (shunt, $\dot{V}_A/\dot{Q} = 0$) complete this clinically useful three-compartment model (2).

The multiple inert gas elimination technique (MIGET) extends this model to contain 50 virtual compartments defined by characteristic $\dot{V}_A/\dot{Q}$ ratios. The steady-state distribution of six biologically inert gases of characteristic blood solubility between arterial blood and mixed expired gas is analyzed using gas chromatography (3) or mass spectrometry (4). The matching of ventilation and perfusion, the scatter and distribution of $\dot{V}_A/\dot{Q}$ ratios, the size of intrapulmonary shunt, alveolar dead space, and the resulting oxygenation may be derived from these data. MIGET still contributes much to the understanding of pulmonary physiology and pathophysiology, but it does not allow for regional allocation of functional lung compartments.

In today's clinical routine, regional $\dot{V}_A/\dot{Q}$ analysis is performed by ventilation–perfusion mapping using radioisotope single photon emission computed tomography (SPECT). This concept is rooted in the seminal work studying regional $\dot{V}_A/\dot{Q}$ ratios by projectional radioisotope ventilation and perfusion scintigraphy (5). Even today, however, the spatial resolution of three-dimensional SPECT in the lung does not approach the dimensions of a pulmonary acinus (3–4 mm), which is considered the terminal respiratory unit. Specifically, the technique's long acquisition time does not allow for breath-hold imaging. This shortcoming reduces resolution, which is most felt in the periphery where respiratory movement is greatest. Unfortunately, these scans represent a temporal and spatial average of ventilation and perfusion over many respiratory cycles.

In recent years, positron emission tomography (PET) with radioactive $^{13}N_2$ as a tracer has emerged into a potent technique to measure the regional $\dot{V}_A/\dot{Q}$ distributions in the lung (6). Images of pulmonary perfusion are acquired during a 30 s breath-hold, following bolus infusion and equilibration of the dissolved tracer. After perfusion-dependent deposition of the inert gaseous tracer in the apnoeic alveolar space, ventilation mapping is derived from washout kinetics of the inert gas during respiration. With latest technology PET scanners, spatial resolution is on the order of 2–3 mm. Meanwhile, the technique has been used in large animals and in models of pulmonary embolism and bronchoconstriction (7–9), in healthy human volunteers (10), and more recently in patients with asthma (11) and acute respiratory distress syndrome (ARDS).

The PET technique can be used to indirectly assess, and image, regional oxygen balance in the lung. Using PET-derived local $\dot{V}_A/\dot{Q}$ data together with mass transfer equations, which assume alveolar-capillary gas equilibration, regional intrapulmonary pO_2, pCO_2, and pH can be modeled mathematically. In an experimental sheep model of pulmonary macroembolism, embolized high $\dot{V}_A/\dot{Q}$ regions became apparent by exhibiting low local pCO_2 values (12). With a spatial resolution of $6 \times 6 \times 6 \text{ mm}^3 = 216 \text{ mm}^3$, this technique now approaches the resolution required to probe human acinar, that is, functional lung unit volumes, which have been measured in adult human lung casts to average $187 \pm 79 \text{ mm}^3$ (13). The temporal resolution is limited by the measurement times of 30 s and 3 min for perfusion and ventilation data acquisition, respectively.

Computed tomography (CT) and magnetic resonance imaging (MRI) have recently undergone enormous technical improvements. With CT, rapid imaging of lung ventilation (14,15) and perfusion (16,17) has become feasible. New MRI methods for assessment of ventilation using both hyperpolarized ^3He (18–20) and fluorinated gases (20–23) as well as perfusion (24–26) have been developed.

Ventilation MRI using gases as exogenous contrast agents has led to a wide variety of new functional imaging methods including methods to measure the regional oxygen partial pressure in the lungs' airspaces. This chapter will describe these exciting new approaches, initial studies in this rapidly evolving research field, and inherent limitations of the methodology. The basics of most proton and non-proton MRI techniques have been described in Chapters 6, 7, and 12). Therefore, we will focus only on those aspects relevant for a quantitative analysis of the regional oxygen balance in the lung.

II. Basic Physiology of Regional Oxygen Balance

Each respiratory cycle moves gas to and fro through common conducting airways and exchanges, by diffusive mixing in the very distal airspaces, a portion of alveolar gas with humidified dead space gas and fresh gas. Pulmonary perfusion, on the other hand, is a pulsatile and continuous process. The alveolar-capillary gas exchange of healthy lungs is extremely efficient. Partial pressures of oxygen and carbon dioxide in pulmonary capillary blood and alveolar gas equilibrate so rapidly that hemoglobin is able to saturate completely within a quarter of the red blood cells' average transit time (~ 1 s) through pulmonary capillaries, even under conditions of exercise with much faster transit times. The structural alveolocapillary diffusion barrier is minute, and is estimated to result in a pO_2 difference of only 4 mmHg between mixed alveolar gas and arterial blood. Thus, it is assumed that in the normal lung exchange of the respiratory gases is not limited by alveolocapillary diffusion but rather by perfusion (27). Models to derive alveolar gas partial pressures from measured $\dot{V}_A/\dot{Q}$ ratios, therefore, conveniently assume complete diffusion equilibrium at the end of the alveolar-capillary transit of blood. This assumption may not hold true in certain pathologic conditions like congestive heart failure or pulmonary edema.

Within a healthy model alveolus, gas composition is determined by the balance between oxygen supplied by ventilation and oxygen removed by perfusion (Fig. 16.1), and by carbon dioxide delivery by perfusion and its elimination by expiration. At a given ventilation and perfusion, and in a steady state of inspired gas mixture and whole-body metabolism, alveolar gas composition is assumed to be fairly constant and quite homogeneous throughout a functional lung unit. In reality, the functional lung unit is composed of an acinus, representing a group of about 10,000 alveoli supplied by a respiratory bronchiole, with a size of about 3.5 mm in diameter (28). In each individual functional lung unit with its diffusion equilibrium, the alveolar pO_2 (p_AO_2) equals the endcapillary pO_2, and according to laws of mass balance, both are uniquely defined by the ratio of this individual unit's alveolar ventilation to its perfusion ($\dot{V}_A/\dot{Q}$ ratio) (1).

In the lung of a normal individual breathing room air (20.9% O_2 in nitrogen), approximately 30,000 of such functional lung units transfer their individual alveolar gas partial pressures across their alveolocapillary membranes to the pulmonary capillary blood. Even in healthy lungs, however, there is a nonuniform distribution of $\dot{V}_A/\dot{Q}$ ratios with some scatter around the normal value of 0.8. Effects of gravitation upon pulmonary blood flow distribution and of lung biomechanics upon gas mixing and ventilation distribution have been invoked to explain this scatter, which also increases with age (even in healthy lungs).

In many types of pulmonary disease, a significant number of lung units with abnormal $\dot{V}_A/\dot{Q}$ ratio contribute to mixed alveolar and arterial gas composition. Alveolar-arterial pO_2 difference increases, and hypoxemia ensues with or without hypercapnia. Particularly during early stages of disease, however, compensatory mechanisms are activated to counteract $\dot{V}_A/\dot{Q}$ maldistribution to some degree. Most prominently, hypoxic pulmonary vasoconstriction efficiently reduces blood flow to hypoventilated lung regions. This reflex compensates regional hypoventilation, for example, in emphysema, atelectasis, and cystic fibrosis or during single-lung ventilation, and will support oxygenation for long periods of time. Recently, this targeted response of perfusion to regionally induced

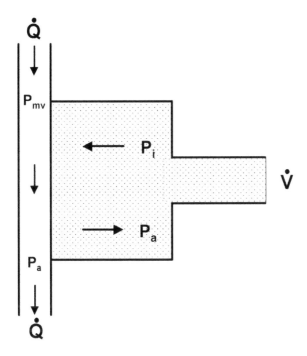

Figure 16.1 Model of a functional lung unit. Under steady-state conditions, respiratory gas composition is determined by the equilibrium between supply of oxygen by ventilation ($\dot{V}$) and its removal by perfusion ($\dot{Q}$). Mixed venous blood with low oxygen partial pressure (Pmv) equilibrates with oxygen from inspired air (Pi). During the passage of blood along the alveolus, capillary and alveolar oxygen partial pressures equilibrate and end-capillary partial pressure equals alveolar partial pressure (Pa). Under normal conditions, the ratio between ventilation and perfusion is on the order of unity. [Adapted with permission from Wagner et al. (1).]

hypoventilation could be demonstrated in bronchoconstricted asthmatics, using the technique of $^{13}N_2$-PET mentioned above (11). By similar means, another reflex mechanism, denoted hypocapnic bronchoconstriction, has been shown to shift alveolar ventilation away from acutely embolized lung regions towards perfused areas, again redressing $\dot{V}_A/\dot{Q}$ maldistribution to a measurable degree (7,8).

III. Methods Based on Hyperpolarized Helium-3

A. Physical Principles

It is not currently possible to obtain spatially resolved, direct measurement of alveolar and end-capillary gas concentrations. However, hyperpolarized noble gases have physical properties that may be exploited to determine these values.

Certain hyperpolarized noble gases such as Helium-3 (^{3}He), or Xenon-129, yield a strong MR signal. This signal is well suited for high-resolution MR imaging of the lungs but, at the same time, is highly sensitive to paramagnetic influences from its molecular environment.

Molecular O_2 is the most abundant paramagnetic molecule in inspired and alveolar gas. The oxygen molecule has two unpaired electrons, which causes a local magnetic field within its vicinity. Due to Brownian motion of both the oxygen molecules and nearby ^{3}He atoms, the ^{3}He atoms experience a rapidly varying magnetic field from the presence of oxygen. This varying magnetic field results in an increase of the longitudinal ($1/T_1$) relaxation rate of ^{3}He. In the early days of hyperpolarized gas imaging using ^{3}He, this relaxation effect was considered disadvantageous to MR imaging because it reduces the available magnetization and, thus, signal intensity. Subsequently, however, these nuclear physical characteristics were to be exploited for measurement of the influence of paramagnetic O_2 on the decay rate of non-equilibrium polarization of the hyperpolarized gas to its equilibrium value. As the hyperpolarized noble gases are inert and nonradioactive, they may be inhaled and act as reporters of intra-alveolar pO_2.

Saam et al. (29) have shown *in vitro* that the T_1 relaxation rate of ^{3}He depends on the oxygen content of the gas mixture:

$$\frac{1}{T_1} = \kappa \, pO_2 \tag{16.1}$$

where pO_2 denotes the oxygen partial pressure in the gas mixture and $\kappa = 3.8 \times 10^{-6} \, \text{s}^{-1} \, \text{Pa}^{-1}$ is the proportionality constant at 37°C and at a magnetic field strength of 1.41 T (Fig. 16.2).

This relationship has been confirmed in *in vivo* experiments by several authors (Figs. 16.3 and 16.4) (30–32). However, it is not only the amount of oxygen which influences the magnetization of hyperpolarized ^{3}He but also the MR measurement itself. Each radiofrequency (RF) pulse with flip angle α reduces the available longitudinal magnetization by a factor of $\cos(\alpha)$. Therefore, after acquisition of an MR image with NP phase encoding steps, the available magnetization is reduced by a factor of $\cos^{NP}(\alpha)$. Measurement of the oxygen concentration on the basis of its influence on the ^{3}He T_1 relaxation time thus requires consideration of RF pulse effects.

B. Techniques of Measurement

If hyperpolarized ^{3}He gas is used as a tracer substance to determine alveolar pO_2, the inhaled amount of ^{3}He should be as small as possible to reduce the disturbance of the physiologic alveolar gas composition. In recent pO_2-sensitive ^{3}He MRI studies of large animals and humans, ~3–4 mL/kg body weight of ^{3}He was administered at the beginning of normal or vital capacity inspirations.

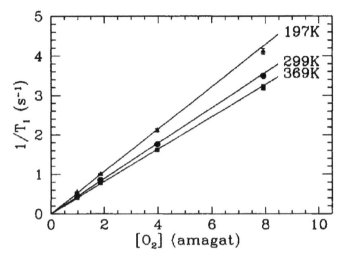

Figure 16.2 Relaxation rate T_1^{-1} of ^{3}He vs. [O_2] (amagat) at various temperatures (in K). Amagat is a unit of density equal to the number of molecules per unit volume of an ideal gas at 0°C and normal atmospheric pressure. [From Saam et al. (29), with permission.]

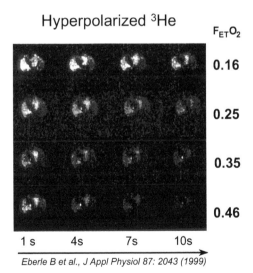

Figure 16.3 Serial ^{3}He images of porcine lungs in axial orientation (slice thickness, 20 mm). Concentration-dependent acceleration of ^{3}He signal decay by molecular oxygen in the lung (40 mL ^{3}He). The first, third, fifth, and seventh images are shown, together with duration of breath-hold and fractional end-tidal oxygen concentration ($F_{ET}O_2$). [From Eberle et al. (30), with permission.]

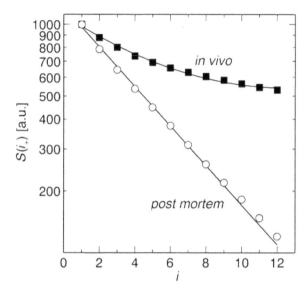

Figure 16.4 ^{3}He-spectroscopy experiment in a guinea pig to assess relaxivity of intrapulmonary oxygen upon ^{3}He signal intensity. Logarithmic plot of the signal intensity, S(i1), measured in arbitrary units after the ith RF pulse of a spectroscopic progressive-saturation sequence ($\alpha = 7°$, TR = 2 s) *in vivo* and post mortem. Both experiments were performed in the same animal with $F_IO_2 = 0.22$. [From Möller et al. (32), with permission.]

Sufficient MR signal intensity is obtained despite the low dosage by using gas with polarization levels as high as 50%. Gas dosage and administration benefit from computer-controlled applicator devices (30,33,34). As an alternative adminis-tration technique, replacement of a fraction of the inspired N_2 by hyperpolarized ^{3}He has been used in small animals under controlled ventilation (32). After admin-istration of the bolus of hyperpolarized ^{3}He, two series of rapid gradient echo images are acquired during two breath-holds. The measurements in the two breath-holds are performed with either different flip angles and/or with different interscan delays. A variation of the interscan delay varies the exposure time to O_2. A subsequent mathematical analysis then separates RF- and O_2-induced depolar-ization (35). As a result, regional values for α and pO_2 are extracted (30), and the time course of regional intrapulmonary pO_2 during short breath-holds can be determined with relative errors of 3% (for pO_2 at onset of breath-hold) and 7% (for decrease rate of pO_2) at an in-plane resolution of 1 cm $\times$ 1 cm (31).

　　In order to circumvent the problem of reproducibility of the double breath-holding maneuver, a single-acquisition imaging sequence for O_2-sensitive ^{3}He-MRI has been developed. It systematically varies both the interscan delay and the flip angle within one and the same serial image acquisition, that is, during one breath-hold of about 15 s duration (Fig. 16.5) (34). This improves temporal

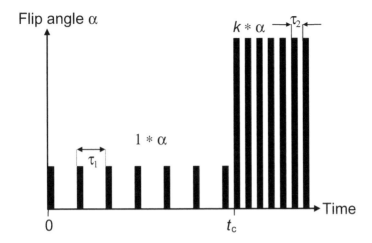

Figure 16.5 Timing diagram for the RF pulses used for pO_2 measurements by the single acquisition technique. Each bar represents one image. α, flip angle; τ, interscan interval; k, multiplication factor for α. [From Deninger et al. (36), with permission.]

resolution, and reduces the error introduced by inadequately reproduced inspirations. A beneficial side effect of the single breath-hold technique is the reduction of ^{3}He dose requirement for the study (36). Further improvements in data analysis methodology allow for mapping of the regional pO_2 distribution within the lung (Fig. 16.6).

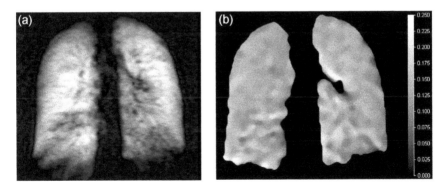

Figure 16.6 Measurement of pO_2 with the double-acquisition ^{3}He technique in a healthy volunteer. (a) The first ^{3}He image demonstrates a homogenous ^{3}He distribution characteristic of a healthy subject. The image was obtained without slice selection and, thus, presents a projection through the lung. (b) Map of oxygen partial pressure from the same volunteer as calculated from two ^{3}He pO_2-MR measurements with equal flip angles. The first image series was obtained with an interscan delay of 1 s, the second series with an interscan delay of 5 s. A relatively homogenous distribution of pO_2 values is observed. The colorbar ranges from 0 to 250 mbar.

C. Validation Studies

Image based determination of intrapulmonary pO_2 has been validated in phantom and in animal measurements (30,31). In pigs, MR imaging sequences of small amounts of ^{3}He inspired within various oxygen fractions demonstrated that the alveolar O_2 fractions measured in peripheral lung regions correlated closely with those measured in end-expiratory gas (30). Using repetitive NMR spectroscopy of inhaled hyperpolarized ^{3}He, Möller et al. (32) also demonstrated in guinea pigs that the longitudinal relaxation rate $1/T_1$ correlates well with the fractional concentration of oxygen in the inspired gas both *in vivo* and post mortem (Fig. 16.7). Moreover, the proportionality constant κ between $1/T_1$ and pO_2 [Eq. (16.1)] predicted by Saam et al. (29) was confirmed to be $(4.1 \pm 0.3) \times 10^{-6} \, \mathrm{s}^{-1} \, \mathrm{Pa}^{-1}$ at 2.0 T and under *in vivo* conditions. A postmortem study of T_1 in porcine lungs, which were deoxygenated by prolonged washout with pure N_2, demonstrated that longitudinal relaxation at the intraalveolar surfaces can be neglected because of the surprisingly long relaxation time of $T_1 \geq 4.3 \, \mathrm{min}$ (31). Therefore, the longitudinal relaxation rate within the healthy lung is dominated by alveolar pO_2.

Thus, kinetics of alveolar gas relaxation offer noninvasive ways to determine, by appropriate imaging routines, regional and global oxygen uptake $\dot{V}_{O_2}$ in the lung and to assess pulmonary perfusion. At barometric pressure P_B and a breath-hold at a continuous positive airway pressure P_{aw}, intrapulmonary

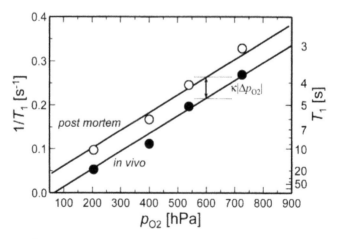

Figure 16.7 ^{3}He spin–lattice relaxation rates $1/T_1$ inside the lung of a guinea pig measured *in vivo* (filled circles) and postmortem (open circles) as a function of the O_2 partial pressure in the inspired gas mixture. Due to pulmonary gas exchange, reduced alveolar pO_2 is observed in the *in vivo* experiments as indicated by prolonged T_1. Solid lines show results from linear regression to Eq. (16.1). The offset between both graphs corresponds to a difference in pO_2 of 64 h Pa. [From Möller et al. (37), with permission.]

pO_2 decreases at a rate R_{O_2} within the intrapulmonary gas volume. The latter is given by the sum of functional residual capacity FRC and inspired tidal volume V_T (corrected for apparatus deadspace V_{Dapp} and anatomical dead space fraction V_D/V_T). Thus,

$$\dot{V}_{O_2} = \frac{R_{O_2}}{(P_B + P_{aw})} \times \left(FRC + (V_T - V_{Dapp}) \times \left(1 - \frac{V_D}{V_T}\right) \right) \qquad (16.2)$$

In a series of 11 pigs (27 ± 2 kg), we found $R_{O_2} = -3.9 \pm 1.2$ mbar/s in parenchymal regions-of-interest (ROI) [data combined from Refs. (31,38)]. At measured values for $P_B = 1004$ mbar, $P_{aw} = 20$ mbar, $V_T = 486 \pm 83$ mL, an apparatus dead space of 150 mL, $V_D/V_T = 0.3$, and assumed values for FRC = 30 mL/kg [from published data for pigs (39,40)], this can be extrapolated to an estimated global $\dot{V}_{O_2} = 9.0 \pm 3.2$ mL O_2 kg^{-1} min^{-1}. These measurements are in the range of published data for swine (41).

In spectroscopy studies of small animals, Möller et al. (32) demonstrated that the decay of signal intensity during consecutive measurements in apnea becomes mono-exponential only after termination of oxygen consumption by cardiac arrest (Fig. 16.4). As long as the animal was alive but apneic, ongoing oxidative metabolism and subsequent hypoxemia reduced the relaxivity of alveolar gas. The initial fractional inspiratory-to-alveolar O_2 difference, extrapolated right to the onset of apnea after a period of constant ventilation and combined with an estimate of alveolar ventilation, allowed to determine values for oxygen uptake $\dot{V}_{O_2}$ (29 mL min^{-1} kg^{-1}) and cardiac output (400 mL min^{-1} kg^{-1}), which were quite consistent with reference data reported for this species in the literature (32). After a step-down of the inspiratory fractional oxygen concentration (F_IO_2) from 1.0 to 0.21, washout characteristics of relaxivity and hence, alveolar pO_2, also allowed to obtain estimates for functional residual capacity.

Diffusional limitations do not apply in spectroscopy experiments and the previously described projection MR imaging, which encompass the entire lung but may become critical in slice-selective MRI pO_2 measurements. Here, convective and diffusive motion of ^{3}He in and out of the imaged slice may systematically bias the observed signal intensities. Diffusion of ^{3}He atoms in the lung is rapid. Measured apparent diffusion coefficients ranged from 0.2 cm^2/s in healthy subjects to 0.9 cm^2/s in severe emphysema (42). Diffusion may limit the accuracy of thin two-dimensional slice-selective measurement, as—during subsequent measurements—less-depolarized ^{3}He may diffuse into the imaged slice from adjacent nonimaged regions (and vice versa). Spins from those regions have not been depolarized by previous RF pulses and, thus, may introduce a systematic overestimation of the MR signal within the slice. To minimize this problem, nonslice selective two-dimensional imaging pulse sequences have been used in most recent studies (30,31,34–37,43). Three-dimensional MRI sequences may be useful to increase the spatial resolution in slice direction by keeping the systematic bias of the signal intensities from diffusion low. Unfortunately, incomplete breath-holding, particularly in dyspneic patients, as well as cardiac oscillations or diaphragmatic motion appear as further potential sources of measurement artifacts.

Intrapulmonary pO_2 measurement using low-field ^{3}He MR imaging has been also shown to be feasible in small animals (44). This technique may be particularly interesting because the developments of low-field MR systems dedicated for low-cost ^{3}He lung MRI appears to be feasible in the future.

D. Studies in Humans

First human applications of the described technique demonstrated a very homogeneous pO_2 distribution in healthy young subjects, its mean being in good agreement with end-tidal pO_2 measured at the mouth. During breath-holding at an inspiratory reserve capacity of the lungs ($\sim$3000 mL), pO_2 decrease rates of ~ -1.6 mmHg/s were observed (31,35) (Fig. 16.9). This value agrees well with an oxygen consumption of $\sim$400 mL O_2/min estimated for such subjects using standard reference data (27,45).

In patients with pulmonary fibrosis after unilateral lung transplantation, alveolar pO_2 was quite heterogeneously distributed. Specifically, it was higher in functioning grafts than in native fibrotic lungs. Mean MRI-determined alveolar pO_2 of these patients ranged quite consistently between the pO_2 levels found in end-tidal gas and arterial blood (43). More recent animal and human data indicate that regional alveolar hypoperfusion and dead space generated by pulmonary artery branch obstruction is correctly detected by pO_2 ^{3}He MRI (Fig. 16.8) (37,46,47).

In perspective, functional ^{3}He-MRI techniques to measure regional alveolar pO_2 and its kinetics may offer a noninvasive and easily repeatable route to assess regional ventilation and, simultaneously, also perfusion-driven local oxygen uptake into pulmonary capillary blood, at least in those parts of the lung reached by inhaled ^{3}He (Fig. 16.9).

IV. Methods Based on Fluorine-19

Fluorine (^{19}F), the only stable isotope of fluorine, has spin $1/2$ and a magnetic moment almost as large as that of ^{1}H. These properties as well as the normal absence of ^{19}F in the body makes fluorine compounds good candidates for ^{19}F MRI of the lung because—in principle—a high signal intensity can be achieved from the intrapulmonary air space without any background signal.

For functional assessment of the oxygen balance, two ^{19}F MRI approaches based on biologically inert fluorine-containing substances are of particular interest. One is based on the use of fluorinated gases such as tetrafluoromethane (CF_4) (48), hexafluoroethane (C_2F_6) (22), and sulfur hexafluoride (SF_6) (20,21,23). These gases are administered with the inspired gas mixture and can be detected

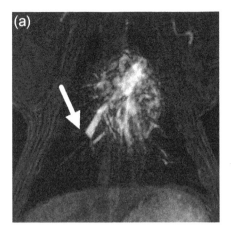 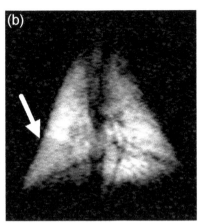

Figure 16.8 MR angiogram (a) and breath-hold ^{3}He-MR projection image (b) of a pig's lungs following acute balloon obstruction of the right lower lobar artery and a short period of steady-state ventilation ($F_IO_2 = 0.29$). (a) The arrow depicts site of vascular obstruction. (b) Enhanced relaxivity of alveolar gas in hypo- and nonperfused parenchyma is evident from regionally increased ^{3}He signal decay, which is due to impaired alveolar-capillary oxygen transfer. Arrow marks region of oxygen-enriched and hence, signal-depleted alveolar deadspace.

by ^{19}F MRI. The other approach uses perfluorocarbons (PFC) (49–51), oxygen-carrying liquids which have been studied in total or partial liquid ventilation, for example, for respiratory support in ARDS (52) and respiratory insufficiency in preterm neonates (53,54). The signal from PFCs can be measured by ^{19}F MRI pulse sequences as well.

Both approaches have in common that the substances used contain a large number of ^{19}F atoms with all of them (in fluorinated gases) or at least part of them (PFCs) resonating at the same Larmor frequency. In consequence, they induce in the receive coil a relatively large MR signal at the ^{19}F Larmor frequency.

A. MRI Techniques Using Fluorinated Gases

It is known since the early days of MRI that biologically inert fluorinated gases can be used for MRI of the lung (48). These gases have extremely short T_1 relaxation times (on the order of milliseconds). Therefore, a large number of signal averages can be obtained within relatively short imaging times. The high number of averages can be used to compensate for the relatively low density of the gases in the lung. In small animals, scan times on the order of hours down to 30 min are feasible (22,48,55). Cyclical lung volume measurements in rats with elastase-induced emphysema have been demonstrated using that approach (23). Recent studies have shown that in larger animals (e.g., pigs) single breath-hold acquisition is feasible if modern gradient technology is

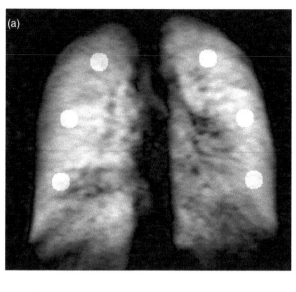

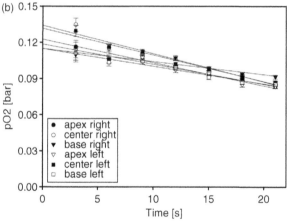

Figure 16.9 Measurement of the pO$_2$ variation during breath-holding. (a) Anatomical image demonstrating the six ROIs used for data analysis. (b) Temporal evolution of the pO$_2$ in the individual ROIs. Little variations are observed both in the initial pO$_2$ values and in the decrease rates.

used, and if the animal is ventilated with a mixture of 79% SF$_6$ and 21% O$_2$ (Fig. 16.10a) (21). Acquisition times with two-dimensional short echo-time gradient-echo pulse sequences are short enough even for the assessment of the wash-in and wash-out kinetics of the gas (Fig. 16.10b) (20).

Spin-rotation relaxation of fluorinated gases is so rapid that dipolar coupling to the paramagnetic oxygen has no effect (56). In consequence, direct

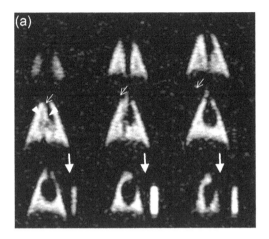

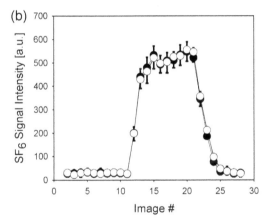

Figure 16.10 ^{19}F image MRI of a pig ventilated with SF_6 gas. (a) Morphologic information obtained after ventilation with a mixture of 79% SF_6 gas and 21% O_2 using a three-dimensional gradient echo pulse sequence. Nine slices from a three-dimensional breath-hold acquisition are shown. Arrowheads point to the mainstem bronchi, small arrows to the trachea, and large arrows to a phantom containing 100% SF_6. (b) Measurement of the wash-in and wash-out kinetics of SF_6. The data were obtained with a two-dimensional gradient-echo pulse sequence without slice selection. One ^{19}F image was obtained after each breath of 100% SF_6 gas. Wash-out was subsequently performed by breathing 100% oxygen. [Reprinted with permission from Schreiber et al. (20).]

imaging of the influence of oxygen on the T_1 relaxation time of the ^{19}F nuclei is not feasible. Instead, the concentration effect due to oxygen uptake into pulmonary capillary blood during a breath-hold (57,58) can be used as a contrast mechanism. If a high inspired fraction of O_2 (e.g., $F_IO_2 = 0.75$) and low inspired SF_6 fraction (e.g., $F_ISF_6 = 25\%$) is administered, the inhaled SF_6 gas concentrates preferentially in lung regions with low $\dot{V}_A/\dot{Q}$ because oxygen is taken up by the blood (and the missing gas volume is replaced by SF_6), and because the SF_6 gas is almost insoluble in blood. In consequence, the signal intensity in that region is higher than in a region with high $\dot{V}_A/\dot{Q}$. In a reference image acquired at low F_1O_2 (e.g., $F_1O_2 = 0.20$) and high F_ISF_6 (e.g., $F_ISF_6 = 80\%$), the concentration effect due to oxygen uptake is smaller (Fig. 16.11). From the ratio of the signal intensities in images taken at these two different conditions, an estimate of the regional $\dot{V}_A/\dot{Q}$ distribution can be obtained (55). Initial results in a rat model of partial bronchial obstruction have been demonstrated recently. Low $\dot{V}_A/\dot{Q}$ areas induced by the partial bronchial obstruction were detected in the calculated $\dot{V}_A/\dot{Q}$ maps (see insert of Fig. 16.11) (55).

B. MRI Techniques Using Liquid PFCs

PFCs denote a group of biologically inert, organic fluid compounds whose hydrogen atoms have been replaced by halogens, that is, mostly fluoride. In these liquids, molecular oxygen and carbon dioxide are highly soluble and diffuse

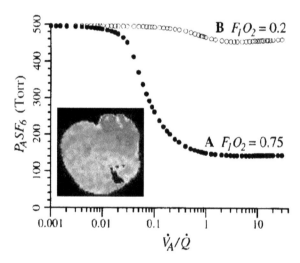

Figure 16.11   Alveolar SF_6 partial pressure as a function of the ventilation–perfusion ratio. The two curves give the alveolar concentration for two different inspiratory oxygen concentrations. With increasing ventilation more oxygen remains in the alveolar space and, thus, alveolar SF_6 concentration is low. This effect is markedly pronounced at high inspiratory oxygen concentrations. A body temperature of 37°C, venous pO_2 of 40 torr, and venous pCO_2 of 46 torr was assumed for the simulations. From the ratio of the SF_6 partial pressures obtained under two different inspiratory conditions, the ventilation–perfusion ratio can be calculated. The insert shows such a ratio image obtained in a rat with partially obstructed left bronchus. Low signal intensity denotes a low ventilation–perfusion ratio in the anatomical region of partial obstruction. [Adapted with permission from Kuethe et al. (55).]

reasonably well. In addition, surface tension of these hydrophobic compounds is very low. PFC emulsions are studied as heme-free oxygen-carrying blood substitutes (59) and as emulsified oxygen carriers in percutaneous coronary interventions. Instilled into the lung, a second-generation PFC (Perflubron) is under evaluation for partial liquid ventilation in ARDS, to improve oxygen transport by reopening the surfactant-depleted atelectatic alveolar space at high $F_{PFC}O_2$ (59). Results also indicate anti-inflammatory effects upon lung parenchyma (60). Despite promising data from animal studies, clinical trials of Perflubron (PFOB) have failed so far to improve the outcome in patients with acute lung injury (53).

PFCs have fluorine atoms in different carbon groups (e.g., $-CF_2$, $-CF_3$, $CBrF_7$) and, therefore, do not all resonate at the same Larmor frequency. Techniques such as the use of chemical shift selective saturation (CHESS) presaturation (50,51) or deconvolution techniques (61) are required to suppress chemical shift artifacts in the MRI images of PFOB instilled into the lung of animals (Fig. 16.12a). Double-resonant $^1H/^{19}F$ MR coils even allow for a correlation between the high-resolution visualization of ^1H MRI and the fluorine distribution (62).

The T_1 relaxation time of PFCs is reduced by the presence of molecular oxygen (Fig. 16.12b). Using this effect, an increase of the MR signal intensity of up to 90% has been demonstrated under conditions of pure oxygen breathing in PFC-filled mice and rat lungs (51). Quantitative measures of the intra-alveolar (intra-PFC) oxygen content can be obtained using the linear relation between $1/T_1$ and the oxygen concentration (50,51,63–65). This O_2-sensitive PFC MRI technique measures the intra-alveolar (intra-PFC) concentration of oxygen established by an equilibrium between ventilation, diffusion within PFC, and perfusion. In ARDS lungs, partial liquid ventilation has been shown to improve oxygenation, lung mechanics, and hence, ventilation, whereas it impairs them in healthy lungs (53).

One mechanism discussed for this behavior is redistribution of pulmonary blood flow to nondependent parts of the lungs due to the high specific gravity of PFB. This will redress the pathological $\dot{V}_A/\dot{Q}$ distribution in ARDS to some degree, but it has been shown to increase shunt and also $\dot{V}_A/\dot{Q}$ heterogeneity in healthy lungs (40). Moreover, diffusion limitation of respiratory gases within PFC may also play an important role, which is difficult to differentiate from the former mechanism (40).

In recent studies of partial liquid ventilation in a healthy porcine model, pO_2 in the PFOB phase ($P\text{-}pO_2$) has been determined, by measuring the T_1 relaxation time, using a series of rapid gradient images followed by a single inversion pulse. By analysis of the signal intensities in that image series regional oxygen concentration estimates were obtained. A PFC- and temperature-specific gauge curve was determined simultaneously using a ventilated PFC phantom placed inside the thoracic cavity (49,50). In addition, regional $P\text{-}pO_2$ was analyzed within isogravitational layers (Fig. 16.12) as a function of the end-tidal $P\text{-}etO_2$.

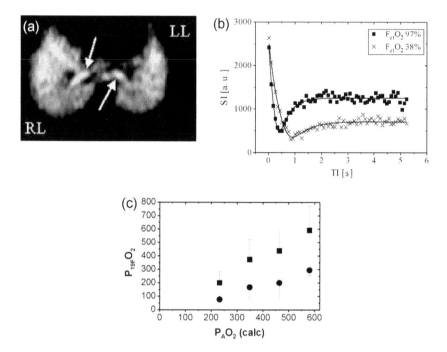

Figure 16.12 ^{19}F MRI of liquid ventilation. (a) Axial ^{19}F image of a pig lung filled with a second generation liquid perfluorocarbon (PFOB). Arrows indicate the two mainstem bronchi. The lungs are homogenously filled with PFOB. Elevated signal intensity in the less dependent parts of the lung indicates higher oxygen concentration. (b) T_1 relaxation curve of PFOB following a single inversion pulse. High oxygen concentrations shorten the T_1 relaxation time. A measurement of the T_1 relaxation time of PFOB therefore leads to estimates of regional oxygen concentration. (c) Variation of regional oxygen partial pressure in the left lung. The dependent (dorsal, circles) regions demonstrate lower oxygen partial pressures than less dependent (ventral, squares) regions. [Adapted with permission from Heussel et al. (49).]

In the uppermost (nondependent layer), the regression line between P-pO$_2$ and P-etO$_2$ closely approached the line of identity. Progressively lower P-pO$_2$ values were observed in more dependent (dorsal) lung regions when compared with nondependent (ventral) regions (Fig. 16.12c). With increasing P-etO$_2$, P-pO$_2$ rose proportionally in all regions; the slope, however, became progressively flatter in the more dependent parts (49). As the amount of PFB inside the lung as well as hemodynamics and ventilation were kept constant, it can be assumed that the oxygen content extracted from the PFB phase also remained constant during the variation of P-etO$_2$ (above normoxic levels). A constant isogravitational reduction of pulmonary blood flow within the PFB-filled lung would be expected to exhibit a behavior similar to that shown in the cardiac arrest experiment of Fig. 16.7. Thus, the pattern of F_IO_2 dependency of the gravitational P-pO$_2$ gradient observed by Heussel et al. (49) is quite compatible with a significant diffusion limitation within the PFC.

Nevertheless, no direct measurement of $\dot{V}_A/\dot{Q}$ appears possible with this technique of PFC-based ^{19}F-MRI. Theoretically, an observation of the decrease of P-pO$_2$ during a breath-hold could provide an indication of regional perfusion. As an alternative, oxygen-sensitive PFC imaging may be combined with quantitative lung perfusion MRI (24) to further analyze $\dot{V}_A/\dot{Q}$ conditions.

V. Comparison of Methods

A. Helium-3 vs. Fluorine-19

When compared with hyperpolarized gas MRI of the lung, the advantage of ^{19}F MRI approaches is that no complicated, costly, and time-consuming hyperpolarization procedure is required, and that there are no biological side effects. Availability and handling of both fluorinated gases (SF$_6$) and PFC compounds is technically much less demanding and also less expensive than that of hyperpolarized ^{3}He. On the other hand, ^{19}F-containing substances are polarized only to the thermal (Boltzmann) level, which is several orders of magnitude smaller than that of hyperpolarized gases. These differences cannot be completely compensated by the number of signal averages in ^{19}F MRI. Thus, the signal-to-noise, and in particular the temporal resolution, is usually lower than that in hyperpolarized noble gas MRI. This limits the use of ^{19}F MRI in functional imaging.

Hyperpolarized ^{3}He MRI currently appears to be the most rapid MR technique for imaging the lung. Subsecond scan times can be reached (18,66–69). Moreover, it is the pO$_2$ measurement technique developed furthest and with most clinical applications until now. Besides the enormous progress made in hyperpolarized gas imaging made in recent years, it must be considered that the hyperpolarization procedure currently can be performed only by a few groups worldwide, and that the amount of total amount of ^{3}He available worldwide may be limited (although a production of 60,000 L per year for many decades should not pose a problem: J Faught, Spectra Gases, personal communication).

B. Other Nuclei

With regard to imaging of the oxygen balance in the lung, a few other techniques exist, which may have the potential to be used for quantitative analysis in the future. However, direct pO$_2$ measurements have neither been demonstrated with hyperpolarized ^{129}Xe nor with oxygen enhanced ^{1}H-MRI.

Hyperpolarized Xenon-129

^{129}Xe is another inert noble gas that can be hyperpolarized (70). When compared with ^{3}He, disadvantages of ^{129}Xe are a magnetic moment, which is <40% of the magnetic moment of ^{3}He, and that the achievable level of hyperpolarization

(30%) is currently lower than that of ^{3}He (80%). These factors limit the achievable signal-to-noise of ^{129}Xe-MRI to lower levels when compared with ^{3}He-MRI. Applications of ^{129}Xe for MRI of the lung can be found in Chapter 7. Here we will focus only on those aspects relevant for the measurement of oxygen balance.

A significant difference of ^{129}Xe to ^{3}He is its relatively high solubility in blood, tissue, and fat. After inhalation, $\sim$2% is dissolved into lung parenchyma and blood. Moreover, the chemical shift of ^{129}Xe depends strongly on its chemical environment, which makes it feasible to simultaneously observe ^{129}Xe in the gas phase and blood. Resonances of xenon in gas, fat, and tissue were observed 192, 199, and 210 ppm downfield the gas phase resonance, respectively, in rats at 2.0 T (71,72) (Fig. 16.13). *In vitro* studies of human blood samples at higher fields demonstrated resonances at 216 and 192 ppm, which were assigned to

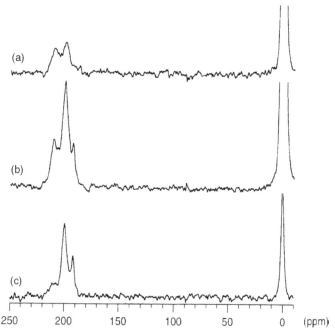

Figure 16.13 ^{129}Xe spectra obtained in rat lung (a) at the beginning, (b) during, and (c) at the end of xenon gas delivery. Signal at 0 ppm corresponds to xenon in the gas phase, resonances at 192, 199, and 210 ppm correspond to fat, tissue, and blood, respectively. (a) At the onset of xenon delivery, signals from gas, tissue, and blood are observed. The tissue component is probably caused by xenon in lung epithelium. (b) All three resonances are near equilibrium. The epithelium resonance is clearly larger than the blood and the fat resonance. (c) At the end of xenon delivery, the blood and gas signals are relatively small. The resonances in fat and tissue remain. [Reprinted with permission from Swanson et al. (72).]

xenon in red blood cells and xenon in blood plasma (71,73). It was hypothesized that differences between studies in rats and studies in humans can be explained by different red blood cell size in the two species, and by rapid exchange of xenon between the blood plasma compartment and the intracellular space of the erythrocytes (72).

Relaxation of ^{129}Xe in gas space is influenced by oxygen due to the intermolecular spin-rotation mechanism. At the oxygen concentrations of interest *in vivo*, $1/T_1$ of ^{129}Xe is proportional to the amount of oxygen, and an equation similar to Eq. (1) can be written. The proportionality constant κ at 4.7 T is $0.388(T/300)^{-0.03}$ s^{-1} amagat^{-1}, where T denotes the absolute temperature (74). Therefore, oxygen-sensitive imaging of the ^{129}Xe gas phase appears feasible but it has not yet been demonstrated.

In principle, hyperpolarized ^{129}Xe would permit the simultaneous examination of the gas and the blood phase in the lung because longitudinal relaxation of ^{129}Xe in blood is also affected by oxygen dissolved in blood (75–81). However, the results of these studies are somewhat conflicting and the proof of the feasibility of simultaneous pO_2 measurements in gas space and in blood by MRI of hyperpolarized ^{129}Xe requires study.

O_2-Sensitive ^{1}H MRI

The weak paramagnetic properties of the oxygen molecule can be used to modify the signal intensity of the lung in ^{1}H MRI (82). Despite the low signal intensity of lung parenchyma at 1.5 T, a signal increase can be measured on T_1-weighted single-shot fast spin-echo images if the oxygen-content in inspired air is increased from 21% to 100% (Fig. 16.14). Depending on the imaging parameters and the duration of the inversion delay the image contrast can be optimized. A signal increase of up to 18% can be obtained (83–85). However, to achieve sufficiently high signal changes, an oxygen flow rate of at least 15 L/min is required (86). The T_1 relaxation time of lung parenchyma is reduced due to the breathing of 100% oxygen by 9–12% (82,87), and $1/T_1$ of the lung correlates linearly with arterial oxygen partial pressure (88). Details of qualitative O_2-sensitive MRI are shown in Chapter 9.

The signal variation observed in O_2-sensitive MRI depends on a variety of factors: (i) regional ventilation, (ii) diffusion of oxygen from the alveolar space to the pulmonary capillaries, and (iii) effect of increased oxygen concentration in blood. Oxygen influences the MR signal in a lung region as soon as it enters from gas space into solid tissue and, subsequently, blood. The influence of oxygen on the MR signal from lung parenchyma is unclear. The T_1 relaxation time of blood and, hence, its signal intensity is affected not only by its oxygenation, but also by a variety of other factors such as the hematocrit (Fig. 16.15). Because of this complex situation a quantitative analysis of pulmonary pO_2 from O_2-sensitive MRI currently appears difficult.

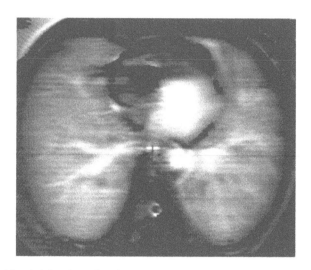

Figure 16.14 Axial subtraction image obtained in a healthy volunteer using O_2-sensitive ^{1}H MRI. The image was obtained by subtraction of two images, one obtained during breathing of 100% O_2 and the other image obtained during breathing of normal air. A marked signal can be appreciated in lung parenchyma, oxygenated lung vessels, and blood in the left ventricle of the heart.

Nevertheless, a few studies have compared O_2-sensitive MRI with the pulmonary diffusion capacity for CO (DL_{CO}), a conventional test for pulmonary function. In dynamic O_2-sensitive measurements the upslope of the ^{1}H signal was significantly smaller in patients with emphysema when compared with that observed in healthy volunteers. A linear correlation of the upslope with the DL_{CO} value was observed in these subjects (Fig. 16.16b) (89–91). Moreover, the upslope was strongly correlated with forced expiratory volume in 1 second (FEV1) (Fig. 16.16c) (88). These results may indicate that O_2-sensitive MRI is a method for assessment of transmembraneous diffusion of oxygen rather than a method for estimation of regional pO_2 in gas space or in the blood stream.

C. Specific Uses and Current Limitations

The described methods allow fascinating new insights into different aspects of the regional oxygen balance. However, inherent to all of the methods are some advantages and limitations. The ^{3}He-technique and the ^{19}F-method use gases with a low solubility. In consequence, these methods allow for a direct analysis of the gas space rather than perfusion. Information from the latter component is available only from an indirect observation of gas space, for example, from the decrease of alveolar pO_2 because of oxygen uptake in blood, that is, perfusion. O_2-sensitive MRI appears to be more sensitive to a combination of ventilation (which cannot be directly assessed with that method), transmembraneous

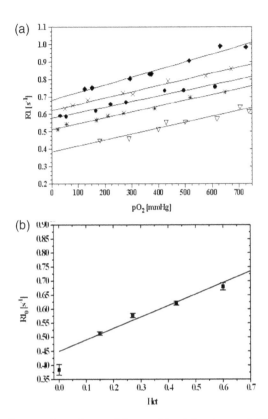

Figure 16.15 Oxygen dependence of human blood *in vitro* at 1.5 T. Human blood samples were exposed to N_2/O_2 gas mixtures of varying oxygen content. (a) Influence of oxygen concentration on the T_1 relaxation rate $1/T_1$ of blood. Symbols denote varying blood hematocrit (◆ 0.60, ×0.43, • 0.27, * 0.15, ▽ 0.00). Oxygen relaxivity in blood is strongly affected by the hematocrit (b).

diffusion of oxygen, and perfusion. [129]Xe may have the potential to quantitatively assess pO_2 both in gas space and blood. However, a variety of methodological challenges need to addressed before the latter application will become possible.

One inherent limitation of all methods relying on a substance which is measured directly (i.e., [3]He, ^{19}F in fluorinated gases or PFCs, and [129]Xe) is that the oxygen content can be assessed only in those lung regions, which are reached by the reporting substance. No information is available for regions not reached by the reporter substance. Hence, in patients with ventilation deficits, mean values over larger areas may probably always be given per ventilated area and not per lung.

The latter argumentation is particularly true for the PFC in partial ventilation. Moreover, liquid ventilation is an experimental technique not used on a routine basis and, thus, that method will almost certainly remain limited to animal studies addressing the physiologic aspects of liquid ventilation.

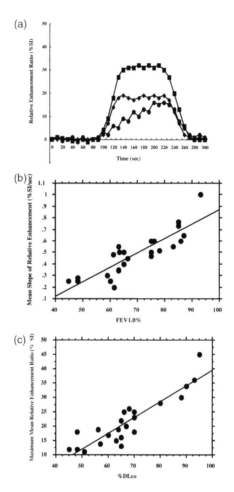

Figure 16.16 (a) Dynamic O_2-sensitive MRI in a healthy volunteer's lung (squares), in lung emphysema (diamonds), and in a lung tumor (circles). Substantial differences can be appreciated between the signal intensity–time curves of the different groups. (b) The upslope of the signal–time curve after start of 100% O_2-breathing shows a good correlation with (b) forced expiratory volume in 1 s and (c) diffusion lung capacity. [Reprinted with permission from Ohno et al. (89).]

Hyperpolarized ^{3}He is probably the most sophisticated technique, but suffers from various limitations. The complicated hyperpolarization procedure as well as the limited amount of ^{3}He available worldwide may reduce its dissemination to a wider clinical (research) community. Moreover, in hyperpolarized ^{3}He MRI, the available polarization decays within 20–30 s after inhalation. No physiologic information is available from a later time, for example, from uptake of oxygen in the blood stream.

Although rapid repetition of the RF excitation is possible in imaging of fluorinated gases, scan times are at least by one or two orders of magnitude longer in ^{19}F MRI than in [3]He MRI. Therefore, single breath-hold imaging measurement of oxygen content currently appears to be impossible with the ^{19}F gas method.

The signal variation in O_2-sensitive MRI depends on a variety of parameters such as ventilation, diffusion across the alveolar wall and lung parenchyma, and blood content. Therefore, quantitative analysis in terms of physiologic parameters like ventilation or perfusion appears difficult. However, it is currently the first MRI technique to estimate pulmonary diffusion capacity.

The O_2-sensitive technique is the only method for assessment of regional oxygen balance, which can be used on a standard clinical scanner. For all other methods described here, additional equipment is required, such as a non-proton MR-scanner, coils and pulse sequences ([3]He, ^{19}F, and [129]Xe) to complex hyperpolarization apparatus ([3]He and [129]Xe).

VI. Summary

Fascinating new methods are now available for regional assessment of pulmonary oxygen balance. Analysis of pO_2 concentrations with hyperpolarized [3]He is probably the most quantitative and most well-developed technique. [19]F MRI of alveolar oxygen content is an interesting quantitative method without the need for a hyperpolarization procedure, but its clinical feasibility still has to be demonstrated. O_2-sensitive ^{1}H MRI is the technically least demanding technique with the benefit that it can be used—in principle—on almost any clinical MR system, and it can be used to assess the pulmonary diffusion capacity semiquantitatively. [129]Xe may have, in theory, the potential for simultaneous quantification of oxygenation in both gas space and blood. However, proof of its feasibility remains to be delivered. [19]F MRI of PFCs is a new research instrument, which can be used for the development of a deeper understanding of the physiologic processes involved in liquid ventilation.

With the invention of these exciting methods, new windows into living organisms have been opened. They permit an almost noninvasive assessment of regional oxygen balance in the lung. Depending on the scientific or diagnostic issue to be answered, the appropriate tool can be selected from a range of newly developed methods. Although the results presented in this chapter are preliminary and, for some of the described methods, hypothetical, they do suggest that these methods may have the potential to become powerful research and diagnostic tools for a quantitative assessment of regional oxygen balance in the lung.

Acknowledgments

This work was supported by Deutsche Forschungsgemeinschaft DFG Grant FOR 474/1 (Eb 247/1 and Schr 687/2), Th 315/8, Th 315/11. We would like to thank Nycomed Amersham plc and Amersham Health.

References

1. Wagner PD. Ventilation, pulmonary blood flow, and ventilation–perfusion relationships. In: Fishman AP, ed. Pulmonary Diseases and Disorders. Vol. 1. New York: McGraw-Hill, 1998:177–192.
2. Riley RL, Cournand A. "Ideal" alveolar air and the analysis of ventilation–perfusion relationships in the lungs. J Appl Physiol 1949; 1:825–847.
3. Wagner PD, Laravuso RB, Uhl RR, West JB. Continuous distributions of ventilation–perfusion ratios in normal subjects breathing air and O_2. J Clin Invest 1974; 54:54–68.
4. Baumgardner JE, Choi IC, Vonk-Noordegraaf A, Frasch HF, Neufeld GR, Marshall BE. Sequential $V(A)/Q$ distributions in the normal rabbit by micropore membrane inlet mass spectrometry. J Appl Physiol 2000; 89:1699–1708.
5. West JB, Dollery CT. Distribution of blood flow and ventilation–perfusion ratio in the lung, measured with radioactive CO_2. J Appl Physiol 1960; 15:405–410.
6. Venegas JG. Noninvasive measurement of local VA, Q, and VA/Q distributions by PET. In: Hlastala MP, Robertson HT, eds. Complexity in Structure and Function of the Lung. Vol. 121. New York: Marcel Dekker Inc., New York, Basel, Hong Kong, 1998:483–508.
7. Simon BA, Tsuzaki K, Venegas JG. Changes in regional lung mechanics and ventilation distribution after unilateral pulmonary artery occlusion. J Appl Physiol 1997; 82:882–891.
8. Vidal Melo MF, Harris RS, Layfield D, Musch G, Venegas JG. Changes in regional ventilation after autologous blood clot pulmonary embolism. Anesthesiology 2002; 97:671–681.
9. Vidal Melo MF, Harris RS, Layfield D, Venegas JG. Contribution of inter- and intraregional V/Q heterogeneity to gas exchange impairment during bronchoconstriction assessed by PET. Anesthesiology 2002; 96:A1311.
10. Musch G, Layfield JD, Harris RS et al. Topographical distribution of pulmonary perfusion and ventilation, assessed by PET in supine and prone humans. J Appl Physiol 2002; 93:1841–1851.
11. Musch G, Harris RS, Vidal Melo MF, Layfield D, Venegas JG. Regional distribution of pulmonary perfusion and ventilation in bronchoconstricted asthmatics, imaged by PET. Anesthesiology 2002; 96:A-1360.
12. Vidal Melo MF, Call DM, Harris RS, Layfield JDH, Venegas JG. Mapping of regional pulmonary PaO_2, $PaCO_2$ and pH through mathematical modeling of positron emission tomography (PET) data. Anesthesiology 2000; 93:A-1339.
13. Haefeli-Bleuer B, Weibel ER. Morphometry of the human pulmonary acinus. Anat Rec 1988; 220:401–414.
14. Hoffman EA, Olson LE. Characteristics of respiratory system complexity captured via X-ray computed tomography: image acquisition, display, and analysis. In: Hlastala MP, Robertson HT, eds. Complexity in Structure and Function of the Lung. Vol. 121. New York: Marcel Dekker Inc., New York, Basel, Hong Kong, 1998:325–378.
15. Markstaller K, Eberle B, Kauczor HU et al. Temporal dynamics of lung aeration determined by dynamic CT in a porcine model of ARDS. Br J Anaesth 2001; 87:459–468.
16. Schoepf UJ, Bruening R, Konschitzky H et al. Pulmonary embolism: comprehensive diagnosis by using electron-beam CT for detection of emboli and assessment of pulmonary blood flow. Radiology 2000; 217:693–700.

17. Screaton NJ, Coxson HO, Kalloger SE et al. Detection of lung perfusion abnormalities using computed tomography in a porcine model of pulmonary embolism. J Thorac Imaging 2003; 18:14–20.

18. Schreiber WG, Weiler N, Kauczor HU et al. Ultrafast MRI of lung ventilation using hyperpolarized helium-3. Rofo Fortschr Geb Rontgenstr Neuen Bildgeb Verfahr 2000; 172:129–133.

19. Salerno M, Altes TA, Mugler JP III, Nakatsu M, Hatabu H, de Lange EE. Hyperpolarized noble gas MR imaging of the lung: potential clinical applications. Eur J Radiol 2001; 40:33–44.

20. Schreiber WG, Eberle B, Laukemper-Ostendorf S et al. Dynamic ^{19}F-MRI of pulmonary ventilation using sulfur hexafluoride (SF_6) gas. Magn Reson Med 2001; 45:605–613.

21. Schreiber WG, Markstaller K, Weiler N et al. ^{19}F-MRT of pulmonary ventilation in the breath-hold technique using SF_6 gas. Rofo Fortschr Geb Rontgenstr Neuen Bildgeb Verfahr 2000; 172:500–503.

22. Kuethe DO, Caprihan A, Fukushima E, Waggoner RA. Imaging lungs using inert fluorinated gases. Magn Reson Med 1998; 39:85–88.

23. Kuethe DO, Behr VC, Begay S. Volume of rat lungs measured throughout the respiratory cycle using ^{19}F NMR of the inert gas SF_6. Magn Reson Med 2002; 48:547–549.

24. Viallon M, Schreiber WG, Heussel CP et al. Absolute quantification of pulmonary perfusion using dynamic T1 contrast enhanced MRI: estimation of regional pulmonary blood flow (rPBF) and blood volume (rPBV). 9th Annual Meeting, Glasgow, 2001. Vol. 1. International Society for Magnetic Resonance in Medicine.

25. Hatabu H, Tadamura E, Levin DL et al. Quantitative assessment of pulmonary perfusion with dynamic contrast-enhanced MRI. Magn Reson Med 1999; 42:1033–1038.

26. Berthezene Y, Croisille P, Bertocchi M et al. Lung perfusion demonstrated by contrast-enhanced dynamic magnetic resonance imaging. Application to unilateral lung transplantation. Invest Radiol 1997; 32:351–356.

27. Lumb A. Nunn's Applied Respiratory Physiology. Oxford: Butterworth Heinemann, 2000.

28. Weibel ER. Anatomical distribution of air channels, blood vessels, and tissue in the lung. In: Arcangeli P, ed. Normal Values for Respiratory Function in Man. Milano: Panminerva Medica, 1970:242.

29. Saam B, Happer W, Middleton H. Nuclear relaxation of ^{3}He in the presence of O_2. Phys Rev 1995; A52:862–865.

30. Eberle B, Weiler N, Markstaller K et al. Analysis of intrapulmonary O_2 concentration by MR imaging of inhaled hyperpolarized helium-3. J Appl Physiol 1999; 87:2043–2052.

31. Deninger AJ, Eberle B, Ebert M et al. Quantification of regional intrapulmonary oxygen partial pressure evolution during apnea by ^{3}He MRI. J Magn Reson 1999; 141:207–216.

32. Möller HE, Hedlund LW, Chen XJ et al. Measurements of hyperpolarized gas properties in the lung. Part III: ^{3}He T(1). Magn Reson Med 2001; 45:421–430.

33. Weiler N, Eberle B, Ebert M, Grossmann T, Heil W, Kauczor H-U, Lauer LO, Markstaller K, Otten EW, Surkau R. Vorrichtung zur Applikation von Fluiden (Gasen und/oder Flüssigkeiten) oder von in einem Fluid transportierten Substanzen. PCT/EP/98/07516. Germany, UK, USA, 2000.

34. Deninger AJ, Mansson S, Petersson JS et al. Quantitative measurement of regional lung ventilation using ^{3}He MRI. Magn Reson Med 2002; 48:223–232.

35. Deninger AJ, Eberle B, Ebert M et al. ^{3}He-MRI-based measurements of intra-pulmonary p(O$_2$) and its time course during apnea in healthy volunteers: first results, reproducibility, and technical limitations. NMR Biomed 2000; 13:194–201.

36. Deninger AJ, Eberle B, Bermuth J et al. Assessment of a single-acquisition imaging sequence for oxygen-sensitive ^{3}He-MRI. Magn Reson Med 2002; 47:105–114.

37. Möller HE, Chen J, Saam B et al. MRI of the Lungs using hyperpolarized noble gases. Magn Reson Med 2002; 47:1029–1051.

38. Eberle B, Markstaller K, Stepniak A et al. ^{3}He-MRI-based assessment of regional gas exchange impairment during experimental pulmonary artery occlusion. Anesthesiology 2002; 96:A1309.

39. Fuhrman BP, Paczan PR, DeFrancisis M. Perfluorocarbon-associated gas exchange. Crit Care Med 1991; 19:712–722.

40. Mates EA, Hildebrandt J, Jackson JC, Tarczy-Hornoch P, Hlastala MP. Shunt and ventilation–perfusion distribution during partial liquid ventilation in healthy piglets. J Appl Physiol 1997; 82:933–942.

41. Kvarstein G, Mirtaheri P, Tonnesen TI. Detection of organ ischemia during hemor-rhagic shock. Acta Anaesthesiol Scand 2003; 47:675–686.

42. Saam BT, Yablonskiy DA, Kodibagkar VD et al. MR imaging of diffusion of ^{3}He gas in healthy and diseased lungs. Magn Reson Med 2000; 44:174–179.

43. Eberle B, Markstaller K, Lill J et al. Oxygen-sensitive ^{3}He magnetic resonance imaging of the lungs in patients after unilateral lung transplantation. Am J Resp Crit Care Med 2000; 161:A-718.

44. Olsson L, Magnusson P, Deninger AJ et al. Intrapulmonary pO$_2$ measured by low field MR imaging of hyperpolarized ^{3}He. Proc Intl Soc Magn Reson Med 2002; 10:2021.

45. Ciba-Geigy L. Geigy Scientific Tables. Basel: Ciba-Geigy Ltd., 1990.

46. Eberle B, Herweling A, Gast KK et al. Detection of of regional gas exchange impairment in patients with chronic thromboembolic pulmonary hypertension (CTEPH) by functional ^{3}He-MR imaging of the lung. Anesthesiology 2003; 96: (abstract).

47. Roberts D, Rizi R, Lipson DA et al. Functional nonspecificity of T$_1$-weighted MRI of laser-polarized helium-3 gas. In: Proceedings of 9th ISMRM Scientific Meeting, 2001; 946.

48. Rinck PA, Petersen SB, Lauterbur PC. NMR imaging of fluorine-containing substances. 19-Fluorine ventilation and perfusion studies. Rofo Fortschr Geb Rontgenstr Nuklearmed 1984; 140:239–243.

49. Heussel CP, Scholz A, Schmittner M et al. Measurements of alveolar pO$_2$ using ^{19}F-MRI in partial liquid ventilation. Invest Radiol 2003; 38:635–641.

50. Laukemper-Ostendorf S, Scholz A, Burger K et al. ^{19}F-MRI of perflubron for measurement of oxygen partial pressure in porcine lungs during partial liquid venti-lation. Magn Reson Med 2002; 47:82–89.

51. Thomas SR, Clark LC Jr, Ackerman JL et al. MR imaging of the lung using liquid perfluorocarbons. J Comput Assist Tomogr 1986; 10:1–9.

52. Quintel M, Heine M, Hirschl RB, Tillmanns R, Wessendorf V. Effects of partial liquid ventilation on lung injury in a model of acute respiratory failure: a histologic and morphometric analysis. Crit Care Med 1998; 26:833–843.

53. Kaisers U, Kelly KP, Busch T. Liquid ventilation. Br J Anaesth 2003; 91:143–151.
54. Greenspan JS, Wolfson MR, Rubenstein SD, Shaffer TH. Liquid ventilation of preterm baby. Lancet 1989; 4:1095.
55. Kuethe DO, Caprihan A, Gach HM, Lowe IJ, Fukushima E. Imaging obstructed ventilation with NMR using inert fluorinated gases. J Appl Physiol 2000; 88:2279–2286.
56. Mohanty S, Bernstein HJ. Fluorine relaxation by NMR absorption in gaseous CF_4, SiF_4, and SF_6. J Chem Phys 1970; 53:461–462.
57. Fenn WO, Rahn H, Otis AB. A theoretical study of the composition of alveolar air at altitude. J Appl Physiol 1946; 146:637–653.
58. Canfield RE, Rahn H. Arterial-alveolar N_2 gas pressure differences due to ventilation–perfusion variations. J Appl Physiol 1957; 10:165–172.
59. Lowe KC. Perfluorochemical respiratory gas carriers: applications in medicine and biotechnology. Sci Prog 1997; 80:169–193.
60. Croce MA, Fabian TC, Patton JHJ, Melton SM, Moore M, Trenthem LL. Partial liquid ventilation decreases the inflammatory response in the alveolar environment of trauma patients. J Trauma 1998; 45:280–282.
61. Busse LJ, Thomas SR, Pratt RG, et al. Deconvolution techniques for removing the effects of chemical shift in ^{19}F nuclear magnetic resonance imaging of perfluorocarbon compounds. Med Phys 1986; 13:518–524.
62. Samaratunga RC, Pratt RG, Zhu Y, Massoth RJ, Thomas SR. Implementation of a modified birdcage resonator for ^{19}F/^{1}H MRI at low fields (0.14 T). Med Phys 1994; 21:697–705.
63. Fishman JE, Joseph PM, Floyd TF, Mukherji B, Sloviter HA. Oxygen-sensitive ^{19}F NMR imaging of the vascular system *in vivo*. Magn Reson Imaging 1987; 5:279–285.
64. Fishman JE, Joseph PM, Carvlin MJ, Saadi-Elmandjra M, Mukherji B, Sloviter HA. *In vivo* measurements of vascular oxygen tension in tumors using MRI of a fluorinated blood substitute. Invest Radiol 1989; 24:65–71.
65. Pratt RG, Zheng J, Stewart BK et al. Application of a 3D volume ^{19}F MR imaging protocol for mapping oxygen tension (pO_2) in perfluorocarbons at low field. Magn Reson Med 1997; 37:307–313.
66. Wild JM, Paley MN, Kasuboski L et al. Dynamic radial projection MRI of inhaled hyperpolarized [3]He gas. Magn Reson Med 2003; 49:991–997.
67. Salerno M, Altes TA, Brookeman JR, de Lange EE, Mugler JP III. Dynamic spiral MRI of pulmonary gas flow using hyperpolarized [3]He: preliminary studies in healthy and diseased lungs. Magn Reson Med 2001; 46:667–677.
68. Gierada DS, Saam B, Yablonskiy D, Cooper JD, Lefrak SS, Conradi MS. Dynamic echo planar MR imaging of lung ventilation with hyperpolarized [3]He in normal subjects and patients with severe emphysema. NMR Biomed 2000; 13:176–181.
69. Saam B, Yablonskiy DA, Gierada DS, Conradi MS. Rapid imaging of hyperpolarized gas using EPI. Magn Reson Med 1999; 42:507–514.
70. Albert MS, Cates GD, Driehuys B et al. Biological magnetic resonance imaging using laser-polarized [129]Xe. Nature 1994; 370:199–201.
71. Albert MS, Schepkin VD, Budinger TF. Measurement of [129]Xe T1 in blood to explore the feasibility of hyperpolarized [129]Xe MRI. J Comput Assist Tomogr 1995; 19:975–978.

72. Swanson SD, Rosen MS, Coulter KP, Welsh RC, Chupp TE. Distribution and dynamics of laser-polarized [129]Xe magnetization *in vivo*. Magn Reson Med 1999; 42:1137–1145.

73. Bifone A, Song YQ, Seydoux R et al. NMR of laser-polarized xenon in human blood. Proc Natl Acad Sci USA 1996; 93:12932–12936.

74. Jameson C, Jameson AK, Hwang JK. Nuclear spin relaxation by intermolecular dipol coupling in the gas phase. J Chem Phys 1988; 89:4074–4081.

75. Tseng CH, Peled S, Nascimben L, Oteiza E, Walsworth RL, Jolesz FA. NMR of laser-polarized [129]Xe in blood foam. J Magn Reson 1997; 126:79–86.

76. Sakai K, Bilek AM, Oteiza E et al. Temporal dynamics of hyperpolarized [129]Xe resonances in living rats. J Magn Reson B 1996; 111:300–304.

77. Wolber J, Cherubini A, Dzik-Jurasz AS, Leach MO, Bifone A. Spin-lattice relaxation of laser-polarized xenon in human blood. Proc Natl Acad Sci USA 1999; 96:3664–3669.

78. Albert MS, Kacher DF, Balamore D, Venkatesh AK, Jolesz FA. T_1 of [129]Xe in blood and the role of oxygenation. J Magn Reson 1999; 140:264–273.

79. Albert MS, Balamore D, Kacher DF, Venkatesh AK, Jolesz FA. Hyperpolarized [129]Xe T_1 in oxygenated and deoxygenated blood. NMR Biomed 2000; 13:407–414.

80. Wolber J, Cherubini A, Leach MO, Bifone A. On the oxygenation-dependent [129]Xe T_1 in blood. NMR Biomed 2000; 13:234–237.

81. Wolber J, Cherubini A, Leach MO, Bifone A. Hyperpolarized [129]Xe NMR as a probe for blood oxygenation. Magn Reson Med 2000; 43:491–496.

82. Edelman RR, Hatabu H, Tadamura E, Li W, Prasad PV. Noninvasive assessment of regional ventilation in the human lung using oxygen-enhanced magnetic resonance imaging. Nat Med 1996; 2:1236–1239.

83. McAdams HP, Hatabu H, Donnelly LF, Chen Q, Tadamura E, MacFall JR. Novel techniques for MR imaging of pulmonary airspaces. Magn Reson Imaging Clin N Am 2000; 8:205–219.

84. Chen Q, Jakob PM, Griswold MA, Levin DL, Hatabu H, Edelman RR. Oxygen enhanced MR ventilation imaging of the lung. Magma 1998; 7:153–161.

85. Ohno Y, Chen Q, Hatabu H. Oxygen-enhanced magnetic resonance ventilation imaging of lung. Eur J Radiol 2001; 37:164–171.

86. Mai VM, Liu B, Li W et al. Influence of oxygen flow rate on signal and T_1 changes in oxygen-enhanced ventilation imaging. J Magn Reson Imaging 2002; 16:37–41.

87. Löffler R, Muller CJ, Peller M et al. Optimization and evaluation of the signal intensity change in multisection oxygen-enhanced MR lung imaging. Magn Reson Med 2000; 43:860–866.

88. Hatabu H, Tadamura E, Chen Q et al. Pulmonary ventilation: dynamic MRI with inhalation of molecular oxygen. Eur J Radiol 2001; 37:172–178.

89. Ohno Y, Hatabu H, Takenaka D, Adachi S, Van Cauteren M, Sugimura K. Oxygen-enhanced MR ventilation imaging of the lung: preliminary clinical experience in 25 subjects. AJR Am J Roentgenol 2001; 177:185–194.

90. Ohno Y, Hatabu H, Takenaka D, Van Cauteren M, Fujii M, Sugimura K. Dynamic oxygen-enhanced MRI reflects diffusing capacity of the lung. Magn Reson Med 2002; 47:1139–1144.

91. Müller CJ, Schwaiblmair M, Scheidler J, et al. Pulmonary diffusing capacity: assessment with oxygen-enhanced lung MR imaging preliminary findings. Radiology 2002; 222:499–506.

Part IV: Nuclear Medicine

17

PET Imaging of Infection and Inflammatory Lung Disease

HONGMING ZHUANG, JUSTIN W. KUNG, and ABASS ALAVI

Hospital of the University of Pennsylvania,
Philadelphia, Pennsylvania, USA

I. Imaging in Infectious and Inflammatory Lung Disease

Diagnostic imaging plays a prominent role in the management of infectious and inflammatory pulmonary processes as the detection and localization of disease is important when initiating therapy. Imaging modalities provide insight into disease progression as well as response to therapy. For example, chest radiography is commonly used in the diagnostic evaluation of patients with sarcoidosis, pulmonary tuberculosis, and pneumonia. Computed tomography (CT) is beneficial in patients with atypical findings. Despite improvements in the resolution of these techniques, many disorders still go unnoticed for extended periods of time and some may never manifest as detectable abnormalities using these modalities until the irreversible anatomical damages have been formed.

Imaging techniques relying on functional changes rather than on structural changes may detect disease at earlier stages. Nuclear medicine procedures offer advantages in that they can both localize and quantify diseases on the basis of metabolic activity. Traditionally, 67-Gallium citrate-, 111-Indium-, or 99m-Technetium-labeled leukocyte scans have been used to evaluate lung infection. Recent attention has focused on the potential of positron emission tomography (PET) for imaging inflammatory/infectious lung diseases. Its utility in this area was brought to light because of the large number of false-positive cases seen during the evaluation of malignancies. What was originally believed to be a potential disadvantage has been exploited in a number of recent studies, resulting in a profound interest for the use of PET in the imaging of inflammatory/infectious conditions.

II. Background of 18-Fluorodeoxyglucose Imaging

18-Fluorodeoxyglucose (FDG) is a glucose analog and the most commonly used diagnostic tracer in PET. This radiopharmaceutical is transported across the cell membrane by the glucose transporters (GLUT). Like glucose, FDG is phosphorylated by hexokinase to FDG-6-phosphate. However, unlike glucose-6-phosphate, FDG-6-phosphate is not a substrate for glucose-6-phosphate dehydrogenase, preventing progression down the glycolytic pathway. Therefore, deoxyglucose-6-phosphate and its derivatives are trapped in tissues long enough to allow imaging with modern PET instruments.

III. FDG-PET Imaging in Infection and Inflammation

There have been multiple reports in the literature of incidental findings of increased FDG uptake in inflammatory and infectious processes when FDG-PET was utilized in the evaluation of a variety of malignancies. FDG accumulation has been noted in a variety of infectious and inflammatory disorders (Table 17.1) (1–31).

These incidental findings of increased FDG uptake by active inflammatory cells have been validated experimentally. Resting inflammatory cells typically

Table 17.1 18-FDG Uptake in Infectious and Inflammatory Processes (Nonmalignant)

Infectious processes	Inflammatory processes
Abdominal abscess (1)	Inflammatory pancreatic disease (20)
Lung abscess (3)	Asthma (25)
Lobar pneumonia (5,6)	Myositis (27)
Tuberculosis (11–13)	Sclerosing mediastinitis (29)
Mastitis (15)	Gastritis (31)
Dental infection (18)	Sarcoidosis (21–24)
Brain abscess (2)	Sinusitis (26)
Renal abscess (4)	Thyroiditis (28)
Osteomyelitis (7–10)	Deep venous thrombosis (30)
Mycobacterium avium-intracellulare infection (14)	
Acute enterocolitis (16,17)	
Infectious mononucleosis (19)	

demonstrate low levels of FDG uptake. However, glucose metabolic activity increases dramatically on stimulation. In a mouse skin transplantation model, FDG uptake was 1.5–2.0 times higher in allografts than in syngeneic grafts and the increase in uptake correlated with the levels of T-cell infiltrate seen histologically (32). In the examination of patients with acute lobar pneumonia, microautoradiography of lavage fluid demonstrated FDG activity localized to >90% of the neutrophils (5). Interestingly, inflammatory cells have been found to contribute to the "tumor" FDG uptake seen in malignancy. Microautoradiography demonstrated that the newly formed granulation tissue around the tumor and corresponding high concentration of macrophages showed a higher uptake of FDG than the viable tumor cells (32).

There are several possible mechanisms for inflammatory cells to increase glucose uptake. Inflammatory cells are known to increase the expression of GLUT when they are activated (33–35). In addition, the affinity of GLUT in inflammatory cells for deoxyglucose has been shown to increase upon exposure to multiple cytokines and growth factors and may also involve both tyrosine kinases and protein kinase C activity (36). Therefore, activated inflammatory cells have enhanced ability to transport FDG into the cells. As most findings of increased FDG uptake at sites of infection and inflammation have been incidental, this may prove to be a powerful approach to the diagnosis and management of patients with these disorders.

IV. PET Advantages over Traditional Nuclear Medicine Techniques in the Evaluation of Lung Infection and Inflammation

Currently, leukocyte imaging is the most commonly used nuclear medicine imaging modality for the detection of lung infection. However, there are limitations to leukocyte imaging. Labeled leukocyte imaging is limited in that only inflammatory/infectious processes that attract predominantly neutrophils are likely to have a positive result. In chronic inflammatory/infectious lesions, lymphocytes, monocytes, or both are the dominant inflammatory cells attracted to sites of acute infection. Therefore, the labeled leukocyte method does not detect lymphocyte-dominant infection (e.g., tuberculosis) and inflammation (e.g., sarcoidosis), whereas both pathologies can be effectively detected by FDG-PET (12,13,21,22). The detection of infection by the labeled leukocyte method also depends on the migration of neutrophils to the infected site. Therefore, when chemotactic signals are reduced (e.g., following antibiotic therapy), the labeled leukocyte method may be ineffective. FDG-PET offers a significant theoretical advantage in that the signal reflects a postmigratory neutrophil event (5) and, probably, the respiratory burst. Thus, PET may prove to be a non-invasive approach to the *in vivo* study of neutrophil activity at otherwise-inaccessible sites. 67-Gallium citrate has been used in some pulmonary diseases, including inflammation without significant neutrophils, such as sarcoidosis. However, its sensitivity is significantly lower than FDG-PET in this setting. In addition, the gallium uptake does not correlate well with other indices of disease activity and is presently not generally recommended or used as part of the routine evaluation in patients suspected of having sarcoidosis.

V. Potential Clinical Applications

While PET is not currently widely used for the detection of inflammatory or infectious processes, recently published studies highlight its great potential in the evaluation of pulmonary inflammatory or infectious processes.

A. Sarcoidosis

Sarcoidosis is a disease of unknown origin characterized by the formation of non-caseating granulomas. The pulmonary, mediastinal, and hilar lymph nodes are the most common sites of involvement, but sarcoidosis is regarded as a systemic disorder that can affect virtually any organ in the body. As the etiology of sarcoidosis is unknown, it is suggested that immune mechanisms are important in the disease pathogenesis. The disease affects the young, with a peak incidence in the 20s and 30s. Women are affected more often than men. In the United States, blacks are affected more frequently than whites. The natural history of the disease is variable. If untreated, most patients will have a self-limited course; however, sarcoidosis may progress and is associated with a mortality rate of ~5%. Because of this, proper initiation of therapy is important. However, owing to the variable natural history of the disease, initiating therapy is difficult. Assessment of the functional status of the involved organ can provide a general framework for monitoring the natural history of the disease. Chest radiography, serum angiotensin-converting enzyme levels, gallium scanning, bronchoalveolar lavage, and pulmonary function tests are used for this purpose but do not give an indication of the inflammatory activity of the disease. Conventional X-ray or CT will detect structural lung changes over a period of time and can thus detect progressive disease. 67-Gallium imaging is currently the most frequently used nuclear medicine technique in the evaluation of sarcoidosis (37–41). However, Gallium scan has limited sensitivity and specificity. Somatostatin receptor scintigraphy has also been proposed to be useful in the assessment of patients with sarcoidosis (42,43). However, the utility of somatostatin receptor imaging in the setting of sarcoidosis has not been widely accepted.

FDG uptake in sarcoidosis was first observed incidentally during the evaluation of lymphoma (21). The typical "lambda sign" (bihilar and mediastinal lymphadenopathy) on gallium scan is usually better imaged on FDG-PET study (Fig. 17.1). It has since been reported to be easily confused with malignancy (23,44,45). FDG uptake levels may reflect disease activity (22). Interestingly, PET is also able to detect recurrent sarcoidosis in transplanted lungs (46). FDG-PET's utility may lie in its ability to monitor disease activity (Fig. 17.2). Although FDG-PET has higher sensitivity than Gallium scan in the evaluation of patients with sarcoidosis (Fig. 17.3), it is unlikely at this moment to play a major role in the initial diagnosis of sarcoidosis. Instead, PET might provide prognostic value. Carbon-11-labeled methionine (Met) has been proven to be an infection/inflammation seeking agent in patients with brain abscess (47). Yamada et al. examined 31 patients with pulmonary sarcoidosis with both FDG and Met as PET tracers. Patients were divided into an FDG-dominant group and a Met-dominant group on the basis of the FDG/Met uptake ratio in

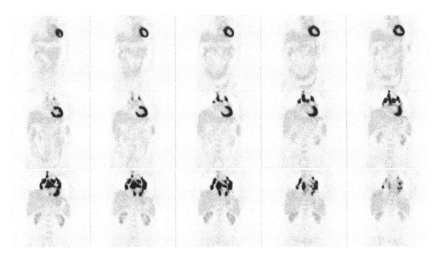

Figure 17.1 Attenuation-corrected FDG-PET images of a 36-year-old male patient with sarcoidosis. The disease activity in both hilar regions of the lung and mediastinum is clearly visualized.

the sarcoid lesions. The authors found that the rate of improvement assessed by clinical status and chest radiographs was considerably higher in the FDG-dominant group (78%) than in the Met-dominant group (33%) (24).

As both sarcoid lesions and malignant lesions can have significant FDG uptake, it can be challenging to interpret the PET images when both these lesions might exist (21–24). However, to evaluate sarcoidosis and malignancy, Oriuchi et al. (48) compared the uptake of ^{18}F-fluoro-a-methyl-tyrosine (FMT) and FDG in patients with sarcoidosis and lung cancer. While both processes

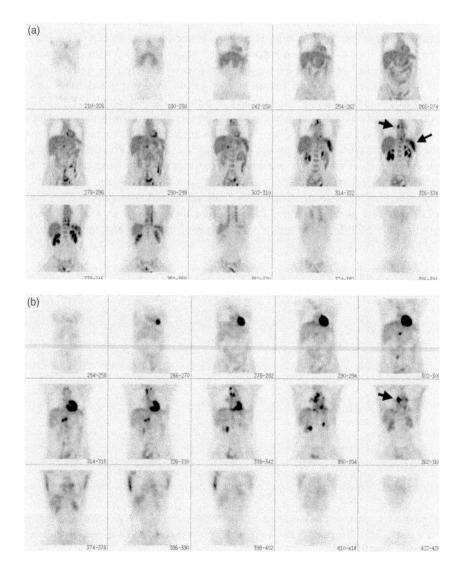

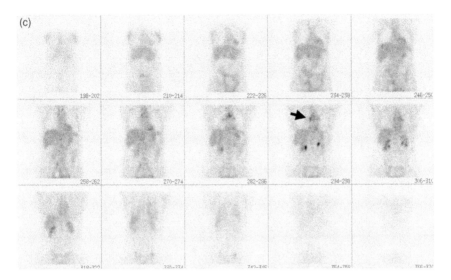

Figure 17.2 *Continued.*

increased the accumulation of FDG, only malignant processes have increased FMT metabolism. The use of this tracer following FDG-PET in patients suspected of having sarcoidosis may provide a means of distinguishing malignancy from sarcoidosis.

B. Chronic Granulomatous Disease

Chronic granulomatous disease (CGD) is a rare hereditary immunodeficiency disorder characterized by the absence or malfunction of phagocytes. The onset

---

Figure 17.2 A 47-year-old female patient presented with dry cough, fatigue, weakness, fever, and weight loss, shortness of breath, and mild chest discomfort. Chest X-ray and CT were unremarkable. However, possible splenic lesions were identified by CT scan. FDG-PET was acquired to evaluate possible tumor of unknown origin. (a) Initial PET images revealed significant abnormal activity in the spleen (long arrow), mediastinum (short arrow), and upper abdomen. As no biopsy was performed at the time of the initial PET imaging, a malignant process was not excluded. In fact, non-Hodgkin's lymphoma was considered. The patient subsequently underwent splenectomy. Pathological examination revealed sarcoidosis. The patient then received her second FDG-PET scan (b) to evaluate residual disease activity before further treatment. The images showed no abnormal activity in the region of the spleen, consistent with the history of splenectomy. However, the abnormal activity in the mediastinum (arrow) and upper abdomen became more prominent. Corticosteroid therapy was initiated and a follow-up PET scan (c) demonstrated a total resolution of the lesion in the upper abdomen and a significant deduction of disease activity in the mediastinum (arrow).

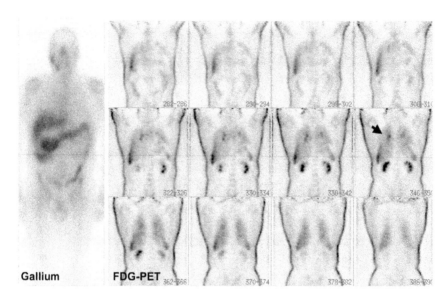

Figure 17.3   A 47-year-old patient with biopsy proven pulmonary sarcoidosis. Follow-ing the therapy, a gallium study was performed to evaluate the disease activity. The images of the gallium scan were essentially normal. However, a concurrent FDG-PET study (non-attenuation-corrected images) demonstrated increased activity in both hilar regions, consistent with residual disease activity (arrow).

of clinical signs and symptoms begins early. Pneumonias, lymphadenitis, and skin infections are most commonly encountered; however, the sequelae of chronic infections are large. Treatment involves antimicrobial activity. In patients with severe recurrent infections, autologous bone marrow transplantation is sometimes indicated. However, transplantation cannot be performed if there is active infection. Although traditional imaging modalities like CT are sensitive for detection of infectious foci, they cannot distinguish active disease from quiescent disease. Gungor et al. (49) investigated the ability of FDG-PET to distinguish between active and quiescent infective lesions in children with CGD. Five children with CGD and signs of infection of unknown origin were examined. FDG-PET imaging was able to detect 102 confirmed lesions, 53 more than what is detected on CT imaging alone. In addition, 20 lesions suspected as active on CT imaging were excluded by FDG-PET.

C.   Cystic Fibrosis

Cystic fibrosis (CF) is an autosomal recessive disease caused by mutations in the CF transmembrane conductance regulator (CFTR) gene on chromosome 7. The disease affects multiple organs; however, the majority of morbidity arises from recurrent pulmonary infections and the development of bronchiectasis. A chronic neutrophil-dominated inflammatory process has been implicated in the destruction of the lung in CF (50). Neutrophils produce and release cytotoxic enzymes and toxic oxygen metabolites that contribute to pulmonary destruction. Monitoring inflammation through WBCs, bronchoalveolar lavage, sputum, and lung biopsy cannot localize regional variations of inflammation. FDG-PET should theoretically be able to determine the degree of lung inflammation and the progression of disease and assess local tissue response to antibiotics and other therapies. Labiris et al. (51) studied FDG-PET for this purpose in 10 adult CF patients. Seven patients were found to have sputum at a normal or slightly depressed glucose utilization rate (mean 1.3 μmol/g h). The authors concluded that despite high-sputum neutrophil levels, lung glucose utilization was not elevated in patients with CF. Similar findings were reported by Jones et al. (5), who examined neutrophil activity by PET in bronchiectasis. It is possible that the findings of Labiris and Jones can be explained by impaired neutrophil activation in patients with CF and bronchiectasis. *Pseudomonas* is known to chronically infect CF patients. It is a well-known cause of morbidity and mortality in patients with CF and is associated with chronic neutrophilic inflammation. *Pseudomonas* produces hemolytic phospholipase-C (PLC) molecules. Hemolytic PLC has been demonstrated to potently suppress the neutrophil respiratory burst response to bacteria (52) which would inhibit glucose uptake. However, contrary to this theory, Schuster et al. (53) reported imaging of lung inflammation in a murine model of *Pseudomonas* infection using FDG-PET. Lung uptake of FDG correlated significantly with the dose of bacteria instilled in mice infected with the M57-15 strain of *Pseudomonas*. The role of PET in imaging patients with CF and bronchiectasis still needs to be defined.

D. Asthma and Chronic Obstructive Pulmonary Disease

Asthma and chronic obstructive pulmonary disease (COPD) are both chronic pulmonary diseases that affect a significant portion of the population in the United States. Both are thought to have an inflammatory component as part of their underlying pathophysiology. Monitoring disease progression *in vivo* may play an important role in designing and studying therapeutic interventions. Current techniques including lung biopsy, chest radiographs, lavage, and high-resolution CT all have limitations. PET may prove useful in imaging the inflammatory component of the disease. A group of 9 men with atopic asthma were studied to determine the ability of FDG-PET to detect airway inflammation in asthma (25). Five were challenged by segmentally administering allergen. In the remaining 4 patients, aerosolized allergen was administered. There was a four-fold increase in FDG uptake in patients who had allergen segmentally administered. Aerosolized administration of allergen did not significantly increase FDG uptake. This study was the first to demonstrate that local allergen-invoked inflammation can be visualized with FDG. Recently, a study by Jones et al. (54) examined the ability of FDG and the radiotracer ^{11}C-labeled

PK11195 to detect inflammation in both COPD and asthma. The mean slope of FDG uptake was higher in COPD (4.0 vs. 1.5 min^{-1}) patients compared with control subjects. Surprisingly, uptake of FDG in asthmatics (1.7 min^{-1}) did not demonstrate a dramatic increase. Mean ^{11}C-labeled PK11195 uptake (plateau tissue/plasma) was higher in four out of six COPD patients (10.8) and three out of five asthmatics (11.8) than the maximum value in control subjects. Further studies will help to demonstrate the applicability of PET in providing indices of disease activity for future therapeutic studies.

E. Silicosis

Occupational pneumoconiosis presents significant health risks to workers in certain occupations, for example, surface mining, and has contributed to 3000 deaths in the United States in 1996 (55). Even in the initial stages of disease, when pulmonary fibrosis is not clinically evident, excess collagen is found in the parenchymal wall. *Cis*-4-fluoro-L-proline (FP) is a proline analog, which can be incorporated into collagen. In a recent study, a rabbit silicosis model was examined to test for the potential use of 18F-FP for the detection of pulmonary fibrosis. The authors showed that 95% of animals with elevated PET scores had evidence of fibrosis (18/19 rabbits). Localization of activity to specific lung areas was less specific. These results suggest that PET imaging with this tracer has the potential sensitivity to detect active fibrosis in silicosis.

VI. Monitoring Disease Processes and Response to Therapy

The ability of PET to quantify the amount of FDG uptake through standardized uptake value (SUV) allows monitoring of the disease process. This may be especially helpful in determining the efficacy of therapy. PET imaging has been used to monitor the course of disease following treatment of aspergillosis (56,57). Similarly, 12 patients with alveolar echinococcosis were monitored with FDG-PET before and after chemotherapy. Three of eight patients with metabolically active lesions demonstrated clear improvement on PET (58). Finally, O'Doherty et al. (59) reported that following effective treatment of *Mycobacterium avium-intracellulare* infection, there is reduction in FDG uptake by the lesions.

VII. Differentiating Between Malignant and Inflammatory Processes

One potential pitfall in the use of FDG-PET for detecting inflammatory and infectious lung diseases is the difficulty in distinguishing between inflammation and malignancy. Inflammatory lesions are known to cause false-positive PET results in patients suspected of harboring cancer. There is a report in the literature describing bone metastasis that was mistakenly interpreted to represent acute osteomyelitis (60). Distinguishing between malignancy and inflammation is obviously of great importance in the management and prognosis of a patient.

Dual-time point PET imaging and delayed PET imaging have been suggested as a possible method of making this distinction. Traditionally, a threshold SUV of between 2.5 and 3.8 (11,61) has been used to distinguish malignancy from inflammation. This presents problems, however, as there is a wide range of FDG uptake among malignant lesions. Non-small cell lung carcinoma has an average SUV of 8, whereas the average SUV for breast cancer is only 3 (62). Because of the potential for overlap, using a concrete threshold value can lead to false-positives. Instead, it has been reported that FDG uptake in tumor and inflammatory cells differs over time. In a turpentine-induced inflammation rat model, uptake of FDG in inflammatory tissue peaked at 60 min after injection and then decreased gradually. The results of several studies demonstrate that tumors generally behave differently. Nakamoto et al. (63) obtained SUV at 60 and 120 min after FDG injection and showed that the SUV in 23 of 31 malignant lesions increased over time, whereas the SUV in 12 of 13 benign lesions decreased over time. Kubota et al. (64) noted similar increases in FDG uptake at 1 and 2 h. Herzog et al. (65) found a 180% increase in SUV between 90 and 180 min in patients with breast cancer. In a recent investigation involving 80 patients with lung nodule on chest CT, both early 1 h and delayed 3 h FDG-PET images were acquired and the findings were correlated with histopathological examinations. The results demonstrated that all malignant lesions showed higher SUV levels at 3 h than at 1 h, and benign lesions revealed the opposite results (66). The different behavior of FDG uptake by malignant and benign lesions has been attributed to dephosphorylation of FDG-6-phosphate (67). These differences can explain why dual-time point PET imaging or delayed PET imaging may play a role in the distinction between malignant and benign lesions. However, because malignant cells do not uniformly increase FDG uptake over time and benign cells do not uniformly decrease FDG uptake over time, further investigation is needed to determine the efficacy of this promising technique.

VIII. Conclusions

PET imaging as a functional imaging modality appears to hold great promise for the diagnosis and management of a number of pulmonary inflammatory and infectious disorders. PET offers unique information because of its reliance on functional changes rather than structural changes. Thus, it may detect the early stages of pulmonary disease and allow prompt therapeutic intervention. FDG is currently the tracer of choice in PET and will likely remain so for the near future. However, other compounds such as ^{11}C-labeled Met and 18F-FP may eventually be widely used. Finally, advances in the field may broaden its future indications.

References

1. Tahara T, Ichiya Y, Kuwabara Y et al. High [18F]-fluorodeoxyglucose uptake in abdominal abscesses: a PET study. J Comput Assist Tomogr 1989; 13:829–831.
2. Meyer MA, Frey KA, Schwaiger M. Discordance between F-18 fluorodeoxyglucose uptake and contrast enhancement in a brain abscess. Clin Nucl Med 1993; 18:682–684.
3. Yen RF, Chen ML, Liu FY et al. False-positive 2-[F-18]-fluoro-2-deoxy-D-glucose positron emission tomography studies for evaluation of focal pulmonary abnormalities. J Formos Med Assoc 1998; 97:642–645.
4. Kaya Z, Kotzerke J, Keller F. FDG PET diagnosis of septic kidney in a renal transplant patient. Transpl Int 1999; 12:156.
5. Jones HA, Sriskandan S, Peters AM et al. Dissociation of neutrophil emigration and metabolic activity in lobar pneumonia and bronchiectasis. Eur Respir J 1997; 10:795–803.
6. Kapucu LO, Meltzer CC, Townsend DW, Keenan RJ, Luketich JD. Fluorine-18-fluorodeoxyglucose uptake in pneumonia. J Nucl Med 1998; 39:1267–1269.
7. Sugawara Y, Braun DK, Kison PV, Russo JE, Zasadny KR, Wahl RL. Rapid detection of human infections with fluorine-18 fluorodeoxyglucose and positron emission tomography: preliminary results. Eur J Nucl Med 1998; 25:1238–1243.
8. Guhlmann A, Brecht-Krauss D, Suger G et al. Chronic osteomyelitis: detection with FDG PET and correlation with histopathologic findings. Radiology 1998; 206:749–754.
9. Guhlmann A, Brecht-Krauss D, Suger G et al. Fluorine-18-FDG PET and technetium-99m antigranulocyte antibody scintigraphy in chronic osteomyelitis. J Nucl Med 1998; 39:2145–2152.
10. Zhuang H, Duarte PS, Pourdehand M, Shnier D, Alavi A. Exclusion of chronic osteomyelitis with F-18 fluorodeoxyglucose positron emission tomographic imaging. Clin Nucl Med 2000; 25:281–284.
11. Patz EF Jr, Lowe VJ, Hoffman JM et al. Focal pulmonary abnormalities: evaluation with F-18 fluorodeoxyglucose PET scanning. Radiology 1993; 188:487–490.
12. Bakheet SM, Powe J, Ezzat A, Rostom A. F-18-FDG uptake in tuberculosis. Clin Nucl Med 1998; 23:739–742.
13. Goo JM, Im JG, Do KH et al. Pulmonary tuberculoma evaluated by means of FDG PET: findings in 10 cases. Radiology 2000; 216:117–121.
14. Zhuang H, Pourdehnad M, Yamamoto AJ, Rossman MD, Alavi A. Intense F-18 fluorodeoxyglucose uptake caused by mycobacterium avium intracellulare infection. Clin Nucl Med 2001; 26:458.
15. Bakheet SM, Powe J, Kandil A, Ezzat A, Rostom A, Amartey J. F-18 FDG uptake in breast infection and inflammation. Clin Nucl Med 2000; 25:100–103.
16. Hannah A, Scott AM, Akhurst T, Berlangieri S, Bishop J, McKay WJ. Abnormal colonic accumulation of fluorine-18-FDG in pseudomembranous colitis. J Nucl Med 1996; 37:1683–1685.

17. Meyer MA. Diffusely increased colonic F-18 FDG uptake in acute enterocolitis. Clin Nucl Med 1995; 20:434–435.
18. Kao CH. Incidental findings of FDG uptake in dental caries. Clin Nucl Med 2003; 28:610.
19. Tomas MB, Tronco GG, Karayalcin G, Palestro CJ. FDG uptake in infectious mononucleosis. Clin Positron Imaging 2000; 3:176.
20. Shreve PD. Focal fluorine-18 fluorodeoxyglucose accumulation in inflammatory pancreatic disease. Eur J Nucl Med 1998; 25:259–264.
21. Lewis PJ, Salama A. Uptake of fluorine-18-fluorodeoxyglucose in sarcoidosis. J Nucl Med 1994; 35:1647–1649.
22. Brudin LH, Valind SO, Rhodes CG et al. Fluorine-18 deoxyglucose uptake in sarcoidosis measured with positron emission tomography. Eur J Nucl Med 1994; 21:297–305.
23. Cook GJ, Fogelman I, Maisey MN. Normal physiological and benign pathological variants of 18-fluoro-2-deoxyglucose positron-emission tomography scanning: potential for error in interpretation. Semin Nucl Med 1996; 26:308–314.
24. Yamada Y, Uchida Y, Tatsumi K et al. Fluorine-18-fluorodeoxyglucose and carbon-11-methionine evaluation of lymphadenopathy in sarcoidosis. J Nucl Med 1998; 39:1160–1166.
25. Taylor IK, Hill AA, Hayes M et al. Imaging allergen-invoked airway inflammation in atopic asthma with [18F]-fluorodeoxyglucose and positron emission tomography. Lancet 1996; 347:937–940.
26. Yasuda S, Fujii H, Takahashi W, Takagi S, Ide M, Shohtsu A. Elevated F-18 FDG uptake in the psoas muscle. Clin Nucl Med 1998; 23:716–717.
27. Gysen M, Stroobants S, Mortelmans L. Proliferative myositis: a case of a pseudo-malignant process. Clin Nucl Med 1998; 23:836–838.
28. Yasuda S, Shohsu A, Ide M, Takagi S, Suzuki Y, Tajima T. Diffuse F-18 FDG uptake in chronic thyroiditis. Clin Nucl Med 1997; 22:341.
29. Imran MB, Kubota K, Yoshioka S et al. Sclerosing mediastinitis: findings on fluorine-18 fluorodeoxyglucose positron emission tomography. Clin Nucl Med 1999; 24:305–308.
30. Chang KJ, Zhuang H, Alavi A. Detection of chronic recurrent lower extremity deep venous thrombosis on fluorine-18 fluorodeoxyglucose positron emission tomography. Clin Nucl Med 2000; 25:838–839.
31. Nunez RF, Yeung HW, Macapinlac H. Increased F-18 FDG uptake in the stomach. Clin Nucl Med 1999; 24:281–282.
32. Kubota R, Yamada S, Kubota K, Ishiwata K, Tamahashi N, Ido T. Intratumoral distribution of fluorine-18-fluorodeoxyglucose *in vivo*: high accumulation in macrophages and granulation tissues studied by microautoradiography. J Nucl Med 1992; 33:1972–1980.
33. Chakrabarti R, Jung CY, Lee TP, Liu H, Mookerjee BK. Changes in glucose transport and transporter isoforms during the activation of human peripheral blood lymphocytes by phytohemagglutinin. J Immunol 1994; 152:2660–2668.
34. Gamelli RL, Liu H, He LK, Hofmann CA. Augmentations of glucose uptake and glucose transporter-1 in macrophages following thermal injury and sepsis in mice. J Leukoc Biol 1996; 59:639–647.
35. Sorbara LR, Maldarelli F, Chamoun G et al. Human immunodeficiency virus type 1 infection of H9 cells induces increased glucose transporter expression. J Virol 1996; 70:7275–7279.

36. Ahmed N, Kansara M, Berridge MV. Acute regulation of glucose transport in a monocyte-macrophage cell line: Glut-3 affinity for glucose is enhanced during the respiratory burst. Biochem J 1997; 327(Pt 2):369–375.

37. Savolaine ER, Schlembach PJ. Gallium scan diagnosis of sarcoidosis in the presence of equivocal radiographic and Ct findings—value of lacrimal gland biopsy. Clin Nucl Med 1990; 15:198–199.

38. Israel HL, Albertine KH, Park CH, Patrick H. Whole-body Ga-67 scans—role in diagnosis of sarcoidosis. Am Rev Respir Disease 1991; 144:1182–1186.

39. Myslivecek M, Husak V, Kolek V, Budikova M, Koranda P. Absolute quantitation of Ga-67-citrate accumulation in the lungs and its importance for the evaluation of disease—activity in pulmonary sarcoidosis. Eur J Nucl Med 1992; 19:1016–1022.

40. Sulavik SB, Spencer RP, Palestro CJ, Swyer AJ, Teirstein AS, Goldsmith SJ. Specificity and sensitivity of distinctive chest radiographic and or Ga-67 images in the noninvasive diagnosis of sarcoidosis. Chest 1993; 103:403–409.

41. Bradvik I, Wollmer P, Evander E et al. Lung function and disease activity in sarcoidosis—disease activity in sarcoidosis. ACP—Appl Cardiopulm Pathophysiol 1996; 6:61–70.

42. Lebtahi R, Crestani B, Daou D et al. Detection of mediastinal and lung lesions of sarcoidosis by somatostatin receptor and/or gallium scintigraphy: additional value of thoracic SPECT compared to planar imaging. Eur J Nucl Med 1999; 26:1115.

43. Lebtahi R, Crestani B, Belmatoug N et al. Somatostatin receptor scintigraphy and gallium scintigraphy in patients with sarcoidosis. J Nucl Med 2001; 42:21–26.

44. Gotway MB, Storto ML, Golden JA, Reddy GP, Webb WR. Incidental detection of thoracic sarcoidosis on whole-body 18fluorine-2-fluoro-2-deoxy-D-glucose positron emission tomography. J Thorac Imaging 2000; 15:201–204.

45. Joe A, Hoegerle S, Moser E. Cervical lymph node sarcoidosis as a pitfall in F-18 FDG positron emission tomography. Clin Nucl Med 2001; 26:542–543.

46. Kiatboonsri C, Resnick SC, Chan KM et al. The detection of recurrent sarcoidosis by FDG-PET in a lung transplant recipient. West J Med 1998; 168:130–132.

47. Tsuyuguchi N, Sunada I, Ohata K et al. Evaluation of treatment effects in brain abscess with positron emission tomography: comparison of fluorine-18-fluorodeoxyglucose and carbon-11-methionine. Ann Nucl Med 2003; 17:47–51.

48. Oriuchi N, Inoue T, Tomiyoshi K et al. F-18-fluoro-alpha-methyl-tyrosine (FMT) and F-18-fluorodeoxyglucose (FDG) PET in patients with sarcoidosis [abstr]. J Nucl Med 1999; 40:196P.

49. Gungor T, Engel-Bicik I, Eich G et al. Diagnostic and therapeutic impact of whole body positron emission tomography using fluorine-18-fluoro-2-deoxy-D-glucose in children with chronic granulomatous disease. Arch Dis Child 2001; 85:341–345.

50. Konstan MW, Berger M. Current understanding of the inflammatory process in cystic fibrosis: onset and etiology. Pediatr Pulmonol 1997; 24:137–142; discussion 159–161.

51. Labiris NR, Nahmias C, Freitag AP, Thompson ML, Dolovich MB. Uptake of 18fluorodeoxyglucose in the cystic fibrosis lung: a measure of lung inflammation? Eur Respir J 2003; 21:848–854.

52. Terada LS, Johansen KA, Nowbar S, Vasil AI, Vasil ML. Pseudomonas aeruginosa hemolytic phospholipase C suppresses neutrophil respiratory burst activity. Infect Immun 1999; 67:2371–2376.

53. Schuster DP, Kozlowski J, Hogue L. Imaging lung inflammation in a murine model of pseudomonas infection: a positron emission tomography study. Exp Lung Res 2003; 29:45–57.

54. Jones HA, Marino PS, Shakur BH, Morrell NW. *In vivo* assessment of lung inflammatory cell activity in patients with COPD and asthma. Eur Respir J 2003; 21:567–573.

55. Wallace WE, Gupta NC, Hubbs AF et al. *Cis*-4-[(18)F]fluoro-L-proline PET imaging of pulmonary fibrosis in a rabbit model. J Nucl Med 2002; 43:413–420.

56. Ozsahin H, von Planta M, Muller I et al. Successful treatment of invasive aspergillosis in chronic granulomatous disease by bone marrow transplantation, granulocyte colony-stimulating factor-mobilized granulocytes, and liposomal amphotericin-B. Blood 1998; 92:2719–2724.

57. Franzius C, Biermann M, Hulskamp G et al. Therapy monitoring in aspergillosis using F-18 FDG positron emission tomography. Clin Nucl Med 2001; 26:232–233.

58. Reuter S, Schirrmeister H, Kratzer W, Dreweck C, Reske SN, Kern P. Pericystic metabolic activity in alveolar echinococcosis: assessment and follow-up by positron emission tomography. Clin Infect Dis 1999; 29:1157–1163.

59. O'Doherty MJ, Barrington SF, Campbell M, Lowe J, Bradbeer CS. PET scanning and the human immunodeficiency virus-positive patient. J Nucl Med 1997; 38:1575–1583.

60. Salem SS, Heiba S, Santiago J et al. Unusual presentation of solitary bone metastasis from breast carcinoma mimicking acute osteomyelitis of the left midtibial shaft. Clin Nucl Med 2000; 25:480–481.

61. Hubner KF, Buonocore E, Gould HR et al. Differentiating benign from malignant lung lesions using "quantitative" parameters of FDG PET images. Clin Nucl Med 1996; 21:941–949.

62. Torizuka T, Zasadny KR, Recker B, Wahl RL. Untreated primary lung and breast cancers: correlation between F-18 FDG kinetic rate constants and findings of *in vitro* studies. Radiology 1998; 207:767–774.

63. Nakamoto Y, Higashi T, Sakahara H, Tamaki N, Imamura M, Konishi J. Delayed FDG-PET scan for the differentiation between malignant and benign lesions [abstr]. J Nucl Med 1999; 40:247P.

64. Kubota K, Yamaguchi K, Itoh M, Ohira H, Yamada K, Fukuda H. Whole body FDG-PET for tumor detection should be imaged at 2 hr after injection [abstr]. J Nucl Med 1999; 40:141P.

65. Herzog HR, Borner AR, Weckesser M, Muller-Gartner HW. Delayed scan time for FDG-PET in breast cancer [abstr]. J Nucl Med 1999; 40:140P.

66. Demura Y, Tsuchida T, Ishizaki T et al. F-18-FDG accumulation with PET for differentiation between benign and malignant lesions in the thorax. J Nucl Med 2003; 44:540–548.

67. Ishizu K, Nakamura S, Shiozaki T et al. Inceasing rate of FDG uptake from early to delayed PET images in lung tumors [abstr]. J Nucl Med 2000; 41:76P.

18

Metabolic Imaging for Assessing Solitary Pulmonary Nodules

HONGMING ZHUANG, NARESH GUPTA, and ABASS ALAVI

Hospital of the University of Pennsylvania,
Philadelphia, Pennsylvania, USA

I. Investigation of Pulmonary Nodules

Solitary pulmonary nodules (SPNs) are common findings on chest radiographs and computed tomography (CT). Primary bronchogenic carcinoma and benign granulomas constitute >80% of pulmonary nodules with equal distribution of ~40% in each category. Primary bronchogenic carcinoma is thought to be the leading cause of cancer mortality worldwide and is currently the leading cause of cancer deaths in males in all European countries (1). The goal of imaging evaluation is to distinguish between benign and malignant SPNs.

Of the nearly 130,000 new SPNs found each year in the US, ~50–60% would be benign and could be spared the surgical resection. Plain film and CT may not be able to differentiate malignant from benign lesions in two-thirds of nodules based on pattern of calcification or even CT densitometry.

II. What is the Current Diagnostic Approach in Lung Nodules?

Although there is no universally accepted definition of an SPN, this term is usually defined as a lung lesion that is well defined, round or oval, and <4.0 cm in diameter. A variety of diagnostic procedures have been used to evaluate patients with SPNs. Currently, plain radiography and CT scanning are the most commonly used modalities. The probability of malignancy of an SPN depends on several clinical factors and radiographic features of the SPN. Clinical factors associated with a high probability of malignancy are as follows: age and history of smoking or previous malignancy (2). Some of the important radiographic appearances that may suggest a malignant process are the thickness of the cavity wall, a spicular nodular edge, and a diameter of >4 cm (2). The risk of malignancy is decreased on CT scans based on following criteria:

1. calcification characterized as central, laminated, or diffuse;
2. stability of the size of the nodule for ≥2 years.

These so-called "typical patterns of benign calcification," which can exclude malignancy, are only seen in a minority of SPNs on plain radiography. The value of change of volume of the lesion (which for spherical lesions is defined as a 25% increase in diameter) is based on the observation that nodules with doubling times of <30 days or >450 days can reliably be considered as benign (3). Most noncalcified SPNs may remain indeterminate on the basis of CT and plain radiographic findings.

In addition, it is equally difficult to distinguish between diffuse benign and malignant parenchymal abnormalities that cannot be classified as SPNs on radiographic studies. Among the nonmalignant causes of SPNs or other radiographic abnormalities are benign tumors, infectious and inflammatory processes, and vascular disorders.

The optimal management of a patient with an SPN depends on the probability estimates of cancer based on the established criteria for this purpose (4) and on the availability of previous studies. If no previous radiographic examinations are available, or such images were acquired close in time to the detection of SPN, subsequent serial follow up radiographs may be adequate if the patient is <30 years of age and has no history of extra thoracic malignancies and the SPN appears benign radiographically. Otherwise, further investigation should be undertaken to determine the nature of the nodule.

Early detection of lung cancer in a resectable stage should improve survival rate, especially in high-risk population groups. Additionally, within the resectable group, the size of tumor (<3 cm vs. >3 cm) also correlates with the survival rate. Patients with large lesions usually have poor prognosis.

Sputum cytology is a noninvasive method that can establish the diagnosis with a very low false-positive rate but with a relatively low sensitivity, particularly for peripheral malignancies. Bronchoscopic biopsy and transthoracic needle aspiration (TTNA) are both semi-invasive methods that can be employed for further characterization of indeterminate SPNs. The former is preferred for centrally located lesions and its diagnostic yield is up to 80% in most hands (5,6). TTNA is preferred for peripherally located SPNs with a sensitivity of 85–90%. For both methods, the false-positive rate is sufficiently low and the diagnosis of malignancy can be made with confidence with a positive result. However, the sensitivity is not sufficiently high to confidently exclude malignancy. In addition, transbronchial biopsy is associated with a small but not insignificant risk of intrabronchial bleed. TTNA is associated with ~24.5% risk of pneumothorax and 6.8% risk of requiring chest tube placement (5,6). Video-assisted thoracoscopic surgery and thoracotomy are also invasive procedures and are usually considered for lesions with a high likelihood of malignancy based on combination of examinations performed for characterizing the lesion.

CT scanning still remains the mainstay in providing anatomic details, for example, detection of all lung parenchymal lesions, tumor size as well as relationship, and involvement of mediastinal structures or pleura as described eloquently in this report. However, studies over the last decade have shown that Fluorodeoxyglucose positron emission tomography (FDG-PET) may actually provide a reliable noninvasive alternative for diagnosis of malignancy in SPNs (<4 cm size) or even in patients with multiple pulmonary nodules. A negative FDG-PET study indicates only <5% probability of cancer in SPN (7). Small lesions (<1 cm) and/or low-grade bronchoalveolar or adenocarcinoma account for majority of false-negative findings on FDG-PET. The major causes of false negative PET findings include lesions which are smaller than the spatial resolution of the instrument employed or low-grade tumors such as carcinoid or necrotic tumor foci.

III. Role of FDG-PET in SPN

FDG-PET is a noninvasive modality that has recently become gold standard for the evaluation of pulmonary nodules. Lowe et al. (8,9), for the first time, described the value of this modality for the differentiation between benign and malignant solitary lung lesions by demonstrating that malignant lesions have higher FDG uptake than benign nodules (Figs. 18.1 and 18.2). Soon thereafter,

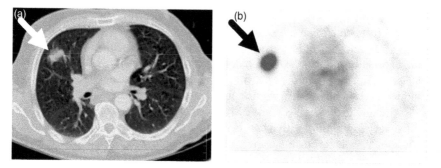

Figure 18.1   A 73-year-old male with CT evidence of right lung nodule (white arrow)
(a). FDG-PET demonstrated significant hypermetabolism (black arrow) (b) of this nodule,
indicating active neoplastic process.

other investigators further confirmed the valuable role of FDG-PET for the evaluation of SPNs with high sensitivity and specificity values (8,9). Dewan et al. (10)
applied the Bayesian analysis for the evaluation of SPNs. On the basis of this
analysis, the likelihood ratios for malignancy in an SPN with increased FDG
uptake were 7.11, suggesting a high probability for malignancy, and 0.06 when
the PET scan was normal, suggesting a high probability for a benign process
(11). An additional advantage of FDG-PET in the evaluation of SPN is that
FDG-PET imaging, in contrast to anatomical imaging, usually scans from the
base of the skull to the upper thigh. Therefore, FDG-PET can frequently detect
unexpected lesions in this setting (12) (Fig. 18.3).

   Many investigators have adopted a semiquantitative method to characterize
the degree of FDG uptake by the lesion by employing the so-called standardized

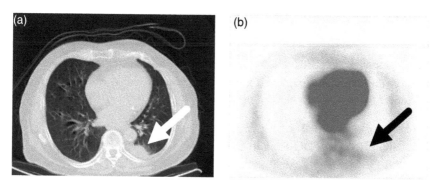

Figure 18.2   A 76-year-old male had a left posterior lung nodule on CT (white arrow)
(a). However, the FDG-PET revealed only minimally increased metabolic activity (black
arrow) (b), which does not meet PET criteria for malignancy and suggests a benignity of
the nodule.

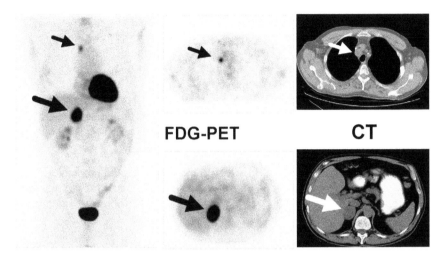

FDG-PET   CT

Figure 18.3 A 58-year-old male had FDG-PET scan to evaluate lung nodule. There were no abnormalities identified in the lungs. However, there were two foci of hypermetabolism in the paratracheal region (small arrow) and right adrenal region (large arrow), suggesting active malignancy. These lesions were confirmed by subsequent CT scan.

uptake value or SUV. This value can be defined as follows:

$$\text{SUV} = \frac{\text{mean ROI activity (MBq/mL)}}{\text{injected dose (MBq)/body weight (g)}} \times \frac{1}{\text{decay factor of }^{18}\text{F}}$$

Several studies have shown that most infectious or inflammatory pulmonary disorders have relatively lower FDG uptake than malignant lung lesions. A threshold of a single-time point SUV of 2.5–3.8 has been proposed as the optimal measure for separating malignant from benign tumor or inflammatory lung nodules. However, there is considerable overlap between the levels of FDG uptake of malignant and benign lesions. Among malignant lesions, there is a wide range of FDG uptake. For example, nonsmall cell lung carcinoma has an average SUV of 8, whereas the average SUV for breast cancer is substantially lower (9). In the chest, some malignant lesions such as bronchioalveolar carcinoma (13) and small nodules may appear with low uptake values. On the other hand, the degree of FDG uptake varies considerably among different classes of inflammatory cells. Sugawara et al. (14) reported that the SUV of infectious lesions could be as high as 6.69. Optimal interpretation of PET images in patients with suspected malignancies requires knowledge of behavior of FDG in such settings (15). Thus, in majority of cases, visual assessment of the pattern of uptake combined with quantitative analysis, clinical presentation and radiological findings may allow accurate assessment of benign and malignant

SPNs. For example, bilateral, symmetrical hilar/mediastinal uptake without lung parenchymal abnormality usually represents inflammatory or other nonmalignant lymphadenopathies. Factors such as body habitus, timing of imaging after FDG injection, and plasma glucose level are important factors that are known to influence the image quality and SUV measurement.

Increased FDG activity has been observed in a variety of benign conditions that are mostly due to infectious or inflammatory processes. These disorders can result in inaccurate interpretation of FDG-PET studies of SPNs. Pathological states in the chest with increased FDG accumulation include

1. infectious processes (16,17), such as an abscess and tuberculosis;
2. noninfectious inflammatory processes (18–21), such as sarcoidosis;
3. iatrogenic disorders (22–24), such as radiation pneumonitis and foreign body.

It has been shown that certain active inflammatory disorders tend to show higher FDG uptake than others. We have noted that some active granulomatous infections such as histoplasmosis have very intense FDG concentration, whereas minimally active or healed granulomas appear negative on the scan. Thus, there is a wide range of variability of FDG uptake in inflammatory lesions, which makes the PET images unpredictable with regard to the degree of metabolic activity of these lesions.

IV. Dual-Time Point Imaging for Differentiating Benign from Malignant Nodules

Dual-time FDG-PET has been effectively employed for differentiating benign from malignant lung nodules. This technique was first described for head and neck malignancies (25). Hustinx et al. performed dual-time point scanning in 21 patients with head and neck malignant tumors. These authors noted that malignant tumors had an average increase of SUVs between the first and second scan of 12%, whereas inflammatory lesions and structures with physiologic uptake of FDG (tongue, larynx) showed essentially stable uptake over time or a slight decline. Another important finding was that the SUV changes in tumors were larger, when >30 min had elapsed between the first and second emission scans. A study by Zhuang et al. (26) suggested that lesions with increasing SUVs over time are likely to be malignant and that dual-time point FDG-PET imaging appears to be a promising method for distinguishing malignant from benign lesions. Increase in FDG uptake over time on dynamic imaging in malignant lesions was also observed by other investigators (27,28). In a study using a turpentine-induced inflammation model on rats, Yamada et al. (29) found that FDG uptake in inflammatory tissue increased gradually until 60 min after injection and thereafter it decreased gradually. There is, however, increasing evidence suggesting that malignant tumor uptake of FDG increases for hours after injection (29,30). In a study to compare the accuracy of early imaging and dual-time

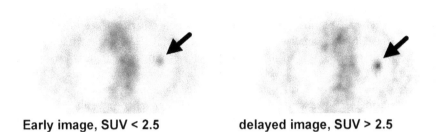

Early image, SUV < 2.5   **delayed image, SUV > 2.5**

Figure 18.4 A 86-year-old female patient with history of renal cell carcinoma and nephrectomy developed left lung nodule. The early images of FDG-PET revealed mild hypermetabolism in the left lung nodule, suggesting inflammation. However, the activity of this nodule was significantly higher on the delayed images, indicating malignancy. The follow-up demonstrated that this lesion is caused by metastasis from renal cell carcinoma.

imaging of FDG-PET in the evaluation of lung nodule, Matthies et al. (31) reported dual-time imaging can further increase the accuracy of FDG-PET in the evaluation of lung nodule (Fig. 18.4).

It is unclear why inflammatory and malignant lesions exhibit a differential FDG uptake pattern over time. Several factors may contribute to this phenomenon on a cellular basis. Although it is well known that many cancer cells express increased number of glucose transporters (Glut1), metabolic trapping through phosphorylation of FDG appears more likely as the rate-determining step in retention of FDG in the cells. Hexokinase and glucose-6-phosphatase (G6Pase) mediate the phosphorylation and dephosphorylation of intracellular FDG, respectively. It has been reported that the rate of dephosphorylation of FDG-6-P may be responsible for the different behavior of FDG uptake between malignant and benign lesions in dual-time FDG-PET imaging (32). Unless FDG-6-phosphate is dephosphorylated by glucose-6-phosphatase, it is unable to leave the cell. On the basis of this theory, FDG is trapped inside cells via 6-phosphorylation. High levels of G6Pase would reduce the intracellular residence of FDG-6-phosphate time by dephosphorylation and subsequent gradual transport of this compound out of cells. In contrast, low levels of G6Pase would allow continuous intracellular FDG accumulation over time as there is no or minimal dephosphorylation. In order to determine whether the levels of G6Pase in different normal and malignant tissues contribute to dynamics of FDG uptake by these tissues, we analyzed FDG-PET studies of 43 patients with confirmed malignancy that underwent FDG-PET dual-time point imaging and also showed cardiac, skeletal muscle, and bone marrow uptake on the images. The data determined that statistically there was no significant difference in the SUV measurement between the first and second time points for skeletal muscle and bone marrow FDG uptake ($p > 0.05$). In contrast, there was significant change for such measurements for both tumor and heart tissue ($p < 0.01$).

Our data demonstrate that organs with low levels of G6Pase (tumor and heart) reveal increasing SUV over time in dual-time imaging, whereas organs with normal level of G6Pase (skeletal muscle and bone marrow) do not. As it is known that G6Pase is present at high concentrations in most normal organs (except heart) and is low in most cancer cells, it would be logical to suggest that the differences in the levels of G6Pase and ratios of hexokinase/G6Pase between these two types of tissues can, at least partially, explain why dual-time point imaging is useful in differentiating malignant from benign disorders (32). Thus, the differential ratio of hexokinase/phosphatase may contribute to the distinct FDG uptake patterns (time course) observed between inflammatory and malignant lesions over time. On the basis of these observations, we believe that dual-time point imaging has the potential to distinguish malignant from benign lesion in some cancers.

Varying levels of G6Pase activity among different tumor cell types may also explain the wide range of FDG retention over time. Tumor types with lower G6Pase activity are more likely to be categorized as malignant by dual-time point FDG-PET imaging than those with higher levels of this enzyme. Zhuang et al. (26) reported that nonsmall cell lung cancer and mesotheliomas appear to have rising levels of FDG uptake over time, whereas ovarian cancers do not show such an increase. Unfortunately, not all malignant lesions reveal increasing levels of FDG uptake with time. Ovarian cancers have been found to express a relatively low ratio of hexokinase/phosphatase. This may explain why ovarian cancer cells behave differently when compared with other types of malignant cells. Similarly, not all inflammatory lesions are noted to show washout of FDG over time. Dynamic image and compartmental model analysis may be an appropriate next step to further understand the role of dual point imaging for separating benign from malignant disorders.

Uptake of FDG in benign lesions can be influenced by the underlying cause (infection vs. inflammation) and the state of inflammation (acute vs. chronic). Differences in FDG uptake may also be related to the type of inflammatory cells in the lesion and the extent of activation of these cells at the time of examination. Furthermore, FDG uptake can be influenced by the physiological and immunological state of the cells. In malignant disease, even among those with similar hexokinase/G6Pase ratios, the combination of coexisting chronic or acute inflammation, necrosis, hypoxia, and degree of angiogenesis can complicate the pattern of FDG uptake. For example, hypoxia can increase FDG uptake by tumor cells due to enhanced anaerobic glycolytic pathway (33).

V. Effects of Partial Volume Correction on Accurate Measurement of SUV

The spatial resolution of the PET systems varies substantially among models and is typically between 5 and 10 mm for most clinical machines. There is a significant difference between resolving powers of modern CT and MRI scanners and those of PET and SPECT instruments, which poses a challenge when structural abnormalities are compared with metabolic findings for the assessment of the nature of the disease process. This results in low sensitivities for the diagnosis of small malignant lesions when instruments with limited resolutions are used (34). The measured SUV underestimates the true metabolic activity of lesions measuring less than twice the spatial resolution of the camera.

One method to correct for the resolution effect is to consider the use the lesion size, which is determined on CT scan, as the basis to calculate the SUV. Hickeson et al. (35) reported an increase of accuracy from 58% to 89% with the use of this technique for lung nodules measuring <2 cm in 42 patients when a SUV threshold of 2.5 was used to characterize benign vs. malignant lesions. In this study, each lesion's SUV was determined by using two different methods. The maximum voxel SUV (maxSUV) was determined in a circular region of interest (ROI) with a diameter of 0.8 cm (2 voxels) at the plane with maximal FDG uptake of the lesion. In the second method, the SUV was corrected for underestimation of true metabolic activity of the entire lesion due to the resolution and partial volume effects (corSUV). Two ROIs were drawn around the lesion. The smaller of two included all the voxels associated with the lesion. In practice, this was drawn at least 0.8 cm outside the 50% uptake level of the maximum pixel to include all of the counts resulting from the SPN. The second larger ROI surrounds the smaller ROI which include the surrounding background. Thus, the background activity could be determined from the average uptake outside the smaller ROI and inside the larger ROI. The halfway point between the maximum lesion activity and surrounding background activity was frequently used as the true size of the lesion. The background uptake was then subtracted from the average uptake in the small ROI. Therefore, the corSUV was calculated by including the injected dose, patient's weight, and time after injection and using the following formula:

$$
\text{corSUV} = \frac{(\text{region's activity (MBq)} - \text{background activity (MBq)})/\text{lesion's size on CT scan (cm}^3)}{\text{injected dose (MBq)}/\text{patient's weight (g)}}
$$

where background activity = activity/volume in background × (region's volume − lesion's size on CT scan in cm^3).

Measuring the SUV using the CT size to correct for resolution effect offers potential value in distinguishing malignant from benign lesions in this population. This semiquantitative approach appears to improve considerably the sensitivity and accuracy in characterizing malignant small lung nodules in this population.

VI. Anatomo-Functional Imaging: PET/CT Combined Scanners

Over the past few years combined PET/CT scanners have been employed for assessing a variety of disorders including malignant disease of the lung. The use of CT scanners in conjunction with PET scanners enhances anatomical localization of sites of abnormalities noted on PET image. Additionally, by using high-resolution CT machines for attenuation correction of PET images improves the quality of whole body scans and enables accurate and instant fusion of functional and anatomical images. Several reports have shown that combined PET/CT fusion images not only allow better anatomical delineation of the PET abnormalities but also improve the sensitivity, specificity, and accuracy of detection of parenchymal and lymph node abnormalities. Combined PET/CT imaging may achieve accuracy approaching 95% for detection of mediastinal adenopathy in patients with lung malignancies. Use of CT scanning for attenuation correction also increases patient throughput. Sequential CT and PET image acquisition within short period of time facilitate accurate alignment and fusion of CT and PET images, which is essential for radiation treatment planning of lung cancer patients.

VII. Other Tracers

Over last several years, various studies have demonstrated that FDG-PET is highly effective in differentiating malignant from benign lesions either in the lung parenchymal or in the lymph nodes. By now, it is well established that inflammatory diseases including several lung conditions such as pneumoconiosis, sarcoidosis, silicosis as well as progressive massive fibrosis (PMF) show FDG activity and therefore are potential sources of false-positive results on PET scan. In pursuit of other tracers, F-18 fluoro proline has been synthesized and has been shown to demonstrate encouraging results in the diagnosis of active pulmonary fibrosis. Other tracers such as C-11 methionine, and C-11 or F-18 labeled tyrosine have been shown to have uptake in inflammatory lesions and therefore appear less specific than F-18 FDG in separating malignant disorders from inflammatory diseases of the lung.

VIII. Role of Somatostatin Scintigraphy in SPN

Somatostatin is a peptide secreted primarily by the hypothalamus and the pancreas, which naturally exists in two forms: one with 14 amino acids and the other with 28 amino acids. It acts as the universal endocrine inhibitor and can also inhibit the growth of neuroendocrine tumors containing somatostatin receptors (SSTRs). Human SSTRs are expressed on many cells of neuroendocrine origin and also on lymphocytes. In addition, many tumors, including bronchogenic carcinomas, express high densities of SSTRs. Therefore, another class of radiopharmaceuticals used for the evaluation of SPN is somatostatin analogs.

One such radiopharmaceutical is ^{111}In-octreotide, which contains eight amino acids. It has variable binding affinities to SSTRs. Five subtypes of SSTRs have been indentified so far (36). ^{111}In-octreotide has the highest binding affinity to SSTR2, followed by SSTR5 and SSTR3. Typically, the administered dose is ~222 MBq (6 mCi) containing at least 10 μg of the peptide. Because of the relatively long effective half-life, images are acquired 24–48 h later. Tomographic images of the thorax are also acquired for SPN imaging. If indicated, a repeat image at 48 h after injection is acquired. Kwekkeboom et al. (37) and other investigators have reported encouraging results in the imaging of lung cancers with ^{111}In-octreotide.

Depreotide is another synthetic peptide which contains 10 amino acids which also binds SSTRs. Unlike with octreotide, depreotide can be easily labeled with ^{99m}Tc, resulting in improved imaging characteristics, lower radiation burden, and lower costs than with ^{111}In-octreotide. In addition, SPECT imaging is possible with ^{99m}Tc-depreotide (NeoTect). Clinically, ~90 min after the intravenous injection of about 20 mCi of ^{99m}Tc-depreotide, whole body planar images in the anterior and posterior projections and SPECT images of the thorax are performed. The anatomic landmarks are provided by the photopenic zones of blood pool regions of the mediastinum.

[99m]Tc-depreotide imaging allows a rapid, effective, and noninvasive method for the evaluation of SPNs. Blum et al. (38) reported a sensitivity and specificity of 93% and 88%, respectively, in 30 patients with SPNs >1 cm. This study was also significant in that there were 18 SPNs that were subsequently proven to be benign. This method of characterizing SPNs as benign or malignant was later confirmed with a larger, multicenter trial with 114 patients in whom the state of all nodules was confirmed by tissue analysis. SPNs as small as 0.8 cm was visualized by ^{99m}Tc scintigraphy. Furthermore, all bronchioalveolar carcinomas in this series were correctly demonstrated with this agent. There were 88 pulmonary nodules that were proven to be malignant. Among these nodules, 85 were correctly characterized with a sensitivity of 96.6%. The three false-negative results were from small SPNs measuring <2 cm. Among the 26 benign pulmonary nodules, 19 were correctly characterized with a specificity of 73.1%. Six of these seven false-positive studies were seen granulomatous processes. The efficacy of this modality for characterizing SPNs was subsequently confirmed by other studies. Several benign conditions have been reported to reveal increased Tc-derpreotide uptake. The underlying mechanism that account for false-positive ^{99m}Tc-depreotide activity is not well understood. However, Krenning et al. (39) reported significantly increased ^{111}In-octretide activity in Graves' disease, sarcoidosis, and tuberculosis, which suggests the possibility of increased SSTR expression or increased somatostatin binding sites in activated lymphocytes.

SSTR-binding radiopharmaceuticals may offer potential for labeling with a therapeutic isotope such as ^{90}Y or ^{188}Re, and administrated as unsealed agent. This can provide an alternate treatment modality to external beam radiotherapy, chemotherapy, or surgery for these frequently fatal lung malignancies.

Previous reports have failed to demonstrate clinical advantage of using Tc-neotect imaging over FDG-PET in the assessment of lung nodules (40,41). Thus far, PET-FDG imaging is considered the gold standard and has been established as the noninvasive test of choice in the differential diagnosis of SPNs.

IX. Conclusions

Functional imaging has emerged as a very effective technique for the noninvasive characterization of SPNs and differentiating benign from malignant lesions. FDG-PET has been proven to be very useful for this purpose, providing an excellent sensitivity and specificity in this setting. Advances in instrumentation have improved the accuracy of detecting small malignant lesions. Image fusion utilizing PET/CT fusion imaging has further enhanced the role of this very powerful modality. Future may further improve upon the efficacy of PET-FDG imaging in differentiating benign from malignant SPNs by synthesis of more specific PET ligands.

References

1. Valanis BG. Epidemiology of lung cancer: a worldwide epidemic. Semin Oncol Nurs 1996; 12:251–259.
2. Webb WR. Radiologic evaluation of the solitary pulmonary nodule. AJR Am J Roentgenol 1990; 154:701–708.
3. Khouri NF, Meziane MA, Zerhouni EA, Fishman EK, Siegelman SS. The solitary pulmonary nodule. Assessment, diagnosis, and management. Chest 1987; 91:128–133.
4. Gupta NC, Maloof J, Gunel E. Probability of malignancy in solitary pulmonary nodules using fluorine-18-FDG and PET [see comments]. J Nucl Med 1996; 37:943–948.
5. Klein JS, Zarka MA. Transthoracic needle biopsy. Radiol Clin North Am 2000; 38:235–266, vii.
6. Klein JS, Zarka MA. Transthoracic needle biopsy: an overview. J Thorac Imaging 1997; 12:232–249.
7. Cummings SR, Lillington GA, Richard RJ. Estimating the probability of malignancy in solitary pulmonary nodules. A Bayesian approach. Am Rev Respir Dis 1986; 134:449–452.
8. Lowe VJ, Hoffman JM, DeLong DM, Patz EF, Coleman RE. Semiquantitative and visual analysis of FDG-PET images in pulmonary abnormalities. J Nucl Med 1994; 35:1771–1776.

9. Valk PE, Pounds TR, Hopkins DM, Haseman MK, Hofer GA, Greiss HB et al. Staging non-small cell lung cancer by whole-body positron emission tomographic imaging. Ann Thorac Surg 1995; 60:1573–1581.

10. Dewan NA, Shehan CJ, Reeb SD, Gobar LS, Scott WJ, Ryschon K. Likelihood of malignancy in a solitary pulmonary nodule: comparison of Bayesian analysis and results of FDG-PET scan. Chest 1997; 112:416–422.

11. Gupta NC, Frank AR, Dewan NA, Redepenning LS, Rothberg ML, Mailliard JA et al. Solitary pulmonary nodules: detection of malignancy with PET with 2-[F-18]-fluoro-2-deoxy-D-glucose. Radiology 1992; 184:441–444.

12. Zhuang H, Hickeson M, Chacko TK, Duarte PS, Nakhoda KZ, Feng Q et al. Incidental detection of colon cancer by FDG positron emission tomography in patients examined for pulmonary nodules. Clin Nucl Med 2002; 27:628–632.

13. Higashi K, Ueda Y, Seki H, Yuasa K, Oguchi M, Noguchi T et al. Fluorine-18-FDG PET imaging is negative in bronchioloalveolar lung carcinoma. J Nucl Med 1998; 39:1016–1020.

14. Sugawara Y, Fisher SJ, Zasadny KR, Kison PV, Baker LH, Wahl RL. Preclinical and clinical studies of bone marrow uptake of fluorine-1-fluorodeoxyglucose with or without granulocyte colony-stimulating factor during chemotherapy. J Clin Oncol 1998; 16:173–180.

15. Zhuang H, Alavi A. 18-Fluorodeoxyglucose positron emission tomographic imaging in the detection and monitoring of infection and inflammation. Semin Nucl Med 2002; 32:47–59.

16. Bakheet SM, Saleem M, Powe J, Al Amro A, Larsson SG, Mahassin Z. F-18 fluorodeoxyglucose chest uptake in lung inflammation and infection. Clin Nucl Med 2000; 25:273–278.

17. Zhuang H, Pourdehnad M, Yamamoto AJ, Rossman MD, Alavi A. Intense F-18 fluorodeoxyglucose uptake caused by *Mycobacterium avium* intracellulare infection. Clin Nucl Med 2001; 26:458.

18. Lewis PJ, Salama A. Uptake of fluorine-18-fluorodeoxyglucose in sarcoidosis. J Nucl Med 1994; 35:1647–1649.

19. Talwar A, Mayerhoff R, London D, Shah R, Stanek A, Epstein M. False-positive PET scan in a patient with lipoid pneumonia simulating lung cancer. Clin Nucl Med 2004; 29:426–428.

20. Yu JQ, Zhuang H, Xiu Y, Talati E, Alavi A. Demonstration of increased FDG activity in Rosai–Dorfman disease on positron emission tomography. Clin Nucl Med 2004; 29:209–210.

21. Kung J, Zhuang H, Yu JQ, Duarte PS, Alavi A. Intense fluorodeoxyglucose activity in pulmonary amyloid lesions on positron emission tomography. Clin Nucl Med 2003; 28:975–976.

22. Lin P, Delaney G, Chu J, Kiat H, Pocock N. Fluorine-18 FDG dual-head gamma camera coincidence imaging of radiation pneumonitis. Clin Nucl Med 2000; 25:866–869.

23. Zhuang H, Cunnane ME, Ghesani NV, Mozley PD, Alavi A. Chest tube insertion as a potential source of false-positive FDG-positron emission tomographic results. Clin Nucl Med 2002; 27:285–286.

24. Bhargava P, Zhuang H, Kumar R, Charron M, Alavi A. Iatrogenic artifacts on whole-body F-18 FDG PET imaging. Clin Nucl Med 2004; 29:429–439.

25. Hustinx R, Smith RJ, Benard F, Rosenthal DI, Machtay M, Farber LA et al. Dual time point fluorine-18 fluorodeoxyglucose positron emission tomography: a potential

method to differentiate malignancy from inflammation and normal tissue in the head and neck. Eur J Nucl Med 1999; 26:1345–1348.

26. Zhuang H, Pourdehnad M, Lambright ES, Yamamoto AJ, Lanuti M, Li PY et al. Dual time point F-18-FDG PET imaging for differentiating malignant from inflammatory processes. J Nucl Med 2001; 42:1412–1417.

27. Conrad GR, Sinha P. Narrow time-window dual-point F-18-FDG PET for the diagnosis of thoracic malignancy. Nucl Med Commun 2003; 24:1129–1137.

28. Lai CH, Huang KG, See LC, Yen TC, Tsai CS, Chang TC et al. Restaging of recurrent cervical carcinoma with dual-phase F-18 fluoro-2-deoxy-D-glucose positron emission tomography. Cancer 2004; 100:544–552.

29. Yamada S, Kubota K, Kubota R, Ido T, Tamahashi N. High accumulation of fluorine-18-fluorodeoxyglucose in turpentine-induced inflammatory tissue. J Nucl Med 1995; 36:1301–1306.

30. Hamberg LM, Hunter GJ, Alpert NM, Choi NC, Babich JW, Fischman AJ. The dose uptake ratio as an index of glucose metabolism: useful parameter or oversimplification? J Nucl Med 1994; 35:1308–1312.

31. Matthies A, Hickeson M, Cuchiara A, Alavi A. Dual time point F-18-FDG PET for the evaluation of pulmonary nodules. J Nucl Med 2002; 43:871–875.

32. Ponzo F, Zhuang HM, Liu FM, Pourdehnad M, Ghesani NV, Alavi A. Can the difference of the levels of glucose-6-phosphatase explain the mechanism of FDG-PET dual time point imaging? [abstr]. Eur J Nucl Med 2001; 28:OS399.

33. Burgman P, Odonoghue JA, Humm JL, Ling CC. Hypoxia-induced increase in FDG uptake in MCF7 cells. J Nucl Med 2001; 42:170–175.

34. Weber W, Young C, Abdel-Dayem HM, Sfakianakis G, Weir GJ, Swaney CM et al. Assessment of pulmonary lesions with F-18-fluorodeoxyglucose positron imaging using coincidence mode gamma cameras. J Nucl Med 1999; 40:574–578.

35. Hickeson M, Yun MJ, Matthies A, Zhuang H, Adam LE, Lacorte L et al. Use of a corrected standardized uptake value based on the lesion size on CT permits accurate characterization of lung nodules on FDG-PET. Eur J Nucl Med Mol Imaging 2002; 29:1639–1647.

36. Patel YC, Greenwood MT, Panetta R, Demchyshyn L, Niznik H, Srikant CB. The somatostatin receptor family. Life Sci 1995; 57:1249–1265.

37. Kwekkeboom DJ, Kho GS, Lamberts SW, Reubi JC, Laissue JA, Krenning EP. The value of octreotide scintigraphy in patients with lung cancer. Eur J Nucl Med 1994; 21:1106–1113.

38. Blum JE, Handmaker H, Rinne NA. The utility of a somatostatin-type receptor binding peptide radiopharmaceutical (P829) in the evaluation of solitary pulmonary nodules. Chest 1999; 115:224–232.

39. Krenning EP, Kwekkeboom DJ, de Jong M, Visser TJ, Reubi JC, Bakker WH et al. Essentials of peptide receptor scintigraphy with emphasis on the somatostatin analog octreotide. Semin Oncol 1994; 21:6–14.

40. Nguyen DT, Morakinyo T. Discordant Tc-99m depreotide and F-18FDG imaging in a patient with poorly differentiated small-cell neuroendocrine carcinoma. Clin Nucl Med 2002; 27:373–375.

41. Kahn D, Menda Y, Kernstine K, Bushnell D, McLaughlin K, Miller S et al. The utility of ^{99m}Tc depreotide compared with F-18 fluorodeoxyglucose positron emission tomography and surgical staging in patients with suspected non-small cell lung cancer. Chest 2004; 125:494–501.

Part V: Clinical Imaging

19

Acute Respiratory Distress Syndrome (ARDS)

HANS-ULRICH KAUCZOR

Deutsches Krebsforschungszentrum,
Heidelberg, Germany

TOBIAS ACHENBACH

Johannes Gutenberg University
Medical School,
Mainz, Germany

I. Definition

The term "acute respiratory distress syndrome" (ARDS) was coined in 1967 by Asbaugh et al. (1), who described a syndrome of severe dyspnea, tachypnea, hypoxemia refractory to oxygen therapy, decreased pulmonary compliance, and diffuse alveolar opacities on chest radiography. Autopsy findings consisted of atelectasis, vascular congestion, hemorrhage, and pulmonary edema. Histology revealed diffuse alveolar damage with hyaline membrane formation. Although this description reflected clinical and pathological findings, the clinical entity of the ARDS at the time was still poorly defined. As similar findings were also observed in children and adolescents, the term "acute respiratory distress syndrome" was adopted and is preferred to the initial name, "adult respiratory distress syndrome". ARDS is characterized by a general inflammatory reaction of the lung, which results in severe pulmonary capillary permeability with the subsequent development of interstitial and alveolar edema. The production of mediators, such as leukotrienes, prostaglandins, and proteolytic enzymes, leads to severe alterations in normal pulmonary physiology and respiratory failure. The primary clinical finding is hypoxemia with an oxygenation index [arterial oxygen partial pressure (PaO_2)/inspiratory oxygen concentration (FiO_2)] of less than 200. The hypoxemia is also associated with reduced pulmonary compliance due to interstitial edema, depletion of surfactant, atelectasis, formation of hyaline membranes, and eventually, the development of fibrosis.

Although patients with ARDS may have a component of hydrostatic edema, patients with volume overload or heart failure (left atrial hypertension) are not considered to have the disorder. To differentiate noncardiogenic from a cardiogenic pulmonary edema, the pulmonary capillary occlusion pressure (PCOP) is measured and should be <18 mmHg in ARDS. If the PCOP is not measured, there would be no clinical evidence of congestive heart failure. The edema possibly contributes to the development of posterior and basal atelectasis observed in some patients with ARDS and may be associated with pulmonary right-to-left shunting and an increase of the pulmonary vascular resistance that is observed in some patients.

ARDS was defined by an American–European consensus conference in 1994 (Table 19.1) (2) as a syndrome characterized by hypoxemia with an altered and inhomogeneous distribution of ventilation and perfusion (oxygenation index [PaO_2/FiO_2] $\leq$ 200) and bilateral alveolar infiltrates on radiography, without cardiac dysfunction (PCOP $\leq$ 18 mmHg). Acute lung injury (ALI) was introduced as a superordinate term for a spectrum of diseases characterized by gas exchange disorders. ARDS is on the severe end of this spectrum.

Since 1994, most ARDS studies have refered to this definition. However, it has limited discriminatory power to define meaningful subgroups for comparative evaluations of outcome across studies or institutions. Many different underlying diseases and disorders may cause ARDS. Additionally, these may be either pulmonary (i.e., infection, toxic inhalation) or nonpulmonary (trauma, sepsis,

Table 19.1 Criteria for ALI and ARDS

Diagnosis	Timing	Oxygenation	Chest radiograph	PCPW
ALI	Acute onset	$PaO_2/FiO_2 \leq 300$ mmHg, regardless of PEEP	Bilateral infiltrates	≤ 18 mmHg or clinical absence of pulmonary venous hypertension
ARDS	Acute onset	$PaO_2/FiO_2 \leq 200$ mmHg, regardless of PEEP	Bilateral infiltrates	≤ 18 mmHg or clinical absence of pulmonary venous hypertension

renal or hepatic failure) in origin. Table 19.2 lists the major risk categories for the development of ARDS according to the 1994 consensus conference (2).

The incidences of ALI and ARDS as reported in American and European studies are variable and range from 18 to 89 per 100,000 inhabitants for ALI, and from 3 to 13 per 100,000 inhabitants for ARDS. Patients with sepsis syndrome have the highest incidence, followed by aspiration, with a 30% incidence, massive transfusion for emergency resuscitation (24%), and pulmonary contusion (17%). The measurement of contusion volume, described in percentage of total lung volume, helps to estimate the individual risk of developing ARDS, because patients with severe pulmonary contusion (>20% of total lung volume) have been found to have a higher rate of development of ARDS than patients with moderate pulmonary contusion (<20%) (3). The mortality of ARDS is highly variable; a range between 0% and 95% can be found in the literature. A meta-analysis reported a mean mortality rate of ~50% (4).

Table 19.2 Major Risk Categories for ALI/ARDS

Direct injury
  Aspiration
  Diffuse pulmonary infection
  Near-drowning
  Toxic inhalation
  Lung contusion
Indirect injury
  Sepsis syndrome
  Severe nonthoracic trauma
  Hypertransfusion for emergency resuscitation
  Cardiopulmonary bypass (rare)

Source: From Bernard et al. (2).

The underlying inflammatory processes of ARDS are reflected by a rather typical time course. In the initial, very early exudative stage of ARDS, there is a small amount of fluid leakage into the interstitium and sequestration of neutrophils. Hypoxemia and pulmonary hypertension are often present. Soon there is an increased leakage of fluid into the interstitial space that is referred to as permeability edema. It is diffuse alveolar damage that permits the proteinaceous permeability edema to leak out into the alveoli (5) and result in alveolar collapse. Microscopic hyaline membranes can be found within respiratory bronchioles and alveolar ducts. Soon, the other manifestations of diffuse alveolar damage dominate: cellular necrosis, epithelial hyperplasia, inflammation, and eventual fibrosis (6). The pathological picture is dominated by epithelial damage, which overwhelms any manifestation of capillary endothelial damage.

Traditionally, the pathological findings of ARDS are divided in four stages: (1) an initial, early exudative phase with swelling and damage of the endothelial cells, microatelectasis, and subtle interstitial edema; (2) a severe exudative phase with massive alveolar edema, accumulation of fibrin, and formation of hyaline membranes; (3) a proliferative phase with an increase of alveolar cells, accumulation of collagen, destruction of microvasculature, and hyperplasia of pneumocytes type II; and finally, (4) a fibrotic phase.

II. Radiologic Findings

The conventional chest radiograph is the most frequently used radiologic examination in an intensive care unit (ICU). Its major indications include determination of cardiac size, evaluation of pulmonary congestion and edema, identification of pulmonary infiltrates or effusion, as well as determination of the position of central venous or pulmonary arterial catheters, tracheal, and chest tubes. Radiologists and clinicians are well aware of the limitations of portable chest radiography in an ICU when compared with standard chest radiography: mandatory anterior–posterior projection, supine positioning, shorter film-to-focus distance leading to magnification of the heart, and increased motion artifacts caused by longer exposure times due to the limited power output of the portable units. The introduction of digital radiography, for example, storage phosphor radiography, has resulted in a significant improvement of image quality for chest radiography in the ICU, but major limitations still prevail.

The classic radiographic findings of ARDS include patchy or diffuse airspace disease combined with normal heart size and normal vascular pedicle [Fig. 19.1(a)]. Additional abnormalities such as septal lines, peribronchial cuffing, and thickening of the fissures are reported with varying frequencies.

Although ARDS was already described as an entity in the late 1960s and the first clinical CT scanners appeared in the mid-1970s, ARDS was not in the

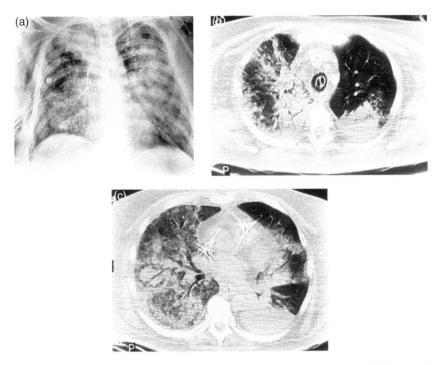

Figure 19.1 A 58-year-old patient with ARDS due to septic shock, renal failure, and bacterial pneumonia. (a) Chest radiograph obtained on day 5 of ARDS shows bilateral patchy and diffuse infiltrates and peribronchial cuffing combined with normal heart size and vascular pedicle. Note also the chest tube for pneumothorax on the right. (b,c) CT obtained on day 4 of ARDS shows heterogeneous distribution of consolidation and ground glass opacities in both lungs, indicating atelectasis and lung infiltration. Ventilation with PEEP leads to patent peripheral airways (air-bronchograms) and hyperlucent areas in the left lung, suggesting overdistension.

focus of cross-sectional imaging techniques until the mid-1980s. The common belief based on the findings from chest radiography that ARDS represented a homogeneous alteration of the lung parenchyma was significantly changed by the application of CT in these critically ill patients [Fig. 19.1(b) and (c)]. With the introduction of CT, the knowledge about ARDS morphology has expanded. To accurately describe the morphological CT findings, an appropriate terminology is recommended (Table 19.3) (7,8).

The typical clinical course of ARDS from the acute onset of respiratory insufficiency to complete recovery or a fibrotic end-stage is reflected by a typical time course of pathological stages which correspond to the changes in the observed radiological patterns. It is important to notice that the different, partly nonuniform pathological stages are not sharply separated from each

Table 19.3 Appropriate Terminology to Describe CT Morphology

Ground glass opacification	Hazy increase in lung attenuation with preservation of bronchial and vascular margins
Consolidation	Homogeneous increase in lung attenuation that obscures bronchovascular margins; air bronchograms may be present
Reticular pattern	Innumerable interlacing line shadows that may be fine, intermediate, or coarse

other, but that transitions are fluent. The following classification serves as a helpful guideline:

A. Initial, Early Exudative Stage/Stage I (1st–24th Hour)

The first chest radiograph of an ARDS patient with acute onset of dyspnea and hypoxemia may not show any abnormalities. There may be a time gap of ~12 h between onset of respiratory failure and the appearance of radiographic abnormalities characteristic for ARDS. CT, being more sensitive, may demonstrate subtle ground glass opacities with a predilection in the middle and perihilar or even peripheral subpleural regions of the lung if CT is performed in this very early phase (Fig. 19.2). Fluid leakage into the peripheral interstitium is minimal, but occasionally there will be signs of interstitial edema, such as the appearance of septal lines. Over time, the findings will become more obvious and convert to patchy and ill-defined opacities. They will show a more homogeneous

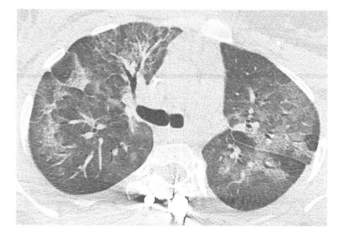

Figure 19.2 A 19-year-old patient developed ARDS after pelvic surgery and atypical pneumonia. Early CT shows patchy ground glass opacities indicative of early exudative ARDS.

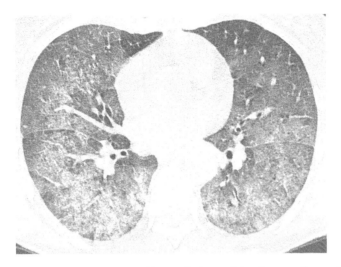

Figure 19.3 A 57-year-old patient with ARDS after peripheral stem cell transplantation. Early CT shows a homogeneous ground glass appearance with some patchy denser areas.

appearance throughout both lungs combined with broadening of the peribronchovascular interstitial tissue (Fig. 19.3). These findings indicate the transition to stage II.

B. Exudative Stage/Stage II (2nd–7th Day)

In this stage, the chest radiograph shows ill-defined hazy opacities, yet the vessels remain visible, probably because the disease is inhomogeneous and some lung areas remain aerated (Fig. 19.1). As alveolar leakage and collapse progress, the opacities become denser and more homogeneous (Fig. 19.4). Air bronchograms may become a prominent feature. They are helpful for the differentiation of the increased permeability edema encountered in ARDS from edema caused by cardiac failure. CT scanning will reveal ground glass opacities and consolidation with a patchy, peripheral distribution. The heterogeneity of mild or moderate ARDS is much better revealed on CT scans than on plain radiographs (Fig. 19.1). This may reflect the heterogeneous nature of the disease with subsequent differences in local compliance and aeration also influenced by the ventilator settings. Often the nondependent lung regions have a normal or ground glass appearance and the dependent and dorsal lung regions will exhibit consolidation and atelectasis. Thus, a ventrodorsal and a cephalocaudal gradient of lung attenuation may be observed. CT scanning demonstrating pleural effusions frequently accompanies these findings. Depending on the severity of ARDS, massive airspace consolidation and bilateral alveolar opacities eventually develop, corresponding to "full-blown ARDS." Later, the consolidation becomes inhomogeneous and more reticular in appearance (Fig. 19.4).

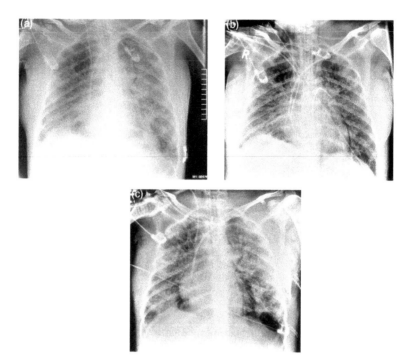

Figure 19.4 A 24-year-old patient who developed postpartal ARDS. (a–c) Repeated chest radiographs show (a) rather homogeneous dense opacities throughout both lung with air bronchograms (exudative ARDS), (b) a mixture of ground glass opacities and reticulation as well as pneumothorax on the left and pneumomediastinum (proliferative ARDS), and (c) patchy consolidation and reticulation with bilateral pneumothoraces (chest tube on the left) (proliferative/fibrotic ARDS).

The development of persistent patchy infiltrates may correspond to secondary infection. Mechanical ventilation may cause typical changes in lung morphology or even cause complications such as baro- and volutrauma with overdistension of the lung or pneumothorax and/or pneumomediastinum (Figs. 19.1 and 19.4). Sometimes these findings are very subtle and difficult to detect, for example, with the patient supine, a pneumothorax leads to an air collection anteriorly and often must be large to be detected. Careful inspection for lung density differences or paramediastinal double lines is necessary, but often hampered by the underlying imaging findings of ARDS and the overlying tubes and wires found on patients in ICUs. A film with the patient in lateral decubitus position and horizontal beam may increase the sensitivity to detect small pneumothoraces. CT is very helpful in this phase, as lung pathology can be detected with greater ease and with higher confidence than with plain radiography.

C. Proliferative and Fibrotic Stages/Stages III and IV (>7th Day)

After a week, the exudative or alveolar phase of ARDS evolves into an organizing and proliferative phase. The overall lung density decreases as consolidation gives way to a mixture of ground glass opacities and parenchymal distortion later developing into a coarser reticular, occasionally "bubbly" pattern due to the development of fibrosis (Figs. 19.4 and 19.5). Cysts may form ranging from a few millimeters to several centimeters in diameter. They can be subpleural or deep in the parenchyma. Rupture of a cyst can cause pneumothorax and/or pneumomediastinum (Fig. 19.4) (5). Follow-up studies have shown a relationship between late-stage fibrosis and areas with cyclic recruitment and collapse due to insufficient positive-end expiratory pressure (PEEP) levels. Atelectatic areas of lung parenchyma in the acute phase seem to be protected from ventilator-induced overdistension (9). It is important to realize, of course, that not every patient will evolve through all these phases in the same way (10).

III. CT Scan Protocols

There are no general standard CT scan protocols for ARDS patients. A contrast-enhanced spiral CT with contiguous 5 mm slices is helpful to obtain an overview of the thorax. For the minute evaluation of the lung parenchyma a "classic" HRCT with 1 mm slice thickness at 10 mm interval is often recommended.

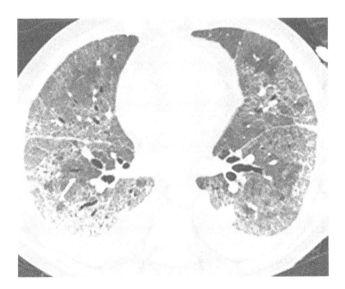

Figure 19.5 A 52-year-old patient with ARDS following an aspiration pneumonia. CT shows a mild reticular pattern representing the fibrotic phase, consolidation, and dilated peripheral airways due to PEEP ventilation and pleural effusion.

With multidetector CT (MDCT) becoming more widely available, volume scanning with high resolution is becoming reality. Thus, the advantages of spiral CT and HRCT can be combined within a single scan, using several reconstruction settings. Obviously, respiratory movement is associated with a severe degradation of image quality that significantly hampers image interpretation. It is preferable to acquire the scans during a breath-hold. For adequate image interpretation, the radiologist should be aware of the ventilation parameters, such as airway pressure and PEEP ventilation (Figs. 19.1 and 19.5). Accurate assessment of recruitment, atelectasis, alveolar collapse and consolidation as well as risk of a barotrauma is feasible only when these parameters are known. If particular breathing maneuvers have been performed directly prior to or during CT scanning, a functional evaluation is possible.

A. Advantages and Indications of CT

When CT imaging of ARDS was introduced, the heterogeneous distribution of density patterns with preference for the gravity-dependent regions was a new discovery. CT also demonstrated that small to moderate-sized pleural effusions were a frequent finding in ARDS (Fig. 19.5), whereas former descriptions on the basis of chest radiography described typical infiltrates without pleural effusion as characteristic. Comparative studies demonstrated the shortcomings of chest radiography in the ICU, for example, only 42% of bed-side chest radiographs were found to assess lung morphology correctly (11). CT brought about a massive improvement in the detection of abscesses, pneumothoraces, and malpositioned catheters. Overall, CT yielded additional diagnostic information over chest radiography in 66% of patients examined, which influenced therapeutic strategies in 22% (12).

Despite the well-known and accepted advantages of CT, its routine application in ARDS patients is still not general practice. Important reasons are the potential risks associated with the transport of a critically ill patient to the scanner room, cost, and radiation dose. In some centers with a clinical or scientific focus on ARDS, CT has been incorporated into routine clinical practice. There are even dedicated, mobile CT scanners available in some centers that have a high number of ICU beds. In many general hospitals, the use of CT in ARDS patients has risen during the last years and CT has become a frequently used imaging modality for patients from the ICU. The emergency indication for CT imaging of an ICU patient is the clinical dilemma of a deteriorating or nonimproving condition. Obviously, in such a devastating state, the whole procedure including transport, change of ventilation regime, apnea phase, and contrast media administration poses an imminent risk to the patient. Thus, there is still some controversy in the optimum approach regarding the clinical indications of CT in ARDS patients (13,14). One of the important factors that should be taken into consideration is workflow. This includes fast access of ICU patients to a high-performance, subsecond CT scanner (10,15), with everything prepared for the arrival of the critically ill patient. A well-trained team of radiologists, technicians, and anesthesiologists strongly enhances the quality of patient management and shortens the time needed for the set-up of the examination and scanning itself. Here, workflow issues which are already well-known from the diagnostic work-up of multitrauma patients referred from the emergency room and the role of the "golden hour" apply accordingly.

With regard to the difficulties in image interpretation of ARDS patients in the proliferative phase, CT scanning of patients with respiratory failure right at the onset, for example, on their way to the ICU, would significantly enhance the diagnostic and therapeutic impact of CT. It would also greatly facilitate the interpretation of repeated CT scans during follow-up such as the development of ARDS, complications (e.g., barotrauma), analysis of pre-existing pathologies, as well as the evaluation of treatment effects [e.g., the ventilation regime (PEEP)].

The main problem in the evaluation of different treatment options in ARDS—even by means of imaging—is the heterogeneity of individual patients. Treatment of the underlying disease is a determinant factor—an optimized ventilator regime cannot compensate for general sepsis caused by an intra-abdominal focus. The heterogeneity of patients also includes the morphology of ARDS as imaged by CT. This heterogeneity has an important impact on therapeutic strategies and might also contribute to the negative results derived from multicenter randomized studies for the evaluation of new therapies (14). Again, early referral for initial CT and follow-up studies would possibly improve the diagnostic impact.

IV. Pulmonary or Extrapulmonary ARDS

In the early phase, morphological differences of the appearance of the lung have been described between pulmonary and extrapulmonary causes of ARDS. Extrapulmonary ARDS (ARDS with a nonpulmonary etiology) reveals the typical symmetric distribution of normally aerated lung parenchyma, ground glass opacities, and posterior consolidation, whereas intrapulmonary ARDS (ARDS with a pulmonary etiology) may have a more asymmetric morphology with a combination of dense consolidation and ground glass opacities (Figs. 19.1, 19.3, and 19.6). This has been described in several studies, but most of them suffer from a small sample size and subject heterogeneity, which limit their value (9,11,16,17). Interestingly, lobectomy or pneumonectomy is classified as an extrapulmonary cause of ARDS causes in certain studies, but only the morphology of the nonoperated lung was evaluated (13). This particular entity of ARDS is called postpneumonectomy or postlobectomy edema. In a study focused on 17 of 583 patients developing ARDS following lobectomy or segmentectomy for neoplasms, an asymmetric ARDS morphology was described (18). Lung density was measured in corresponding regions of interest with a ventral and a dorsal localization. Astonishingly, the typical density increase in dependent

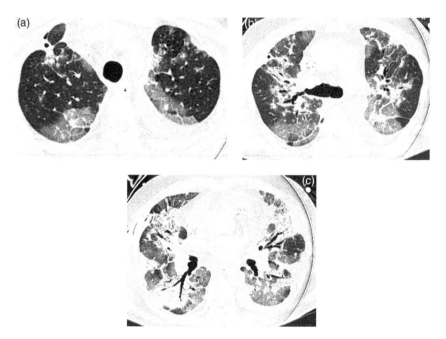

Figure 19.6 A 51-year-old patient with ARDS. CT shows asymmetric morphology with both consolidation and ground glass opacities (exudative ARDS). Note chest tube for pneumothorax on the right.

lung regions was found predominantly in the nonoperated, contralateral lung. The underlying pathophysiological mechanism remains unclear, and established models like impaired lymphatic drainage or hilar dissection causing inflammatory reactions do not completely explain these findings. Possible reasons may be the preferential contralateral influence of inflammatory mediators released in the operated lung, transfusion-related ALI (TRALI), and single lung ventilation during the operation with subsequent hyperinflation and increased alveolar oxygen tensions in the nonoperated lung. Another explanation may be the increased blood flow in the nonoperated lung during collapse of the operated lung, resulting in shear stress on the pulmonary vascular endothelium (18).

V. Basic Concepts of Therapy and Potential Complications

By definition, ARDS patients have an oxygenation index (PaO_2/FIO_2 ratio) of less than 200. However, the oxygenation index is not only used to define ARDS, but it is also one of the most important indicators of the efficacy of therapy and the settings on the ventilator. Various authors have proposed different scoring systems, such as the Murray score, (19) to grade ARDS severity. It grades the following clinical parameters on a scale of 0–4: the extent of chest infiltration on radiographs, the ratio of arterial oxygen tension to inspired oxygen concentration, the PEEP, and pulmonary compliance. The overall lung injury score is derived by dividing the total score by the number of criteria evaluated. Then, a score of 0 represents "no lung injury"; 0.1–2.5, "mild-to-moderate lung injury"; and >2.5, "severe lung injury." The CT Scan ARDS Study Group introduced the results of CT scanning in such a score and suggested oxygenation index as well as parameters derived from the pressure–volume (P/V) curve and CT scans (11). Such scoring systems are not widely established, because meta-analysis could not establish a correlation between outcome, PaO_2/FIO_2, and different lung injury scores (20).

The "open lung concept" plays a central role in ventilator therapy of ARDS. Its paradigm, "open the lung, and keep it open," aims to assure adequate gas exchange by recruitment of atelectatic lung with the least damage to pulmonary tissue and hemodynamics as possible. The use of PEEP is an important procedure in therapy, although the selection of the optimum PEEP is still a challenge and controversial. The individual PEEP requirement for a specific patient is often selected on the basis of a "trial and error" procedure, using repeated adjustments of the respirator pressures and blood gas analysis. Formal "peep trials" measuring cardiac output, oxygenation, and hemodynamics, with a pulmonary artery catheter, have also been described. Preliminary studies show a homogeneous distribution of ventilation with rising PEEP (0–20 cmH$_2$O) at a constant tidal volume, although there is still a lack of evidence for the benefit of PEEP on clinical outcome (21).

Prospective randomized multicenter studies were designed to address the contribution of different ventilatory strategies on the outcome of artificially ventilated patients in ARDS, which demonstrated a significantly improved outcome for low tidal volumes, avoidance of high peak airway pressures, and permissive hypercapnia (22). These "lung protective strategies" have gained wide clinical acceptance and use; however, their applicability to lung disorders other than ARDS remains controversial (23).

A. Prone Positioning

Another very simple means in respiration therapy of ARDS is prone positioning. The main physiological aims are (1) to improve oxygenation; (2) to improve respiratory mechanics; (3) to homogenize pleural pressure gradient, alveolar inflation, and ventilation distribution; (4) to increase lung volume and reduce atelectasis; (5) to facilitate the drainage of secretions; and (6) to reduce ventilator-associated lung injury (VALI). Prone positioning does not affect overall mortality, but studies of "proning" have shown that (1) oxygenation temporarily improves in ∼70–80% of ARDS patients; (2) the etiology of ARDS may affect the response to prone positioning; (3) extreme care is necessary when the maneuver is performed; and (4) ICU and hospital stay and mortality still remain high despite prone positioning (24). After repositioning from supine to prone position, CT demonstrates a redistribution of dense pulmonary opacities. This is associated with an improvement in oxygenation. Dependent opacities that resolve possibly represent atelectasis, whereas consolidation that does not change may represent pneumonia or hemorrhage. Unfortunately, there are no distinctive CT morphological features that have been identified, which predict response to prone positioning (25).

VI. Ventilator-Associated Lung Injury

Several mechanisms in current respiratory therapy can also lead to or aggravate lung damage. Termed "ventilator-associated lung injury," this entity relates to four major aspects of lung injuries: (1) gross air leaks induced by large transpulmonary pressures (barotrauma); (2) overdistention of aerated lung parenchyma which manifests as increased alveolo-capillary permeability (volutrauma); (3) cyclical recruitment and collapse of atelectasis which leads to high shear forces between collapsed and aerated alveoli as well as varying shunt fractions during the respiratory cycle (atelectrauma); and (4) release of various cytokine mediators (biotrauma) (23).

The cyclic recruitment and collapse of healthy lung compartments by mechanical ventilation can damage alveolar walls and their associated pulmonary capillaries. Because of many microscopic ruptures, alveolar air collects within lung parenchyma, interstitial emphysema develops, and pneumatoceles can result. These may be difficult to differentiate from postpneumonic cavitations. Early and subtle CT signs are regional or diffuse areas of low attenuation. Density measurements and a comparison with a previous scan are helpful in this situation. In addition, imaging may reveal pneumothorax, pneumomediastinum, pneumoperitoneum, or pneumoretroperitoneum. In theory, the localization of such air collections could give hints to its pathogenesis. Bullae in nondependent areas could be supported by overdistension of normally aerated lung regions, whereas bullae in middle or dependent regions may be attributed to shear forces from repetitive opening and closing of air spaces. These alveoli are recruited in inspiration but will collapse in expiration if the PEEP settings are too low.

VII. Long-Term CT Findings

In many ARDS survivors, reticular or cystic patterns may prevail, though there may be complete resolution of lung opacities and fibrosis. There seems to be a relationship between mechanical ventilation and the localization of fibrosis, air cysts, and bronchiectasis (Fig. 19.5). As cyclic recruitment and collapse as well as overdistension of pulmonary units cause lung tissue damage, lung areas which were exposed to high shear stress or high levels of inflammatory mediators during mechanical ventilation are prone to the development of fibrosis or air cysts. The most dependent (posterior) areas that were not recruited for ventilation and not exposed to the trauma of mechanical ventilation and toxic FiO_2 levels, do not tend to develop fibrosis. The better-ventilated, nondependent anterior areas more frequently show more pronounced fibrosis (26). The severity of the changes may be associated with higher inspiratory peak pressures (>30 mmHg), longer exposure to higher oxygen concentrations ($FiO_2 > 0.7$) (26), and the duration of mechanical ventilation (27).

VIII. Deeper Insights in ARDS and Mechanical Ventilation by Functional CT

Novel diagnostic approaches to further optimize mechanical ventilation and respiratory therapies in ARDS to decrease the high mortality and morbidity rates are urgently needed. There is continuous interest to determine and measure the effects of mechanical ventilation and the effects of PEEP on lung parenchyma, within the "open lung concept" (28). The main goal is to find the best compromise between overdistension caused by high peak pressures or large tidal volumes on one hand and cyclic recruitment and collapse of alveoli caused by very low PEEP levels on the other hand. In order to approach this dilemma, one focus of interest is the "lower inflection point" (LIP), which is a critical point of the P/V curve (29). It represents the pressure required to reopen distal bronchioles and alveoli.

The lung is sometimes referred to as a "sponge model," where the spaces within the "sponge" are either fluid- or air-filled (Fig. 19.7). In ARDS, a large amount of normally aerated lung parenchyma often coexist with other parts of

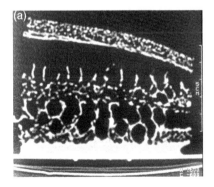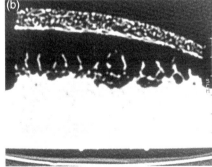

Figure 19.7 "Sponge model" of alveolar opening and collapse. CT of a sponge with little (a) and a large amount of (b) fluid representing alveolar flooding or collapsed alveoli on the bottom and air-filled spaces representing recruited alveoli on the top. Note that there are only two different states, fluid- or air-filled.

lung that are nonaerated. The patient is then at risk of lung overdistension at higher PEEP levels due to preferential ventilation to nonaffected alveolar units. This theory was confirmed by CT findings when well-aerated lung areas were shown to coexist with nonaerated areas, and an increase of PEEP resulted in additional alveolar recruitment and in overdistension (Fig. 19.8) (30). At the LIP on the lung P/V curve, air and tissue are more homogeneously distributed within the lungs, and increasing levels of PEEP result in additional alveolar recruitment without lung overdistension (31,32). At the same time, care should be taken that the tidal volume does not reach a peak pressure exceeding the

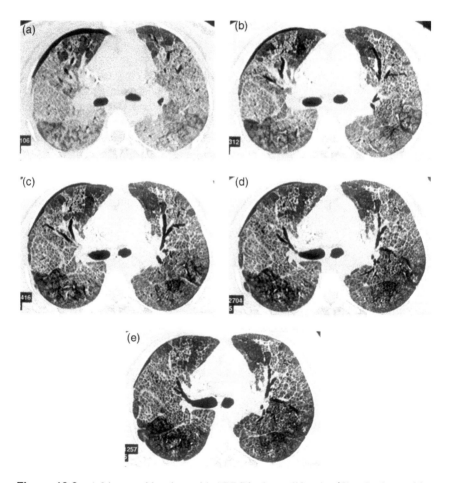

Figure 19.8 A 24-year-old patient with ARDS in the proliferative/fibrotic phase with a right-sided pneumothorax. CT was performed at different PEEP levels: (a) 10, (b) 15, (c) 20, (d) 25, and (e) 30 cmH$_2$O. The sequence illustrates the inhomogeneous behavior of aerated and nonaerated areas leading to both alveolar recruitment and overdistension.

upper inflection pressure, because further increases in tidal volume at this point results in overdistension of alveolar units without additional alveolar recruitment.

Early functional CT studies aiming at dynamic visualization of PEEP effects in ARDS were often limited to one to three slices $\sim$1 cm above the diaphragm covering a large lung area. The main advantage of this minimal slice technique is the limited radiation exposure compared with protocols scanning the entire lung volume. Low-dose protocols also allow for scanning at different respirator settings. Although these slices were thought to be representative of the entire lung, the inhomogeneous distribution of PEEP-induced reopening of collapsed lung regions has to be taken into consideration (33), as single slices may not be representative if density patterns are heterogeneously distributed.

The recent introduction of MDCT will improve spatial resolution and minimize acquisition time in lung imaging, but increase radiation exposure. Dedicated MDCT low-dose protocols have already been developed and tested in animal experiments and may lead to important insights into the pathogenesis and pathophysiologic alteration in ARDS. Although subjective image quality is rated inferior for low-dose CT as compared with standard-dose scans because of increased noise, information about extent, localization, and distribution of lung opacities is equally well provided by low-dose MDCT (34). With the use of low-dose MDCT, radiation exposure for ICU patients can be reduced significantly. Another new technique is dynamic cine CT, which can be performed with a temporal resolution of 100–250 ms (35). This temporal resolution is appropriate to observe attenuation changes during mechanical ventilation and has been applied to porcine ARDS models. Two of the more common porcine models include slow intravenous injection (>20 min) of oleic acid and repeated lung lavage with isotonic saline to wash out surfactant. The procedure is repeated until a low but stable PaO_2 between 50 and 100 mmHg is obtained. Other groups have injected intravenous endotoxin (*Escherichia coli* lipopolysaccharide) to induce ARDS. Obviously, different degrees of endothelial damage are associated with these three models (36), but imaging is fairly straightforward once the model has been developed.

Dynamic cine CT carries the already mentioned disadvantage that only a single slice at a subcarinal/supradiaphragmatic level is scanned. As imaging is performed during the whole respiratory cycle the lung will move, preferentially along the cranio–caudal axis, CT will look at slightly different parts of the lung all the time. At the present time there is no tool available to correct respiratory motion. Dynamic CT confirms that recruitment takes place during the whole inspiratory phase; different compartments with different opening pressures and recruiting characters as well as end-expiratory prevention of collapse by PEEP have been observed (37).

Several quantitative tools based on CT have been developed to image the lung in ARDS. Although CT is not able to visualize individual alveoli and their recruitment due to limited spatial resolution, the air content of the lung is represented by its CT attenuation. The density patterns of lung CT scans can be quantified if we assume a close correlation of the Hounsfield units (HU) of a voxel and the physical density of the volume of tissue that it represents. Depending on the respiratory level or whether the alveoli are collapsed or filled with fluid, a single voxel includes many alveoli, and thus a voxel with normal attenuation can consist of a heterogeneous mixture of atelectatic and overdistended alveoli instead of only normally aerated lung (15). The general concept of quantitative CT accepts the earlier mentioned imprecision to generalize the different densities of the depicted volume into one density value. As the total volume (volume$_{gas}$ + volume$_{tissue}$) of the ROI is known, the mean density within the ROI can be extracted from the image data, and as standard CT densities of gas and water are known, the following parameters can be calculated: volume of gas, volume of tissue, and the gas/tissue ratio. This calculation assumes that a linear relation of the CT density exists between 0 HU for water and − 1000 HU for pure gas. It has been demonstrated that ground glass opacification can be detected as soon as extravascular lung water increases. In the oleic acid-induced ARDS, there is a high correlation between the extravascular lung water and lung attenuation as in hydrostatic edema but the gravitational gradient is almost absent (38).

A basic precondition for an accurate classification is the segmentation of the lung fields, which is done manually by many authors. Accurate segmentation is crucial for evaluation to prevent misclassification of pleural effusion or portions of the chest wall. Semiautomatic or automatic algorithms have been successfully implemented. Intelligent software tools combine different density masks with anatomic knowledge and have shown a high correlation with an interactive manual segmentation procedure ($r^2 = 0.99$) (39). As the differences of such software tools do not affect our general understanding of recruitment, further details will not be discussed; however, all evaluation techniques, either lung segmentation or placement of regions of interests, are not standardized and may be affected by a high degree of intra- and interobserver variability.

The definition of specific density ranges related to different ventilatory states plays a pivotal role in the evaluation of functional and/or dynamic cine CT in ARDS. The appropriate density range will most clearly exhibit the biggest area change to mirror volumetric changes of lung between inspiration and expiration. There is some variety between different scanners from different manufacturers and different examination protocols, that is, slice thickness or reconstruction algorithms. It is generally accepted to separate well-ventilated lung (−910 to −700 or −900 to −501 HU) from hypoventilated lung or parenchyma with a maximum of 50% gas (−700 to −300 or −200 or −100, or −500 to −101 HU), from atelectasis or parenchyma with a maximum of 10% gas (−300 or −200 or −100 to 100 or 200 HU) and also from hyperinflated/overdistended lung as well as airways (−1024 to −910 or −1000 to −901 HU) (35,40,41). Markstaller et al. (42) were the first to describe different density ranges appropriate for largest increase in area during inspiration for healthy lungs and diseased (i.e., ARDS) lungs. Thus, a well-ventilated lung in a healthy subject corresponds to the density range -910 to -700 HU, whereas in ARDS it corresponds to -910 to -300 HU (35). Studies show a good correlation between nonaerated tissue and hypoxemia or shunt fraction.

Dynamic cine CT in a porcine model demonstrates lung collapse and reopening within the first seconds of expiration and inspiration, respectively (43). From such dynamic cine CT studies, pulmonary time constants of different compartments can be calculated. The detection of compartments with a different compliance can be used successfully to optimize the respirator settings (43). Dynamic cine CT has been applied in humans to visualize a "recruitment maneuver," with rising short-time PEEP up to $30-40$ cmH$_2$O for $3-6$ min in 10 ARDS patients. Recruitment improves oxygenation by expanding collapsed alveoli, without leading to severe hyperinflation (41).

The analysis of gravity-dependent gradients is also important in any functional CT study of ARDS. This analysis can be performed by dividing the anterior–posterior height of the lung into 10 equal intervals (21). In early ARDS, the "tissue" portion of the lung, most probably representing edema, was doubled in all compartments when compared with normal lungs. This finding of diffuse, homogeneous consolidation indicates the nongravitational distribution of edema. At the same time, the diffuse damage increases the weight of the lung, which results in an anterior–posterior pressure gradient, termed the "superimposed pressure". It causes compression of dependent portions and collapse of alveoli. Volume loss (especially in the caudal lung regions) is probably also related to heart weight and increased abdominal pressure. Prone positioning and PEEP can effectively counteract this mechanism (15).

Impaired gas exchange in ARDS is not only a problem of ventilation, but it is also a problem of perfusion, which is very difficult to measure by CT technology. Some studies showed a close correlation between lung tissue in excess, impairment of PaO_2, and increase in pulmonary artery pressure (44). Redistribution of pulmonary blood flow toward the upper lobes or uneven distribution of pulmonary edema are discussed as possible causes observed for the more pronounced excess lung tissue in the upper lobes at expiratory CT when compared with healthy subjects (14). Another reason for this finding may be a selection bias with different ARDS morphologies (lobar attenuation, diffuse attenuation, or patchy attenuation).

IX. Alternative to Radiological Imaging: Electrical Impedance Tomography

Electrical impedance tomography (EIT) represents a novel functional imaging technique for transthoracic visualization of changes in lung aeration. It is noninvasive, does not use ionizing radiation, and can be employed as a bedside test. The principle of EIT is the measurement of electrical impedance at the surface of the chest during continuous breathing (45).

The changes in impedance are produced by continuous electrical impulses measured by skin surface electrodes (16–32 in number) that are placed around the thorax. The technique is based on the different electrical properties of lung tissue compared with other thoracic tissues and their changes that are related to ventilation. One measurement cycle is finished once each single electrode has served as transmitter of such an electrical impulse. This leads to 208 different data points for changes in impedance during one measurement cycle. The measured impedances are then normalized using the impedance of a reference scan (46). Finally, these normalized changes in impedance and their regional distribution are used to generate a two-dimensional image. This map represents the relative time-dependent changes of intrathoracic gas volumes during inspiration and expiration. Temporal resolution is higher than 10 scans per second and thus better than MDCT. Spatial resolution, however (32 × 32 matrix) is far below CT. Obviously, only processes which influence the impedances at the surface of the thoracic wall, such as aeration, are visible by this technique. EIT was recently compared with different imaging techniques. Regional hypoventilation and enhanced ventilation in dependent lung areas can be assessed (47). As EIT detects changes in lung aeration it allows measurement of inspired tidal volumes with good correlation to plethysmography (48) and the estimation of alveolar collapse and recruitment in ARDS (49). EIT can also be applied to generate an image-based P/V curve. In an experimental setting, no differences in the LIP were found compared with a conventional P/V curve in healthy animals, whereas in a lavage ARDS model, the LIP determined by EIT demonstrated regional differences: LIP was significantly higher in the dependent lung than in the aerated nondependent lung (48). When EIT was compared with quantitative CT, changes in lung aeration are equally well depicted with both modalities (50).

X. Conclusion

CT plays a major role in the imaging approach to structure and function in ARDS. ARDS is characterized by a marked increase in lung consolidation and a massive, but heterogeneous, loss of aeration. In its earliest phases, ground glass opacities possibly correspond to alveolar and interstitial edema. Later in the course of ARDS widespread consolidation and atelectasis develop. As the disease progresses, the proliferative phase may lead to fibrotic changes. These fibrotic changes may partially improve over time.

CT has an impact on the optimization of the ventilatory strategies and allows for an accurate assessment of the volumes of gas and lung tissue and of lung aeration. Quantitative analysis requires delineation of lung parenchyma and dedicated postprocessing for calculation and color-coding of overdistended, normally aerated, poorly aerated, and nonaerated lung regions. Dynamic CT provides visualization of recruitment and collapse during the respiratory cycle, as well as the basis for the calculation of pulmonary ventilation time constants.

CT can also support the selection of the optimal PEEP level. EIT is a novel technique that may develop as an attractive bedside method to measure changes in ventilation.

References

1. Ashbaugh D, Bigelow D, Petty T, Levine B. Acute respiratory distress in adults. Lancet 1967; 2:319–323.
2. Bernard G, Artigas A, Brigham K, Carlet J, Falke K, Hudson L, Lamy M, Legall J, Morris A, Spragg R. The American–European consensus conference on ARDS. Definitions, mechanisms, relevant outcomes, and clinical trial coordination. Am J Respir Crit Care Med 1994; 149:818–824.
3. Miller P, Croce M, Bee T, Qaisi W, Smith C, Collins G, Fabian T. ARDS after pulmonary contusion: accurate measurement of contusion volume identifies high-risk patients. J Trauma 2001; 51:223–228.
4. Krafft P, Fridrich P, Pernerstorfer T, Fitzgerald R, Koc D, Schneider B, Hammerle A, Steltzer H. The ARDS: definitions, severity and clinical outcome. Intensive Care Med 1996; 22:519–529.
5. Ketai LH, Godwin JD. A new view of pulmonary edema and acute respiratory distress syndrome. J Thoracic Imaging 1998; 13:147–171.
6. Tomashefski J. Pulmonary pathology of the adult respiratory distress syndrome. Clin Chest Med 1990; 11:593–619.
7. Austin JHM, Müller NL, Friedman PJ, Hansell DM, Naidich DP, Remy-Jardin M, Webb WR, Zerhouni EA. Glossary of terms for CT of the lungs: recommendations of the nomenclature committee of the Fleischner Society. Radiology 1996; 200:327–331.
8. Kauczor H-U, Heussel C-P, Mildenberger P, Thelen M. Was heißt wie? Ansatz und Glossar zu Befundung und Verständnis in der HRCT der Lunge. Fortschr Röntgenstr 1996; 165:428–437.
9. Desai S, Wells A, Rubens M, Evans T, Hansell DM. Acute respiratory distress syndrome: CT abnormalities at long-term follow up. Radiology 1999; 210:29–35.
10. Desai S, Hansell D. Lung imaging in the ARDS: current practice and new insights. Intensive Care Med 1997; 23:7–15.
11. Rouby J, Puybasset L, Cluzel P, Richecoeur J, Lu Q, Grenier P. Regional distribution of gas and tissue in ARDS. II. Physiological correlations and definition of an ARDS severity score. Intensive Care Med 2000; 26:1046–1056.
12. Tagliabue M, Casella T, Zincone G, Fumagalli R, Salvini E. CT and chest radiography in the evaluation of adult respiratory distress syndrome. Acta Radiol 1994; 35:230–234.
13. Desai S, Wells A, Suntharalingam G, Rubens M, Evans T, Hansell D. Acute respiratory distress syndrome caused by pulmonary and extrapulmonary injury: a comparative CT study. Radiology 2001; 218:689–693.
14. Puybasset L, Cluzl P, Gusman P, Grenier P, Preteux F, Rouby J, Group aCss. Regional distribution of gas and tissue in acute respiratory distress syndrome. I. Consequences for lung morphology. Intensive Care Med 2000; 26:857–869.
15. Gattinoni L, Caironi P, Pelosi P, Goodman L. What has CT taught us about the ARDS? Am J Respir Crit Care Med 2001; 164:1701–1711.

16. Winer-Muram H, Steiner R, Gurney J, Shah R, Jennings S, Arheart K, Eltorky M, Meduri G. Ventilator-associated pneumonia in patients with adult respiratory distress syndrome: CT evaluation. Radiology 1998; 208:193–199.
17. Goodman L, Fumagalli R, Tagliabue P, Tagliabue M, Ferrario M, Gattinoni L, Pesenti A. Adult respiratory distress syndrome due to pulmonary and extra-pulmonary causes: CT, clinical, and functional correlation. Radiology 1999; 213:545–552.
18. Padley S, Jordan S, Goldstraw P, Wells A, Hansell DH. Asymmetric ARDS follow-ing pulmonary resection: CT findings—initial observations. Radiology 2002; 223:468–473.
19. Murray J, Matthay M, Luce J, Flick M. An expanded definition of the adult respir-atory distress syndrome. Am Rev Respir Dis 1988; 138:720–723.
20. Krafft P, Fridrich P, Pernerstorfer T, Fitzgerald R, Koc D, Schneider B, Hammerle A, Steltzer H. The acute respiratory distress syndrome: definitions, severity and clinical outcome. An analysis of 101 clinical investigations. Intensive Care Med 1996; 22:519–529.
21. Gattinoni L, Pelosi P, Crotti S, Valenza F. Effects of positive end-expiratory pressure on regional distribution of tidal volume and recruitment in adult respiratory distress syndrome. Am J Respir Crit Care Med 1995; 151:1807–1814.
22. The Acute Respiratory Distress Syndrome Network. Ventilation with lower tidal volumes as compared with traditional tidal volumes for acute lung injury and the acute respiratory distress syndrome. N Engl J Med 2000; 342:1301–1308.
23. Slutsky A, Ranieri V. Mechanical ventilation: lessons from the ARDSNet trial. Respir Res 2000; 1:73–77.
24. Pelosi P, Brazzi L, Gattinoni L. Prone position in acute respiratory distress syn-drome. Eur Respir J 2002; 20:1017–1028.
25. Papazian L, Paladini M, Bregeon F, Thirion X, Durieux O, Gainnier M, Huiart L, Agostini S, Auffray J. Can the tomographic aspect characteristics of patients presenting with acute respiratory distress syndrome predict improvement in oxygenation-related response to the prone position? Anesthesiology 2002; 97:599–607.
26. Nobauer-Huhmann I, Eibenberger K, Schaefer-Prokop C, Steltzer H, Schlick W, Strasser K, Fridrich P, Herold C. Changes in lung parenchyma after acute respiratory distress syndrome (ARDS): assessment with high-resolution computed tomography. Eur Radiol 2001; 11:2436–2443.
27. Treggiari M, Romand J, Martin J, Suter P. Air cysts and bronchiectasis prevail in nondependent areas in severe acute respiratory distress syndrome: a computed tomo-graphic study of ventilator-associated changes. Crit Care Med 2002; 30:1747–1752.
28. Valente-Barbas C. Lung recruitment maneuvers in acute respiratory distress syn-drome and facilitating resolution. Crit Care Med 2003; 31:S265–S271.
29. Richard J, Brochard L, Vandelet P, Breton L, Maggiore S, Jonson B, Clabault K, Leroy J, Bonmarchand G. Respective effects of end-expiratory and end-inspiratory pressures on alveolar recruitment in acute lung injury. Crit Care Med 2003; 31:89–92.
30. Lim C, Soon-Lee S, Seoung-Lee L, Koh Y, Sun-Shim T, Do-Lee S, Sung-Kim K, Kim D, Dong-Kim W. Morphometric effects of the recruitment maneuver on saline-lavaged canine lungs—a computed tomographic analysis. Anesthesiology 2003; 99:71–80.

31. Vieira S, Puybasset L, Lu Q, Richecoeur J, Cluzel P, Coriat P, Rouby J. A scanographic assessment of pulmonary morphology in acute lung injury. Significance of the lower inflection point detected on the lung pressure–volume curve. Am J Respir Crit Care Med 1999; 159:1612–1623.

32. Rouby J, Puybasset L, Nieszkowska A, Lu Q. Acute respiratory distress syndrome: lessons from computed tomography of the whole lung. Crit Care Med 2003; 31 (suppl 4):S285–S295.

33. Lu Q, Malbouisson L, Mourgeon E, Goldstein I, Coriat P, Rouby J. Assessment of PEEP-induced reopening of collapsed lung regions in acute lung injury: are one or three CT sections representative of the entire lung? Intensive Care Med 2001; 27:1504–1510.

34. Wildberger J, Max M, Wein B, Mahnken A, Weiss C, Dembinski R, Katoh M, Schaller S, Rossaint R, Gunther R. Low-dose multislice spiral computed tomography in acute lung injury: animal experience. Invest Radiol 2003; 38:9–16.

35. Markstaller K, Kauczor H-U, Eberle B, Weiler N, Siebertz D, Birkenkamp K, Heinrichs W, Thelen M. Multi-rotation CT during continuous ventilation: comparison of different density areas in healthy lungs and in the ARDS lavage model. Fortschr Roentgenstr 1999; 170:575–580.

36. Neumann P, Berglund J, Mondejar E, Magnusson A, Hedenstierna G. Dynamics of lung collapse and recruitment during prolonged breathing in porcine lung injury. J Appl Physiol 1998; 85:1533–1543.

37. Richard J, Maggiore S, Jonson B, Mancebo J, Lemaire F, Brochard L. Influence of tidal volume on alveolar recruitment. Respective role of PEEP and a recruitment maneuver. Am J Respir Crit Care Med 2001; 163:1609–1613.

38. Scillia P, Kafi S, Melot C, Keyzer C, Naeije R, Gevenois P. Oleic acid-induced lung injury: thin-section CT evaluation in dogs. Radiology 2001; 219:724–731.

39. Markstaller K, Arnold M, Döbrich M, Heitmann K, Karmrodt J, Weiler N, Uthmann T, Eberle B, Thelen M, Kauczor H-U. Software zur automatischen Quantifizierung von Belüftungszuständen bei akutem Lungenversagen in dynamischen CT-Aufnahmen der Lunge. Fortschr Röntgenstr 2001; 173:830–835.

40. Neumann P, Berglund J, Mondejar E, Magnusson A, Hedenstierna G. Effect of different pressure levels on the dynamics of lung collapse and recruitment in oleic acid-induced lung injury. Am J Respir Crit Care Med 1998; 158:1636–1643.

41. Bugedo G, Bruhn A, Hernandez G, Rojas G, Varela C, Tapia J, Castillo L. Lung computed tomography during a lung recruitment maneuver in patients with acute lung injury. Intensive Care Med 2003; 29:218–225.

42. Markstaller K, Kauczor H-U, Weiler N, Karmrodt J, Doebrich M, Ferrante M, Thelen M, Eberle B. Lung density distribution on dynamic CT correlates with oxygenation in ventilated pigs with lavage ARDS. Br J Anaesth 2005; 91:699–708.

43. Markstaller K, Eberle B, Kauczor H-U, Scholz A, Bink A, Thelen M, Heinrichs W, Weiler N. Temporal dynamics of lung aeration determined by dynamic CT in a porcine model of ARDS. Brit J Anaesth 2001; 87:459–468.

44. Gattinoni L, Pesenti A, Bombino M, Baglioni S, Rivolta M, Rossi F, Rossi G, Fumagalli R, Marcolin R, Mascheroni D. Relationships between lung computed tomographic density, gas exchange, and PEEP in acute respiratory failure. Anesthesiology 1988; 69:824–832.

45. Frerichs I, Schiffmann H, Hahn G, Hellige G. Non-invasive radiation-free monitoring of regional lung ventilation in critically ill infants. Intensive Care Med 2001; 27:1385–1394.

46. Barber D. A review of image reconstruction techniques for electrical impedance tomography. Med Phys 1989; 16:162–169.

47. Frerichs I, Hahn G, Hellige G. Gravity-dependent phenomena in lung ventilation determined by functional EIT. Physiol Meas 1996; 7(suppl 4A):A149–A157.

48. Kunst P, Bohm S, VazquezdeAnda G, Amato M, Lachmann B, Postmus P, deVries P. Regional pressure volume curves by electrical impedance tomography in a model of acute lung injury. Crit Care Med 2000; 28:178–183.

49. Kunst P, VazquezdeAnda G, Bohm S, Faes T, Lachmann B, Postmus P, deVries P. Monitoring of recruitment and derecruitment by electrical impedance tomography in a model of acute lung injury. Crit Care Med 2000; 28:3891–3895.

50. Frerichs I, Hinz J, Herrmann P, Weisser G, Hahn G, Dudykevych T, Quintel M, Hellige G. Detection of local lung air content by electrical impedance tomography compared with electron beam CT. J Appl Physiol 2002; 93:660–666.

20

Asthma: Assessment of Lung Ventilation with Hyperpolarized Helium-3 MR Imaging

EDUARD E. DE LANGE and **TALISSA A. ALTES**

University of Virginia Health Sciences Center,
Charlottesville, Virginia, USA

I. Introduction

Asthma is a chronic inflammatory disorder characterized by airway inflammation, recurrent episodes of wheezing, breathlessness, chest tightness, and cough. The symptoms are usually associated with widespread but variable airflow obstruction, caused by changes such as bronchoconstriction, edema, mucus plug formation, and airway remodeling (defined as a process of sustained disruption and modification of structural cells and tissues leading to the development of new airway wall morphology). There is an increase in airway hyperresponsiveness to a variety of stimuli such as allergens, irritants, cold air, and viruses (1).

The disease is relatively common with more than 17 million people affected in the United States. Asthma is the most common chronic respiratory disease of childhood, with more than two-thirds of patients being younger than 16 years (2,3). Over the last several decades there has been a steady increase in prevalence of asthma, and this trend is seen in all age groups, with the greatest increase in children (4). The rate of remission of asthma in children has been suggested to be ~50% (5,6). Asthma that begins after age 50 is thought to be more severe and less reversible than asthma that begins in childhood (7). In the United States, the disease is more common in African-Americans than in Whites. The disease is more prevalent among inner-city children when compared with those who live in the country, and in poor communities, asthma is generally more severe (8–10). In children born prematurely, the risk of developing the disease appears to be increased when compared with those who were born at full term (11).

Histopathologically, asthma is characterized by widespread plugging of the segmental, subsegmental, and smaller conducting airways by mucus and cellular debris. Although the material that plugs the airways may extend to the bronchioles, it usually does not fill the alveolar airspaces. The findings are caused by inflammation of the mucus-secreting airway epithelium leading to a mixture of mucus, inflammatory cells, plasma protein, and sloughed epithelium. In addition, there is an increase of the bronchial wall thickness, caused by thickening of the epithelial basement membrane from deposition of collagen fibrils and extracellular matrix, increase in size of the bronchial glands, and hypertrophy and hyperplasia of the airway smooth muscle (12–14). The inflammatory process is thought to be important in the pathogenesis of both bronchial hyperresponsiveness and reversible airflow obstruction. The end result is abnormal airway function and obstruction, leading to gas trapping and hyperinflation, with the result that asthmatics often have an elevated residual lung volume (12).

II. Diagnosis of Asthma

The diagnosis of asthma is usually straightforward in a young, atopic, nonsmoking subject with recurrent dyspnea, wheezing or chest tightness, and variable reversible airflow limitation. The symptoms may vary throughout the day and worsen at night or are triggered by factors such as exposure to allergens, exercise, viral infections, or fumes. Allergic rhinitis or atopic dermatitis may be present. Frequently, the patient has a family history of asthma, allergy, sinusitis, or rhinitis. Essential for the diagnosis is the presence of reversible airflow limitation or bronchial hyperresponsiveness. The diagnosis of asthma is more difficult to make when the patient is older, or there is a history of cigarette smoking or when airflow limitation is only partially reversible. In these cases, differentiation with other chronic obstructive pulmonary diseases may be difficult.

During physical examination, there may be hyperinflation of the thorax, wheezing, a prolonged expiratory phase, nasal secretions, sinusitis, rhinitis, nasal polyps, atopic or allergic dermatitis, or eczema. However, the diagnosis of asthma is not excluded when these symptoms are absent. Typically, there is bronchial hyperresponsiveness, which is characterized by a marked airway constrictor response to a variety of nonspecific inhaled stimuli such as methacholine, histamine, cold and dry air, hypertonic or hypotonic solutions, and pollutants in the atmosphere. The precise mechanism of the hyperresponsiveness is not known, although it is likely multifactorial. The increased airway hyperresponsiveness may be present even when the airway function is normal. There is no definite correlation between the degree of inflammation and the severity of the clinical symptoms. Interestingly, the degree of inflammation may be related to the airway hyperresponsiveness as measured by histamine or methacholine challenge (15).

Pulmonary function testing plays a crucial role in the diagnosis of asthma. Reversibility of lung function requires a 200 cc or 15% change in the forced expiratory volume in 1 s (FEV$_1$) following treatment with β-agonist such as Albuterol. The severity of asthma has been classified by the National Asthma Education and Prevention Program of the National Institutes of Health into mild intermittent, mild persistent, moderate persistent, and severe persistent, based on the clinical symptoms and the FEV$_1$ or peak expiratory flow (PEF) (Table 20.1) (1).

III. Treatment of Asthma

Asthma is treated using a variety of approaches. There are many allergens that have been associated with asthma including mites, cats, dogs, and cockroaches, and avoidance of these allergens is helpful. Although it may be difficult to achieve a low-allergen environment in the patient's homes, such an environment may lead to substantial improvement of clinical symptoms (16). Cigarette smoking causes exacerbations of the disease, and asthmatics who smoke may have a more rapid decline in their FEV$_1$ than those who do not smoke. Furthermore, there appears to be an association between passive smoking and the severity of asthma (17). Thus, cessation of smoking and avoidance of second-hand smoke are important for treatment of the disease. The most commonly used medical treatment for the bronchoconstrictive aspect of asthma consists of the use of short or long acting β_2-agonists brochodilator agents. These agents bind to the β_2-adrenoceptor present in the cell membrane of many of the cells of the

Table 20.1 Classification of Asthma Severity

Severity	Symptoms	Nighttime symptoms	PEF or FEV$_1$	PEF variability (%)
Mild intermittent	Symptoms ≤2 × per week Asymptomatic and normal PEF between exacerbations Exacerbations brief	≤2 × per month	≥80% predicted	<20
Mild persistent	Symptoms >2 × per week but <1 × per day Exacerbations may affect activity	>2 × per month	≥80% predicted	20–30
Moderate persistent	Symptoms daily Daily use of short acting β$_2$-agonist Exacerbations affect activity Exacerbations ≥2 × per week; may last days	>1 × per week	>60% to <80% predicted	>30
Severe persistent	Continual symptoms Limited physical activity Frequent exacerbations	Frequent	≤60% predicted	>30

Note: The presence of one of the features of severity is sufficient to place a patient in that category. An individual is assigned to the most severe grade in which any feature occurs. Patients at any level can have mild, moderate, or severe exacerbations. FEV$_1$, forced expiratory volume in 1 min; PEF, peak expiratory flow.
Source: Adapted and modified from National Asthma Education and Prevention Program; Expert Panel Report 2. (1).

airways. The greatest effect is on the smooth muscle of the airways leading to their relaxation that, in turn, leads to a reversal of the airflow obstruction. These agents also produce a bronchodilator effect in healthy, nonasthmatic individuals, although the extent of this effect is usually much smaller. Other treatments include anticholinergic bronchodilators, theophylline, leukotriene inhibitor agonists, and inflammatory mediator antagonists. Inhaled corticosteroids are considered to be the most effective treatment of asthma and are commonly used with moderate or severe disease (18).

IV. Radiologic Examination in Asthma

Chest radiography has played a limited role for the diagnosis or monitoring of the disease. In patients with uncomplicated asthma, chest radiography usually shows no discernible abnormalities (19). However, hyperinflation is the most common finding during an acute exacerbation of the disease (20). Standard chest radiographs are useful in excluding pneumonia or similar pathology in patients with an asthma exacerbation. In 30–42% of the patients with asthma bronchial wall thickening of the large airways may be seen on chest radiographs. Lung structures are better depicted with computed tomography (CT) than with radiography, and changes in lung and airway morphology are, therefore, demonstrated with increased sensitivity (21). However, neither CT nor lung radiography provides direct information about lung function. Changes in ventilation can only be inferred from morphological abnormalities such as hyperinflation, bronchial wall thickening, or air trapping. It is not clear whether these findings correlate with disease severity in asthmatics (22,23). Therefore, chest radiography and CT are limited in assessing functional abnormalities of the lung, and because both methods also have low sensitivity in demonstrating the asthma-induced morphologic lung changes, the techniques are of limited value in asthma. Although there have been studies with CT for studying the lung ventilation following inhalation of xenon gas, whereby well-ventilated regions of the lung show greater radiodensity due to increased concentrations of the gas when compared with poorly ventilated regions, xenon-inhaled CT has not gained broad acceptance as a method for assessing lung function. Pulmonary radionuclide ventilation/perfusion (V/Q) studies are also used to evaluate regional lung ventilation and have been used in asthmatics (24,25). However, radionuclide scanning is not routinely used in the clinical assessment of the disease because of its poor spatial resolution and exposure to ionizing radiation.

V. Hyperpolarized Noble Gas MR Imaging

Conventional ^{1}H MR imaging of the lung is limited because of respiratory motion artifact and low lung proton density, which provides a weak MR signal. In traditional proton MR, the nuclear spins of hydrogen atoms are aligned by the large static magnetic field of the MR scanner, but because of low proton density within the lung, this yields extremely low net magnetizations. In addition, in the lung, there are considerable susceptibility artifacts caused by numerous air/tissue interfaces. As a result, the airspaces are poorly depicted with ^{1}H MR imaging. Hyperpolarized noble gas MR imaging is a relatively new method that allows visualization of the lung airspaces following inhalation of hyperpolarized gas. Using specialized laser polarizers, two nonradioactive isotopes of noble gases can be polarized, helium-3 (^{3}He) and xenon (^{129}Xe), allowing the nuclear spins of the gas atoms to be brought into alignment outside the MR scanner. The resulting large nonequilibrium polarization of the nuclei, which can be 10^4 to 10^5 times greater than that of the thermal equilibrium polarization of water protons in conventional MR systems, is the key feature of the hyperpolarized gases and allows for sufficient signal to image airspaces despite the low physical density of the gases in the lung (26,27). A particular advantage of ^{3}He is that its magnetic moment is larger than that of ^{129}Xe leading to MR signal intensity which is more than several times greater than that of ^{129}Xe for a given polarization density (28,29). Other advantages of ^{3}He over ^{129}Xe are that it does not have anesthetic effects and it has no biological activity. For these reasons, ^{3}He gas has been primarily used for imaging of the lung in humans. However, in the United States, the Food and Drug Administration has not yet approved ^{3}He gas for medical use, and at present, it is used as an investigational contrast agent for MR imaging of the lungs.

When hyperpolarized ^{3}He gas is inhaled, the gas quickly fills the lung airspaces. When MR imaging is performed immediately following the gas inhalation, the well-ventilated, gas-filled regions of the lung display high signal intensity. Regions with diminished ventilation show decreased signal intensity and those regions that do not fill with the gas, and thus are not ventilated, show as areas with no signal intensity and are referred to as ventilation defects. On the basis of these findings, it is assumed that hyperpolarized ^{3}He MR imaging of the lung provides a visual display of the pulmonary gas distribution (ventilation) without the use of ionizing radiation. In a recent study, while comparing hyperpolarized ^{3}He MR findings with those of ventilation xenon-133 scintigraphy, the standard imaging technique for assessing the lung ventilation, there was a good correlation in findings between the two modalities, supporting the assumption that with hyperpolarized MR imaging, the ventilatory changes of the lung are visualized (30). A major advantage of hyperpolarized ^{3}He MR imaging compared to xenon-133 scintigraphy is that images are obtained with much higher spatial resolution, and thus ventilatory changes of the lung are visualized with greater detail. Hyperpolarized ^{3}He MR has been performed in normal volunteers for investigation of a variety of lung diseases, such as emphysema, asthma, and cystic fibrosis, and for assessment of patients after lung transplantation and cancer (31–42).

In asthma, hyperpolarized ^{3}He MR imaging has the potential to provide direct visualization of the pulmonary functional impairment that characterizes the disease as a result of airway inflammation, bronchoconstriction, mucus plug formation, and airway remodeling. In particular, the technique appears to be ideal for visualization of the subsegmental obstructional changes of the small airways that are common with the disease. Hyperpolarized ³He MR may provide insight into the changes that occur in the lung with disease progression and treatment. In the following sections, we will present, on the basis of our initial experiences, the findings of hyperpolarized ³He MR imaging in subjects with treated and untreated asthma and those undergoing asthma provocation testing.

VI. Hyperpolarized Helium-3 MR of Untreated Asthma

There is great variation in extent and size of the ³He MR ventilation defects in patients with asthma. However, there appears to be a correlation between the severity of the imaging findings and severity of disease. Mild asthmatics usually have small defects, with the lesions typically being pleural-based at the periphery of the lung, likely resulting from closure of the subsegmental bronchi, either by bronchoconstriction or by mucus plugging, or both (Fig. 20.1). In patients with more severe disease, there are an increased number of defects that may also involve the more central portions of the lung, although the pleural-based appearance is still present.

Although a correlation between the severity of defects and disease severity as measured by spirometry appears to be present, the correlation between clinical symptoms and number of defects is less obvious. For instance, in an investigation involving subjects with varying asthma severity and age-matched nonasthmatic volunteers, we found that the asthmatics had significantly greater number of ventilation defects than the normal volunteers (42,43). However, when comparing the imaging findings of the asthmatics according to their disease severity (mild intermittent, mild persistent, moderate persistent, severe persistent), the number of defects correlated poorly, and there was marked overlap between the groups (43). Most likely, the poor correlation is because the recording of clinical symptoms is based on subjective, self-reporting by the patients and not on objective measures. However, when comparing the number of ventilation defects with the findings of spirometry, much better correlations were found, with best correlation for FEV_1/FVC ($r = -0.78$) followed by percent predicted FEV_{25-75} ($r = -0.65$) and FEV_1 ($r = -0.55$).

We have also noted in few asthmatics who were imaged over a period of several days to weeks that some ventilation defects spontaneously resolved and new defects appeared (Fig. 20.2). It seems likely that the variation of defects relates to the natural behavior of the disease, whereby over time, varying airways close and open, likely from the combination of bronchospasm, airway edema, and mucous plugging. In many cases, we have also observed that some defects remained in the same location, suggesting that persistence of the

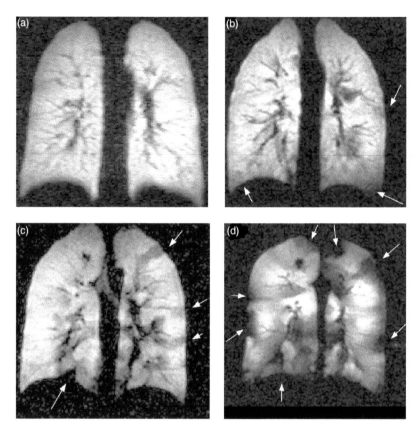

Figure 20.1 Coronal hyperpolarized helium-3 MR images of the lungs obtained in a (a) healthy nonasthmatic volunteer and subjects with (b) mild (FEV_1 132% of predicted), (c) moderate (FEV_1 83% of predicted), and (d) severe asthma (FEV_1 34% of predicted). There is homogenous distribution of the gas signal in the lungs without ventilation defects. In the asthmatics, ventilation defects are observed (arrows). There are fewer defects in the subject with mild asthma and greater in the subject with severe disease.

defects over time represents a chronic feature of the disease. This is currently being studied.

VII. Hyperpolarized Helium-3 MR Following Provocation of Asthma

As described earlier, the clinical symptoms of asthma and changes in the pulmonary function can be triggered by numerous stimuli. We have performed studies to determine how hyperpolarized ^{3}He MR imaging depicts the ventilatory changes

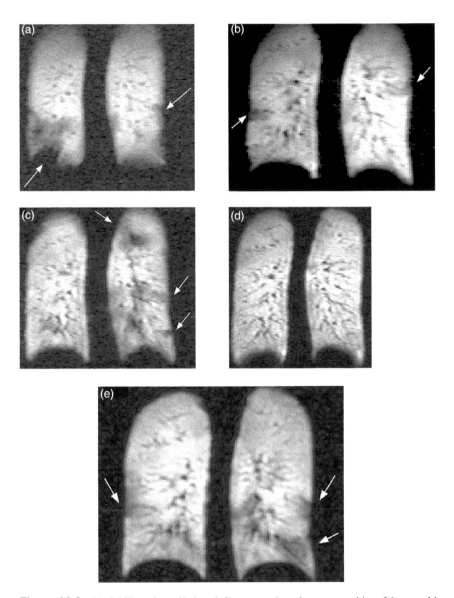

Figure 20.2 Variability of ventilation defects over time demonstrated in a 26-year-old asthmatic. Coronal images are depicted at the same anatomical level. (a) Image obtained at baseline (FEV$_1$ 82% of predicted) shows relatively large, bilateral defects (arrows), predominantly at the lung bases. (b) After 3 weeks (FEV$_1$ 84% of predicted), most defects have resolved and new small defects (arrows) are observed bilaterally. (c) After 4 months (FEV$_1$ 83% of predicted), there are new defects on the left (arrows) and no increase in the number of defects on the right. (d) After 4 months (FEV$_1$ 83% of predicted), there are no defects at all. (e) Two and a half years later (FEV$_1$ 73% of predicted), there is heterogeneity of the signal at the lung bases bilaterally and several relatively large defects are present (arrows).

that occur in the lung following disease provocation with exercise and methacholine.

A. Exercise Challenge Testing

In asthmatics, exercise may act to trigger airflow obstruction. However, there does not appear to be a strong correlation between the clinical severity of asthma and the severity of exercise-induced asthma. As a result, the exercise challenge test is a poor tool for distinguishing differences in clinical severity between asthmatics (44). Asthma symptoms can be induced in many asthmatics if they exercise at a high level, and thus prevent continued exercise because of symptom severity. Asthmatic patients may notice that different types of exercise provoke symptoms. With swimming in an out-door pool, for example, exercise-induced asthma is far less severe than with running, and this is thought to be related to the fact that air is breathed when swimming is humid, whereas the air inhaled when running is drier (45,46). The changes in lung function which occur in response to $\sim$6 min of exercise are quite characteristic. With the beginning of exercise, there is little change or some improvement of lung function. With further exertion, however, lung function begins to deteriorate. There may be a plateau effect as increasing the duration or severity of exercise, usually, does not lead to further airflow obstruction. After stopping exercise lung function falls, with the major decrease usually occurring 5–10 min after completion of exertion. Lung function then returns spontaneously to baseline, or higher, over the next 30–45 min (47).

Studies have shown that after the initial exercise, asthmatics can become refractory to subsequent exercise challenges repeated over a short period (48). The refractoriness may be caused by inhibitory prostaglandins that are released during the first exercise period (49). This initial exercise may be in the form of a brief warming-up period or a single, more prolonged period of exercise. Continued refractoriness to airflow obstruction depends upon the time between the exercise challenges. The half-life of this effect is $\sim$45 min, so that after $\sim$2–3 h the asthmatic is again fully responsive to an exercise challenge (50).

In a recent study in which we performed hyperpolarized ^{3}He MR imaging in six subjects with exercise-induced asthma and one healthy volunteer, we found that in four, who had ventilation defects at baseline and normal spirometry, the initial ventilation defects improved in some cases after exercise, while new defects also appeared (51). However, overall there was a significant increase in the number of defects and a decrease in the lung function (FEV_1). Two of the subjects had extensive changes in their ventilation patterns with the development of large defects. No ventilation defects developed in the healthy volunteer. In some asthmatics with exercise-induced asthma, we have seen improvement of the ventilation defects with delayed imaging, paralleling the improvement of the lung function after the initial deterioration (Fig. 20.3).

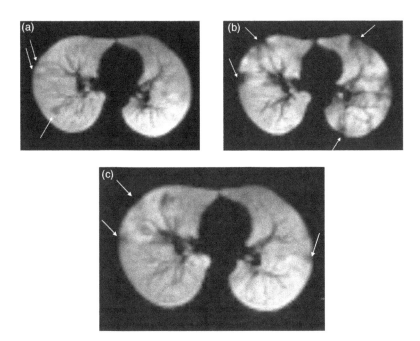

Figure 20.3   Exercise-induced asthma. (a) Axial image obtained in 22-year-old patient with exercise induced asthma. A few small ventilation defects (arrows) are seen (FEV$_1$ 107% of predicted). (b) After exercising for 6 min on a treadmill, a large number of defects (several indicated with arrows) have developed bilaterally as demonstrated in the lung image obtained 5 min after exercise (FEV$_1$ 65% of predicted). (c) On the delayed image obtained 90 min after stopping with exercise, most of the defects have resolved with few small remaining (arrows), and lung function has improved (FEV$_1$ 99% of predicted).

B.   Methacholine Challenge Testing

Bronchial challenge tests with inhaled methacholine are often used to determine whether a patient has airway hyperresponsiveness. This test is most useful in a patient with atypical asthmatic symptoms. Increasing concentrations of the methacholine are inhaled, while the effect on FEV$_1$ is monitored. The most commonly used index of response is the provoking concentration (PC$_{20}$) or dose (PD$_{20}$) causing a reduction in FEV$_1$ of 20%. The level of responsiveness correlates with the severity of asthma as assessed by current symptoms or treatment requirements (52).

Hyperpolarized ^{3}He imaging in three asthmatics following administration of the PC$_{20}$ dose of methacholine demonstrated a marked increase in the number and size of defects compared with the baseline studies (Fig. 20.4) (51). A marked decrease in the FEV$_1$ also developed after methacholine

---

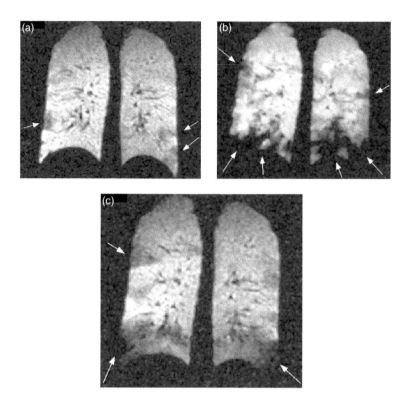

Figure 20.4 Methacholine challenge. (a) Coronal ventilation image obtained in a 25-year-old mild asthmatic shows a few small defects (arrows) in the periphery of the lung bilaterally (FEV$_1$ 118% of predicted). (b) After administration of the PC$_{20}$ dose of methacholine, there is marked increase in the number of ventilation defects (arrows) and deterioration of lung function (FEV$_1$ 73% of predicted). (c) After subsequent inhalation of a short acting β-agonist, lung function normalizes again (FEV$_1$ 123% of predicted), and there is improvement of the observed ventilation defects (arrows).

administration. In contrast, methacholine administered to a healthy volunteer did not result in development of defects or a significant decrease in FEV$_1$.

VIII. Hyperpolarized Helium-3 MR Following Treatment of Asthma

Hyperpolarized ^{3}He imaging has been performed in asthmatics immediately before and 20–40 min following treatment with an inhaled, short-acting β_2-agonist (Albuterol). In each case, pleural-based ventilation defects were noted on the initial MR scan. In some subjects, the defects resolved completely following inhalation of the bronchodilator (Fig. 20.5). However, in other subjects, there

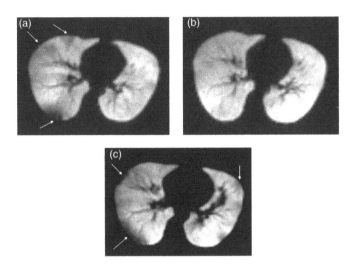

Figure 20.5   Effect of inhalation of a bronchodilator. (a) Axial hyperpolarized helium-3 image of 28 year patient with mild persistent asthma shows several defects (arrows) at baseline (FEV$_1$ 88% of predicted). (b) Image obtained 40 min after inhalation of a short acting β-agonist bronchodilator shows marked improvement of the defects (FEV$_1$ 103% of predicted). (c) Image obtained 5 h later demonstrates re-occurrence of several of the defects (arrow) as lung function diminished (FEV$_1$ 93% of predicted).

was a decrease in the number and size of the observed defects without their complete resolution. Ventilation defects recurred on delayed imaging when the bronchodilator effect diminished. Although only a small number of subjects were investigated, the findings indicate that the response to treatment can be assessed with hyperpolarized ^{3}He imaging; however, more experience will be needed to determine the effects of various forms of treatment.

IX. Summary

Asthma is a common chronic inflammatory disorder of the airways characterized by airflow obstruction and variable clinical symptoms. Bronchial hyperresponsiveness is a key feature of the disease causing marked airway constriction in response to a variety of stimuli. Chest radiography and CT play little role in the diagnosis and monitoring of the disease. Hyperpolarized ^{3}He MR imaging is a new technique for imaging of lung ventilation without the use of ionizing radiation. Although initial studies of hyperpolarized helium-3 gas in asthmatics have shown relatively poor correlation with the clinical symptoms, the extent of the ^{3}He ventilation defects appears to correlate with spirometry. Furthermore, the changes in ^{3}He ventilation caused by stimuli that trigger an asthma attack such as methacholine or exercise, as well as the effects of a bronchodilator, are well visualized. Hyperpolarized ^{3}He MR imaging may become an important tool in the assessment of the ventilatory changes that occur in the lungs of asthmatics. The technique may also become a valuable method to diagnose and monitor the disease. The imaging method also holds promise for evaluating the efficacy of various asthma treatments.

Acknowledgments

Supported partly by NIH 1R01 HL66479, Virginia Commonwealth Technology Research Fund, Siemens Medical Solutions, Iselin, NJ, and Amersham Health, Durham, NC.

References

1. National Asthma Education and Prevention Program Expert Panel Report 2. Guidelines for the Diagnosis and Management of Asthma, National Institutes of Health, National Heart, Lung, and Blood Institute. NIH Publication No. 97–4051, 1997.
2. Yunginger JW, Reed CE, O'Connell EJ, Melton LJ III, O'Fallon WM, Silverstein MD. A community-based study of the epidemiology of asthma: incidence rates, 1964–1983. Am Rev Respir Dis 1992; 146:888–894.
3. McWhorter WP, Polis MA, Kaslow RA. Occurrence, predictors, and consequences of adult asthma in NHANESI and follow-up survey. Am Rev Respir Dis 1989; 139:721–724.
4. National Health Lung and Blood Institute. Morbidity and Mortality Chartbook, 2000. http://www.nhlbi.nih.gov/resources/docs/cht-book.htm.
5. Strachan DP, Butland BK, Anerson HR. Incidence and prognosis of asthma and wheezing illness from early childhood to age 33 in a national British cohort. Br Med J 1996: 312:1195–1199.
6. Johnson JA, Boe J, Berlin E. The longterm prognosis of childhood asthma in predominantly rural Swedish county. Acta Paediatr Scand 1987; 76:950–954.
7. Vergnenegre A, Antonini MT, Bonnaud F, Melloni B, Mignonat G, Bousquet J. Comparison between late onset and childhood asthma. Allergol Immunopathol Madr 1992; 20:190–196.
8. Crain EF, Weiss KB, Bijur PE, Hersh M, Westbrook L, Stein RE. An estimate of the prevalence of asthma and wheezing among inner-city children. Pediatrics 1994; 94: 356–362.
9. Duran-Tauleria E, Rona RJ. Geographical and socioeconomic variation in the prevalence of asthma symptoms in English and Scottish children. Thorax 1999; 54:476–481.
10. Mielck A, Reitmeir P, Wjst M. Severity of childhood asthma by socioeconomic status. Int J Epidemiol 1996; 25:388–393.
11. Von Mutius E, Nicolai T, Martinez FD. Prematurity as a risk factor for asthma in preadolescent children. J Pediatr 1993; 123:223–229.

12. Hogg JC. Airway pathology. In: Barnes P, Drazen JM, Rennard S, Thomson NC, eds. Asthma and COPD. Basic Mechanisms and Clinical Management. London: Academic Press, 2002:57–66.

13. Huber HL, Koessler KK. The pathology of bronchial asthma. Arch Int Med 1922; 30:689–760.

14. Messer J, Peters GA, Bennet WA. Cause of death and pathological findings in 304 cases of bronchial asthma. Dis Chest 1960; 38:616–624

15. Barnes PJ, Drazen JM. Pathophysiology of asthma. In: Barnes P, Drazen JM, Rennard S, Thomson NC, eds. Asthma and COPD. Basic Mechanisms and Clinical Management. London: Academic Press, 2002:343–359.

16. Custovic A, Woodcock A. Allergen avoidance. In: Barnes P, Drazen JM, Rennard S, Thomson NC, eds. Asthma and COPD. Basic Mechanisms and Clinical Management. London: Academic Press, 2002:489–507.

17. Larsson ML, Frisk M, Hallstrom J, Kiviloog J, Lundback B. Environmental tobacco smoke exposure during childhood is associated with increased prevalence of asthma in adults. Chest 2001; 120:711–717.

18. Barnes PJ. Corticosteroids. In: Barnes P, Drazen JM, Rennard S, Thomson NC, eds. Asthma and COPD. Basic Mechanisms and Clinical Management. London: Academic Press, 2002:547–564.

19. Hodson ME, Simon G, Batten JC. Radiology of uncomplicated asthma. Thorax 1974; 29:296–303.

20. Petheram IS, Kerr IH, Collins JV. Value of chest radiographs in severe acute asthma. Clin Radiol 1981; 32:281–282.

21. Paganin F, Trussard V, Seneterre E, Chanez P, Giron J, Godard P, Senac JP, Michel FB, Bousquet J. Chest radiography and high resolution computed tomography of the lungs in asthma. Am Rev Respir Dis 1992; 146:1084–1087.

22. Paganin F, Seneterre E, Chanez P, Daures JP, Bruel JM, Michel FB, Bousquet J. Computed tomography of the lungs in asthma: influence of disease severity and etiology. Am J Respir Crit Care Med 1996; 153:110–114.

23. Newman KB, Lunch DA, Newman LS, Ellegood D, Newell J Jr. Quantitative computed tomography detects air trapping due to asthma. Chest 1994; 106:105–109.

24. Agnew JE, Bateman JR, Pavia D, Clarke SW. Radionuclide demonstration of ventilatory abnormalities in mild asthma. Clin Sci 1984, 66:525–531.

25. Vernon P, Burton GH, Seed WA. Lung scan abnormalities in asthma and their correlation with lung function. Eur J Nucl Med 1986; 12:16–20.

26. Middleton H, Black RD, Saam B, Cates GD, Cofer GP, Guenther R, Happer W, Hedlund LW, Johnson GA, Juvan K et al. MR imaging with hyperpolarized ^{3}He gas. Magn Reson Med 1995; 33:271–275.

27. MacFall JR, Charles HC, Black RD, Middleton H, Swartz JC, Saam B, Driehuys B, Erickson C, Happer W, Cates GD, Johnson GA, Ravin CE. Human lung airspaces: potential for MR imaging with hyperpolarized ^{3}He. Radiology 1996; 200:553–558.

28. Albert MS, Cates GD, Driehuys B et al. Biological magnetic resonance imaging using laser-polarized ^{129}Xe. Nature 1994; 370:199–201.

29. Mugler JP, Driehuys B, Brookeman JR, Cates GD, Berr SS, Bryant RG, Daniel TM, de Lange EE, Downs JH III, Erickson CJ, Happer W, Hinton DP, Kassel NF, Maier T, Phillips CD, Saam BT, Sauer KL, Wagshul ME. MR imaging and spectroscopy using hyperpolarized ^{129}Xe gas: preliminary human results. Magn Reson Med 1997; 37:809–815.

30. Altes TA, Rehm PK, Harrell F, Salerno M, Daniel TM, de Lange EE. Ventilation imaging of the lung: comparison of hyperpolarized helium-3 MR imaging with Xe-133 scintigraphy. Acad Radiol 2004; 11:729–734.
31. MacFall JR, Charles HC, Black RD, Middleton H, Swartz JC, Saam B, Driehuys B, Erickson C, Happer W, Cates GD, Johnson GA, Ravin CE. Human lung airspaces: potential for MR imaging with hyperpolarized ^{3}He. Radiology 1996; 200:553–558.
32. Kauczor HU, Hofmann D, Kreitner KF, Nilgens H, Surkau R, Heil W, Potthast A, Knopp MV, Otten EW, Thelen M. Normal and abnormal pulmonary ventilation: visualization at hyperpolarized ^{3}He MR imaging. Radiology 1996; 201:564–568.
33. Kauczor HU, Ebert M, Kreitner KF, Nilgens H, Surkau R, Heil W, Hofmann D, Otten EW, Thelen M. Imaging of the lungs using ^{3}He MRI: preliminary clinical experience in 18 patients with and without lung disease. J Magn Reson Imaging 1997; 7:538–543.
34. de Lange EE, Mugler JP III, Brookeman JR, Knight-Scott J, Truwit JD, Teates CD, Daniel TM, Bogorad PL, Cates GD. Lung air spaces: MR imaging evaluation with hyperpolarized ^{3}He gas. Radiology 1999; 210:851–857.
35. Donnelly LF, MacFall JR, McAdams HP, Majure JM, Smith J, Frush DP, Bogonad P, Charles HC, Ravin CE. Cystic fibrosis: combined hyperpolarized ^{3}He-enhanced and conventional proton MR imaging in the lung-preliminary observations. Radiology 1999; 212:885–889.
36. Moller HE, Chen XJ, Saam B, Hagspiel KD, Johnson GA, Altes TA, de Lange EE, Kauczor HU. MRI of the lungs using hyperpolarized noble gases. Magn Reson Med 2002; 47:1029–1051.
37. McAdams HP, Palmer SM, Donnelly LF et al. Hyperpolarized ^{3}He-enhanced MR imaging of lung transplant recipients: preliminary results. Am J Roentgenol 1999; 173:955–959.
38. Salerno M, Altes TA, Mugler JP III, Nakatsu M, Hatabu H, de Lange EE. Hyperpolarized noble gas MR imaging of the lung: potential clinical applications. Eur J Radiol 2001; 40:33–44.
39. de Lange EE, Altes TA, Jones DR, Daniel TM, Dalerno MS, Brookeman JR, Mugler JP. Bronchiolitis obliterans following lung transplantation: evaluation with hyperpolarized helium-3 MR imaging. In: Proceedings of the International Society for Magnetic Resonance in Medicine, 9th Meeting, 2001.
40. Salerno M, de Lange EE, Altes TA, Truwit JD, Brookeman JR, Mugler JP III. Emphysema: hyperpolarized helium 3 diffusion MR imaging of the lungs compared with spirometric indexes-initial experience. Radiology 2002; 222:252–260.
41. Gast KK, Viallon M, Eberle B, Lill J, Puderbach MU, Hanke AT, Schmiedeskamp J, Kauczor HU. MRI in lung transplant recipients using hyperpolarized ^{3}He: comparison with CT. J Magn Reson Imaging 2002; 15:268–274.
42. Altes TA, Powers PL, Knight-Scott J, Rakes G, Platts-Mills TAE, de Lange EE, Alford BA, Mugler JP, Brookeman JR. Hyperpolarized ^{3}He MR lung ventilation imaging in asthmatics: preliminary findings. J Magn Reson Imaging 2001; 13:378–384.
43. de Lange EE, Altes TA, Alford BA, Mugler JP. Hyperpolarized helium-3 MR imaging of the lung in asthmatics: correlation of imaging findings with clinical symptoms and spirometry. European Society of Thoracic Imaging Annual Meeting, Lausanne, Switzerland, June 2003.

44. Godfrey S. Exercise as a trigger. In: Barnes P, Drazen JM, Rennard S, Thomson NC, (eds). Asthma and COPD. Basic Mechanisms and Clinical Management. London: Academic Press, 2002:421–429.

45. Fitch KD, Morton AR. Specificity in exercise-induced asthma. Br Med J 1971; 4:577–581.

46. Godfrey S, Siverman M, Anderson SD. Problems of interpreting exercise induced asthma. J Allergy Clin Immunol 1973; 52:199–209.

47. Silverman M, Anderson SD. Standardization of exercise tests in asthmatic children. Arch Dis Child 1972; 47:882–889.

48. McNeill RS, Nairn JR, Millar JS, Ingram CG. Exercise induced asthma. Q J Med 1966; 35:55–67.

49. Manning PJ, Watson RM, O'Byrne PM. Exercise-induced refractoriness in asthmatic subjects involves leukotriene and prostaglandin interdependent mechanisms. Am Rev Respir Dis 1993; 148:950–954.

50. Edmunds AT, Tooley M, Grodfrey S. The refractory period after exercise-induced asthma, its duration and relation to severity of exercise. Am Rev Respir Dis 1978; 117:247–254.

51. Samee S, Altes TA, Powers P, de Lange EE, Knight-Scott J, Rakes G, Mugler JP, Ciambotti JM, Alford BA, Brookeman JR, Platts-Mills TAE. Imaging the lungs in asthmatics using hyperpolarized helium-3 MR: assesment of response to methacholine and exercise challenge. J Allergy Clin Immunol 2003; 111:1205–1211.

52. Josephs LK, Gregg I, Mullee MA, Holgate ST. Nonspecific bronchial reactivity and its relationship to the clinical expression of asthma. A longitudinal study. Am Rev Respir Dis 1989; 140:350–357.

21

The Role of Computed Tomography in Emphysema and Lung Volume Reduction Surgery

KEVIN R. FLAHERTY and **FERNANDO J. MARTINEZ**

University of Michigan Health System,
Ann Arbor, Michigan, USA

I. Introduction

Over 11 million people in the United States were estimated to have chronic obstructive pulmonary disease (COPD) in the year 2000 (1). Approximately

9.4 million patients have chronic bronchitis and 3.1 million patients have emphysema (1). In the United States, COPD is the fourth leading cause of death and the leading pulmonary cause of death (1). Worldwide, COPD is expected to rank fifth in terms of morbidity and mortality by the year 2020 (2). Recent reviews have defined the current pharmacological and nonpharmacological therapies in COPD (3). Unfortunately, despite medical advances, significant limitation in quality of life persists. As such, much effort has been devoted to the identification of surgical options for selected patients, including lung volume reduction surgery (LVRS) (4). LVRS has been identified as a viable treatment for selected patients with advanced emphysema (5). An understanding of imaging for emphysema is crucial to understand the appropriate role of LVRS in selected patients.

Traditionally, emphysema has been defined anatomically as the abnormal permanent enlargement of the air spaces distal to the terminal bronchioles accompanied by the destruction of their walls and without obvious fibrosis (6). Over the past decade, it has become apparent that computed tomography (CT) can readily identify the areas of low attenuation that pathologically represent emphysema. In this chapter, we will review chest imaging, including CT, for emphysema, how radiographically detected emphysema compares to pathologic specimens and pulmonary physiology, and lastly review the role of CT to aid in the selection of patients for LVRS.

II. Detection of Emphysema by Chest Radiograph

Before the advent of CT, the clinical imaging of emphysema relied on the chest radiograph (CXR). Scoring systems for emphysema used signs of lung destruction or hyperinflation such as irregular radiolucency of the lungs, arterial deficiency or increased perivascular markings, flattening or depression of the diaphragm, enlargement of the retrosternal air space, increased lung height, and depressed position of the right hemidiaphragm (7). Although CXRs are widely available and relatively inexpensive, they lack specificity for discriminating emphysema from other types of obstructive lung disease (7,8). Furthermore, although the amount of emphysema detected by CXR correlates with the amount of emphysema quantified by high resolution CT (HRCT) (9), studies also suggest that CXRs lack the sensitivity to detect *mild* emphysema as seen in pathologic specimens (10) or HRCT (11,12).

III. Quantification of Emphysema from Pathologic Specimens

Several methods have been proposed and utilized to quantify the extent of emphysema present in pathologic specimens (13–15). The most commonly used are the point counting technique (15) and the panel grading system (14). The point counting technique uses a transparent grid that is placed over a section of lung. Points on this grid are arranged as equilateral triangles with 1 cm sides (Fig. 21.1). The percentage of lung occupied by emphysema is calculated by counting the number of points overlying emphysema, multiplying by 100, and then dividing by the total number of points on the lung section (15). The panel grading method compares paper mounted lung sections to standards scoring emphysema from 0 to 100 at intervals of 5–10. Emphysema is scored as mild (5–15), moderate (30–50), or severe ($\geq$60). This method is not quantitative (unlike the point counting method) but does give the severity based on previous derived milestones (14).

IV. CT Methodology for Detecting Emphysema

The methodology for assessing emphysema with CT has been extensively reviewed by others (7,13,16). Briefly, images displayed by CT comprise pixels (each picture element), which represent the radiographic attenuation of a defined volume of tissue (voxel) (13). The pixel density is determined by the relative amounts of air, tissue, and blood present (17). The radiographic attenuation (tissue density) is expressed in Hounsfield units (HU). The range of attenuation spans from -1000 (corresponding to air) to 3000 HU; 0 HU has been defined as the attenuation of water (13). The collimation refers to the CT slice thickness, with thinner sections having less volume averaging and, therefore, better

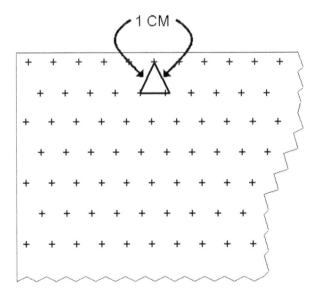

Figure 21.1 Point-counting grid used for the estimation of volume proportions of emphysema on a gross specimen. The points are arranged at the angles of equilateral triangles with 1 cm sides. [From Dunnill (15) with permission.]

resolution. HRCT typically has collimation around 1 mm, whereas conventional CT scans have collimation around 10 mm. Modern CT techniques provide excellent visual resolution and the opportunity to quantify the volume of tissue within a certain range of HU. These features make CT well suited for the diagnosis and quantification of emphysema. CT technique is described in more detail in Chapter 2.

The amount of emphysema, as determined by CT, can be quantified by using visual grading systems or by using computer software that calculates the volume below a certain HU threshold. Goddard et al. (18) published a visual scoring system for the quantification of emphysema, which has been used by most subsequent studies (Table 21.1). Visual scoring is assessed using 2D image slices; computerized methods can be performed on 3D images using helical CT technology or on 2D images (16).

V. Relationship Between CT Detected Emphysema and Pathologically Defined Emphysema

Emphysema is visualized on CT scans as abnormally low attenuation areas (LAAs) (19). CT displays several attributes regarding the assessment of emphysema. First, the extent of emphysema detected by CT correlates well with anatomically defined emphysema (20–27). Secondly, CT has excellent sensitivity (87–100%) for detecting pathologically defined emphysema (24,28), although localized areas of destruction that are <5 mm may be missed (25). Finally, HRCT is likely more sensitive than conventional CT for detecting mild degrees of emphysema (25,26).

The quantity of emphysema, as determined by CT, may also vary depending on the method of assessment. Visual scoring methods tend to overestimate the

Table 21.1 Visual Scoring System for the Quantity of Emphysema

Scoring	Degree of parenchymal abnormality
0	Normal
1	LAAs up to 25%
2	LAAs between 26% and 50%
3	LAAs between 51% and 75%
4	LAAs >75%

Note: A score is assigned to each lung on each CT image. The total score is the sum of each lung's score on each CT image. For example, a patient having eight CT slices (images) could have a maximum score of 64. A patient with three CT images could have a maximum score of 24.
Source: Scoring adapted from Goddard et al. (18).

amount of emphysema in pathologic specimens compared with morphometric (23) or densitonometric methods using thresholds of -950 HU (23) and 2D or 3D analysis with thresholds of -900, -910, -950 HU (29). Interestingly, a threshold of -950 HU appears to have the best correlation with anatomically defined emphysema (17). Thresholds of < -950 HU tend to overestimate the amount of emphysema, while thresholds > -950 HU tend to underestimate the amount of emphysema in pathologic specimens (Fig. 21.2) (17). Finally, the amount of emphysema appears less on expiratory images compared with inspiratory images (26,30).

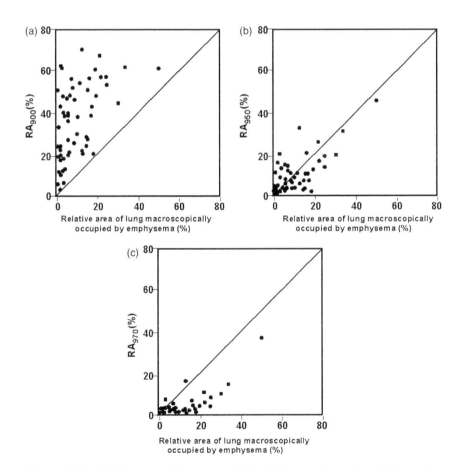

Figure 21.2 Relative area of lung occupied by CT attenuation values (a) lower than -900, (b) -950, and (c) -970 HU (RA_{900}, RA_{950}, and RA_{970}, respectively) against the relative area of lung macroscopically occupied by emphysema. The diagonal represents the line of identity, circles represent lungs resected for tumor, and squares represent lungs resected before transplantation. [From Gevenois et al. (17) with permission.]

VI. Relationship Between CT Detected Emphysema and Pulmonary Function

The presence of emphysema has classically been suggested by pulmonary function studies that reveal obstruction, hyperinflation, and a decrease in gas transfer. Overall, CT is more sensitive than pulmonary function studies for the detection of emphysema (31,32) and correlates better with pathologically quantified emphysema than pulmonary function testing (33). CT correlates well with pulmonary function testing in most studies (18,29,30,34–36), but not all (37,38). Similarly, the amount of emphysema has been shown to correlate with walk distance by some investigators (38), but not by others (39). Some investigators have successfully identified patients with severe obstruction without significant emphysema (37) and other patients with significant emphysema, despite a lack of obstructive lung disease (12,32). The CT methodology utilized to quantify emphysema does not seem to significantly impact the correlation with pulmonary function test results, although expiratory films may show better correlation and less interpatient variability (35). In general, smokers and more symptomatic patients are more likely to have significant amounts of emphysema and worse lung function (32,40).

It is clear that although a good correlation exists between CT quantified emphysema and pulmonary function, the correlation is not perfect. This likely relates to the contribution of airway disease in COPD patients. In fact, Nakano et al. (36) demonstrated that the best correlation with pulmonary function testing was obtained using a multivariable model that considered both LAAs and airway wall features. It is important to remember the importance of evaluating the entire lung as a functional unit and not completely separate the impact of the distal airspaces and central airways. It is also critical to remember that the lung is only one component of exercise capacity, which may explain the discrepancy between the quantification of emphysema and functional (walk distance) outcome between studies.

VII. Role of CT in LVRS

LVRS has become an increasingly accepted surgical therapy in highly selected patients with emphysema (4,5,41). As such, it is not surprising that thoracic imaging has assumed a primary role in the evaluation of patients for LVRS (41). CT imaging, in particular, has been the predominant technique utilized. It has the advantage of identifying additional features that may alter the decision to perform LVRS or change the approach to LVRS. For example, the National Emphysema Treatment Trial (NETT), a multi-center study that randomized 1218 patients to maximal medical therapy vs. maximal medical therapy plus bilateral LVRS, excluded patients with clinically significant bronchiectasis, pleural or interstitial disease, a pulmonary nodule suspicious for malignancy, or a giant bulla; these were predominantly identified by CT imaging (42).

Several groups have identified lung nodules during evaluation for LVRS (43–48). In the report of Hazelrigg et al. (46), at least one lung nodule was identified in 39.5% of 281 patients prospectively evaluated for LVRS. Of these 111 patients with nodules, 52 were felt to have benign lesions by radiographic imaging. Of the remaining nodules, 78 were resected and 17 of these proved malignant. Interestingly, of the neoplastic lesions, three were identified by CT only, five by both CXR and CT, four in the operating room (not seen radiographically), and five incidentally by the pathologist. This low sensitivity by CT could (in part) be explained by the technique of HRCT, which does not yield a total volume assessment of the chest. The overall incidence of cancer was 6.4%.

CT imaging has also assumed a pivotal role in the assessment of the severity and distribution of emphysema. These concepts have become accepted as important variables influencing patient selection and in predicting response to therapy (41). These latter concepts will be discussed subsequently.

VIII. Prediction of Outcome

A. Presence of Emphysema

Numerous investigators have examined the role of imaging in identifying the presence of emphysema. As such, Hunsaker et al. (49) evaluated the impact of the quantity and distribution of emphysema along with physiology to predict outcomes in 20 patients with severe obstructive lung disease [forced expiratory volume in 1 s (FEV_1) <36% predicted] undergoing LVRS. The quantity and heterogeneity of emphysema were subjectively graded from CT scans. Although all patients had severe obstructive lung disease, only four patients had mild emphysema by CT grading. Although none of the four patients with mild emphysema improved following LVRS, the quantity of emphysema in the entire cohort did not correlate with improvement in FEV_1 following LVRS ($r = 0.30$, $p = 0.20$). Rogers et al. (50) analyzed the relationship between outcome after LVRS and CT morphometry in 30 patients. The quantity of preoperative severe emphysema (< -910 HU) correlated better with improved maximal achieved wattage during cycle ergometry ($r = 0.595$) than with FEV_1 ($r = 0.366$). Severe emphysema correlated with TLC, mild/moderate emphysema, surface area, and surface area/volume variables. However, in multivariate models, severe emphysema accounted for the effect of the other variables (50).

Slone et al. (51) evaluated 50 consecutive patients undergoing LVRS and retrospectively examined the relationship between emphysema as visualized by CT and outcome (FEV_1, PaO_2, and 6 min walk distance). Severity of emphysema was graded on a 5-point subjective scale (0 = normal, 1 = mild, 2 = moderate, 3 = marked, and 4 = severe). Heterogeneity was also scored from 0 (uniform) to 4 (extreme differences). Overall, there was greater improvement in patients with greater regional heterogeneity, lung compression, and upper lobe predominant emphysema. In a multivariate model quantifying heterogeneity, compressed lung, hyperinflation, severity, and global distribution, the three most predictive variables were distribution (upper vs. lower), lung compression, and the percentages of normal and mildly emphysematous lung (51).

B. Emphysema Distribution—Craniocaudal

The importance of heterogeneity in the distribution of emphysema has been suggested to be an important factor in predicting a favorable outcome following LVRS by numerous authors. In an early study, Brenner et al. (52) confirmed greater spirometric improvement in patients with upper lobe predominant emphysema. Similar results were reported by McKenna et al. (43) in patients undergoing unilateral LVRS. In a more detailed analysis, this group examined results in 138 patients surviving bilateral LVRS (53). One hundred and six patients (77%) had upper lobe predominant emphysema whereas 10 (7%) had lower lobe predominant and 22 (16%) had diffusely homogenous emphysema. Patients with upper lobe predominant disease had a significantly greater improvement in FEV_1 [73%, preoperative 0.64 L (95% CI 0.59, 0.70) to postoperative 1.07 L (95% CI 0.98 to 1.16) vs. 38%, preoperative 0.70 L (95% CI 0.63 to 0.78) to postoperative 0.93 L (95% CI 0.85 to 1.01)]. There were no differences in outcome (FEV_1) based on preoperative FEV_1, prednisone use, hypoxemia, or hypercarbia (53). Furthermore, patients older than 70 years and/or patients on >4 L of supplemental oxygen had a lesser benefit compared with younger patients and/or patients on less oxygen. There were no differences in outcome (FEV_1) based on preoperative FEV_1, prednisone use, hypoxemia, or hypercarbia (53).

As noted earlier, Slone et al. (51) confirmed that greater improvement was noted in patients with greater regional heterogeneity, lung compression, and upper lobe predominant emphysema. In a multivariate model, emphysema distribution (upper vs. lower) was one of the most predictive variables. Similarly, Weder et al. (54) examined the correlation between emphysema distribution and heterogeneity on CT and outcomes following LVRS. These investigators assessed the degree of heterogeneity (marked, intermediate, homogeneous) and distribution (upper, lower, bullae), noting improvement in pulmonary function, walking distance, and dyspnea in all groups. The effect on FEV_1 was most pronounced in upper lobe predominant and heterogeneous emphysema, as was the greatest decrease in RV/TLC (54). This same group described outcomes 24 months after bilateral LVRS (55). A greater initial improvement was noted in patients with heterogeneous disease although these patients also experienced a greater decline over time. A worsening in dyspnea was noted in all groups although it was not significant between the 3 and 24 months time points; dyspnea at both of these time points was improved compared with baseline. Furthermore, survival was improved in the markedly heterogeneous group although this group had better initial pulmonary function and a preponderance of males, which limited interpretation. Finally, these investigators presented results of 115 patients who were followed for a median of 37 months (56). Patients with markedly heterogeneous emphysema experienced a greater early gain in $FEV_1\%$ predicted (Fig. 21.3). Interestingly, the decline in FEV_1 over the subsequent years was similar for all morphologic types.

In a study described earlier, Hunsaker et al. (49) noted that disease heterogeneity, among patients with moderate to severe emphysema, tended to correlate with change in FEV_1 following LVRS ($r = 0.47$, $p = 0.07$). Similarly, Wisser et al. (57) examined the relationship between the morphologic grading of emphysema and outcome following bilateral LVRS in 47 consecutive patients. Regression analysis demonstrated a significant correlation between increased heterogeneity and post-LVRS FEV_1 ($r^2 = 0.11$, $p = 0.04$) (57). In a subsequent study, these investigators followed 70 patients for 12 months after LVRS (58). Those patients with the greatest improvement in FEV_1 exhibited the greatest emphysema heterogeneity on preoperative CT. Qualitatively similar results have been presented by Pompeo et al. (59).

The most compelling data supporting the value of visual grading of emphysema distribution have been provided by the NETT (60). Radiologists at participating clinical centers classified HRCT scans as predominantly upper lobe vs. non-upper lobe emphysema on the basis of visual scoring of disproportionate

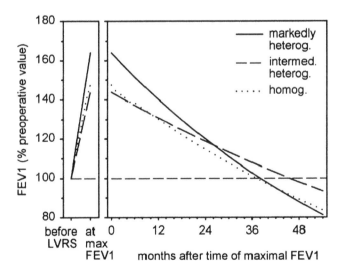

Figure 21.3 Gain in FEV_1 following LVRS in 60 patients. The left panel represents the medians of measured gains in FEV_1 for patients with markedly heterogeneous, intermediately heterogeneous, and homogeneous emphysema distribution. The right panel represents the exponential decay function of FEV_1 with origins and time constants corresponding to respective median values of the different heterogeneity groups. The absolute and relative gain in FEV_1 is greater in patients with markedly heterogeneous emphysema than in the other two groups, the subsequent decline is similar for the three groups ($p =$ not significant). [Reproduced from Bloch et al. (56) with permission.]

disease between non-anatomic thirds divided equally from apex to the base (41). In addition, patients were stratified by their post-pulmonary rehabilitation maximal-achieved exercise capacity (low exercise capacity: <25 W for women; <40 W for men). Using these methods, NETT investigators have published two sentinel studies which clarify the role of CT imaging in the evaluation of patients for LVRS. An early manuscript identified an increased risk of surgical mortality in patients with severe obstruction ($FEV_1 < 20\%$ predicted) and either diffuse emphysema on HRCT or a $DL_{CO} < 20\%$ predicted (RR 3.9, 95% CI 1.9, 9.0) (61). In an analysis of all patients during a mean follow-up of 29 months, patients with upper lobe predominant emphysema and a low post-rehabilitation exercise tolerance exhibited a decreased risk of mortality (RR 0.47, $p = 0.005$) after LVRS; patients with non-upper lobe predominant emphysema and a high post-rehabilitation exercise capacity exhibited an increased risk of death during follow-up after LVRS (RR 2.06, $p = 0.02$) (Table 21.2) (60). Patients with upper lobe predominant emphysema and a high post-rehabilitation exercise capacity or patients with non-upper lobe predominant emphysema and a low post-rehabilitation exercise capacity did not have a survival advantage or disadvantage (60). In addition, patients with upper lobe predominant emphysema undergoing LVRS were more likely to improve their exercise capacity compared with medically treated patients (Table 21.2). Similarly, with the exception of non-upper lobe disease and high exercise capacity patients, LVRS patients experienced improved quality of life (60). Figure 21.4 and Table 21.2 illustrate an approach to the evaluation of patients based on NETT data.

Unfortunately, the definition of emphysema heterogeneity has varied widely among the published literature (41). To overcome the difficulty in subjective assessment of emphysema heterogeneity, some investigators have utilized quantitative CT methodology to define disease heterogeneity. In 46 patients undergoing LVRS, Gierada et al. (62) quantified emphysema by measuring lung attenuation on preoperative CT scans. These investigators noted moderately strong correlations between several quantitative CT values and outcome measures (magnitude of $r = 0.31–0.47$, $P < 0.05$). As such, postoperative outcome was better with 75% or greater of upper lung < -900 HU (emphysema index), a ratio of upper- and lower-lung emphysema indexes 1.5 or greater, and full width at half maximum of attenuation–frequency distribution of ≤ 80 HU, among others.

Flaherty et al. (63) evaluated the predictive ability of CT and LVRS outcomes in 65 patients undergoing bilateral LVRS. The amount of emphysema was determined as the volume < -900 HU with the ratio of upper to lower lobe emphysema, the CT emphysema ratio (CTR), calculated as:

$$CTR = \frac{\text{emphysema volume in upper lung/total volume of upper lung}}{\text{emphysema volume in lower lung/total volume of lower lung}}$$

A higher CTR (heterogeneous, upper lung predominant emphysema) exhibited a good positive predictive value for improved FEV_1 (defined as a 12% and 200 cc

Table 21.2 Results of Bilateral LVRS Compared with Medical Therapy in Patients with Severe Emphysema

Patients	LVRS	Medical therapy	Risk ratio[a]	*p* Value
		Total mortality		
Group A	42/70	30/70	1.82	0.06
Group B	26/139	51/151	0.47	0.005
Group C	34/206	39/213	0.98	0.70
Group D	28/84	26/65	0.81	0.49
Group E	27/109	14/111	2.06	0.02
Patients	LVRS	Medical therapy	Odds ratio	*p* Value
		Improvement in exercise capacity[b]		
Group A	4/58 (7)	1/48 (2)	3.48	0.37
Group B	25/84 (30)	0/92 (0)	—	<0.001
Group C	17/115 (15)	4/138 (3)	5.81	0.001
Group D	6/49 (12)	3/41 (7)	1.77	0.50
Group E	2/65 (3)	2/59 (3)	0.90	1.00
		Improvement in health-related quality of life[c]		
Group A	6/58 (10)	0/48 (0)	—	0.03
Group B	40/84 (48)	9/92 (10)	8.38	<0.001
Group C	47/115 (41)	15/138 (11)	5.67	<0.001
Group D	18/49 (37)	3/41 (7)	7.35	0.001
Group E	10/65 (15)	7/59 (12)	1.35	0.61

[a]Risk ratio for total mortality in surgically vs. medically treated patients during a mean follow-up of 29.2 months.
[b]Increase in the maximal workload of >10 W from the patient's post-rehabilitation base-line value (24 months after randomization).
[c]Decrease in the score on the St. George's Respiratory Questionnaire of more than eight points (on a 100 point scale) from the patient's post-rehabilitation base-line score (24 months after randomization).
Note: Values in parentheses indicate percentage. Groups A–E refer to the patients as defined in Fig. 21.4.
Source: Adapted from American Thoracic Society (75).

absolute increase) but low sensitivity. Table 21.3 enumerates the sensitivity, specificity, and predictive values of various CTR thresholds for an FEV_1 improvement 3–36 months after bilateral LVRS. These data suggest that patients with upper lobe predominant, heterogeneous emphysema are most likely to benefit from bilateral LVRS, although some patients with a low CTR may still benefit from LVRS. Importantly, CTR was not consistently able to predict significant improvements in walk distance or dyspnea (63).

Some investigative groups have suggested the positive predictive value of identifying heterogeneous perfusion during ventilation/perfusion scanning in predicting outcome after LVRS (64–66). Others have contrasted the findings of CT with those of ventilation/perfusion imaging in predicting outcome after

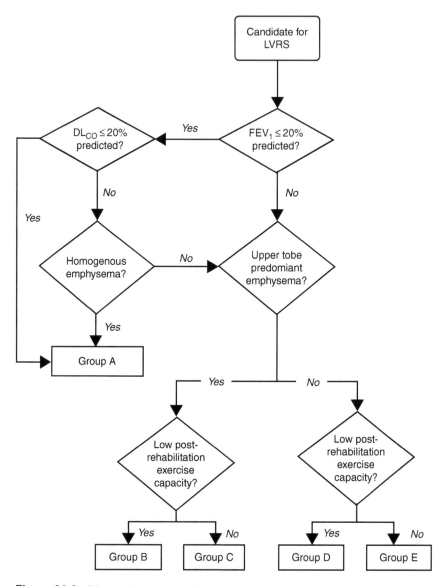

Figure 21.4 Diagnostic algorithm for patients being considered for LVRS based on data from the NETT (60,61). [Reproduced with permission from American Thoracic Society (75).]

LVRS. Thurnheer et al. (67). categorized perfusion scans and CT images as markedly heterogeneous, intermediately heterogeneous, and homogeneous; a visual analog scale was also employed. The lobes primarily affected by emphysema were also determined. Functional improvement was better correlated with

Table 21.3 Test Characteristics for the CTR and Prediction of FEV₁ Following Bilateral LVRS

	CTR	Sensitivity (%)	Specificity (%)	PPV	NPV
3 months					
	>1.5	69	50	76	50
	>2.0	41	78	76	39
	>2.5	23	94	100	40
6 months					
	>1.5	82	52	61	72
	>2.0	56	82	71	64
	>2.5	33	96	100	60
12 months					
	>1.5	67	42	53	61
	>2.0	46	73	58	58
	>2.5	33	92	89	63
18 months					
	>1.5	61	0	48	62
	>2.0	44	78	57	63
	>2.5	39	96	78	68
24 months					
	>1.5	73	48	48	71
	>2.0	47	78	58	68
	>2.5	40	96	75	41
36 months					
	>1.5	42	20	56	13
	>2.0	38	89	75	62
	>2.5	25	100	100	60

Note: CT, computed tomography; FEV₁, forced expiratory volume in 1 s; CTR, CT emphysema ratio (see text for details), PPV, positive predictive value; NPV, negative predictive value.
Source: Adapted from Flaherty et al. (63).

physiologic hyperinflation and emphysema heterogeneity as assessed by CT compared with perfusion heterogeneity assessed by scintigraphy (67). Hunsaker et al. (68) evaluated the correlation of LVRS outcomes and indexes of CT and ventilation/perfusion (V/Q) imaging. Thirty-nine patients had subjective grading of emphysema from 1 mm collimation at 20 mm intervals performed; 17 patients also had computer determined quantification of emphysema (−910 HU). Twenty-one patients had upper lobe predominant disease, 14 patients had homogeneous disease, and 4 patients had lower lobe predominant disease. As noted by previous investigators, there was a good correlation between subjective and computer generated scoring of emphysema. Patients with more heterogeneous disease, as determined by CT or V/Q, tended to show a greater magnitude and likelihood for improved FEV₁. The indexes of disease distribution accounted for 18–23% of the variance in postoperative FEV₁. The outcomes were similar for CT and V/Q and for scores that were obtained by subjective or computer generated methods (68). Most recently, Cederlund et al. (69) examined the qualitative assessment of emphysema heterogeneity using CT, perfusion scintigraphy, or the combination of the two in 45 patients evaluated for LVRS. There was little difference in emphysema heterogeneity classification based on CT or scintigraphy alone; the combination of the two was superior when contrasted with quantitative methodology as the "gold standard (Table 21.4)." Interestingly, these results are somewhat different than that of Cleverley et al. (70), who noted similar extent of normal pulmonary vasculature on HRCT and scintigraphy in 30 patients with emphysema. Neither of the two studies examined outcome of LVRS. As such, it is likely that CT and scintigraphy demonstrate similar predictive ability in suggesting outcome after LVRS.

C. Emphysema Distribution—Novel Methodologies

Recently, several groups have attempted to increase the predictive ability of CT by performing novel analyses of emphysema distribution in emphysema patients evaluated for LVRS. Nakano et al. (71) evaluated the core to rind distribution of emphysema and its relationship to outcomes following LVRS in 21 patients. The rind region was defined as the peripheral 50% of the lung area and the remaining area was defined as the core area (Fig. 21.5). There was a positive correlation between the amount of the upper lung expanded beyond < -910 HU and the change in watts following LVRS; the amount of normal lung and the amount of mild/moderate emphysema (< -856 HU) in the upper lung correlated negatively with change in watts following surgery. Stepwise multiple regression analysis demonstrated that the addition of percentage of voxels with severe emphysema in the upper rind had a better prediction of watts ($r^2 = 0.462$, $p < 0.005$) compared with the total amount of emphysema ($r^2 = 0.266$) (71). This same group recently examined the relationship between the number and size of emphysematous lesions and the short term response to LVRS in 21 patients (72). The power law exponent (D) in this analysis represents the slope of the relationship between the log of the cumulative number of emphysematous lesions and the log of the emphysema lesion size; a steep slope and thus large

Table 21.4 Statistical Results of Visual Classification of Emphysema Heterogeneity Between CT and Lung Perfusion Scintigraphy (LPS)

	Markedly heterogeneous	Intermediately heterogeneous	Homogeneous
CT vs. LPS	NS	NS	NS
CT + LPS vs. CT	NS	NS	$p < 0.01$
CT + LPS vs. LPS	$p < 0.05$	NS	$p < 0.01$

Source: Adapted from Cederlund et al. (69).

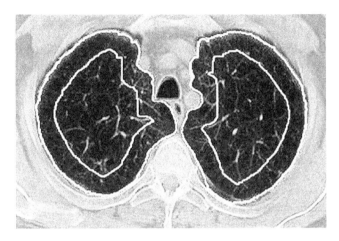

Figure 21.5   Illustration of the division of the lung into an inner (core) and outer (rind) region as described by Nakano et al. (71). [Reproduced from Nakano et al. (71) with permission.]

D represents lungs with predominantly small lesions, whereas a shallow slope and small *D* suggests lungs with larger emphysematous lesions. In the 21 patients studied before and 3 months after LVRS, a positive correlation was noted between the change in *D* and the change in maximal wattage achieved during cycle ergometry. The authors suggest that patients with larger, upper lobe lesions respond better to surgery than patients with small, uniformly distributed lesions. Further data are required to better define the role of such novel imaging methods in predicting response to LVRS.

IX.   CT Volumes as an Outcome or Correlate with Outcomes

Holbert et al. (73) evaluated the change in lung volume, determined by CT, in 28 patients who underwent unilateral LVRS. Patients underwent a CT scan (5 or 10 mm collimation) pre-operatively and 3 months post-LVRS. Using a threshold of −910 HU to define emphysema, patients experienced an average of 14% decrease in emphysema in the surgical lung. These were associated with an improved TLC (−13 ± 14% predicted), RV (−45 ± 43% predicted), and FEV_1 (7 ± 8% predicted) (73). Bae et al. (74) examined the relationship between changes in emphysema volume and physiologic outcomes in 10 patients who underwent LVRS. All patients exhibited a decrease in emphysema volume following LVRS (inspiratory mean pre vs. post, 60% vs. 38%; expiratory mean pre vs. post, 60% vs. 27%). In general, increased emphysema was associated with worse pulmonary function; however, many correlations did not reach statistical significance. Similarly, a decrease in the amount of emphysema tended to correlate with improved pulmonary function and improved hall walk distance, although, many of the correlations were not statistically significant (74). These data suggest that changes in emphysema volume, as measured by CT, may correlate with functional outcomes, although the small number of patients in this study may have limited statistical significance.

X. Conclusion

LVRS has proven to be an effective therapy for highly selected patients with severe emphysema. Thoracic imaging studies, particularly novel CT techniques, have assumed a crucial role in the preoperative assessment of patients considered candidates for such surgical intervention. Patients with severe emphysema, predominating in the upper lung zones appear to have the greatest chance of a positive response to surgery. Unfortunately, the predictive ability of current techniques is far from ideal and further study is required to better characterize which patients are most likely to benefit from LVRS.

References

1. National Heart Lung and Blood Institute. Morbidity and mortality chartbook, 2002. Web page available at www.nhlbi.nih.gov/resources/docs/cht-book.htm.
2. Pauwels RA, Buist AS, Calverley PMA, Jenkins CR, Hurd SS, Committee GOLD Scientific. Global strategy for the diagnosis, management, and prevention of chronic obstructive pulmonary disease. NHLBI/WHO global initiative for chronic obstructive lung disease (GOLD) workshop summary. Am J Respir Crit Care 2001; 163:1256–1276.
3. Martinez FJ, Gay SE, Flaherty KR. Management of non-bronchiectatic chronic obstructive pulmonary disease. In: Maurer J, ed. Management of Non-neoplastic Advanced Lung Disease. New York: Marcel Dekker, 2003:271–337.
4. Flaherty KR, Martinez FJ. Lung volume reduction surgery for emphysema. Clin Chest Med 2000; 21:819–848.
5. Meyers BF, Patterson GA. Chronic obstructive pulmonary disease. 10: Bullectomy, lung volume reduction surgery, and transplantation for patients with chronic obstructive pulmonary disease. Thorax 2003; 58:634–638.
6. Murray JF, Nadel JA, eds. Textbook of Respiratory Medicine. 3rd ed. Philadelphia: W.B. Saunders Company, 2000.
7. Kazerooni EA. Radiologic evaluation of emphysema for lung volume reduction surgery. Clin Chest Med 1999; 20:845–861.
8. Slone RM, Gierada DS. Radiology of pulmonary emphysema and lung volume reduction surgery. Semin Thorac Cardiovasc Surg 1996; 8:61–82.
9. Miniati M, Filippi E, Falaschi F, Carrozzi L, Milne EN, Sostman HD, Pistolesi M. Radiologic evaluation of emphysema in patients with chronic obstructive pulmonary

disease: chest radiography versus high resolution computed tomography. Am J Respir Crit Care Med 1995; 151:1359–1367.

10. Hayhurst MD, MacNee W, Flenley DC, Wright D, McLean A, Lamb D, Wightman AJ, Best J. Diagnosis of pulmonary emphysema by computerised tomography. Lancet 1984; 2:320–322.

11. Klein JS, Gamsu G, Webb WR, Golden JA, Muller NL. High-resolution CT diagnosis of emphysema in symptomatic patients with normal chest radiographs and isolated low diffusing capacity. Radiology 1992; 182:817–821.

12. Sanders C, Nath PH, Bailey WC. Detection of emphysema with computed tomography. Correlation with pulmonary function tests and chest radiography. Invest Radiol 1988; 23:262–266.

13. Madani A, Keyzer C, Gevenois PA. Quantitative computed tomography assessment of lung structure and function in pulmonary emphysema. Eur Respir J 2001; 18:720–730.

14. Thurlbeck WM, Dunnill MS, Hartung W, Heard BE, Hepplestn AG, Ryder RC. A comparison of three methods of measuring emphysema. Hum Pathol 1970; 1:215–226.

15. Dunnill MS. Quantitative methods in the study of pulmonary pathology. Thorax 1962; 17:320–328.

16. Goldin JG. Quantitative CT of the lung. Radiol Clin North Am 2002; 40:45–58.

17. Gevenois PA, de Maertelaer V, De Vuyst P, Zanen J, Yernault JC. Comparison of computed density and macroscopic morphometry in pulmonary emphysema. Am J Respir Crit Care Med 1995; 152:653–657.

18. Goddard PR, Nicholson EM, Laszlo G, Watt I. Computed tomography in pulmonary emphysema. Clin Radiol 1982; 33:379–387.

19. Thurlbeck WM, Müller NL. Emphysema: definition, imaging, and quantification. Am J Roentgenol 1994; 163:1017–1025.

20. Murata K, Itoh H, Kanaoka M, Noma S, Itoh T, Furuta M, Asamoto H, Torizuka K. Centrilobular lesions of the lung: demonstration by high-resolution CT and pathologic correlation. Radiology 1986; 161:641–645.

21. Bergin CJ, Müller NL, Miller RR. CT in the qualitative assessment of emphysema. J Thorac Imaging 1986; 1:94–103.

22. Foster WL Jr, Pratt PC, Roggli VL, Godwin JD, Halvorsen RA Jr, Putman CE. Centrilobular emphysema: CT-pathologic correlation. Radiology 1986; 159:27–32.

23. Bankier AA, De Maertelaer V, Keyzer C, Gevenois PA. Pulmonary emphysema: subjective visual grading versus objective quantification with macroscopic morphometry and thin-section CT densitometry. Radiology 1999; 211:851–858.

24. Hruban RH, Meziane MA, Zerhouni EA, Khouri NF, Fishman EK, Wheeler PS, Dumler JS, Hutchins GM. High resolution computed tomography of inflation-fixed lungs. Pathologic–radiologic correlation of centrilobular emphysema. Am Rev Respir Dis 1987; 136:935–940.

25. Miller RR, Müller NL, Vedal S, Morrison NJ, Staples CA. Limitations of computed tomography in the assessment of emphysema. Am Rev Respir Dis 1989; 139:980–983.

26. Kuwano K, Matsuba K, Ikeda T, Murakami J, Araki A, Nishitani H, Ishida T, Yasumoto K, Shigematsu N. The diagnosis of mild emphysema. Correlation of computed tomography and pathology scores. Am Rev Respir Dis 1990; 141:169–178.

27. Gevenois PA, Zanen J, de Maertelaer V, De Vuyst P, Dumortier P, Yernault JC. Macroscopic assessment of pulmonary emphysema by image analysis. J Clin Pathol 1995; 48:318–322.

28. Foster WL Jr, Gimenez EI, Roubidoux MA, Sherrier RH, Shannon RH, Roggli VL, Pratt PC. The emphysemas: radiologic–pathologic correlations. Radiographics 1993; 13:311–328.

29. Park KJ, Bergin CJ, Clausen JL. Quantitation of emphysema with three-dimensional CT densitometry: comparison with two-dimensional analysis, visual emphysema scores, and pulmonary function test results. Radiology 1999; 211:541–547.

30. Nishimura K, Murata K, Yamagishi M, Itoh H, Ikeda A, Tsukino M, Koyama H, Sakai N, Mishima M, Izumi T. Comparison of different computed tomography scanning methods for quantifying emphysema. J Thorac Imaging 1998; 13:193–198.

31. Sanders C. The radiographic diagnosis of emphysema. Radiol Clin North Am 1991; 29:1019–1030.

32. Sashidhar K, Gulati M, Gupta D, Monga S, Suri S. Emphysema in heavy smokers with normal chest radiography. Detection and quantification by HCRT. Acta Radiol 2002; 43:60–65.

33. Bergin C, Müller N, Nichols DM, Lillington G, Hogg JC, Mullen B, Grymaloski MR, Osborne S, Pare PD. The diagnosis of emphysema. A computed tomographic–pathologic correlation. Am Rev Respir Dis 1986; 133:541–546.

34. Baldi S, Miniati M, Bellina CR, Battolla L, Catapano G, Begliomini E, Giustini D, Giuntini C. Relationship between extent of pulmonary emphysema by high-resolution computed tomography and lung elastic recoil in patients with chronic obstructive pulmonary disease. Am J Respir Crit Care Med 2001; 164:585–589.

35. Sandek K, Bratel T, Lagerstrand L, Rosell H. Relationship between lung function, ventilation–perfusion inequality and extent of emphysema as assessed by high-resolution computed tomography. Respir Med 2002; 96:934–943.

36. Nakano Y, Muro S, Sakai H, Hirai T, Chin K, Tsukino M, Nishimura K, Itoh H, Pare PD, Hogg JC, Mishima M. Computed tomographic measurements of airway dimensions and emphysema in smokers. Correlation with lung function. Am J Respir Crit Care Med 2000; 162:1102–1108.

37. Gelb AF, Schein M, Kuei J, Tashkin DP, Müller NL, Hogg JC, Epstein JD, Zamel N. Limited contribution of emphysema in advanced chronic obstructive pulmonary disease. Am Rev Respir Dis 1993; 147:1157–1161.

38. Wakayama K, Kurihara N, Fujimoto S, Hata M, Takeda T. Relationship between exercise capacity and the severity of emphysema as determined by high resolution CT. Eur Respir J 1993; 6:1362–1367.

39. Taguchi O, Gabazza EC, Yoshida M, Yasui H, Kobayashi T, Yuda H, Hataji O, Adachi Y. CT scores of emphysema and oxygen desaturation during low-grade exercise in patients with emphysema. Acta Radiol 2000; 41:196–197.

40. Betsuyaku T, Yoshioka A, Nishimura M, Miyamoto K, Kawakami Y. Pulmonary function is diminished in older asymptomatic smokers and ex-smokers with low attenuation areas on high-resolution computed tomography. Respiration 1996; 63:333–338.

41. Sciurba FC. Preoperative predictors of outcome following lung volume reduction surgery. Thorax 2002; 57(suppl 2):ii47–52.

42. National Emphysema Treatment Trial Research Group. Rationale and design of the National Emphysema Treatment Trial: A prospective randomized trial of lung volume reduction surgery. Chest 1999; 116:1750–1761.

43. McKenna RJ Jr, Fischel RJ, Brenner M, Gelb AF. Combined operations for lung volume reduction surgery and lung cancer. Chest 1996; 110:885–888.

44. Pigula FA, Keenan RJ, Ferson PF, Landreneau RJ. Unsuspected lung cancer found in work-up for lung reduction operation. Ann Thorac Surg 1996; 61.

45. Ojo TC, Martinez F, Paine R III, Christensen P, Curtis JL, Weg JG, Kazerooni EA, Whyte R. Lung volume reduction surgery alters management of pulmonary nodules in patients with severe COPD. Chest 1997; 112:1494–1500.

46. Hazelrigg SR, Boley TM, Weber D, Magee MJ, Naunheim KS. Incidence of lung nodules found in patients undergoing lung volume reduction. Ann Thorac Surg 1997; 64:303–306.

47. DeMeester SR, Patterson GA, Sundaresan RS, Cooper JD. Lobectomy combined with volume reduction for patients with lung cancer and advanced emphysema. J Thorac Cardiovasc Surg 1998; 115:681–688.

48. DeRose JJ, Argenziano M, El-Amir N, Jellen PA, Gorenstein LA, Steinglass KM, Thomashow B, Ginsburg ME. Lung reduction operation and resection of pulmonary nodules in patients with severe emphysema. Ann Thorac Surg 1998; 65:314–318.

49. Hunsaker A, Ingenito E, Topal U, Pugatch R, Reilly J. Preoperative screening for lung volume reduction surgery: usefulness of combining thin-section CT with physiologic assessment. Am J Roentgenol 1998; 170:309–314.

50. Rogers RM, Coxson HO, Sciurba FC, Keenan RJ, Whittall KP, Hogg JC. Preoperative severity of emphysema predictive of improvement after lung volume reduction surgery: use of CT morphometry. Chest 2000; 118:1240–1247.

51. Slone RM, Pilgram TK, Gierada DS, Sagel SS, Glazer HS, Yusen RD, Cooper JD. Lung volume reduction surgery: comparison of preoperative radiologic features and clinical outcome. Radiology 1997; 204:685–693.

52. Brenner M, Kayaleh RA, Milne EN, Della Bella L, Osann K, Tadir Y, Berns MW, Wilson AF. Thoracoscopic laser ablation of pulmonary bullae. Radiographic selection and treatment response. J Thorac Cardiovasc Surg 1994; 107:883–890.

53. McKenna RJ, Brenner M, Fischel RJ, Singh N, Yoong B, Gelb AF, Osann KE. Patient selection criteria for lung volume reduction surgery. J Thorac Cardiovasc Surg 1997; 114:957–964; discussion 964–967.

54. Weder W, Thurnheer R, Stammberger U, Burge M, Russi EW, Bloch KE. Radiologic emphysema morphology is associated with outcome after surgical lung volume reduction. Ann Thorac Surg 1997; 64:313–320.

55. Hamacher J, Bloch KE, Stammberger U, Schmid RA, Laube I, Russi EW, Weder W. Two years' outcome of lung volume reduction surgery in different morphologic emphysema types. Ann Thorac Surg 1999; 68:1792–1798.

56. Bloch KE, Georgescu CL, Russi EW, Weder W. Gain and subsequent loss of lung function after lung volume reduction surgery in cases of severe emphysema with different morphologic patterns. J Thorac Cardiovasc Surg 2002; 123:845–854.

57. Wisser W, Klepetko W, Kontrus M, Bankier A, Senbaklavaci O, Kaider A, Wanke T, Tschernko E, Wolner E. Morphologic grading of the emphysematous lung and its relation to improvement after lung volume reduction surgery. Ann Thorac Surg 1998; 65:793–799.

58. Wisser W, Senbaklavaci O, Ozpeker C, Ploner M, Wanke T, Tschernko E, Wolner E, Klepetko W. Is long-term functional outcome after lung volume reduction surgery predictable? Eur J Cardiothorac Surg 2000; 17:666–672.

59. Pompeo E, Sergiacomi G, Nofroni I, Roscetti W, Simonetti G, Mineo TC. Morphologic grading of emphysema is useful in the selection of candidates for unilateral or bilateral reduction pneumoplasty. Eur J Cardiothorac Surg 2000; 17:680–686.
60. Fishman A, Martinez F, Naunheim K, Piantadosi S, Wise R, Ries A, Weinmann G, Wood DE, for the National Emphysema Treatment Trial Research Group. A randomized trial comparing lung-volume-reduction surgery with medical therapy for severe emphysema. N Engl J Med 2003; 348:2059–2073.
61. National Emphysema Treatment Trial Research Group. Patients at high risk of death after lung-volume-reduction surgery. N Engl J Med 2001; 345:1075–1083.
62. Gierada DS, Slone RM, Bae KT, Yusen RD, Lefrak SS, Cooper JD. Pulmonary emphysema: comparison of preoperative quantitative CT and physiologic index values with clinical outcome after lung-volume reduction surgery. Radiology 1997; 205:235–242.
63. Flaherty KR, Kazerooni EA, Curtis JL, Iannettoni M, Lange L, Schork MA, Martinez FJ. Short-term and long-term outcomes after bilateral lung volume reduction surgery. Prediction by Quantitative CT. Chest 2001; 119:1337–1346.
64. Jamadar DA, Kazerooni EA, Martinez FJ, Wahl RL. Semi-quantitative ventilation–perfusion scintigraphy and single photon emission computed tomography for evaluation of lung volume reduction surgery candidates: description and prediction of clinical outcomes. Eur J Nucl Med 1999; 26:734–742.
65. Kotloff RM, Hansen-Flaschen J, Lipson DA, Tino G, Arcasoy SM, Alavi A, Kaiser LR. Apical perfusion fraction as a predictor of short-term functional outcomes following bilateral lung volume reduction surgery. Chest 2001; 120:1609–1615.
66. Wang SC, Fischer KC, Slone RM, Gierada DS, Yusen RD, Lefrak SS, Pilgram TK, Cooper JD. Perfusion scintigraphy in the evaluation for lung volume reduction surgery: correlation with clinical outcome. Radiology 1997; 205:243–248.
67. Thurnheer R, Hermann E, Weder W, Stannberger U, Laube I, Russi EW, Bloch KE. Role of lung perfusion scintigraphy in relation to chest computed tomography and pulmonary function in the evaluation of candidates for lung volume reduction surgery. Am J Respir Crit Care Med 1999; 159:301–310.
68. Hunsaker AR, Ingenito EP, Reilly JJ, Costello P. Lung volume reduction surgery for emphysema: correlation of CT and V/Q imaging with physiologic mechanisms of improvement in lung function. Radiology 2002; 222:491–498.
69. Cederlund K, Hogberg S, Jorfeldt L, Larsen F, Norman M, Rasmussen E, Tylen U. Lung perfusion scintigraphy prior to lung volume reduction surgery. Acta Radiol 2003; 44:246–251.
70. Cleverley JR, Desai SR, Wells AU, Koyama H, Eastick S, Schmidt MA, Charrier CL, Gatehouse PD, Goldstraw P, Pepper JR, Geddes DM, Hansell DM. Evaluation of patients undergoing lung volume reduction surgery: ancillary information available from computed tomography. Clin Radiol 2000; 55:45–50.
71. Nakano Y, Coxson HO, Bosan S, Rogers RM, Sciurba FC, Keenan RJ, Walley KR, Pare PD, Hogg JC. Core to rind distribution of severe emphysema predicts outcome of lung volume reduction surgery. Am J Respir Crit Care Med 2001; 164:2195–2199.
72. Coxson HO, Whittall KP, Nakano Y, Rogers RM, Sciurba FC, Keenan RJ, Hogg JC. Selection of patients for lung volume reduction surgery using a power law analysis of the computed tomographic scan. Thorax 2003; 58:510–514.

73. Holbert JM, Brown ML, Sciruba FC, Keenan RJ, Landreneau RJ, Holzer AD. Changes in lung volume and volume of emphysema after unilateral lung reduction surgery: analysis with CT densitometry. Radiology 1996; 201:793–797.
74. Bae K, Slone RM, Gierada DS, Yusen RD, Cooper JD. Patients with emphysema: quantitative CT analysis before and after lung volume reduction surgery—work in progress. Radiology 1997; 203:705–714.
75. Standards for the diagnosis and treatment of patients with COPD: a summary of the ATS/ERS position paper. Eur Respir J 2004; 23:932–946.

22

Emphysema/Alpha-1 Antitrypsin Deficiency

TRINE STAVNGAARD and
JAHN MORTENSEN

Copenhagen University Hospital,
Copenhagen, Denmark

ASGER DIRKSEN

Gentofte University Hospital,
Hellerup, Denmark

I. Introduction

Anatomically, emphysema is defined as abnormal permanent enlargement of the airspaces distal to the terminal bronchioles, accompanied by destruction of their walls, without obvious fibrosis (1). The underlying cause of emphysema is believed to be an imbalance in the activities of proteolytic and antiproteolytic enzymes in the lung tissue, resulting in destructions of lung elastin and collagen. Cigarette smoke has been shown to increase this destruction and is the major cause of emphysema worldwide. Another cause is alpha-1 antitrypsin deficiency (A1AD), which was discovered as a cause of emphysema in 1963 (2). This enzyme normally inactivates the neutrophil elastase in the lung. Owing to insufficient quantities of the enzyme, the abundance of activated neutrophil elastase causes destruction of alveolar walls and panacinar emphysema with lower lobe predominance. This is most typical in patients with homozygote phenotype (PiZZ). The gene frequency in white individuals of this phenotype varies among countries, but in the Scandinavian countries and the UK it is 2–3% (3).

II. Plain Radiography Findings

Radiographic examination of the lung for the presence of emphysema is of limited use since the pulmonary lobules cannot be visualized with conventional radiography (4). Chest radiographs are known to underestimate the extent of emphysema, and there is a poor correlation between the extent and severity of emphysema as evaluated by chest X-ray (CXR) and pulmonary function tests (5,6). Despite these shortcomings, the conventional chest radiograph is still the first choice in evaluating lung diseases. Some diagnostic features will be discussed in the following text.

Several early studies have correlated roentgenologic features of emphysema with necropsy-demonstrated disease (7–9), and different signs, such as diaphragmatic flattening and hyperinflation, were found to be variably accurate in diagnosing emphysema. Signs of emphysema can be grouped into two major classes: signs of hyperinflation of the thorax and signs of vascular depletion. However, it is important to recognize that population-based studies of imaging in chronic obstructive pulmonary disease (COPD) do not exist, which means that published frequencies and correlations must be interpreted with caution.

The CXR signs in A1AD are preferentially distributed to the lower lobes. Brantly and co-workers found the typical CXR signs in a population of adults with PiZZ A1AD was: (1) lung hyperinflation; (2) symmetrical loss of parenchymal vascularity, primarily in the bases and commonly associated with bullae; (3) cardiovascular abnormalities consisting of a reduction in the cardiothoracic ratio and a convex main pulmonary artery (5,10).

III. Computed Tomography Findings

In the 1970s, when Hounsfield developed computed tomography (CT) for clinical use, he envisaged the scanner as a measuring device, because it provides precise information on the density of tissues derived from the attenuation of X-rays. Attenuation is expressed in terms of the Hounsfield unit (HU) scale in which water is 0 HU and air is -1000 HU. By approximation, Hounsfield units can be translated into tissue density by adding 1000 to the HU value. Thus, an attenuation value of -950 HU corresponds to a tissue density of 50 g/L.

The pathological correlation of emphysema is loss of lung tissue, and therefore it is logical that CT has greatly improved the diagnosis and especially the quantification of emphysema.

Emphysema was described by CT as early as in the late 1970s and early 1980s (11,12). Since that time, several studies have compared CT and pathologic findings, and with improved resolution, faster scan times, and thinner collimation, the correlation of CT scores and pathologic grading has improved. Because of its tomographic nature and improved contrast resolution, CT is superior to plain radiography in detection (13,14), and characterization and grading of emphysema (15). At present, CT is the imaging method of choice to diagnose emphysema in the clinical setting (16,17).

The CT diagnosis of emphysema is morphologic (18) and based on visual inspection for low attenuation areas (LAA), that is, regions of parenchymal destruction. The density of the emphysematous lung is decreased as compared with the normal lung, and the severity of the disease can be assessed by quantitative analyses of the CT density of the lung.

A. CT Morphology of Emphysema/A1AD

On the basis of the distribution of emphysema within the secondary lobule and more peripherally along interlobular septa and in the subpleural area, it is possible on high resolution computed tomography (HRCT) to separate various subtypes of emphysema (19,20). However, it is important to recognize that with more severe disease, it often becomes difficult to distinguish the different subtypes of emphysema from each other. Commonly, we describe centrilobular, panlobular, and paraseptal emphysema.

- *Centrilobular emphysema*: multiple, small, centrilobular lucencies, patchy in central parts of lobes and predominantly upper lobe distribution. This is the most common type of emphysema in smokers (7) and is associated with airflow limitation (Fig. 22.1).
- *Panlobular emphysema*: uniform destruction of lobules, extensive, predominant lower lobe distribution, classically associated with A1AD (6,7,10,21,22). In addition to panlobular emphysema, bronchiectasis is also frequently identified in patients who have A1AD (2,6,23).

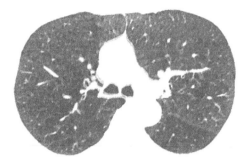

Figure 22.1 Centrilobular emphysema. HRCT (1 mm slices), −600/1500 (window mean/window width). Spotty areas of lucency predominate in the upper lobes.

However, the frequency of alpha-1 antitrypsin alleles is not increased among patients with bronchiectasis (24) (Fig. 22.2).

- *Paraseptal emphysema*: destruction of alveolar duct and sacs, often marginated by interlobular septa, showing subpleural and perihilar bullae and cysts, typically arranged in a single row (17). This form of emphysema is associated with spontaneous pneumothorax (25,26) (Fig. 22.3).
- *Irregular air-space enlargement*: irregular areas of decreased opacity in regions of fibrosis (patients with tuberculosis, sarcoidosis, and sometimes lymphangioleiomyomatosis) (20).

B. Other CT Characteristics of Emphysema

Emphysema is associated with loss of elastic recoil (27), and CT scans taken at full expiration can effectively reveal the abnormal permanent enlargement

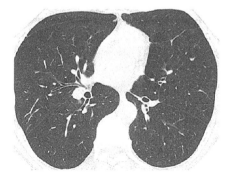

Figure 22.2 Panlobular emphysema. HRCT (1 mm slices), −600/1500 (window mean/window width). Lung volume is increased, the lung appears lucent, and the size of pulmonary vessels is diminished.

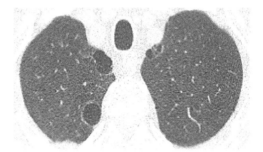

Figure 22.3 Paraseptal emphysema. HRCT (1 mm slices), $-600/1500$ (window mean/window width). Subpleural bullae with visible walls.

of airspaces which defines emphysema (28). Although emphysema scores on expiratory scans correlate better with functional assessment of airway obstruction (FEV$_1$) (29–31), scans obtained in exhalation appear to underestimate the severity of emphysema (32,33). Inspiratory CT scans gated to spirometry may, therefore, be more accurate than expiratory CT for quantifying emphysema (30).

The extent of emphysema diagnosed through inspiratory HRCT cannot predict the elastic properties of the lung (34). Expiratory CT reflects airway obstruction and air trapping (discussed subsequently) more than it does emphysema (35). HRCT is superior to pulmonary function tests (PFTs) for diagnosing emphysema, especially in mild cases. Emphysema in the lower lobes has better correlation with abnormal PFT than emphysema in the upper lobes (20). Furthermore, CT volumetric assessments of abnormally low attenuation of the lung at inspiration and expiration has a high correlation, suggesting that a dedicated expiratory examination may not be needed (36).

C. CT Quantitation of Emphysema

More than 20 years ago it was noted that the CT density of the emphysematous lung was decreased as compared with the normal lung (11,12). Several studies have correlated the quantitative assessment of emphysema by CT with pathologic findings (7,14,30,37–56) and PFT and exercise tests (11,13–15,27–32,36,38, 41–43,47,48,50,52,53,57–81). CT grading of emphysema, whether by visual estimation or by computer analysis, correlates best with decreased diffusing capacity (47,48,58,63) and less well with air-flow obstruction (e.g., FEV$_1$) (11, 13,14,27–30,32,38,42,43,50,52,53,58,59,64–70,72–74,76–83). In centrilobular emphysema, lung destruction is typically concentrated in the upper lobes, where little gas exchange occurs and where even severe destruction may have little effect on lung function (75), and therefore CT is more sensitive than PFT in the diagnosis of mild emphysema (14,37,41,49,57,76).

Quantitation of emphysema by CT can be based on subjective (visual) or objective (computer) scoring. Visual scoring is both time consuming and subject to observer variability (33,40,56,77). Because of their digital nature, CT images lend themselves to objective computer analysis, and software has been developed for semi-automatic calculation of so-called densitometric parameters from the pixel attenuation values of the CT images. At present, such software is available on a limited number of scanners only.

D. CT Quantitation of Emphysema by Densitometric Parameters

Quantitative analysis of CT lung density begins with the delineation of lung in the images. At a given threshold for the soft tissue lung interface, lung tissue can be separated from the thoracic wall and the mediastinum by a semi-automatic contour tracing or region growing algorithm (84,85). From the pixel attenuation values (HU) within the lung, a frequency distribution is generated, called the CT lung density histogram (Fig. 22.4). This histogram is usually unimodal, but in bullous disease the histogram may show a bimodal distribution (53). On the basis of the histogram, various types of densitometric parameters can be calculated. Owing to low reproducibility, simple parameters such as the mean, median, and mode of the histogram have not been implemented for the quantitation of emphysema (78,86–88), whereas two more sophisticated parameters, the percentile density and the relative area, have proven more useful (59,74,81).

The percentile density method was introduced by a group of researchers in Edinburgh (38). The percentile density is the cut-off point, in the histogram, that defines a given percentile of the histogram. For example, the 15th percentile density is extracted from the histogram as the density value (HU) at which 15% of the pixels have lower densities (Fig. 22.4). The percentile density depends on the extent of emphysema and is less influenced by the relative amount of higher attenuation values, corresponding to airway walls, blood vessels, and infiltrate (33).

The other parameter often used is the relative area that indicates the percentage of lung volume affected by emphysema. The relative area is defined as the relative volume of lung for which pixel attenuation values fall below a given threshold. Using the density mask method, it is possible to highlight areas of attenuation below a given threshold, thus making it easy to identify and visualize (even three-dimensionally) the emphysematous regions. Originally, a group in Vancouver used a threshold of -910 HU (40) (Fig. 22.4), and later Gevenois found a better correlation with both microscopic and macroscopic emphysema at a threshold of -950 HU (30,33,50,51). Others found the best correlation with a threshold of -900 (57) and -912 HU (31). The differences in threshold values can be explained by different factors that are influencing lung density (age, CT parameters, number of slices, hardware, lung volume and size) (33,89–91,91–94). There is a need for standardizing all these variables.

In addition to quantitation at static lung volumes, analysis of the rate of change in HU during a forced vital capacity (FVC) maneuver plotted against

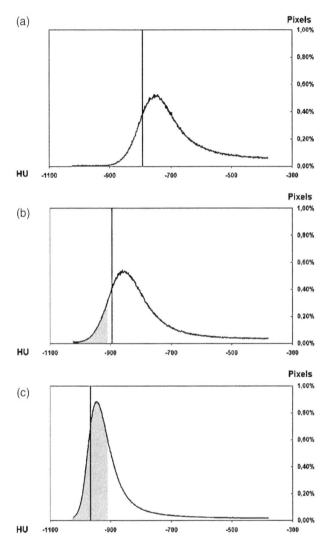

Figure 22.4 CT lung density histograms of three patients. The area under the curves correspond to total lung volumes. The gray area corresponds to the area of the lung below a threshold of −910 HU (the relative area of the lung with emphysematic changes). The solid vertical line in each histogram indicates the 15th percentile. Both relative area and pixel percentile vary much between patients. (a) COPD patient, RA < 1%, 15th percentile = −791 HU; (b) COPD patient, RA = 10%, 15th percentile = −896 HU; (c) A1AD patient, RA = 59%, 15th percentile = −966.

time (*T*) can give additional functional information. In patients with emphysema this HU/*T* curve is flattened, and can be very dissimilar in different patients despite comparable visually apparent extent of structural damage (95).

E. CT Monitoring of the Progress of Emphysema

With the possibility of treatment of some forms of emphysema, for example, augmentation therapy for A1AD, a better measurement of the progress of emphysema than PFT is urgently needed. CT quantitation of emphysema by densitometric parameters seems to be such a test because it is more sensitive for monitoring the progress of emphysema as compared to PFT (e.g., forced expiratory volume in one second, FEV_1) (31,96).

The principal source of variation of lung density measurements is the depth of inspiration. Ranging from full inspiration to full expiration, lung densities more than double (97,98). The volume of air in the lung can be derived from the CT images (i.e., the CT lung density histogram) (59,61,99). Half of the lung density is composed of blood in the microvascular circulation (100), and when taking a deep breath not only the volume of air increases, but blood also enters the thoracic cavity, which makes the relation between inspiratory level and lung density more complicated.

Investigators (29,84,101–103) have tried to standardize the amount of air in the lung by spirometrically controlled CT, with patients breathing through a spirometer during the examination. As soon as a preselected inspiration level is reached, the CT scan is initiated during breath holding. Using this technique, CT lung density measurements were most reproducible at inspiration as compared with expiration (101), but patients with COPD were less able to reproduce the levels of full expiration and inspiration (102,103). Other methods to evaluate the air content in the lung have been developed (99).

Recently, analysis of repeated CT scans at various levels of inspiration has revealed the relationship within an individual between lung density and volume. On the basis of this relationship, densitometric parameters can be standardized by log-transformed lung volume, which corrects for differences in lung volume between scans and eliminates the need for spirometrically controlled CT (104).

Inspiratory CT was superior to expiratory CT for longitudinal estimation of structural abnormalities caused by aging and smoking (31), and the percentile density was more robust than the pixel index for monitoring the progress of emphysema in patients with A1AD. Studies have shown that for the 15th percentile, the annual decline in patients with A1AD is 2–3 HU (104).

The inherent radiation exposure is a serious consideration when using CT for monitoring the progress of emphysema. A reduction of the electrical current (mA) to levels 10 times below standard settings has little influence on lung density measurements (93), and lung density measurements of high quality can be obtained from volume scans of the whole lung using radiation doses <1 mSv.

F. CT Findings in Small Airways Disease

Diseases of the small airways leads to airway obstruction in COPD (105), and the poor correlation between CT emphysema scores and airflow limitation, as found in some studies, may be explained by small airways inflammation of varying extent (52,65,74,106). Therefore, in the evaluation of COPD, CT measurement of emphysema and airway dimensions may be both useful and complementary (107). However, the contribution and role of emphysema and small airways disease in causing expiratory airflow limitation in COPD is still controversial (42).

In healthy adult cigarette smokers, apart from destructive lesions, HRCT may also reveal inflammatory changes such as ill-defined 2–3 mm centrilobular micronodules and patchy ground-glass opacity (108–110). These abnormalities indicate small airways disease and may progress to respiratory bronchiolitis interstitial lung disease (RBILD) (111–113). If smoking is stopped, the changes may show no further progression or slowly resolve.

Reduction of lung volume on expiratory CT scans usually results in a uniform increase in attenuation. Increased resistance to air flow in small airways disease may result in air trapping on expiration leading to decreased attenuation and less volume loss than normal lung (114). Small airways disease is usually patchy in distribution, and expiratory scans accentuate subtle differences between normal and abnormal lung (115).

Expiratory air trapping can be detected in most patients with airway obstruction. In COPD, pulmonary function (FEV_1 and DL_{CO}) was negatively correlated to both an air trapping score (116–119) and a reduction score (66,116,119). The air trapping score was defined as the ratio of the cross-sectional air trapping area vs. the total cross-sectional lung area on expiratory CT, and the reduction score was defined as the change in cross-sectional lung area or mean lung attenuation at inspiration and expiration.

However, limited or focal air trapping is seen in normal subjects (119), particularly in the superior segment of the lower lobe (117), and the frequency of air trapping increases with age, and its severity increases with age and smoking in asymptomatic subjects (120). Furthermore, diffuse air trapping without intervening areas of normal lung may be difficult to appreciate, even on expiratory scans (121).

In many diseases resulting in small airways abnormalities, large airway abnormalities such as bronchiectasis are also visible. Although bronchiectasis is a separate disease entity from COPD, there is a high prevalence of emphysema in patients with bronchiectasis as observed with HRCT (70). The severity and extent of bronchiectasis correlates with severity of airways obstruction (122,123). In bronchiectasis, the airflow obstruction is primarily linked to evidence of small airways disease, such as the extent of decreased attenuation on the expiratory CT, and not so much to bronchiectatic abnormalities in large airways, emphysema, or retained endobronchial secretions (124).

Preliminary studies of airway dimensions in CT suggest that airway thickening and low attenuation areas are independent markers of pulmonary pathophysiology in smokers, that is, the airway and parenchymal components, respectively. Interestingly, in patients with comparable levels of FEV_1, subjects with severe emphysema tend to have less severe airways thickening than patients with less severe emphysema (107).

IV. Scintigraphy Findings

Lung scintigraphy methods are discussed in detail elsewhere in this book. In the current setting, the main findings in emphysema are discussed.

A. Lung Scintigraphy in Emphysema/A1AD

The spatial resolution of scintigraphy is inferior to CT, but nuclear medicine is useful for evaluating pulmonary ventilation because it allows assessment of regional lung function in a physiologic, noninvasive manner. The most widely used radioactive gases are [127]Xe, ^{133}Xe and [81m]Kr (125–127). The ultra fine radiolabeled aerosols [99m]Tc Technegas and [99m]Tc Pertechnegas (particle size 0.02–0.2 μm) distribute within the lung in proportion to regional lung ventilation—almost but not exactly like the gases (128,129). In addition to lung ventilation studies, lung perfusion studies may be performed. The most widely used radiotracer is ^{99m}Tc macro aggregated albumin (MAA). Owing to the different energy of [81m]Kr and ^{99m}Tc, the images can be obtained simultaneously.

The emphysema changes in the lung result in increased airway compliance and resistance, and therefore decreased ventilation to the affected areas. This is typically illustrated as matched inhomogeneous ventilation/perfusion defects, but mismatches also occur (5,60,125,130) (Fig. 22.5).

Many approaches have been made to diagnose and grade the degree of emphysema (125,131–134). The studies have compared the sensitivities of Xenon and Krypton gas (125) for detecting emphysema and also compared them with CXR and CT. Scintigraphic imaging was found superior to CXR and in some studies to CT (60,132). Xenon gas may be more sensitive than [81m]Kr gas for detecting airway obstruction, especially when it is mild in degree (125). Single photon emission computed tomography (SPECT) provides improved contrast resolution and more complete three-dimensional spatial information about the ventilation distribution that can be achieved with planar imaging. SPECT seems superior to planar images in mild and advanced cases of emphysema (135,136).

The emphysematic changes in patients with severe A1AD deficiency have been shown to be associated with panlobular emphysema with characteristic decreased ventilation and perfusion to the lung bases (Fig. 22.6). [133]Xe ventilatory studies have shown delayed ventilatory clearance in patients with homozygous as well as heterozygous A1AD (19,137).

B. Radio-Aerosol Scintigraphy in Emphysema/A1AD

A radio-aerosol is a radiolabeled solid or liquid particle of sufficiently small diameter to maintain some stability as a suspension in air (138). The predominant mechanisms, by which aerosols deposit in the lungs, are inertial impaction, sedimentation, and diffusion. (138). Radio-aerosols are also used for ventilation imaging, and have the advantage of being cheaper and more widely available than the gases described earlier. There are several ^{99m}Tc-radiolabeled aerosols

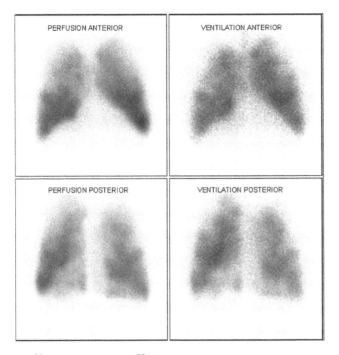

Figure 22.5 [81m]Kr ventilation and ^{99m}Tc MAA perfusion scintigraphy in a patient with COPD/emphysema. Multiple matched inhomogeneous ventilation/perfusion defects.

available, including diethylene triamine penta-acetic acid (^{99m}Tc-DTPA), ^{99m}Tc sulfur colloid, and ^{99m}Tc pyrophosphate (128).

Usually, radio-aerosols deposit centrally in patients with COPD, probably because of airways obstruction and turbulent flow (Fig. 22.7). Therefore, it might not provide an accurate measure of ventilation, yet in milder cases of inhomogenous ventilation distribution radio-aerosols might be more sensitive than the radioactive gases (128,139).

[99m]Tc-phytat-aerosol scans has been applied to distinguish different types of emphysema: panacinar emphysema was characterized by dominant airspace defects in the lower lung with airway deposition in the upper zones. In centrilobular emphysema, the findings were reversed. Similarly, reduced ventilation to obstructed regions can be visualized with the other radio-aerosols and gases (140).

The grading of emphysema using radio-aerosol has also been studied (141). In addition to ventilation imaging, radio-aerosols can be used to investigate drug deposition, mucociliary clearance, and alveolar membrane integrity in emphysema.

C. Drug Deposition

Total deposition in the respiratory tract under various breathing conditions can be determined by measuring the concentration of the aerosol in the inhaled and

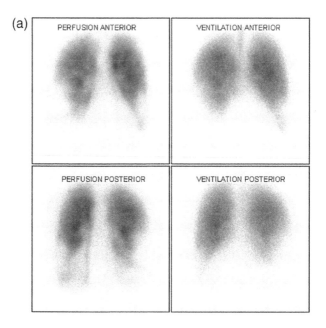

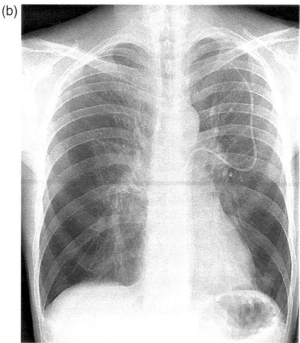

Figure 22.6 (a) [81m]Kr ventilation and ^{99m}Tc MAA perfusion scintigraphy in a patient with A1AD emphysema. Decreased ventilation/perfusion in the lower thirds of the lung. (b) The corresponding CXR.

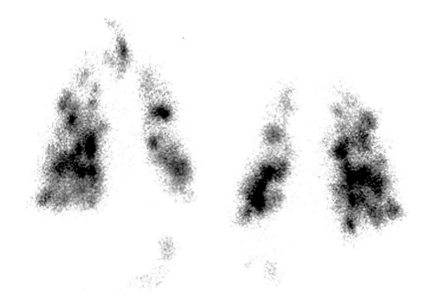

Figure 22.7 Ventilation scintigraphy with radioaerosol (^{99m}Tc-DTPA). The anterior scan at left, and the posterior scan at right, showing inhomogeneous ventilation distribution with hot spot formation. Note the extra-pulmonary activity in the stomach and intestine in the bottom of the illustration.

exhaled air. The regional distribution of aerosol retained within the neck and chest, can be determined by measuring a deposited radio-aerosol with either a gamma camera or a scintillation probe (138).

Drug deposition is interesting from both an environmental point of view and a clinical perspective. Data regarding environmental or occupational aerosol particles suggest that relative to healthy subjects, patients with moderate-to-severe chronic airways obstruction receive an increased dose from ultra-fine particle exposure (particles <0.1 µm in diameter). Some of this increased deposition occurs in the airways, although most deposits in the lung parenchyma. For larger particles, such as applied in clinical drugs like inhaled bronchodilators and steroids, the deposition is also higher in COPD patients than in healthy persons (142). Radiolabeling enables assessment of the deposition of inhaled alpha-one-antitrypsin and other anti-proteases to emphysema patients (143).

D. Mucociliary Clearance

Mucociliary transport can be assessed with a gamma camera after inhalation of insoluble radio-aerosols such as ^{99m}Tc-labeled colloids, that are deposited on the ciliated airways (140). Normally, the transport is unidirectional and continuous and reference values are available (144) (Fig. 22.8). In asymptomatic smokers radio-aerosol clearance is normal, but it is reduced in most patients

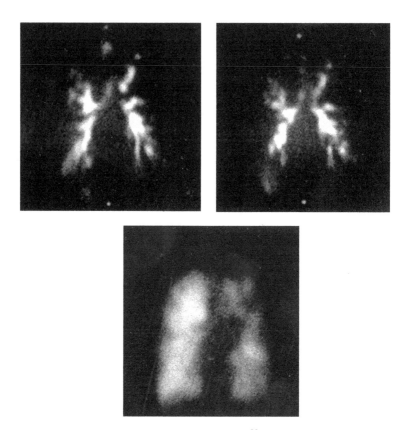

Figure 22.8   Radioaerosol mucociliary clearance ([99m]human albumin colloid) in an emphysema patient. The upper bronchoscintigram represents the initial deposition in the ciliated airways. The middle bronchoscintigram depicts a high retention after 60 min. characterizing slow mucociliary clearance. At the bottom, the corresponding inhomogeneous [81m]Kr ventilation distribution is shown.

with COPD (145,146). In patients with severe emphysema, studies have shown stopping and renewed migrations of mucociliary clearance many times, reversal of mucus flow, and shuttling between the right and left main bronchus. Overall, the lung retention ratio might not be abnormal, but this is explained by the alveolar deposition of aerosols, which is decreased in emphysema patients in comparison with lung healthy persons (147). In a small study of emphysema and A1AD, mucociliary clearance was in the normal range (148).

E.   DTPA Lung Clearance

Clearance of soluble radio-aerosols like ^{99m}Tc-DTPA indicates transepithelial transport, and if ^{99m}Tc-DTPA is preferentially deposited in the alveolar region its removal rate reflects the integrity of the alveolar–capillary membrane. ^{99m}Tc-DTPA clearance is normal in nonsmoking COPD patients, including emphysema patients, but abnormally increased in smokers and patients with interstitial lung disease.

V. Magnetic Resonance Imaging Findings

Magnetic resonance imaging (MRI) has emerged as an important instrument for functional ventilation imaging over the last years. Owing to technical and physical limitations, proton-MRI has been very restricted. Developments in the technique as well as advances in new techniques such as inhaled contrast aerosols, oxygen, hyperpolarized noble gasses ([3]He, [129]Xe), and fluorinated gases (sulfur hexafluoride, SF_6), have improved anatomical and functional ventilation imaging (149,150). The different hyperpolarized gases have various advantages and disadvantages: [3]He is very expensive and limited in amount, but has a greater polarization than [129]Xe. [3]He is not absorbed and is restricted to the airspaces and has no known side effects. [129]Xe is soluble in blood and lipid-rich tissues, which presents the opportunity for additional dissolved-phase imaging, providing a step toward simultaneous ventilation/perfusion studies (151), but the anesthetic effects restrict the use of large amounts.

Using conventional techniques, MRI findings in patients with emphysema have shown reduced and irregular motion of the diaphragm and chest wall, and reduced differences between inspiration and expiration values of wall motion compared with healthy volunteers (149). In preliminary studies using hyperpolarized gases, four different aspects of the lungs have been studied: morphology, dynamic ventilation distribution, apparent diffusion coefficient (a measure of the alveolar size), and partial oxygen tension distribution. These aspects are dealt with separately in different chapters in this book. Preliminary studies of morphology show ventilatory defects characterized by reduced signal intensity or complete lack of signal, corresponding to the affected areas found in scintigraphic evaluations (149,152,153). The defects were round or wedge-shaped, patchy or widespread, small or large, with whole segments or lobes involved. Oval defects are thought to be associated with bronchiolar diseases and alveolar hypoventilation, whereas wedge-shaped ventilatory disturbances are assumed to be associated with bronchial disease (151). In studies of dynamic distribution of ventilation, severely emphysematic parts of the lung show slow or no ventilation at all as well as slow washout (151).

It has been demonstrated that the apparent diffusion coefficient (ADC) is a useful indicator of the relative size of airspaces, and it shows larger values in emphysema patients than in healthy subjects (4,151,154,155). The spatial distribution of the area with highest values of ADC reflects the well-known apical predominance of centrilobular emphysema, and preliminary studies confirm the well-known basilar distribution of A1AD (4,149,156). See Chapter 15 for further details of this technique.

Results from MRI with hyperpolarized ^{3}He show a low degree of specificity, but a very high sensitivity, much higher than CT, nuclear medicine, or PFT (156). The defects seen are in many cases larger than the corresponding abnormalities seen on chest radiographs or CT (157).

Magnetic labeling of blood (arterial spin-tagging) in combination with hyperpolarized helium makes it possible to study ventilation/perfusion abnormalities (153). See Chapters 6 and 14 for further details.

VI. Conclusion

Patients with A1AD often develop panacinar emphysema, primarily located toward the bases. When the disease becomes severe, it becomes more difficult to discriminate this type of emphysema from severe emphysema caused by cigarette smoking.

The first choice for the evaluation of lung diseases is often the chest radiograph. However, CT is superior to both the chest radiograph and pulmonary function testing in detecting the type, distribution, and severity of emphysema. CT also has the advantage of possible monitoring of the progress of emphysema through lung density measurements, in a more sensitive and specific manner than PFTs. The truly functional lung imaging methods, such as nuclear medicine and MR imaging, provide additional information regarding emphysema in patients. For potential inhalation therapy for A1AD and other types of emphysema, information about drug deposition and clearance mechanisms is important and may be obtained using these new imaging methods.

Novel, promising studies with hyperpolarized gas MRI show that it may be superior to CT in detecting emphysema, and also has the potential of monitoring disease progression. Additionally, hyperpolarized gas MRI appears to be safe without significant side effects. Present studies with these novel techniques are further defining their operating characteristics.

References

1. Snider GL, Kleinerman J, Thurlbeck WM, Bengali Z. The definition of emphysema. Report of a National Heart, Lung, and Blood Institute, Division of Lung Diseases Workshop. Am Rev Respir Dis 1985; 132(1):182–185.
2. Eriksson S. Studies in alpha 1-antitrypsin deficiency. Acta Med Scand Suppl 1965; 432:1–85.
3. Hutchison DC. Alpha 1-antitrypsin deficiency in Europe: geographical distribution of Pi types S and Z. Respir Med 1998; 92(3):367–377.

4. Salerno M, de Lange EE, Altes TA, Truwit JD, Brookeman JR, Mugler JP III. Emphysema: hyperpolarized helium-3 diffusion MR imaging of the lungs compared with spirometric indexes—initial experience. Radiology 2002; 222(1):252–260.
5. Fazio F, Lavender JP, Steiner RE. 81 mKr ventilation and 99 mTc perfusion scans in chest disease: comparison with standard radiographs. AJR Am J Roentgenol 1978; 130(3):421–428.
6. Guest PJ, Hansell DM. High resolution computed tomography (HRCT) in emphysema associated with alpha-1-antitrypsin deficiency. Clin Radiol 1992; 45(4):260–266.
7. Foster WL Jr, Gimenez EI, Roubidoux MA, Sherrier RH, Shannon RH, Roggli VL et al. The emphysemas: radiologic–pathologic correlations. Radiographics 1993; 13(2):311–328.
8. Katsura S, Martin CJ. The roenrgenologic diagnosis of anatomic emphysema. Am Rev Respir Dis 1967; 96(4):700–706.
9. Nicklaus TM, Stowell DW, Christiansen WR, Renzetti AD Jr. The accuracy of the roentgenologic diagnosis of chronic pulmonary emphysema. Am Rev Respir Dis 1966; 93(6):889–899.
10. Brantly ML, Paul LD, Miller BH, Falk RT, Wu M, Crystal RG. Clinical features and history of the destructive lung disease associated with alpha-1-antitrypsin deficiency of adults with pulmonary symptoms. Am Rev Respir Dis 1988; 138(2):327–336.
11. Goddard PR, Nicholson EM, Laszlo G, Watt I. Computed tomography in pulmonary emphysema. Clin Radiol 1982; 33(4):379–387.
12. Rosenblum LJ, Mauceri RA, Wellenstein DE, Bassano DA, Cohen WN, Heitzman ER. Computed tomography of the lung. Radiology 1978; 129(2):521–524.
13. Klein JS, Gamsu G, Webb WR, Golden JA, Muller NL. High-resolution CT diagnosis of emphysema in symptomatic patients with normal chest radiographs and isolated low diffusing capacity. Radiology 1992; 182(3):817–821.
14. Sanders C, Nath PH, Bailey WC. Detection of emphysema with computed tomography. Correlation with pulmonary function tests and chest radiography. Invest Radiol 1988; 23(4):262–266.
15. Miniati M, Filippi E, Falaschi F, Carrozzi L, Milne EN, Sostman HD et al. Radiologic evaluation of emphysema in patients with chronic obstructive pulmonary disease. Chest radiography versus high resolution computed tomography. Am J Respir Crit Care Med 1995; 151(5):1359–1367.
16. Thurlbeck WM, Muller NL. Emphysema: definition, imaging, and quantification. Am J Roentgenol 1994; 163(5):1017–1025.
17. Takasugi JE, Godwin JD. Radiology of chronic obstructive pulmonary disease. Radiol Clin North Am 1998; 36(1):29–55.
18. Bonelli FS, Hartman TE, Swensen SJ, Sherrick A. Accuracy of high-resolution CT in diagnosing lung diseases. AJR Am J Roentgenol 1998; 170(6):1507–1512.
19. Webb WR, Müller NL, Naidich DP. High-Resolution CT of the Lung. 3rd ed. Lippincott Williams & Wilkins, 2001.
20. Newell JD Jr. CT of emphysema. Radiol Clin North Am 2002; 40(1):31–42, vii.
21. Guenter CA, Welch MH, Russell TR, Hyde RM, Hammarsten JF. The pattern of lung disease associated with alpha antitrypsin deficiency. Arch Intern Med 1968; 122(3):254–257.

22. Gishen P, Saunders AJ, Tobin MJ, Hutchison DC. Alpha 1-antitrypsin deficiency: the radiological features of pulmonary emphysema in subjects of Pi type Z and Pi type SZ: a survey by the British Thoracic Association. Clin Radiol 1982; 33(4):371–377.

23. King MA, Stone JA, Diaz PT, Mueller CF, Becker WJ, Gadek JE. Alpha 1-antitrypsin deficiency: evaluation of bronchiectasis with CT. Radiology 1996; 199(1):137–141.

24. Cuvelier A, Muir JF, Hellot MF, Benhamou D, Martin JP, Benichou J et al. Distribution of alpha(1)-antitrypsin alleles in patients with bronchiectasis. Chest 2000; 117(2):415–419.

25. Lesur O, Delorme N, Fromaget JM, Bernadac P, Polu JM. Computed tomography in the etiologic assessment of idiopathic spontaneous pneumothorax. Chest 1990; 98(2):341–347.

26. Bense L, Lewander R, Eklund G, Hedenstierna G, Wiman LG. Nonsmoking, non-alpha 1-antitrypsin deficiency-induced emphysema in nonsmokers with healed spontaneous pneumothorax, identified by computed tomography of the lungs. Chest 1993; 103(2):433–438.

27. Gugger M, Gould G, Sudlow MF, Wraith PK, MacNee W. Extent of pulmonary emphysema in man and its relation to the loss of elastic recoil. Clin Sci (Lond) 1991; 80(4):353–358.

28. Knudson RJ, Standen JR, Kaltenborn WT, Knudson DE, Rehm K, Habib MP et al. Expiratory computed tomography for assessment of suspected pulmonary emphysema. Chest 1991; 99(6):1357–1366.

29. Lamers RJ, Thelissen GR, Kessels AG, Wouters EF, van Engelshoven JM. Chronic obstructive pulmonary disease: evaluation with spirometrically controlled CT lung densitometry. Radiology 1994; 193(1):109–113.

30. Gevenois PA, De Vuyst P, Sy M, Scillia P, Chaminade L, de Maertelaer V, Zanen J, Yernault JC. Pulmonary emphysema: quantitative CT during expiration. Radiology 1996; 199(3):825–829.

31. Soejima K, Yamaguchi K, Kohda E, Takeshita K, Ito Y, Mastubara H et al. Longitudinal follow-up study of smoking-induced lung density changes by high-resolution computed tomography. Am J Respir Crit Care Med 2000; 161(4 Pt 1):1264–1273.

32. Nishimura K, Murata K, Yamagishi M, Itoh H, Ikeda A, Tsukino M et al. Comparison of different computed tomography scanning methods for quantifying emphysema. J Thorac Imaging 1998; 13(3):193–198.

33. Madani A, Keyzer C, Gevenois PA. Quantitative computed tomography assessment of lung structure and function in pulmonary emphysema. Eur Respir J 2001; 18(4):720–730.

34. Baldi S, Miniati M, Bellina CR, Battolla L, Catapano G, Begliomini E et al. Relationship between extent of pulmonary emphysema by high-resolution computed tomography and lung elastic recoil in patients with chronic obstructive pulmonary disease. Am J Respir Crit Care Med 2001; 164(4):585–589.

35. Muller NL, Thurlbeck WM. Thin-section CT, emphysema, air trapping, and airway obstruction. Radiology 1996; 199(3):621–622.

36. Mergo PJ, Williams WF, Gonzalez-Rothi R, Gibson R, Ros PR, Staab EV et al. Three-dimensional volumetric assessment of abnormally low attenuation of the

lung from routine helical CT: inspiratory and expiratory quantification. AJR Am J Roentgenol 1998; 170(5):1355–1360.

37. Hayhurst MD, MacNee W, Flenley DC, Wright D, McLean A, Lamb D et al. Diagnosis of pulmonary emphysema by computerised tomography. Lancet 1984; 2(8398):320–322.

38. Gould GA, MacNee W, McLean A, Warren PM, Redpath A, Best JJ et al. CT measurements of lung density in life can quantitate distal airspace enlargement—an essential defining feature of human emphysema. Am Rev Respir Dis 1988; 137(2):380–392.

39. Miller RR, Muller NL, Vedal S, Morrison NJ, Staples CA. Limitations of computed tomography in the assessment of emphysema. Am Rev Respir Dis 1989; 139(4):980–983.

40. Muller NL, Staples CA, Miller RR, Abboud RT. "Density mask." An objective method to quantitate emphysema using computed tomography. Chest 1988; 94(4):782–787.

41. Bergin C, Muller N, Nichols DM, Lillington G, Hogg JC, Mullen B et al. The diagnosis of emphysema. A computed tomographic–pathologic correlation. Am Rev Respir Dis 1986; 133(4):541–546.

42. Gelb AF, Hogg JC, Muller NL, Schein MJ, Kuei J, Tashkin DP et al. Contribution of emphysema and small airways in COPD. Chest 1996; 109(2):353–359.

43. Coxson HO, Rogers RM, Whittall KP, D'yachkova Y, Pare PD, Sciurba FC et al. A quantification of the lung surface area in emphysema using computed tomography. Am J Respir Crit Care Med 1999; 159(3):851–856.

44. Foster WL Jr, Pratt PC, Roggli VL, Godwin JD, Halvorsen RA Jr, Putman CE. Centrilobular emphysema: CT–pathologic correlation. Radiology 1986; 159(1):27–32.

45. Murata K, Itoh H, Todo G, Kanaoka M, Noma S, Itoh T et al. Centrilobular lesions of the lung: demonstration by high-resolution CT and pathologic correlation. Radiology 1986; 161(3):641–645.

46. Hruban RH, Meziane MA, Zerhouni EA, Khouri NF, Fishman EK, Wheeler PS et al. High resolution computed tomography of inflation-fixed lungs. Pathologic–radiologic correlation of centrilobular emphysema. Am Rev Respir Dis 1987; 136(4):935–940.

47. Morrison NJ, Abboud RT, Ramadan F, Miller RR, Gibson NN, Evans KG et al. Comparison of single breath carbon monoxide diffusing capacity and pressure–volume curves in detecting emphysema. Am Rev Respir Dis 1989; 139(5):1179–1187.

48. Morrison NJ, Abboud RT, Muller NL, Miller RR, Gibson NN, Nelems B et al. Pulmonary capillary blood volume in emphysema. Am Rev Respir Dis 1990; 141(1):53–61.

49. Kuwano K, Matsuba K, Ikeda T, Murakami J, Araki A, Nishitani H et al. The diagnosis of mild emphysema. Correlation of computed tomography and pathology scores. Am Rev Respir Dis 1990; 141(1):169–178.

50. Gevenois PA, De Vuyst P, de Maertelaer V, Zanen J, Jacobovitz D, Cosio MG, Yernault JC. Comparison of computed density and microscopic morphometry in pulmonary emphysema. Am J Respir Crit Care Med 1996; 154(1):187–192.

51. Gevenois PA, de Maertelaer V, De Vuyst P, Zanen J, Yernault JC. Comparison of computed density and macroscopic morphometry in pulmonary emphysema. Am J Respir Crit Care Med 1995; 152(2):653–657.

52. Gelb AF, Zamel N, Hogg JC, Muller NL, Schein MJ. Pseudophysiologic emphysema resulting from severe small-airways disease. Am J Respir Crit Care Med 1998; 158(3):815–819.
53. MacNee W, Gould G, Lamb D. Quantifying emphysema by CT scanning. Clinicopathologic correlates. Ann N Y Acad Sci 1991; 624:179–194.
54. Spouge D, Mayo JR, Cardoso W, Muller NL. Panacinar emphysema: CT and pathologic findings. J Comput Assist Tomogr 1993; 17(5):710–713.
55. Hamada T, Sasaguri T, Hisaoka M, Hirakata K, Tanimoto A, Nakata H et al. Mild emphysema: a novel method using formalin-fixed lungs for computed tomography and pathological analyses. Virchows Arch 1995; 426(6):597–602.
56. Bankier AA, de Maertelaer V, Keyzer C, Gevenois PA. Pulmonary emphysema: subjective visual grading versus objective quantification with macroscopic morphometry and thin-section CT densitometry. Radiology 1999; 211(3):851–858.
57. Sashidhar K, Gulati M, Gupta D, Monga S, Suri S. Emphysema in heavy smokers with normal chest radiography. Detection and quantification by HCRT. Acta Radiol 2002; 43(1):60–65.
58. Malinen A, Erkinjuntti-Pekkanen R, Partanen K, Rytkonen H, Vanninen R. Reproducibility of scoring emphysema by HRCT. Acta Radiol 2002; 43(1):54–59.
59. Kinsella M, Muller NL, Abboud RT, Morrison NJ, DyBuncio A. Quantitation of emphysema by computed tomography using a "density mask" program and correlation with pulmonary function tests. Chest 1990; 97(2):315–321.
60. Satoh K, Nakano S, Tanabe M, Nishiyama Y, Takahashi K, Kobayashi T et al. A clinical comparison between Technegas SPECT, CT, and pulmonary function tests in patients with emphysema. Radiat Med 1997; 15(5):277–282.
61. Kauczor HU, Heussel CP, Fischer B, Klamm R, Mildenberger P, Thelen M. Assessment of lung volumes using helical CT at inspiration and expiration: comparison with pulmonary function tests. Am J Roentgenol 1998; 171(4):1091–1095.
62. Crausman RS, Ferguson G, Irvin CG, Make B, Newell JD Jr. Quantitative chest computed tomography as a means of predicting exercise performance in severe emphysema. Acad Radiol 1995; 2(6):463–469.
63. Biernacki W, Gould GA, Whyte KF, Flenley DC. Pulmonary hemodynamics, gas exchange, and the severity of emphysema as assessed by quantitative CT scan in chronic bronchitis and emphysema. Am Rev Respir Dis 1989; 139(6):1509–1515.
64. Fujita J, Nelson NL, Daughton DM, Dobry CA, Spurzem JR, Irino S et al. Evaluation of elastase and antielastase balance in patients with chronic bronchitis and pulmonary emphysema. Am Rev Respir Dis 1990; 142(1):57–62.
65. Gelb AF, Schein M, Kuei J, Tashkin DP, Muller NL, Hogg JC et al. Limited contribution of emphysema in advanced chronic obstructive pulmonary disease. Am Rev Respir Dis 1993; 147(5):1157–1161.
66. Eda S, Kubo K, Fujimoto K, Matsuzawa Y, Sekiguchi M, Sakai F. The relations between expiratory chest CT using helical CT and pulmonary function tests in emphysema. Am J Respir Crit Care Med 1997; 155(4):1290–1294.
67. Watanuki Y, Suzuki S, Nishikawa M, Miyashita A, Okubo T. Correlation of quantitative CT with selective alveolobronchogram and pulmonary function tests in emphysema. Chest 1994; 106(3):806–813.
68. Sakai N, Mishima M, Nishimura K, Itoh H, Kuno K. An automated method to assess the distribution of low attenuation areas on chest CT scans in chronic pulmonary emphysema patients. Chest 1994; 106(5):1319–1325.

69. Beinert T, Brand P, Behr J, Vogelmeier C, Heyder J. Peripheral airspace dimensions in patients with COPD. Chest 1995; 108(4):998–1003.
70. Loubeyre P, Paret M, Revel D, Wiesendanger T, Brune J. Thin-section CT detection of emphysema associated with bronchiectasis and correlation with pulmonary function tests. Chest 1996; 109(2):360–365.
71. Schwaiblmair M, Beinert T, Seemann M, Behr J, Reiser M, Vogelmeier C. Relations between cardiopulmonary exercise testing and quantitative high-resolution computed tomography associated in patients with alpha-1-antitrypsin deficiency. Eur J Med Res 1998; 3(11):527–532.
72. Sakai F, Gamsu G, Im JG, Ray CS. Pulmonary function abnormalities in patients with CT-determined emphysema. J Comput Assist Tomogr 1987; 11(6):963–968.
73. Wakayama K, Kurihara N, Fujimoto S, Hata M, Takeda T. Relationship between exercise capacity and the severity of emphysema as determined by high resolution CT. Eur Respir J 1993; 6(9):1362–1367.
74. Gould GA, Redpath AT, Ryan M, Warren PM, Best JJ, Flenley DC et al. Lung CT density correlates with measurements of airflow limitation and the diffusing capacity. Eur Respir J 1991; 4(2):141–146.
75. Gurney JW, Jones KK, Robbins RA, Gossman GL, Nelson KJ, Daughton D et al. Regional distribution of emphysema: correlation of high-resolution CT with pulmonary function tests in unselected smokers. Radiology 1992; 183(2):457–463.
76. Betsuyaku T, Yoshioka A, Nishimura M, Miyamoto K, Kawakami Y. Pulmonary function is diminished in older asymptomatic smokers and ex-smokers with low attenuation areas on high-resolution computed tomography. Respiration 1996; 63(6):333–338.
77. Bae KT, Slone RM, Gierada DS, Yusen RD, Cooper JD. Patients with emphysema: quantitative CT analysis before and after lung volume reduction surgery. Work in progress. Radiology 1997; 203(3):705–714.
78. Haraguchi M, Shimura S, Hida W, Shirato K. Pulmonary function and regional distribution of emphysema as determined by high-resolution computed tomography. Respiration 1998; 65(2):125–129.
79. Mishima M, Hirai T, Itoh H, Nakano Y, Sakai H, Muro S et al. Complexity of terminal airspace geometry assessed by lung computed tomography in normal subjects and patients with chronic obstructive pulmonary disease. Proc Natl Acad Sci USA 1999; 96(16):8829–8834.
80. Nakano Y, Sakai H, Muro S, Hirai T, Oku Y, Nishimura K et al. Comparison of low attenuation areas on computed tomographic scans between inner and outer segments of the lung in patients with chronic obstructive pulmonary disease: incidence and contribution to lung function. Thorax 1999; 54(5):384–389.
81. Park KJ, Bergin CJ, Clausen JL. Quantitation of emphysema with three-dimensional CT densitometry: comparison with two-dimensional analysis, visual emphysema scores, and pulmonary function test results. Radiology 1999; 211(2):541–547.
82. Kondoh Y, Taniguchi H, Yokoyama S, Taki F, Takagi K, Satake T. Emphysematous change in chronic asthma in relation to cigarette smoking. Assessment by computed tomography. Chest 1990; 97(4):845–849.
83. Wilson JS, Galvin JR. Normal diffusing capacity in patients with PiZ alpha(1)-antitrypsin deficiency, severe airflow obstruction, and significant radiographic emphysema. Chest 2000; 118(3):867–871.

84. Kalender WA, Fichte H, Bautz W, Skalej M. Semiautomatic evaluation procedures for quantitative CT of the lung. J Comput Assist Tomogr 1991; 15(2):248–255.

85. Zagers R, Vrooman HA, Aarts NJ, Stolk J, Schultze Kool LJ, van Voorthuisen E et al. Quantitative analysis of computed tomography scans of the lungs for the diagnosis of pulmonary emphysema. A validation study of a semiautomated contour detection technique. Invest Radiol 1995; 30(9):552–562.

86. Guenard H, Diallo MH, Laurent F, Vergeret J. Lung density and lung mass in emphysema. Chest 1992; 102(1):198–203.

87. Heremans A, Verschakelen JA, van Fraeyenhoven L, Demedts M. Measurement of lung density by means of quantitative CT scanning. A study of correlations with pulmonary function tests. Chest 1992; 102(3):805–811.

88. Zagers H, Vrooman HA, Aarts NJ, Stolk J, Schultze Kool LJ, Dijkman JH et al. Assessment of the progression of emphysema by quantitative analysis of spirometrically gated computed tomography images. Invest Radiol 1996; 31(12):761–767.

89. Hedlund LW, Vock P, Effmann EL. Computed tomography of the lung. Densitometric studies. Radiol Clin North Am 1983; 21(4):775–788.

90. Kemerink GJ, Lamers RJ, Thelissen GR, van Engelshoven JM. CT densitometry of the lungs: scanner performance. J Comput Assist Tomogr 1996; 20(1):24–33.

91. Kemerink GJ, Kruize HH, Lamers RJ, van Engelshoven JM. CT lung densitometry: dependence of CT number histograms on sample volume and consequences for scan protocol comparability. J Comput Assist Tomogr 1997; 21(6):948–954.

92. Naidich DP, Marshall CH, Gribbin C, Arams RS, McCauley DI. Low-dose CT of the lungs: preliminary observations. Radiology 1990; 175(3):729–731.

93. Mishima M, Hirai T, Jin Z, Oku Y, Sakai N, Nakano Y et al. Standardization of low attenuation area versus total lung area in chest X-ray CT as an indicator of chronic pulmonary emphysema. Frontiers Med Biol Engng 1997; 8(2):79–86.

94. Stoel BC, Vrooman HA, Stolk J, Reiber JH. Sources of error in lung densitometry with CT. Invest Radiol 1999; 34(4):303–309.

95. Goldin JG. Quantitative CT of the lung. Radiol Clin North Am 2002; 40(1):145–162.

96. Dirksen A, Dijkman JH, Madsen F, Stoel B, Hutchison DC, Ulrik CS et al. A randomized clinical trial of alpha(1)-antitrypsin augmentation therapy. Am J Respir Crit Care Med 1999; 160(5 Pt 1):1468–1472.

97. Robinson PJ, Kreel L. Pulmonary tissue attenuation with computed tomography: comparison of inspiration and expiration scans. J Comput Assist Tomogr 1979; 3(6):740–748.

98. Rosenblum LJ, Mauceri RA, Wellenstein DE, Thomas FD, Bassano DA, Raasch BN et al. Density patterns in the normal lung as determined by computed tomography. Radiology 1980; 137(2):409–416.

99. Perhomaa M, Jauhiainen J, Lahde S, Ojala A, Suramo I. CT lung densitometry in assessing intralobular air content. An experimental and clinical study. Acta Radiol 2000; 41(3):242–248.

100. Levant MN, Bass H, Anthonisen N, Fraser RG. Microvascular circulation of the lungs in emphysema: correlation of results obtained with Roentgenologic and radioactive-isotope techniques. J Can Assoc Radiol 1968; 19(3):130–134.

101. Lamers RJ, Kemerink GJ, Drent M, van Engelshoven JM. Reproducibility of spirometrically controlled CT lung densitometry in a clinical setting. Eur Respir J 1998; 11(4):942–945.

102. Kalender WA, Rienmuller R, Seissler W, Behr J, Welke M, Fichte H. Measurement of pulmonary parenchymal attenuation: use of spirometric gating with quantitative CT. Radiology 1990; 175(1):265–268.

103. Kohz P, Stabler A, Beinert T, Behr J, Egge T, Heuck A et al. Reproducibility of quantitative, spirometrically controlled CT. Radiology 1995; 197(2):539–542.

104. Dirksen A, Friis M, Olesen KP, Skovgaard LT, Sorensen K. Progress of emphysema in severe alpha 1-antitrypsin deficiency as assessed by annual CT. Acta Radiol 1997; 38(5):826–832.

105. Hogg JC, Macklem PT, Thurlbeck WM. Site and nature of airway obstruction in chronic obstructive lung disease. N Engl J Med 1968; 278(25):1355–1360.

106. Snider GL. CT and COPD. Am J Respir Crit Care Med 1994; 149(2 Pt 1):552–553.

107. Nakano Y, Muro S, Sakai H, Hirai T, Chin K, Tsukino M et al. Computed tomographic measurements of airway dimensions and emphysema in smokers. Correlation with lung function. Am J Respir Crit Care Med 2000; 162(3 Pt 1):1102–1108.

108. Remy-Jardin M, Remy J, Boulenguez C, Sobaszek A, Edme JL, Furon D. Morphologic effects of cigarette smoking on airways and pulmonary parenchyma in healthy adult volunteers: CT evaluation and correlation with pulmonary function tests. Radiology 1993; 186(1):107–115.

109. Remy-Jardin M, Remy J, Gosselin B, Becette V, Edme JL. Lung parenchymal changes secondary to cigarette smoking: pathologic–CT correlations. Radiology 1993; 186(3):643–651.

110. Moon J, du Bois RM, Colby TV, Hansell DM, Nicholson AG. Clinical significance of respiratory bronchiolitis on open lung biopsy and its relationship to smoking related interstitial lung disease. Thorax 1999; 54(11):1009–1014.

111. Heyneman LE, Ward S, Lynch DA, Remy-Jardin M, Johkoh T, Muller NL. Respiratory bronchiolitis, respiratory bronchiolitis-associated interstitial lung disease, and desquamative interstitial pneumonia: different entities or part of the spectrum of the same disease process? Am J Roentgenol 1999; 173(6):1617–1622.

112. Guckel C, Hansell DM. Imaging the "dirty lung"—has high resolution computed tomography cleared the smoke? Clin Radiol 1998; 53(10):717–722.

113. Holt RM, Schmidt RA, Godwin JD, Raghu G. High resolution CT in respiratory bronchiolitis-associated interstitial lung disease. J Comput Assist Tomogr 1993; 17(1):46–50.

114. Sutherland GR, Hume R, James WB, Davison M, Kennedy J. Correlation of regional densitometry patterns, radiological appearances, and pulmonary function tests in chronic bronchitis and emphysema. Thorax 1971; 26(6):716–720.

115. Ng CS, Desai SR, Rubens MB, Padley SP, Wells AU, Hansell DM. Visual quantitation and observer variation of signs of small airways disease at inspiratory and expiratory CT. J Thorac Imaging 1999; 14(4):279–285.

116. Lucidarme O, Coche E, Cluzel P, Mourey-Gerosa I, Howarth N, Grenier P. Expiratory CT scans for chronic airway disease: correlation with pulmonary function test results. Am J Roentgenol 1998; 170(2):301–307.

117. Verschakelen JA, Scheinbaum K, Bogaert J, Demedts M, Lacquet LL, Baert AL. Expiratory CT in cigarette smokers: correlation between areas of decreased lung attenuation, pulmonary function tests and smoking history. Eur Radiol 1998; 8(8):1391–1399.

118. Stern EJ, Webb WR, Gamsu G. Dynamic quantitative computed tomography. A predictor of pulmonary function in obstructive lung diseases. Invest Radiol 1994; 29(5):564–569.
119. Chen D, Webb WR, Storto ML, Lee KN. Assessment of air trapping using post-expiratory high-resolution computed tomography. J Thorac Imaging 1998; 13(2):135–143.
120. Lee KW, Chung SY, Yang I, Lee Y, Ko EY, Park MJ. Correlation of aging and smoking with air trapping at thin-section CT of the lung in asymptomatic subjects. Radiology 2000; 214(3):831–836.
121. Stern EJ, Frank MS. Small-airway diseases of the lungs: findings at expiratory CT. Am J Roentgenol 1994; 163(1):37–41.
122. Lynch DA, Newell J, Hale V, Dyer D, Corkery K, Fox NL et al. Correlation of CT findings with clinical evaluations in 261 patients with symptomatic bronchiectasis. Am J Roentgenol 1999; 173(1):53–58.
123. Wong-You-Cheong JJ, Leahy BC, Taylor PM, Church SE. Airways obstruction and bronchiectasis: correlation with duration of symptoms and extent of bronchiectasis on computed tomography. Clin Radiol 1992; 45(4):256–259.
124. Roberts HR, Wells AU, Milne DG, Rubens MB, Kolbe J, Cole PJ et al. Airflow obstruction in bronchiectasis: correlation between computed tomography features and pulmonary function tests. Thorax 2000; 55(3):198–204.
125. Alderson PO, Line BR. Scintigraphic evaluation of regional pulmonary ventilation. Semin Nucl Med 1980; 10(3):218–242.
126. Fazio F, Jones T. Assessment of regional ventilation by continuous inhalation of radioactive ^{81m}Kr. Br Med J 1975; 3(5985):673–676.
127. Goris ML, Daspit SG, Walter JP, McRae J, Lamb J. Applications of ventilation lung imaging with ^{81m}Kr. Radiology 1977; 122(2):399–403.
128. Worsley D, Gottschalk A. Nuclear medicine techniques and applications. In: Murray J, Nadel J, eds. Textbook of Respiratory Medicine. W.B. Saunders Company, 2000:697–723.
129. Isawa T, Teshima T, Anazawa Y, Miki M, Soni PS. Technegas versus krypton-81m gas as an inhalation agent. Comparison of pulmonary distribution at total lung capacity. Clin Nucl Med 1994; 19(12):1085–1090.
130. Alderson PO, Lee H, Summer WR, Motazedi A, Wagner HN Jr. Comparison of Xe-133 washout and single-breath imaging for the detection of ventilation abnormalities. J Nucl Med 1979; 20(9):917–922.
131. Kaplan E, Mayron LW, Gergans GA, Shponka S, Barnes WE, Friedman AM et al. Pulmonary function and ^{81m}Kr scans in obstructive pulmonary disease. Int J Nucl Med Biol 1981; 8(1):39–51.
132. Alderson PO, Secker-Walker RH, Forrest JV. Detection of obstructive pulmonary disease. Relative sensitivity of ventilation–perfusion studies and chest radiography. Radiology 1974; 112(3):643–648.
133. Xu J, Moonen M, Johansson A, Gustafsson A, Bake B. Quantitative analysis of inhomogeneity in ventilation SPET. Eur J Nucl Med 2001; 28(12):1795–1800.
134. Xu JH, Moonen M, Johansson A, Bake B. Inhomogeneity in planar ventilation scintigraphy of emphysematous patients. Clin Physiol 1998; 18(5):435–440.
135. Satoh K, Tanabe M, Takahashi K, Kobayashi T, Nishiyama Y, Yamamoto Y et al. Assessment of technetium-99 m Technegas scintigraphy for ventilatory impairment

in pulmonary emphysema: comparison of planar and SPECT images. Ann Nucl Med 1997; 11(2):109–113.

136. Suga K, Kume N, Matsunaga N, Ogasawara N, Motoyama K, Hara A et al. Relative preservation of peripheral lung function in smoking-related pulmonary emphysema: assessment with ^{99m}Tc-MAA perfusion and dynamic ^{133}Xe SPET. Eur J Nucl Med 2000; 27(7):800–806.

137. Fallat RJ, Powell MR, Kueppers F, Lilker E. ^{133}Xe ventilatory studies in 1-antitrypsin deficiency. J Nucl Med 1973; 14(1):5–13.

138. Yeates D, Mortensen J. Deposition and clearance. In: Murray J, Nadel J, eds. Textbook of Respiratory Medicine. W.B. Saunders Company, 2000:349–384.

139. Isawa T, Wasserman K, Taplin GV. Lung scintigraphy and pulmonary function studies in obstructive airways disease. UCLA 12–724. UCLA Rep 1969; 60–61.

140. Bahk Y, Kim E, Isawa T. Nuclear Imaging of the Chest. Springer, 1998.

141. Jamadar DA, Kazerooni EA, Martinez FJ, Wahl RL. Semi-quantitative ventilation/perfusion scintigraphy and single-photon emission tomography for evaluation of lung volume reduction surgery candidates: description and prediction of clinical outcome. Eur J Nucl Med 1999; 26(7):734–742.

142. Brown JS, Zeman KL, Bennett WD. Ultrafine particle deposition and clearance in the healthy and obstructed lung. Am J Respir Crit Care Med 2002; 166(9):1240–1247.

143. Hubbard RC, Crystal RG. Augmentation therapy of alpha 1-antitrypsin deficiency. Eur Respir J Suppl 1990; 9:44s–52s.

144. Mortensen J, Lange P, Nyboe J, Groth S. Lung mucociliary clearance. Eur J Nucl Med 1994; 21(9):953–961.

145. Smaldone GC, Foster WM, O'Riordan TG, Messina MS, Perry RJ, Langenback EG. Regional impairment of mucociliary clearance in chronic obstructive pulmonary disease. Chest 1993; 103(5):1390–1396.

146. Ericsson CH, Svartengren K, Svartengren M, Mossberg B, Philipson K, Blomquist M et al. Repeatability of airway deposition and tracheobronchial clearance rate over three days in chronic bronchitis. Eur Respir J 1995; 8(11):1886–1893.

147. Isawa T, Teshima T, Hirano T, Ebina A, Motomiya M, Konno K. Lung clearance mechanisms in obstructive airways disease. J Nucl Med 1984; 25(4):447–454.

148. Mossberg B, Philipson K, Camner P. Tracheobronchial clearance in patients with emphysema associated with alpha1-antitrypsin deficiency. Scand J Respir Dis 1978; 59(1):1–7.

149. Kauczor HU, Chen XJ, van Beek EJ, Schreiber WG. Pulmonary ventilation imaged by magnetic resonance: at the doorstep of clinical application. Eur Respir J 2001; 17(5):1008–1023.

150. Ohno Y, Chen Q, Hatabu H. Oxygen-enhanced magnetic resonance ventilation imaging of lung. Eur J Radiol 2001; 37(3):164–171.

151. Guenther D, Hanisch G, Kauczor HU. Functional MR imaging of pulmonary ventilation using hyperpolarized noble gases. Acta Radiol 2000; 41(6):519–528.

152. de Lange EE, Mugler JP III, Brookeman JR, Knight-Scott J, Truwit JD, Teates CD et al. Lung air spaces: MR imaging evaluation with hyperpolarized ^{3}He gas. Radiology 1999; 210(3):851–857.

153. Lipson DA, Roberts DA, Hansen-Flaschen J, Gentile TR, Jones G, Thompson A et al. Pulmonary ventilation and perfusion scanning using hyperpolarized helium-3 MRI and arterial spin tagging in healthy normal subjects and in pulmonary embolism and orthotopic lung transplant patients. Magn Reson Med 2002; 47(6):1073–1076.

154. Eberle B, Markstaller K, Schreiber WG, Kauczor HU. Hyperpolarised gases in magnetic resonance: a new tool for functional imaging of the lung. Swiss Med Weekly 2001; 131(35–36):503–509.

155. Salerno M, Altes TA, Mugler JP III, Nakatsu M, Hatabu H, de Lange EE. Hyperpolarized noble gas MR imaging of the lung: potential clinical applications. Eur J Radiol 2001; 40(1):33–44.

156. Kauczor HU, Eberle B. Elucidation of structure–function relationships in the lung: contributions from hyperpolarized ^{3}He MRI. Clin Physiol Funct Imaging 2002; 22(6):361–369.

157. McAdams HP, Donnelly LF, MacFall JR. Hyperpolarized gas-enhanced magnetic resonance imaging of the lung. In: Boiselle PM, White CS, eds. New techniques in thoracic imaging. New York: Marcel Dekker, Inc., 2002:265–287.

23

Pulmonary Embolism

MAAIKE SÖHNE, MARIJE TEN WOLDE, and HARRY R. BÜLLER

Academic Medical Center,
Amsterdam, The Netherlands

EDWIN J. R. VAN BEEK

University of Iowa,
Iowa City, Iowa, USA

University of Sheffield,
Sheffield, UK

I. Introduction

In western society, pulmonary embolism is a common disease in both in- and out-patients, with an estimated incidence of one to two per 1000 inhabitants per year. This number increases with age, likely because of the higher prevalence of known risk factors for pulmonary embolism in the elderly. Besides increasing age, many other factors including previous venous thromboembolism, malignancy, immobilization, surgery, pregnancy, the use of oral contraceptives, and genetic risk factors are known to increase the incidence of pulmonary embolism.

It is well known that the clinical diagnosis of pulmonary embolism is inaccurate because of the nonspecificity of the signs and symptoms in patients presenting with a suspicion of this disease. On one hand, overestimation of pulmonary embolism is prevalent, as the disease is confirmed by objective testing in only 25% of the patients. On the other hand, however, the diagnosis is frequently missed in clinical practice as revealed by the high incidence of the disease in autopsy studies. Therefore, objective diagnostic strategies are mandatory to safely confirm or exclude pulmonary embolism. Until recently, pulmonary angiography was the gold standard diagnostic method for establishing and ruling out pulmonary embolism. Nowadays, less invasive diagnostic tests are available to confirm or refute the presence of thrombosis. In this chapter, we will discuss different strategies to exclude or confirm the presence of pulmonary embolism. First, a general overview of the etiology, natural history and treatment will be presented.

II. Etiology

Our understanding of the etiology of venous thromboembolism has markedly improved in the last decades due to many studies that have been exploring the role of inherited and acquired risk factors. Currently, venous thromboembolism is considered to be a multifactorial disease; a result of the interaction between different inherited, genetic, or acquired risk factors. In a majority of patients with deep venous thrombosis or pulmonary embolism, one or more underlying causes can be identified. This knowledge may be helpful in optimizing the duration and intensity of therapy to prevent recurrent venous thromboembolism in the individual patient.

A. Inherited Risk Factors

A number of hereditary abnormalities of the coagulation system are associated with an increased risk for venous thromboembolism. These genetic risk factors can be detected in ~50% of the patients with a first episode of venous thromboembolism.

Antithrombin, Protein C, and Protein S Deficiencies

The first inherited risk factor for venous thrombosis was described by Egeberg in 1965 in a Norwegian family with a tendency for venous thromboembolism (1). This family showed a deficiency of antithrombin, an important physiological inhibitor of activated coagulation factors. Since then, almost all components of the coagulation cascade have been investigated and many risk factors have been identified. The initial studies revealed two more deficiencies of natural anti-coagulants associated with a higher risk of venous thromboembolism, that is, protein C and protein S (2–4). These deficiencies, together with the antithrombin deficiency, are present in 5–10% of the patients diagnosed with thrombosis (5), whereas the prevalence in the general population is <1% (6–8). Patients with heterozygous deficiencies of one or more of these natural anticoagulants are at increased risk of developing thrombosis at a young age, which often occurs spontaneously. Moreover, thrombotic events in these patients have a tendency to recur. Figures on the absolute incidence of venous thromboembolism in subjects with one of these natural anticoagulant deficiencies vary from 3% per year in retrospective family studies (9) to 0.8% per year in a prospective family study (10).

Factor V Leiden

Factor V Leiden is the most common thrombophilic risk factor, with a prevalence varying from 2–15% in the Caucasian population (11) to 15–25% in unselected patients with venous thromboembolism (11–13). A point mutation in the factor V gene causes a hypercoaguable state by slowing the inactivation of factor Va by activated protein C (14). Two large studies show a 2- to 7-fold increased risk of venous thromboembolism for heterozygous carriers over noncarriers (12,15). Homozygous carriers have an approximately 80-fold increased risk when compared with noncarriers (16). The prevalence of the factor V Leiden mutation in patients with primary deep vein thrombosis is twice as high as in those with primary pulmonary embolism (17). Therefore, it is likely that factor V Leiden mutation more often predisposes to deep venous thrombosis than to pulmonary embolism. Furthermore, recent data show that the risk of recurrent venous thromboembolism is similar among carriers and noncarriers of the factor V Leiden mutation (18).

Prothrombin G20210A Mutation

The prothrombin G20210A mutation is found in 2–4% of the Caucasian population (19) and in 6–16% of the patients with unselected deep venous thrombosis

(20). Patients with this mutation have an ~30% increase in plasma prothrombin levels, which therefore likely generates more thrombin. Carriers have a higher risk to develop venous thromboembolism, with an odds ratio of approximately 4 (20).

Furthermore, there are risk factors for which at present it is unknown whether they are congenital. Mild hyperhomocysteinemia, high factor VIII, IX, XI, and thrombin activatable fibrinolysis inhibitor (TAFI) levels, activated protein C resistance without factor V Leiden and dysfibrinogenemia or high levels of fibrinogen belong to this category and are all found to be associated with a higher risk for the development of venous thromboembolism.

B. Acquired Risk Factors

Most of the acquired risk factors are transient. However, increasing age and a history of previous venous thromboembolism are independent and persistent risk factors for life. Estimated incidences of venous thromboembolism in the elderly are 10 times higher than in people under the age of 40 (21). Malignancy and major surgery are probably the strongest risk factors for venous thromboembolism. The association between cancer and venous thromboembolism was already recognized in the 19th century by Trousseau. Thrombosis most commonly occurs in advanced stage of disease with certain types, such as prostatic, pancreatic, ovarian, gastrointestinal, and pulmonary tumors, being most associated (22). Furthermore, in patients with a first episode of idiopathic thrombosis there is a 10–20% probability of having occult cancer at the time of diagnosis or which becomes apparent within the following 2 years (21).

Different surgical procedures carry various risks for the development of deep venous thrombosis and pulmonary embolism. Orthopedic and neurosurgical procedures are associated with the highest risk of developing thrombosis in the postoperative period. For example, incidences of 45–70% (asymptomatic) deep venous thrombosis have been described if no prophylaxis is given after total knee or hip replacement.

Pregnancy and the postpartum period carry a 6- to 10-fold increased thromboembolic risk, with yearly incidences of 0.8 to 1.3 per 1000, with the highest risk during the immediate postpartum period. The presence of antiphospholipid antibodies is another acquired risk factor and is associated with a 9-fold increased risk of venous thrombosis (21). Finally, oral contraceptives are known to increase the risk of venous thromboembolism and use of the second or third generation pills have odds ratios of 4 to 8 towards developing thrombosis as compared with nonusers.

III. Prognosis

Ninety percent of the patients with acute pulmonary embolism will reach hospital to allow a diagnosis to be made, and a classification of massive, submassive, and nonmassive pulmonary embolism has been proposed (23). Massive pulmonary embolism, consisting of patients with hemodynamic instability, is relatively rare, occurring in <5% of the patients. These patients will require aggressive therapy to prevent death. Fibrinolytic therapy is the first line of treatment for this critically ill patient population (24). In the group of hemodynamic stable patients with pulmonary embolism, standard treatment consists of heparin followed by a course of vitamin K antagonists. Recent studies have suggested that patients be then continued on low-dose anticoagulation to diminish the risk of recurrent deep venous thrombosis (34). In the subgroup of patients with echocardiographic signs of right ventricular dysfunction, there is some evidence that more aggressive therapy may be helpful in preventing clinical deterioration (25,26).

Mortality rates over a 3 month observation period in hemodynamically stable patients range from 1% to 7%, with only a small proportion due to recurrent pulmonary embolism. Whether a patient with an adequate blood pressure will die as a result of pulmonary embolism is difficult to predict. Therefore, prognostic parameters are needed to select those patients who might benefit from more aggressive therapy to prevent a bad outcome. Echocardiographic right ventricular dysfunction and laboratory parameters like brain natriuretic peptide (BNP) and cardiac troponin are advocated as prognostic parameters in recent studies.

A. Echocardiography

In patients with acute pulmonary embolism a minimal to severe rise in pulmonary artery pressure can occur, depending on the extent and localization of the embolus, as well as the pre-existing cardiopulmonary status of the patient. With the subsequent increase in right ventricular afterload, the right ventricle may dilate, become hypokinetic, and ultimately fail. Several studies have been performed showing an association between echocardiographic right ventricular dysfunction in patients with pulmonary embolism and a poor prognosis. The prevalence of right ventricular dysfunction in these studies varied from 40% in normotensive patients to 70% in patients with more extensive pulmonary embolism. They suggest an at least 2-fold increased risk of pulmonary embolism related mortality in patients with right ventricular dysfunction. However, this predictive potential seems less strong in hemodynamically stable patients with acute pulmonary embolism. The studies in normotensive patients show a low specificity of 60% and a poor positive predictive value of 5% (24,27). Therefore, it remains unclear whether right ventricular dysfunction is a reliable predictor of adverse outcomes in normotensive patients with acute pulmonary embolism.

B. BNP and Cardiac Troponins

BNP is a plasma neuro-hormone secreted in the cardiac ventricles in response to stretch or pressure increase. Cardiac troponins are released when myocardial injury occurs. Three studies investigating elevated troponin levels in patients with pulmonary embolism have been performed. Elevated levels occur in 20–40% of the patients with acute pulmonary embolism (28–30). These studies show that there is a strong association between elevated troponin levels and mortality in patients with pulmonary embolism, with odds ratios up to 29. However, with small numbers of patients the confidence intervals of these odds ratios are very wide and all the studies included hemodynamically unstable patients. BNP levels are known to correlate with left ventricular dysfunction. One clinical study in 110 hemodynamically stable patients with pulmonary embolism showed an odds ratio of 9 for the risk of death if BNP levels are >21.7 pmol/L (31).

In the future, cardiac troponins, as well as BNP, have the potential to be prognostic indicators and may be useful for optimizing management of patients with acute pulmonary embolism. Prospective studies will be needed to confirm these assumptions.

IV. Therapy

After confirming the diagnosis of pulmonary embolism, treatment is mandatory because the natural history of untreated pulmonary embolism is highly unfavorable. Mortality is as high as 25% as shown by the only randomized, nontreatment controlled trial by Barrit and Jordan in 1960. In patients receiving anticoagulant therapy, mortality varies from 1% to 7%. Standard treatment of patients with hemodynamically stable pulmonary embolism consists of a 5–10 day course of heparin, during which oral vitamin K antagonists are started in a dose to achieve an international normalized ratio (INR) between 2.0 and 3.0. Vitamin K antagonists are then continued for 3–12 months, depending on the presence of risk factors and comorbidity. After this period the treatment is usually stopped, although recurrent venous thromboembolism occurs in 5–10% of the patients in the first year. Extended use of full-dose vitamin K antagonists is associated with reduced rates of recurrent venous thromboembolism (32,33), but this benefit does not outweigh the annual bleeding rate of this therapy in the long term. A recent trial suggested that long-term, low-intensity warfarin therapy given with a target INR of 1.5–2.0 results in a large and significant reduction in the risk of recurrent venous thrombosis and is safe with regard to major bleeding (34). However, this intensity was less effective when compared with an INR of 2–3, while the bleeding rate was similar (35). Hence, the optimal duration and intensity of anticoagulation remains unknown.

Placement of an inferior vena cava filter to prevent lower extremity thrombi from embolizing to the lungs should be considered when a patient cannot be given anticoagulant treatment, when recurrent embolism occurs despite adequate therapy, or if significant bleeding complications are encountered during anticoagulation.

The indication for fibrinolytic therapy in patients with pulmonary embolism is limited to those patients with massive embolism, accompanied by hypotension and/or shock. The use of fibrinolytic therapy in patients with submassive pulmonary embolism and right ventricular dysfunction is still a matter of debate.

V. Diagnostic Strategies

A. Proper Methodological Evaluation of Diagnostic Strategies

Over the last decades many new diagnostic strategies have been introduced in the work-up of patients suspected of pulmonary embolism. In contrast to the development and introduction of new drugs where four subsequent phases must be adequately completed before registration, there are no mandatory guidelines for the evaluation of new diagnostic methods or procedures. To prevent the premature introduction and inappropriate use of new diagnostic techniques, it would be desirable to evaluate a new diagnostic strategy analogs to the four phase hierarchical model for the evaluation of new drugs.

Summary of Phases in Implementing New Diagnostic Strategies

Phase 1

The first phase consists of developing specified technical details of the test. Equipment and use should be defined, as well as physical and/or biochemical parameters specific to the test (e.g., minimal detection level, circadian fluctuation, resolution, and amount of contrast). Objective diagnostic criteria regarding a normal and an abnormal test result should be established and inter-/intraobserver variability needs to be assessed.

Phase 2

In phase two the diagnostic accuracy of the test is assessed. The results of the test under evaluation are compared with the outcome of the gold standard method. This should be performed in sufficiently large numbers of consecutive patients and the readers blinded to the other test results. The accuracy of the test can then be evaluated in terms of sensitivity, specificity, and positive and negative predictive values. If necessary, adjustments of the criteria set in the first phase can be made.

Phase 3

When sufficient accuracy of the test has been proven in the second phase, the third phase can be executed, in which the test will be implemented in the diagnostic process through management studies. Therapeutic decisions will be made, based on the results of the new diagnostic test. Follow-up of all patients will detect false negative test results. In general, a test is considered to be safe if the upper limit of the 95% confidence interval of the number of false negative test results does not exceed 3%. The test can now be introduced into routine clinical practice.

Phase 4

In the fourth and last phase, cost-effectiveness of the new test will be evaluated in comparison to the existing strategies.

B. Criteria in Reviewing Clinical Outcome Studies

Clinical outcome management studies play an important role in the implementation of strategies to exclude or confirm pulmonary embolism. We reviewed different studies to evaluate various diagnostic strategies to exclude or confirm pulmonary embolism. To ensure that the different strategies were safe, we used the following methodological criteria: inclusion of consecutive patients suspected of pulmonary embolism; a predefined diagnostic strategy is used to refute or confirm the diagnosis; whether anticoagulant treatment is withheld or given based on the outcome of the diagnostic strategy; a follow-up of minimum 3 months, with an adequate description of the method of follow-up, and <10% of the patients lost during this time.

C. Clinical Strategies to Exclude or Confirm Pulmonary Embolism

Since <30% of the patients presenting with signs and symptoms suggestive of pulmonary embolism actually have the disease confirmed after objective testing (24,36,37), the diagnostic approach has gradually changed over the years. Strategies range from studies which try to confirm the diagnosis of pulmonary embolism to strategies that try to exclude the diagnosis.

Which Strategies Have Proven to Safely Exclude Pulmonary Embolism?

Strategies to refute pulmonary embolism have been evaluated in numerous clinical outcome studies. Primary outcomes are defined as death due or possibly due to pulmonary embolism and the development of symptomatic deep venous thrombosis or pulmonary embolism in the follow-up period. Sensitivity of these strategies should approach 100%, because with every 2% decrease in sensitivity, 1 per 1000 patients evaluated will die as a result of inappropriately withholding anticoagulant therapy (38). In general, a failure rate with an upper limit of the 95% confidence interval of 3% is considered to be safe. In the next section, we will discuss the diagnostic strategies that have proven to safely exclude pulmonary embolism (Table 23.1).

Clinical Decision Rule, Probability Estimates, and D-Dimer

In excluding pulmonary embolism it is desirable to perform tests that are not invasive. Clinical assessment can be used to identify patients with a low or a high probability for pulmonary embolism. Intuitive clinical probability estimates, as well as structured algorithms are able to achieve a stratification of

Table 23.1 Diagnostic Strategies to Exclude Pulmonary Embolism

Reference	Number of patients	Number of VTE complications	Percentage (upper limit 95% CI)
Normal D-dimer (41,42)	201	0	0 (1.8)
Normal D-dimer and low clinical probability (40,43–45)	894	2	0.2 (0.8)
Normal angiography (36)	480	4	0.8 (2.1)
Normal perfusion lung scintigraphy (51–57)	441	4	0.9 (2.3)
Non-diagnostic V/Q scan and normal serial IPG (51,56,71)	779	13	1.7 (2.8)
Non-diagnostic V/Q scan and normal serial ultrasound (44,72)	875	9	1.0 (2.0)
Normal spiral CT and normal ultrasound (45,65,73)	1264	16	1.3 (2.0)

low, moderate, and high probability categories in patients with suspected pulmonary embolism. According to several studies, the prevalence is expected to be $\leq 10\%$ in patients with a low clinical probability, $\sim 25\%$ in the group with an intermediate probability and $\geq 60\%$ in patients with a high probability (39). However, one may not exclude pulmonary embolism solely on the basis of clinical assessment, because ~ 1 in 10 (40) of the patients with a low clinical probability still have the disease confirmed by objective testing.

D-dimer assay levels have been suggested to be helpful in evaluating whether a patient has developed a deep venous thrombosis or pulmonary embolism. D-dimers are formed when crosslinked fibrin is lysed by plasmin. Therefore, patients with thrombosis usually have elevated D-dimer concentrations. Unfortunately, elevations of D-dimer concentrations are nonspecific (e.g., levels can be increased by aging, inflammation, and cancer). Thus, an abnormal result has a low positive predictive value. The utility of measuring D-dimer concentration in patients suspected of pulmonary embolism is its high negative predictive value. There are many different D-dimer assays available with widely varying sensitivities and negative predictive values. With the current rapid

ELISA test and immunoturbidimetric assay, both sensitivity and negative predictive values are high (90–100% and 94–100%, respectively). Nevertheless, most D-dimer assays do not have a sufficiently high sensitivity to be used as the only method to exclude pulmonary embolism. Two studies have been performed using a normal D-dimer concentration, measured with a rapid ELISA test, as the only step to exclude the disease in all referred patients (41,42). A total of 201 patients were included and none of the patients experienced venous thrombotic events during a 3 month follow-up period (failure rate 0%; upper limit 95% CI 1.8%).

The combination of a normal D-dimer concentration together with a low clinical probability to exclude pulmonary embolism in all referred patients was evaluated in four studies (40,43–45). Of the 894 patients included, there were two venous thrombotic events during follow-up (failure rate 0.2%; upper 95% CI 0.8%). Hence, the combination of low clinical probability and a normal high sensitive D-dimer assay is safe to rule out pulmonary embolism.

Pulmonary Angiography

The procedure for the performance of pulmonary angiography is standardized and criteria for a normal and an abnormal test result are well formulated (46,47). Interobserver variability has been found to be minimal, especially with use of intra-arterial digital subtraction angiography (48,49). As pulmonary angiography is generally accepted as the "gold standard" or reference method in the diagnostic process of pulmonary embolism, sensitivity and specificity of this technique cannot be evaluated formally. Nevertheless, the technique has shown its reliability in several clinical studies where follow-up of patients with normal angiographies revealed a recurrent thromboembolic event rate of 1.9%. In one multicenter study of 931 in- and outpatients, 755 (81%) underwent pulmonary angiography. Results were normal in 480 patients and these patients did not receive anticoagulant treatment. During follow-up 4 patients died of pulmonary embolism (failure rate 0.8%; upper limit 95% CI 2.1%) (36).

Ventilation–Perfusion Scintigraphy and Serial Leg Testing

Ventilation–perfusion scintigraphy (V/Q scan) has completed all phases of a proper methodological evaluation of a diagnostic test. The first phase started with the introduction of the perfusion scan in 1964. The technique is safe (50), but the criteria for interpretation of the scans have long been a matter of debate. Presently, a classification of normal, high probability and nondiagnostic scan outcomes is clinically most applicable and widely accepted. A comprehensive assessment of the sensitivity and specificity of V/Q scans was reported in the PIOPED study (36). In this study, 755 patients suspected of pulmonary embolism underwent V/Q scanning and pulmonary angiography. Two hundred and fifty-one patients (33%) had angiographic proven pulmonary embolism. Ninety-eight percent of these patients had abnormal V/Q scan findings, with 41% having high probability scans. Sensitivity and negative predictive value of the near normal/normal scan were 98% and 91%, respectively. Thus, in using scintigraphy in the management of patients with suspected pulmonary embolism, a normal perfusion scan safely rules out the diagnosis and treatment can be withheld (51–57). Unfortunately, this occurs only in approximately one-fourth of patients. In 40–60% of the patients with a nondiagnostic scan, a second diagnostic test is necessary to exclude pulmonary embolism. For this purpose, serial leg testing (ultrasound or impedance plethysmography) over a period of ~10 days or angiography may be used (44,58).

Helical Computed Tomography

Helical computed tomography (CT), also known as spiral CT, has been developed as a diagnostic tool in confirming and excluding pulmonary embolism since 1992, when the first clinical study with spiral CT was performed (59). Criteria for diagnosing pulmonary embolism have been established. Interobserver variability is demonstrated to be good in several studies, although there is a clear learning curve for reliably interpreting spiral CT (60). Considering pulmonary angiography as the reference standard, the reported sensitivities in different studies with spiral CT ranges from 64% to 93%, with specificity from 89% to 100% (61). These wide ranges may be related to differences in patient selection and other study design aspects (60,61). Recently, a new generation helical CT has become available, the multidetector helical CT, which has a shorter imaging time and thinner collimation. Initial studies with this multidetector helical CT suggest higher sensitivities, especially for subsegmental embolism (62–64), however, management studies have not yet been performed with this newer technology.

Thus far, a few management studies have been performed using single-detector spiral CT. These studies show reasonable operating characteristics. In two studies, single-detector spiral CT was combined with ultrasound to exclude pulmonary embolism in either patients with a low/intermediate clinical probability or in patients with a moderate/high probability. The study of Musset et al. shows venous thromboembolic events during a 3 month follow-up in 1.8% (upper 95% CI 3.3%). Anderson et al. did not observe any thrombotic events during follow-up (upper 95% CI 1.3%) in patients with a moderate/high probability or an abnormal D-dimer and normal spiral CT and ultrasound. The only management study using normal single detector spiral CT and normal serial ultrasound to exclude pulmonary embolism in all referred patients showed a sensitivity >99% (65). Ultrasound was positive in only 2 of these 248 (0.8%) patients. It could be suggested that with new multidetector spiral CT it may even be safe to exclude pulmonary embolism based on the result of a normal scan alone. However, this needs to be confirmed in future prospective studies.

Which Strategies Have Proven to Adequately Confirm Pulmonary Embolism?

In evaluating whether a diagnostic strategy is accurate enough to confirm pulmonary embolism, the most important parameters are the positive predictive value and the specificity of the test. This should be high, because incorrect

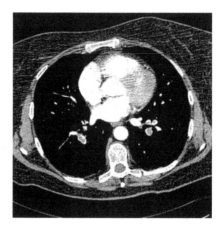

Figure 23.1 Central intravascular filling defects in the lower lobe pulmonary arteries bilaterally consistent with pulmonary embolism. The clot is surrounded by contrast medium.

diagnosis of the condition (false positive) exposes the patient to anticoagulant therapy and therefore to the risk of major bleeding. Several strategies are available to confirm the presence of pulmonary embolism.

Pulmonary Angiography

Pulmonary angiography visualizes emboli through a persistent intraluminal filling defect or an abrupt cut-off in an artery with a diameter of >2 mm (66). Specificity figures are unknown because it is the reference method. Interobserver

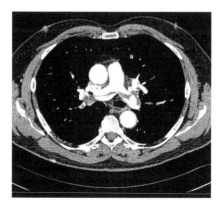

Figure 23.2 Large eccentric central mural defect observed in the pulmonary arteries bilaterally as a sign of pulmonary embolism on spiral CT.

variability is good and nondiagnostic results occur in ~4%. Approximately 10–20% of patients are unable to undergo angiography because of contraindications (46,67). With modern techniques, pulmonary angiography is associated with a 0.1% mortality rate and major nonfatal complications in 0.4% of patients (68,69). Because of this known risk of fatal complications, although minimal, clinicians often hesitate to perform angiography.

Ventilation–Perfusion Scintigraphy

By comparing the distribution of ^{99m}Technetium labeled albumin in the pulmonary vasculature with the distribution of radioactive aerosol in the lung airspace, mismatches can be defined. A high probability lung scan is defined as at least one mismatched perfusion defect that is segmental or larger (36,70). The specificity in the PIOPED study of a high probability scan result was 97% and the positive predictive value was 88%.

Helical Computed Tomography

A central partial intravascular filling defect surrounded by contrast medium, an eccentric or mural defect surrounded by contrast or a complete filling defect in a vessel are all signs of acute pulmonary embolism on spiral CT (60) (Figs. 23.1 and 23.2). Specificity of spiral CT varies widely depending on collimation thickness. For 5 mm collimation scans, specificity ranges from 67% to 100%, while specificities of 94–100% are reported with 2 mm collimation (60). Spiral CT has the additional advantage of providing an alternative diagnosis in a large proportion of patients suspected of pulmonary embolism (61).

Serial Leg Testing

If in the diagnostic work-up of patients with suspected pulmonary embolism the result of a ventilation–perfusion scintigraphy is nondiagnostic, further tests should be performed. Serial leg testing has been used because deep venous thrombosis and pulmonary embolism are both entities of the same disease. About three quarters of all patients who are diagnosed with pulmonary embolism do have deep venous thrombosis. Therefore, the visualization of a deep venous thrombosis in a patient with clinical symptoms of pulmonary embolism is considered to be diagnostic for venous thromboembolism. Positive results of serial leg testing after nondiagnostic ventilation–perfusion scan are found in 5–11% of the patients and almost all within the first 5 days (58,71,72). Furthermore, serial leg testing is used in some studies after a normal spiral CT. Positive ultrasound is found in 1–8% of the patients with a normal spiral CT (45,65,73).

D. Recommended Diagnostic Algorithms

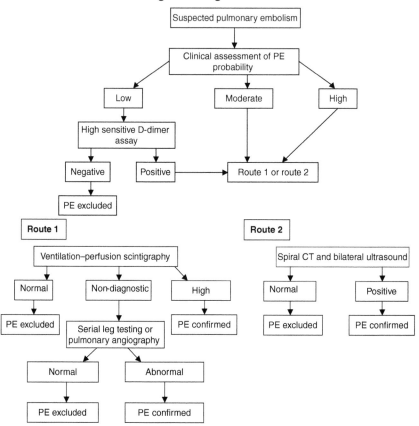

References

1. Egeberg O. Inherited antithrombin deficiency causing thrombophilia. Thromb Diath Haemorrh 1965; 13:516–530.
2. Griffin JH, Evatt B, Zimmerman TS, Kleiss AJ, Wideman C. Deficiency of protein C in congenital thrombotic disease. J Clin Invest 1981; 68(5):1370–1373.
3. Broekmans AW, Veltkamp JJ, Bertina RM. Congenital protein C deficiency and venous thromboembolism. A study of three Dutch families. N Engl J Med 1983; 309(6):340–344.
4. Schwarz HP, Fischer M, Hopmeier P, Batard MA, Griffin JH. Plasma protein S deficiency in familial thrombotic disease. Blood 1984; 64(6):1297–1300.
5. Lensing AW, Prandoni P, Prins MH, Buller HR. Deep-vein thrombosis. Lancet 1999; 353(9151):479–485.
6. Tait RC, Walker ID, Perry DJ, Islam SI, Daly ME, McCall F et al. Prevalence of antithrombin deficiency in the healthy population. Br J Haematol 1994; 87(1):106–112.

7. Miletich J, Sherman L, Broze G Jr. Absence of thrombosis in subjects with hetero-zygous protein C deficiency. N Engl J Med 1987; 317(16):991–996.
8. Tait RC, Walker ID, Reitsma PH, Islam SI, McCall F, Poort SR et al. Prevalence of protein C deficiency in the healthy population. Thromb Haemost 1995; 73(1):87–93.
9. van den Belt AGM, Prins MH, Huisman MV, Hirsh J. Familial thrombophilia: a review analysis. Clin Appl Thromb Hemost 1996; 2:227–236.
10. Sanson BJ, Simioni P, Tormene D, Moia M, Friederich PW, Huisman MV et al. The incidence of venous thromboembolism in asymptomatic carriers of a deficiency of antithrombin, protein C, or protein S: a prospective cohort study. Blood 1999; 94(11):3702–3706.
11. Rees DC, Cox M, Clegg JB. World distribution of factor V Leiden. Lancet 1995; 346(8983):1133–1134.
12. Koster T, Rosendaal FR, de Ronde H, Briet E, Vandenbroucke JP, Bertina RM. Venous thrombosis due to poor anticoagulant response to activated protein C: Leiden Thrombophilia Study. Lancet 1993; 342(8886–8887):1503–1506.
13. Svensson PJ, Dahlback B. Resistance to activated protein C as a basis for venous thrombosis. N Engl J Med 1994; 330(8):517–522.
14. De Stefano V, Finazzi G, Mannucci PM. Inherited thrombophilia: pathogenesis, clinical syndromes, and management. Blood 1996; 87(9):3531–3544.
15. Ridker PM, Hennekens CH, Lindpaintner K, Stampfer MJ, Eisenberg PR, Miletich JP. Mutation in the gene coding for coagulation factor V and the risk of myocardial infarction, stroke, and venous thrombosis in apparently healthy men. N Engl J Med 1995; 332(14):912–917.
16. Rosendaal FR, Koster T, Vandenbroucke JP, Reitsma PH. High risk of thrombosis in patients homozygous for factor V Leiden (activated protein C resistance). Blood 1995; 85(6):1504–1508.
17. Turkstra F, Karemaker R, Kuijer PM, Prins MH, Buller HR. Is the prevalence of the factor V Leiden mutation in patients with pulmonary embolism and deep vein throm-bosis really different? Thromb Haemost 1999; 81(3):345–348.
18. Eichinger S, Weltermann A, Mannhalter C, Minar E, Bialonczyk C, Hirschl M et al. The risk of recurrent venous thromboembolism in heterozygous carriers of factor V Leiden and a first spontaneous venous thromboembolism. Arch Intern Med 2002; 162(20):2357–2360.
19. Rosendaal FR, Doggen CJ, Zivelin A, Arruda VR, Aiach M, Siscovick DS et al. Geographic distribution of the 20210 G to A prothrombin variant. Thromb Haemost 1998; 79(4):706–708.
20. Emmerich J, Rosendaal FR, Cattaneo M, Margaglione M, De Stefano V, Cumming T et al. Combined effect of factor V Leiden and prothrombin 20210A on the risk of venous thromboembolism–pooled analysis of 8 case–control studies including 2310 cases and 3204 controls. Study Group for Pooled-Analysis in Venous Throm-boembolism. Thromb Haemost 2001; 86(3):809–816.
21. Martinelli I. Risk factors in venous thromboembolism. Thromb Haemost 2001; 86(1):395–403.
22. Sorensen HT, Mellemkjaer L, Olsen JH, Baron JA. Prognosis of cancers associated with venous thromboembolism. N Engl J Med 2000; 343(25):1846–1850.
23. Guidelines on diagnosis and management of acute pulmonary embolism. Task Force on Pulmonary Embolism, European Society of Cardiology. Eur Heart J 2000; 21(16):1301–1336.

24. Goldhaber SZ, Haire WD, Feldstein ML, Miller M, Toltzis R, Smith JL et al. Alteplase versus heparin in acute pulmonary embolism: randomised trial assessing right-ventricular function and pulmonary perfusion. Lancet 1993; 341(8844):507–511.

25. Konstantinides S, Geibel A, Heusel G, Heinrich F, Kasper W. Heparin plus alteplase compared with heparin alone in patients with submassive pulmonary embolism. N Engl J Med 2002; 347(15):1143–1150.

26. Konstantinides S, Geibel A, Olschewski M, Heinrich F, Grosser K, Rauber K et al. Association between thrombolytic treatment and the prognosis of hemodynamically stable patients with major pulmonary embolism: results of a multicenter registry. Circulation 1997; 96(3):882–888.

27. Grifoni S, Olivotto I, Cecchini P, Pieralli F, Camaiti A, Santoro G et al. Short-term clinical outcome of patients with acute pulmonary embolism, normal blood pressure, and echocardiographic right ventricular dysfunction. Circulation 2000; 101(24):2817–2822.

28. Konstantinides S, Geibel A, Olschewski M, Kasper W, Hruska N, Jackle S et al. Importance of cardiac troponins I and T in risk stratification of patients with acute pulmonary embolism. Circulation 2002; 106(10):1263–1268.

29. Douketis JD, Crowther MA, Stanton EB, Ginsberg JS. Elevated cardiac troponin levels in patients with submassive pulmonary embolism. Arch Intern Med 2002; 162(1):79–81.

30. Giannitsis E, Muller-Bardorff M, Kurowski V, Weidtmann B, Wiegand U, Kampmann M et al. Independent prognostic value of cardiac troponin T in patients with confirmed pulmonary embolism. Circulation 2000; 102(2):211–217.

31. ten Wolde M, Tulevski II, Mulder JWM, Söhne M, Boomsma F, Mulder BJM, Buller HR. Brain natriuretic peptide (BNP) as a predictor of adverse outcome in patients with pulmonary embolism. Circulation 2003; 107(16):2082–2084.

32. Schulman S, Granqvist S, Holmstrom M, Carlsson A, Lindmarker P, Nicol P et al. The duration of oral anticoagulant therapy after a second episode of venous thromboembolism. The Duration of Anticoagulation Trial Study Group. N Engl J Med 1997; 336(6):393–398.

33. Kearon C, Gent M, Hirsh J, Weitz J, Kovacs MJ, Anderson DR et al. A comparison of three months of anticoagulation with extended anticoagulation for a first episode of idiopathic venous thromboembolism. N Engl J Med 1999; 340(12):901–907.

34. Ridker PM, Goldhaber SZ, Danielson E, Rosenberg Y, Eby CS, Deitcher SR et al. Long-term, low-intensity warfarin therapy for the prevention of recurrent venous thromboembolism. N Engl J Med 2003; 348;1425–1434.

35. Kearon C, Ginsberg JS, Kovacs M, Anderson DR, Wells P. Low-intensity (INR 1.5-1.9) versus conventional-intensity (INR 2.0–3.0) anticoagulation for extended treatment of unprovoked VTE: a randomized double blind trial. Blood 2002; 100(11):150a.

36. PIOPED Investigators. Value of the ventilation/perfusion scan in acute pulmonary embolism. Results of the prospective investigation of pulmonary embolism diagnosis (PIOPED). The PIOPED Investigators. J Am Med Assoc 1990; 263(20):2753–2759.

37. Hull RD, Hirsh J, Carter CJ, Jay RM, Dodd PE, Ockelford PA et al. Pulmonary angiography, ventilation lung scanning, and venography for clinically suspected pulmonary embolism with abnormal perfusion lung scan. Ann Intern Med 1983; 98(6):891–899.

38. van Beek EJ, Schenk BE, Michel BC, van den Ende B, Brandjes DP, van der Heide YT, Bossuyt PM, Buller HR. The role of plasma D-dimers concentration in the exclusion of pulmonary embolism. Br J Haematol 1996; 92(3):725–732.

39. Kearon C. Diagnosis of pulmonary embolism. CMAJ 2003; 168(2):183–194.

40. Kruip MJ, Slob MJ, Schijen JH, van der HC, Buller HR. Use of a clinical decision rule in combination with D-dimer concentration in diagnostic workup of patients with suspected pulmonary embolism: a prospective management study. Arch Intern Med 2002; 162(14):1631–1635.

41. Perrier A, Desmarais S, Miron MJ, de Moerloose P, Lepage R, Slosman D et al. Non-invasive diagnosis of venous thromboembolism in outpatients. Lancet 1999; 353(9148):190–195.

42. Bernier M, Miron MJ, Desmarais S, Berube C. Use of the D-dimer measurement as first step in the diagnosis deep vein thrombosis (DVT) and pulmonary embolism (PE) in an emergency department. Thromb Haemost 7(suppl):P754. 2001.

43. Wells PS, Anderson DR, Rodger M, Stiell I, Dreyer JF, Barnes D et al. Excluding pulmonary embolism at the bedside without diagnostic imaging: management of patients with suspected pulmonary embolism presenting to the emergency department by using a simple clinical model and d-dimer. Ann Intern Med 2001; 135(2):98–107.

44. ten Wolde M, Hagen PJ, Mac Gillavry MR, Pollen IJ, Koopman MMW, Postmus PE, Buller HR. Non-invasive diagnostic work-up of patients with suspected pulmonary embolism: preliminary results of a management study. Thromb Haemost 7(suppl):OC153. 2001.

45. Anderson DR, Wells P, Kovacs M, Dennie C, Kovacs G, Stiell I et al. Use of spiral computerized tomography (CT) to exclude the diagnosis of pulmonary embolism in the emergency department. Thromb Haemost 7(suppl):OC156. 2001 BC.

46. Stein PD, Athanasoulis C, Alavi A, Greenspan RH, Hales CA, Saltzman HA et al. Complications and validity of pulmonary angiography in acute pulmonary embolism. Circulation 1992; 85(2):462–468.

47. Bookstein JJ. Segmental arteriography by pulmonary embolism. Radiology 1969; 93(5):1007–1012.

48. van Beek EJ, Bakker AJ, Reekers JA. Pulmonary embolism: interobserver agreement in the interpretation of conventional angiographic and DSA images in patients with nondiagnostic lung scan results. Radiology 1996; 198(3):721–724.

49. Quinn MF, Lundell CJ, Klotz TA, Finck EJ, Pentecost M, McGehee WG et al. Reliability of selective pulmonary arteriography in the diagnosis of pulmonary embolism. AJR Am J Roentgenol 1987; 149(3):469–471.

50. Wagner HN, Sabiston DC, McAfee JG, Tow D, Stern HS. Diagnosis of massive pulmonary embolism in man by radioisotope scanning. N Engl J Med 1964; 271:377–384.

51. van Beek EJ, Kuyer PM, Schenk BE, Brandjes DP, ten Cate JW, Buller HR. A normal perfusion lung scan in patients with clinically suspected pulmonary embolism. Frequency and clinical validity. Chest 1995; 108(1):170–173.

52. Miron MJ, Perrier A, Bounameaux H, de Moerloose P, Slosman DO, Didier D et al. Contribution of noninvasive evaluation to the diagnosis of pulmonary embolism in hospitalized patients. Eur Respir J 1999; 13(6):1365–1370.

53. Perrier A, Bounameaux H, Morabia A, de Moerloose P, Slosman D, Didier D et al. Diagnosis of pulmonary embolism by a decision analysis-based strategy including

clinical probability, D-dimer levels, and ultrasonography: a management study. Arch Intern Med 1996; 156(5):531–536.

54. Kruit WH, de Boer AC, Sing AK, van Roon F. The significance of venography in the management of patients with clinically suspected pulmonary embolism. J Intern Med 1991; 230(4):333–339.

55. van Beek EJ, Kuijer PM, Buller HR, Brandjes DP, Bossuyt PM, ten Cate JW. The clinical course of patients with suspected pulmonary embolism. Arch Intern Med 1997; 157(22):2593–2598.

56. de Groot MR, van Marwijk KM, Pouwels JG, Engelage AH, Kuipers BF, Buller HR. The use of a rapid D-dimer blood test in the diagnostic work-up for pulmonary embolism: a management study. Thromb Haemost 1999; 82(6):1588–1592.

57. Miniati M, Monti S, Pratali L, Di Ricco G, Marini C, Formichi B et al. Value of transthoracic echocardiography in the diagnosis of pulmonary embolism: results of a prospective study in unselected patients. Am J Med 2001; 110(7):528–535.

58. Hull RD, Raskob GE, Ginsberg JS, Panju AA, Brill-Edwards P, Coates G et al. A noninvasive strategy for the treatment of patients with suspected pulmonary embolism. Arch Intern Med 1994; 154(3):289–297.

59. Remy-Jardin M, Remy J, Wattinne L, Giraud F. Central pulmonary thromboembolism: diagnosis with spiral volumetric CT with the single-breath-hold technique—comparison with pulmonary angiography. Radiology 1992; 185(2):381–387.

60. Ghaye B, Remy J, Remy-Jardin M. Non-traumatic thoracic emergencies: CT diagnosis of acute pulmonary embolism: the first 10 years. Eur Radiol 2002; 12(8):1886–1905.

61. Mullins MD, Becker DM, Hagspiel KD, Philbrick JT. The role of spiral volumetric computed tomography in the diagnosis of pulmonary embolism. Arch Intern Med 2000; 160(3):293–298.

62. Raptopoulos V, Boiselle PM. Multi-detector row spiral CT pulmonary angiography: comparison with single-detector row spiral CT. Radiology 2001; 221(3):606–613.

63. Schoepf UJ, Holzknecht N, Helmberger TK, Crispin A, Hong C, Becker CR et al. Subsegmental pulmonary emboli: improved detection with thin-collimation multi-detector row spiral CT. Radiology 2002; 222(2):483–490.

64. Remy-Jardin M, Tillie-Leblond I, Szapiro D, Ghaye B, Cotte L, Mastora I et al. CT angiography of pulmonary embolism in patients with underlying respiratory disease: impact of multislice CT on image quality and negative predictive value. Eur Radiol 2002; 12(8):1971–1978.

65. Van Strijen MJ, De Monye W, Schiereck J, Kieft GJ, Prins MH, Huisman MV, Pattynama PM. Single-detector helical computed tomography as the primary diagnostic test in suspected pulmonary embolism: a multicenter clinical management study of 510 patients. Ann Intern Med 2003; 138(4):307–314.

66. Lee AY, Hirsh J. Diagnosis and treatment of venous thromboembolism. Annu Rev Med 2002; 53:15–33.

67. van Beek EJ, Reekers JA, Batchelor DA, Brandjes DP, Büller HR. Feasibility, safety and clinical utility of angiography in patients with suspected pulmonary embolism. Eur Radiol 1996; 6(4):415–419.

68. Nilsson T, Carlsson A, Mare K. Pulmonary angiography: a safe procedure with modern contrast media and technique. Eur Radiol 1998; 8(1):86–89.

69. Hudson ER, Smith TP, McDermott VG, Newman GE, Suhocki PV, Payne CS et al. Pulmonary angiography performed with iopamidol: complications in 1434 patients. Radiology 1996; 198(1):61–65.

70. Hull RD, Hirsh J, Carter CJ, Raskob GE, Gill GJ, Jay RM et al. Diagnostic value of ventilation–perfusion lung scanning in patients with suspected pulmonary embolism. Chest 1985; 88(6):819–828.

71. Ginsberg JS, Brill-Edwards PA, Demers C, Donovan D, Panju A. D-dimer in patients with clinically suspected pulmonary embolism. Chest 1993; 104(6):1679–1684.

72. Wells PS, Ginsberg JS, Anderson DR, Kearon C, Gent M, Turpie AG et al. Use of a clinical model for safe management of patients with suspected pulmonary embolism. Ann Intern Med 1998; 129(12):997–1005.

73. Musset D, Parent F, Meyer G, Maitre S, Girard P, Leroyer C et al. Diagnostic strategy for patients with suspected pulmonary embolism: a prospective multicentre outcome study. Lancet 2002; 360(9349):1914–1920.

24

Chronic Thromboembolic Pulmonary Hypertension

LEWIS J. RUBIN

University of California,
La Jolla, California, USA

JOHN DUNNING

Cambridge University School of Medicine,
Cambridge, UK

I. Introduction

Pulmonary artery hypertension (PAH) is increasingly recognized as a source of major morbidity and mortality in the population. A revised classification system for the various causes of PAH has been recently proposed, which highlights the heterogeneous nature of this condition (1) The mainstay of therapy for PAH is medical management, including the use of new potent pulmonary vasodilator and antiproliferative agents (2). When medical therapy fails, lung transplantation has been used to good effect, and pulmonary hypertension from all causes accounts for approximately one-third of all lung transplants performed. However, this surgical therapy carries a significant operative risk, and its effectiveness is limited in the long-term by the side effects of immunosuppressive therapy and allograft rejection (3).

As awareness of PAH has increased, it has become apparent that chronic thromboembolism as a cause of chronic pulmonary hypertension is a more prevalent condition than had been previously considered (4). Recognition of this condition has led to the development and acceptance of pulmonary endarterectomy as a definitive surgical therapy for this group of patients, offering a perioperative risk similar to or lower than transplantation, with the benefit of improved prognosis and function without the restrictions of complex therapeutic regimens.

II. Etiology

The majority of patients with acute pulmonary emboli experience resolution of the emboli with no physiological or functional sequelae. Although the prevalence of chronic thromboembolic pulmonary hypertension (CTEPH) is unknown, a recent report of patients followed after an initial episode of pulmonary embolism found an incidence of 3.8% at 2 years (4). This is likely an underestimate of the incidence, because the majority of patients with CTEPH do not have a prior history of symptomatic or documented acute thromboembolism (5).

Although a clinical history of acute pulmonary embolism is absent in half or more of all patients who develop CTEPH, it is likely that most of these patients have experienced one or more episodes of acute venous thromboembolism in the past. In these patients, failure to resolve these thromboemboli is the presumed cause of the disease, although the exact mechanism responsible for failure of the normal fibrinolytic pathway is unclear. Recent evidence suggests elevations in Factor VIII in patients with CTEPH may be responsible (6).

Thrombotic material will proceed along large vessels until it reaches a bifurcation where the lumenal diameter is less than the diameter of the material resulting in occlusion. At this point, the blood in the distal vessel will demonstrate stasis, with *in situ* thrombosis leading to the development of propagated thrombus, as described by Virchow (7). In addition, the proximal blood flow becomes turbulent with associated development of laminar thrombus. The original occlusive material may now change in one of two ways: first, the organized thrombus may recanalize, producing a variable number of endothelialized channels, which may also demonstrate internal elastic laminae. These channels remain separated by fibrous septa. Secondly, the clot may undergo complete fibrinous organization without canalization, which in turn becomes continuous with the propagated thrombus, forming dense plugs that completely occlude the arterial lumen.

One diagnostic dilemma is that patients may develop *in situ* thrombosis, and there have been isolated reports of patients who have CTEPH as a result of *in situ* thrombosis. Although this may occur in isolation, it may also take place super-imposed on a background of other etiologies of pulmonary hypertension (8); in these cases, the preoperative investigations suggest that surgery will be successful, but no lasting benefit is obtained. Other conditions mimicking CTEPH include patients with embolizing RA myxomas, tumor emboli typically from renal tumors, and emboli from indwelling prostheses such as ventriculoatrial shunts or pacing systems. In addition, pulmonary artery sarcomas may also present with the features of CTEPH (9). Finally, patients with fibrosing mediastinitis and pulmonary artery vasculitis may show similar imaging features, such as stenoses and soft tissue adherent to the pulmonary arteries, which may make these conditions difficult to distinguish from CTEPH (10).

In the minority of patients, specific abnormalities of coagulation may also be present and predispose to CTEPH. These include lupus anticoagulant, the antiphospholipid syndrome, and inherited deficiencies of antithrombin III, protein C, and protein S (5). These conditions may also precipitate *in situ* thrombosis, although they make deep vein thrombosis (DVT) more likely. Similarly, *in situ* thrombosis may further contribute to an altered pulmonary vascular state in connective tissue disorders that may directly affect the pulmonary circulation and produce pulmonary hypertension, such as scleroderma and systemic lupus erythematosus.

Whereas elimination of up to half of the pulmonary vascular bed (e.g., with a pneumonectomy) does not result in the development of PH, pulmonary hypertension is present in many cases of CTEPH in which less than half of the pulmonary vascular bed is obstructed. It has been suggested that the nonobstructed pulmonary capillary beds develop a vasculopathy similar to that seen in other forms of pulmonary hypertension. These changes may persist even after surgical clearance of occlusive material and result in persistent PH.

The factors responsible for this small-vessel arteriopathy remain unknown, although it has been suggested that a variety of locally produced mitogens or vasoactive mediators may be responsible (8). These findings support early intervention, before the vascular changes in other parts of the lung have become established.

III. Prognosis and Natural History

Pulmonary hypertension is a condition that has a poor outlook. Death occurs as a result of right ventricular hypertrophy leading to cardiac dysrhythmias and right ventricular failure. Although the presence of an intracardiac shunt, such as a patent foramen ovale, allows decompression of the right heart with a concomitant increase in systemic blood flow, this is achieved at the expense of systemic oxygen saturation. This phenomenon seems to confer advantage in patients with Eisenmenger's syndrome, in whom long-term survival is more typical.

Riedel et al. (11) followed a cohort of 147 patients with CTEPH using serial right heart catheter studies. They confirmed the dismal prognosis of this condition, demonstrating a 5 year survival of <30% when the mean pulmonary artery pressure was in excess of 30 mmHg, and a 2 year survival of only 20% when the mean pressure reaches 50 mmHg.

Although medical therapy makes a positive impact on prognosis for other forms of PH, it is only recently been explored in inoperable CTEPH, with variable results (12,13).

IV. Patient Assessment and Selection

The diagnosis of chronic thromboembolic pulmonary vascular disease may be difficult to establish, because its clinical presentation is often insidious and it is often confused with other conditions.

The condition has been described in patients at all ages, but is most common in the 40–50-year-old age group; there is no difference in distribution between the sexes.

A history of prior VTE should always be sought, even though less than one half of patients with thromboembolic pulmonary hypertension will give such a history (8). Other predisposing factors for DVT should also be sought, including a history of abdominal or orthopaedic surgery of the lower limb, a familial blood hypercoagulable state, periods of enforced immobility, or dehydration. In addition, a history of leg swelling, chest pain, hemoptysis, or syncope should also be explored.

The most frequent early symptom is progressive exertional dyspnea, which will be present before the development of pulmonary hypertension at rest. However, in patients in whom there is partial occlusion of the pulmonary vascular bed, hypoxemia with exercise may develop, leading to the typical symptoms of dyspnea. This breathlessness is out of proportion to what might be expected on the basis of other investigations for respiratory and cardiac diseases.

More advanced symptoms include exertional chest pain, a chronic nonproductive cough, hemoptysis, palpitations, and exercise-induced syncope or presyncope.

The presentation of dyspnea is often initially interpreted as being due to other pathologies such as airways disease, cardiac disease including either valve or arterial pathologies, or physical deconditioning. Indeed, the average delay from the onset of cardio-pulmonary symptoms to the establishment of the correct diagnosis is typically several years (8).

V. Signs

As with the symptoms, the physical signs seen in patients with CTEPH are often relatively nonspecific and may become apparent only as right-sided heart failure supervenes. Peripheral cyanosis may occur with severe reduction in cardiac output, and central cyanosis may be present if there is a significant intracardiac right to left shunt, for example, through a patent foramen ovale.

Examination of the legs may reveal signs of chronic venous stasis and skin discoloration, gross varicose veins, or even varicose ulceration. Peripheral edema is usually present as right heart failure ensues.

Auscultation of the chest is often unremarkable, although in later stages of the disease the murmur of tricuspid regurgitation may be audible. Auscultation may also reveal the presence of intrapulmonary systolic bruits (5). These bruits resemble those encountered in congenital pulmonary branch stenosis and are assumed to result from turbulent blood flow past a segmental narrowing. These murmurs have not been described in patients with other forms of pulmonary arterial hypertension.

VI. Laboratory Studies

Full blood count and biochemical asides are standard, but are rarely disordered. However, liver function tests may become disordered as a result of hepatic congestion, and secondary polycythemia may develop in cases of long-standing low cardiac output and hypoxemia. Additionally, low cardiac output states may produce prerenal impairment with elevation of serum creatinine levels.

The possibility of a pro thrombotic state should also be investigated, because evidence of a hypercoagulable state is found in 10–15% of patients. Deficiencies of antithrombin 3, protein C, and protein S are found in 5% of patients (5). Other hematological abnormalities that may predispose to pulmonary hypertension, such as sickle cell disease or previous splenectomy, may also be identified.

Chest radiograph, electrocardiogram, and pulmonary function tests are useful investigations to exclude other conditions, but they have little value in differentiating thromboembolic pulmonary hypertension from other forms of pulmonary hypertension. Pulmonary function studies demonstrate either a mild to moderate restrictive lung defect or, on occasion, mild obstructive defects. The presence of a severe obstructive component may be a contraindication to proceeding to endarterectomy. The diffusing capacity for carbon monoxide (DLCO) is typically reduced in CTEPH, as it is in other pulmonary vascular diseases in which the pulmonary capillary blood volume is reduced.

The chest radiograph is often normal in the early stages of pulmonary hypertension, but as the disease progresses several abnormalities may become visible: right ventricular prominence is common, and right-sided venous stasis with widening of the superior vena cava and azygos vein with prominent hilar pulmonary arteries is typical in advanced disease.

The main pulmonary arteries may be markedly enlarged, and unilateral or asymmetrical enlargement is particularly suggestive of thromboembolic disease

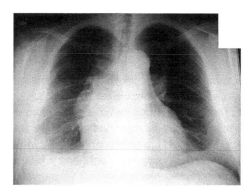

Figure 24.1   Chest radiograph, demonstrating enlargement of cardiac contour (in particular, right heart) and large pulmonary arterial segments (right more than left) in a patient with proven CTEPH.

(Fig. 24.1). In addition, areas of an entire lung field may be avascular; evidence of old or recent pulmonary infarction with peripheral scarring and localized pleural thickening may also be apparent. Atelectasis and small pleural effusions are also common, but nonspecific.

VII.   Echocardiography

Two-dimensional transthoracic echocardiography is a useful investigation, because this helps to define the presence of pulmonary hypertension and excludes underlying cardiac conditions. The typical findings are of right-sided dilatation and right ventricular hypertrophy. The main pulmonary trunk is also enlarged. Interventricular septal motion is paradoxical and the septum may appear flattened, with encroachment of the right ventricle into the left ventricular cavity. Tricuspid regurgitation is usually present in varying degrees. If the changes are subtle, performing echocardiography after exercise should be considered because this tends to accentuate the degree of pulmonary hypertension. It is unusual to identify pulmonary arterial obstructive material echocardiographically.

Radioisotope perfusion scanning is a critical screening investigation. In chronic thromboembolic disease, discreet lower or segmental defects are normally seen (Fig. 24.2), in contrast to the appearance of primary pulmonary hypertension in which the scan is either normal or has a patchy and mottled appearance (14). The presence of an equivocal scan in patients with other features suggestive of chronic thrombo-embolic disease should always prompt additional investigation (15).

CT scanning has also proved to be very useful in helping to identify patients with this disorder (16). The images can confirm occlusion in the main and lobar pulmonary arteries, and on occasion it may be possible to follow

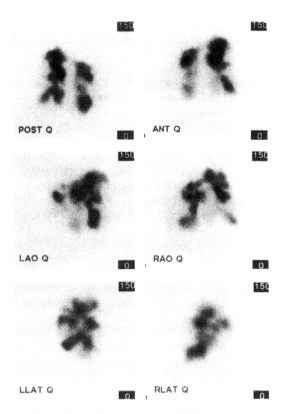

Figure 24.2 Ventilation/perfusion lung scan (V/Q) from a patient with CTEPH demonstrating multiple mismatched perfusion defects.

thrombotic material into segmental vessels (Fig. 24.3). Furthermore, enlargement of the pulmonary arterial trunk in combination with mural thrombus may be present (Fig. 24.4). Occlusion of the main pulmonary arteries is relatively uncommon, and its presence suggests the presence of a pulmonary artery tumor. When viewed on lung settings, a mosaic pattern of lung attenuation on the CT scan represents regional perfusion inhomogeneities that may be suggestive of chronic pulmonary thrombo-embolism (Fig. 24.5). Finally, some patients may demonstrate cavity formation in areas of previous infarction (Fig. 24.6). The gold standard for the diagnosis and planning of surgery, however, remains the standard pulmonary angiogram (17). The combination of right heart catheterization and selective pulmonary artery angiography allows accurate assessment of the level of pulmonary hypertension, permits an assessment of surgical accessibility, and excludes other diagnoses. The pulmonary vascular resistance calculated at right heart catheterization may not be accurate, because the pulmonary capillary wedge pressure does not give an accurate reflection of left atrial pressure if it is

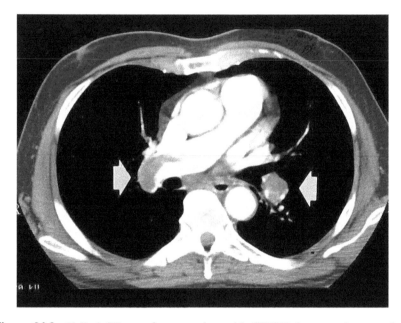

Figure 24.3 Helical CT scan from a patient with CTEPH demonstrating organized thrombotic material in the proximal vasculature.

wedged within an occluded segment. In some patients, the pulmonary artery pressure may be relatively normal despite the presence of substantial obstruction; however, during exercise, the pulmonary artery pressures may rise steeply. When the pulmonary vascular resistance appears to be higher than expected, based on the degree of vascular occlusion, the presence of underlying small-vessel

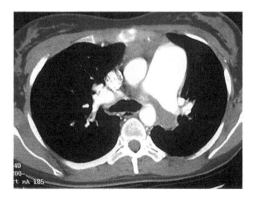

Figure 24.4 CT pulmonary angiogram demonstrating gross enlargement of the pulmonary artery (compared with the ascending aorta) and mural thrombus.

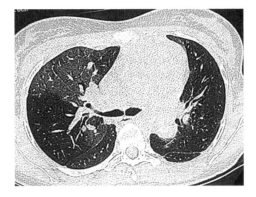

Figure 24.5 High-resolution CT scan demonstrating inhomogeneity of pulmonary parenchyma (mosaic perfusion).

arteriopathic changes should be considered. These patients will carry a higher perioperative risk, and their long-term benefit is unlikely to be as great (18).

Pulmonary angiography has been reported as being a high-risk procedure for patients with pulmonary hypertension, but in our experience this investigation can be performed safely and is performed on an almost daily basis at our centers. We have performed over 3000 angiograms in CTEPH patients without a death and with a minimal morbidity using selective injections with nonionic contrast agents.

The classic signs visible on pulmonary angiography are dilated proximal and main pulmonary arteries with irregular lumens, indicating the attachment of thrombus to the vessel wall (5). Bands or webs may be seen crossing the vascular lumen, sometimes with a poststenotic dilatation, and with failure of filling of branch vessels to the periphery. In addition, there may be abrupt termination of pulmonary vessels with a pouch-like appearance.

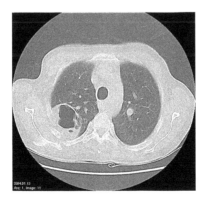

Figure 24.6 CT scan demonstrating a cavity in a patient with CTEPH. The cavity subsequently decreased in size developing into a scar (pulmonary infarct).

In addition to pulmonary angiography, patients over 50 years of age should undergo coronary artery angiography and other cardiac investigations as necessary. If other cardiac pathology is identified, this can be corrected surgically at the time of pulmonary endarterectomy. In addition, it is our practice to perform carotid artery Doppler studies to characterize the presence of peripheral vascular disease. It is important to know this prior to surgery in order to minimize the risks of cardiopulmonary bypass at low flows in association with profound hypothermic circulatory arrest.

Magnetic resonance imaging has also been used recently as a screening technique for the diagnosis of CTEPH (16). This investigation allows three-dimensional assessment of the occluded vessels that is useful in planning surgery (Fig. 24.7). Furthermore, it may yield information on cardiac function, including ventricular hypertrophy (Fig. 24.8), ventricular contractility, and other parameters which can indicate myocardial dysfunction. In addition, it provides a useful technique for following the patients postoperatively and assessing the completeness of the operation.

In some patients, the location and extent of vascular occlusion cannot be assessed sufficiently using the techniques described earlier. Direct visualization of the vasculature using an angioscope inserted into the jugular vein and advanced into the pulmonary arterial tree has been used to provide a more complete assessment of the occluded vasculature, particularly in patients deemed at increased risk for surgery. Angioscopy can also be useful in establishing alternative diagnoses such as pulmonary artery tumors and vasculitis (5).

VIII. Operation: Pulmonary Thromboendarterectomy

The general approach to pulmonary endarterectomy is similar to that of other patients undergoing cardiac surgery. In particular, attention must be paid to

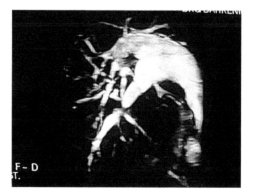

Figure 24.7 MR pulmonary angiogram (maximum intensity projection) demonstrating multiple stenoses and webs in a patient with CTEPH.

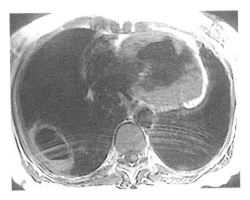

Figure 24.8 MR of the chest demonstrating right ventricular hypertrophy (patient also has a cavitating lung infarct (same patient as in Fig. 24.6).

ensure adequate levels of anticoagulation, initially with heparin and subsequently with warfarin. A detailed discussion is beyond the scope of this chapter, and the reader is referred to detailed descriptions of the procedure published elsewhere (5,19,20).

A. Postoperative Care

Postoperative cardiac dysrhythmias are no more common than would be seen following coronary artery surgery. The patients are mobilized as their postoperative condition permits, with emphasis on early activity and appropriate physiotherapy. The majority of patients are ready for discharge from the hospital within 2 weeks.

B. Results

The majority of patients undergoing pulmonary thromboendarterectomy (PTE) will experience near-normalization of their pulmonary hemodynamic derangement (19,20). Even patients with severe right heart failure exhibit normalization of right heart function when right ventricular afterload is reduced. Further improvement is often observed over the first year after surgery. For the majority of patients, surgery results in effective and complete treatment of their pulmonary hypertension, although some patients require medical therapy for persistent pulmonary hypertension. These patients, who are both high-risk candidates for surgery and are the least likely to benefit from PTE, may now be identifiable preoperatively using novel techniques to differentiate those with proximal (and operable) vascular obstruction from those with distal (inoperable) disease (18). As over a third of perioperative deaths and nearly half of long-term deaths are attributed to persistent pulmonary hypertension (21), implementation of these novel diagnostic techniques will hopefully lead to improved patient selection and reduced operative morbidity and mortality.

C. Medical Therapy

The role of medical therapy for CTEPH remains unclear. Case reports and small series suggest that some patients with CTEPH, who are deemed inoperable due to (1) the distal location of their vascular occlusions, (2) underlying concomitant medical conditions, or (3) the presence of mixed large-vessel and small-vessel diseases, may benefit from medical therapy. Inhaled iloprost, oral beraprost, intravenous prostacyclin, and oral sildenafil have all been used to treat inoperable CTEPH, with mixed results (12,13,22). A course of preoperative treatment for patients with decompensated right heart failure with these agents, which have been used successfully for other forms of pulmonary hypertension, may be helpful in optimizing their status prior to surgery (23).

IX. Conclusions

Pulmonary hypertension caused by thrombo-embolic conditions remains an under-diagnosed condition. Many patients receive inappropriate therapy in the belief that they have some other underlying condition such as asthma or heart failure of unclear origin.

Until recently, the only effective surgical therapy was lung transplantation, but with the associated perioperative mortality, and the long-term complications of immunosuppressive therapy, this is now an obsolete choice for the majority of patients with CTEPH.

With the advent of pulmonary endarterectomy as a treatment option, the responsibility must lie with physicians to recognize this condition. There is now an option for patients that will allow their return to normal levels of activity, with improved life expectancy and without the long-term complications of complex drug regimens. Sustained benefit is seen following an operation that carries a perioperative mortality of not >10%, comparing favorably with the immediate results of transplantation.

References

1. Simonneau G, Galie N, Rubin LJ et al. Clinical classification of pulmonary hypertension. J Am Coll Cardiol 2004; 43:5S–12S.
2. Galie N, Seeger W, Naeije R et al. Comparative analysis of clinical trials and evidence-based treatment algorithm in pulmonary arterial hypertension. J Am Coll Cardiol 2004; 43:81S–88S.
3. Hertz MI, Taylor DO, Trulock EP et al. The registry of the International Society for Heart and Lung Transplantation: Nineteenth Official Report 2002. J Heart Lung Transplant 2002; 21:950–970.

4. Pengo V, Lensing AWA, Prins MH et al. Incidence of chronic thromboembolic pulmonary hypertension after pulmonary embolism. N Engl J Med 2004; 350:2257–2264.

5. Fedullo PF, Auger WR, Kerr KM, Rubin LJ. Chronic thromboembolic pulmonary hypertension. N Engl J Med 2001; 345:1465–1472.

6. Bonderman D, Turecek PL, Jakowitsch J et al. High prevalence of elevated clotting factor VIII in chronic thromboembolic pulmonary hypertension. Thromb Haemost 2003; 90:372–376.

7. Phlogose und thrombose in Gefassystem. In: Virchow R, ed. Gesammelteandlungen zur Wissenschaftlichen Medecin. Berlin: Verlag von Max Hirsch, 1862:458.

8. Lang IM. Chronic thromboembolic pulmonary hypertension—not so rare after all. N Engl J Med 2004; 350:2236–2238.

9. Kerr KM. Pulmonary vascular tumors. In: Peacock AJ, Rubin LJ, eds. The Pulmonary Circulation. Edward Arnold/Oxford University Press, 2004.

10. Bergin CJ, Hauschildt JP, Brown MA, Channick RN, Fedullo PF. Identifying the cause of unilateral hypoperfusion in patients suspected to have chronic pulmonary thromboembolism: diagnostic accuracy of helical CT and conventional angiography. Radiology 1999; 213:743–749.

11. Riedel M, Stanek V, Widimsky J et al. Longterm follow-up of patients with pulmonary thromboembolism: late prognosis and evolution of hemodynamic and respiratory data. Chest 1982; 81:151–158.

12. Ghofrani HA, Schermuly RT, Rose F et al. Sildenafil for long-term treatment of non-operable chronic thromboembolic pulmonary hypertension. Am J Resp Crit Care Med 2003; 167:1139–1141.

13. Ono F, Noritoshi N, Okumura H et al. Effect or orally active prostacyclin analogue on survival in patients with chronic thromboembolic pulmonary hypertension without major vessel obstruction. Chest 2003; 123:1583–1588.

14. Ryan KL, Fedullo PF, Davis GB et al. Perfusion scan findings understate the severity of angiographic and hemodynamic compromise in chronic thromboembolic pulmonary hypertension. Chest 1998; 93:1180–1185.

15. Moser KM, Page GT, Ashburn WL et al. Perfusion lung scans provide a guide to which patients with apparent primary pulmonary hypertension merit angiography. West J Med 1988; 148:167–170.

16. Bergin CJ, Sirlin CB, Hauschildt JP et al. Chronic thromboembolism: diagnosis with helical CT and MR imaging with angiographic and surgical correlation. Radiology 1997; 204:695–702.

17. Doyle RL, McCrory D, Channick RN et al. Surgical treatments/interventions for pulmonary arterial hypertension. An ACCP evidence-based clinical practice guideline. Chest 2004; 126:63S–71S.

18. Kim NHS, Fesler P, Channick RN et al. Pre-operative partitioning of pulmonary vascular resistance correlates with early outcome following thromboendarterectomy for chronic thromboembolic pulmonary hypertension. Circulation 2004; 109:18–22.

19. Jamieson SW, Kapelanski DP, Sakakibara N et al. Pulmonary thromboendarterectomy: experience and lessons learned in 1500 cases. Ann Thorac Surg 2003; 76:1457–1464.

20. Klepetko W, mayer E, Sandoval J et al. Interventional and surgical modalities of treatment for pulmonary arterial hypertension. J Am Coll Cardiol 2004; 43:73S–80S.

21. Archibald CJ, Auger WR, Fedullo PF et al. Long-term outcome after pulmonary thromboendarterectomy. Am J Resp Crit Care Med 1999; 160:523–528.
22. Bresser P, Fedullo PF, Auger WR et al. Continuous intravenous epoprostenol for chronic thromboembolic pulmonary hypertension. Eur Resp J 2004; 23:595–600.
23. Kerr KM, Rubin LJ. Epoprostenol therapy as a bridge to pulmonary thromboendarterectomy for chronic thromboembolic pulmonary hypertension. Chest 2003; 123:319–320.

25

Sleep Apnea

RICHARD J. SCHWAB, RAANAN ARENS, and ALLAN PACK

University of Pennsylvania Medical Center,
Philadelphia, Pennsylvania, USA

I. Introduction

Obstructive sleep apnea is a highly prevalent disorder with major public health ramifications. Upper airway imaging has become a powerful tool to understand the pathogenesis of this disorder in adults and children. Upper airway imaging studies have provided important insights into the anatomical basis of obstructive sleep apnea and the mechanisms by which treatments [continuous positive airway pressure (CPAP), weight loss, oral appliances, upper airway surgery] for this disorder increase upper airway caliber. Upper airway soft tissue and craniofacial structures can be objectively quantified with imaging techniques. Upper airway imaging has been utilized to evaluate the effects of gender and obesity on upper airway structure and function. Three-dimensional volumetric images of the upper airway have been used to phenotype the upper airway. State-dependent and dynamic imaging studies have provided important information on the compliance and collapsibility of the upper airway.

This chapter will examine different aspects of upper airway imaging and how it relates to obstructive sleep apnea. First, normal upper airway anatomy will be reviewed. Second, the advantages and disadvantages of different upper airway imaging modalities [acoustic reflection, fluoroscopy, nasopharyngoscopy, cephalometry, magnetic resonance imaging (MRI)], both conventional and electron beam computed tomography (CT), will be described. Third, insights into the pathogenesis of obstructive sleep apnea obtained from upper airway imaging studies will be discussed, including studies examining dynamic and state-related changes in upper airway caliber. Fourth, data from studies examining the mechanisms by which the therapeutic interventions for sleep apnea increase upper airway caliber will be reviewed. Subsequently, pediatric upper airway imaging studies will be discussed. Finally, the chapter will conclude with clinical indications for upper airway imaging in patients with sleep disordered breathing.

II. Normal Upper Airway Anatomy

The upper airway has been divided into three regions based on a mid-sagittal characterization of upper airway anatomy: (1) the nasopharynx (the nasal turbinates to the hard palate); (2) the oropharynx, subdivided into retropalatal (the hard palate to the caudal margin of the soft palate) and retroglossal (the caudal margin of the soft palate to the base of the epiglottis) regions; and (3) the hypopharynx (the base of the tongue to the larynx) (see Fig. 25.1) (1–3). In the majority of patients with obstructive sleep apnea, upper airway closure/narrowing during sleep occurs in the retropalatal and retroglossal regions (4–6). Therefore, this chapter will focus on studies evaluating data on the oropharyngeal region of the upper airway.

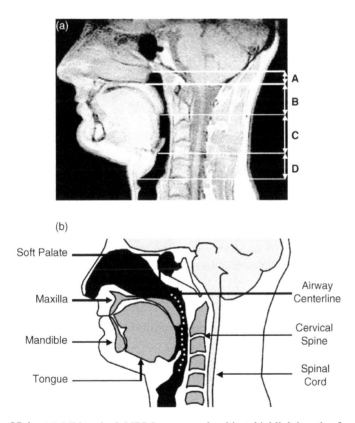

Figure 25.1 (a) Mid-sagittal MRI in a normal subject highlighting the four upper airway regions: (A) nasopharynx; (B) retropalatal (RP); (C) retroglossal (RG); and (D) hypopharynx. SP, soft palate; T, tongue; M, mandible. (b) A diagram demonstrating important upper airway, soft tissue, and craniofacial anatomy on a sagittal MRI.

Most upper airway imaging studies have primarily examined the airway itself rather than the surrounding soft tissue and craniofacial structures. However, the upper airway is formed by the structures that surround it (evaluation of the donut rather than the hole in the donut). Thus, it is important to understand which structures form the walls of the upper airway. The majority of the anterior oropharyngeal wall is formed by the soft palate and tongue, while the posterior wall of the oropharynx is comprises primarily the superior, middle, and inferior constrictor muscles (3,7). The anatomy of the lateral oropharyngeal walls is complicated. The lateral walls are formed by several different structures including oropharyngeal muscles [hyoglossus, styloglossus, stylohyoid, stylopharyngeus, palatoglossus, palatopharyngeus, and the pharyngeal constrictors (superior, middle and inferior) (2,5,8)], lymphoid tissue (primarily the palatine tonsils), and adipose tissue (parapharyngeal fat pads). All the structures that form the lateral walls are bounded by the mandibular rami. MRI has been shown to be an ideal modality to examine the lateral pharyngeal walls (2,5,9–20). On the basis of MRI morphology, the lateral pharyngeal walls traverse the retropalatal and retroglossal regions. In the retropalatal region, the tissue between the lateral edge of the airway and the medial edge of the parapharyngeal fat pads forms the lateral walls [see Fig. 25.2(a) and (b)]. In the retroglossal region the tissue between the lateral edge of the airway and the mandible forms the lateral walls (see Fig. 25.3; the parapharyngeal fat pads disappear in the retroglossal region). The biomechanical relationships between the lateral walls, the tongue, the soft palate, and the mandible, and the roles these structures play in mediating upper airway caliber is not completely understood. It is likely that these upper airway soft tissue and craniofacial structures are interdependent. For instance, changes in the dimensions of the soft palate may directly affect the geometry of the lateral walls since fascicles of the palatopharyngeus muscle, which arise from the soft palate and insert on the thyroid cartilage, form a portion of the lateral pharyngeal walls. Three-dimensional upper airway imaging may allow us to better understand the complex interactions between the upper airway soft tissue and craniofacial structures so that we can better characterize the biomechanics of the upper airway (15,16).

III. Upper Airway Imaging Modalities

The imaging techniques that have been used to examine the upper airway include: acoustic reflection (21–25), fluoroscopy (26–28), nasopharyngoscopy (5,29–31), cephalometry (25,32–40), MRI (2,5,10,41), and both conventional and electron beam CT (4,12,13,42–56). However, each of these upper airway imaging modalities has problems. A perfect upper airway imaging technique would be inexpensive, noninvasive, be performed in the supine position, be free of ionizing radiation, allow for three-dimensional volumetric reconstructions of the upper airway and surrounding soft tissue/craniofacial structures, and

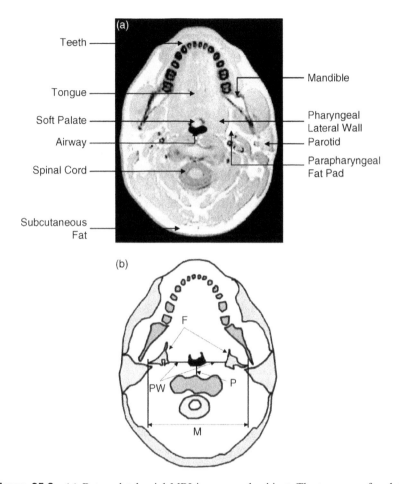

Figure 25.2 (a) Retropalatal axial MRI in a normal subject. The tongue, soft palate, parapharyngeal fat pads (fat is white on an MRI), lateral parapharyngeal walls (muscles between the airway and lateral parapharyngeal fat pads), and mandibular rami can all be visualized on an axial MRI. (b) A diagram demonstrating important soft tissue and craniofacial anatomy on an axial MRI in the retropalatal region. Measurements displayed: PW, lateral pharyngeal wall thickness; M, distance between the mandibular rami; F, distance between the parapharyngeal fat pads; P, posterior airway wall thickness.

permit dynamic and state-dependent imaging. Although such an imaging modality does not yet exist, magnetic resonance scanning may be the best method currently available for assessing the upper airway and surrounding soft tissue and craniofacial structures (5,57). The advantages and disadvantages of acoustic reflection, fluoroscopy, nasopharyngoscopy, cephalometry, MRI, and CT scanning are reviewed in Table 25.1 and are discussed in the following text.

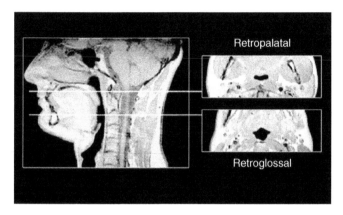

Figure 25.3 Mid-retropalatal (RP) and mid-retroglossal (RG) regions depicted from a mid-sagittal MRI in a normal subject.

A. Acoustic Reflection

Acoustic reflection is a noninvasive imaging technique, usually performed through the mouth, that analyzes sound waves reflected from the upper airway. Calculation of upper airway area as a function of distance from the incisors in the mouth can be performed with acoustic reflections by examining the phase and amplitude of the reflected sound waves (21–25,30). The technique is radiation free, fast (images can be obtained at 0.2 s intervals), and repeatable. Upper airway area has been shown to be smaller in patients with sleep apnea compared with normal subjects in studies using acoustic reflection (23,48). Unfortunately, acoustic reflection only evaluates the lumen of the upper airway in an indirect manner; it does not provide direct images of the airway, surrounding soft tissues, or craniofacial structures. Acoustic reflection measurements are usually performed through the mouth with an oral mouthpiece. This is a problem since opening the mouth alters upper airway geometry. Once the mouth opens, the soft palate elevates from the posterior portion of the tongue. Because nasopharyngoscopy, cephalometry, MRI, and CT scanning are performed with the mouth closed, the measurement of upper airway area with acoustic reflection may not be comparable to these other imaging modalities. Thus far, acoustic reflection has been used primarily as a research tool for the determination of upper airway area and has not been routinely used in clinical settings.

B. Fluoroscopy

Fluoroscopy has also been used to dynamically study upper airway anatomy in patients with sleep apnea during wakefulness and sleep. In the majority of patients with sleep apnea, fluoroscopic studies during sleep have demonstrated that upper airway closure occurs in the retropalatal region (26–28,30). Although

Table 25.1 Advantages and Disadvantages of Different Upper Airway Imaging Modalities

Pros	Cons
Acoustic reflection	
Noninvasive study	Primarily used a research tool; clinical utility not well assessed
Free of ionizing radiation	Generally performed sitting, not supine
Studies can be repeated	Technique is performed through the mouth which will alter upper airway anatomy
Dynamic imaging capability	No direct anatomical representation of the airway and surrounding
No weight restrictions	soft tissue/craniofacial structures
Can be used during pregnancy	
Fluoroscopy	
Dynamic imaging capability	Significant ionizing radiation exposure
Potential for state dependent imaging	Unable to quantify upper airway soft tissue structures
	No cross-sectional (axial or sagittal) imaging
Nasopharyngoscopy	
Widely available	Invasive
Relatively easy to perform	Requires nasal anesthesia
Free of ionizing radiation	Evaluates only airway lumen, not surrounding soft tissue or
No weight limitation	craniofacial structures
Performed sitting or supine	Pressure changes during a Müller maneuver needs to be quantified
State-dependent imaging capability	Aspiration risk
Müller maneuver may provide information into the location of	Nasopharyngoscope needs to be cleaned and sterilized
upper airway closure (Fig. 25.10)	

(continued)

Table 25.1 *Continued*

Pros	Cons
Possibly useful in predicting UPPP outcome by determining site of airway obstruction (retropalatal or retroglossal) during Müller maneuver	
Cephalometry	
Widely available	Radiographic equipment, technique, and interpretative skills must be standardized
Relatively easy to perform	Performed in the sitting or standing position, generally not supine
No weight limitation	Two-dimensional evaluation of skeletal and soft tissue structures, volumetric analysis difficult
Much less expensive than CT or MRI	Provides no information about lateral soft tissue structures and limited information about AP structures
May be useful in evaluating patients with craniofacial abnormalities such as retrognathia	No state-dependent imaging capability
Useful in the evaluation of oral appliances, craniofacial surgery	No dynamic imaging capability
	Radiation exposure
Computed tomography	
Widely available	Relatively expensive
Supine imaging	Weight limitation approximately 300 pounds
Accurate measurement of upper airway cross-sectional area and volume	Radiation exposure limits ability to perform state-dependent imaging
Excellent resolution for the airway and craniofacial structures	Relatively poor resolution for upper airway adipose tissue compared to MRI
Capability of three dimensional reconstruction of craniofacial	

structures (cranium, mandible, hyoid) and airway Potentially useful in the evaluation of apneic patients who undergo maxillomandibular advancement Dynamic imaging (50 ms) with electron beam CT providing excellent temporal resolution Helical CT allows for direct acquisition of three-dimensional images	Should not be performed during pregnancy
Magnetic resonance imaging Supine imaging Accurate measurement of upper airway cross-sectional area and volume Excellent airway, soft tissue, and fat resolution Direct sagittal, coronal, and axial images Potential for state-dependent imaging since no radiation Three-dimensional reconstruction of soft tissue structures (tongue, lateral pharyngeal walls, soft palate lateral parapharyngeal fat pads) and airway (Fig. 25.4) May be useful in the evaluation of patients with sleep apnea who undergo UPPP Dynamic imaging with ultrafast MR imaging Soft tissue characterization with spectroscopic studies and magnetic tagging can be used to study upper airway biomechanics	Not widely available Expensive Weight limitation approximately 300 pounds Claustrophobia is a problem Cannot be performed in patients with pacemakers or ferromagnetic clips Subjects need to be able to lie still in the scanner and not swallow repeatedly

fluoroscopy can provide a dynamic evaluation of the upper airway, radiation exposure makes this study impractical for routine use. In addition, it is difficult to quantify soft tissue measurements with flouroscopy.

C. Nasopharyngoscopy

Nasopharyngoscopy is a commonly used technique by otorhinolaryngologists to examine the nasal passages, the oropharynx, and vocal cords. Although nasopharyngoscopy is invasive, it is easily performed, allows for dynamic imaging of the upper airway, and there is no ionizing radiation. Nasopharnygoscopy has been used to study the physiologic changes in the hypotonic airway (31,58); state-dependent upper airway changes in patients with obstructive and central sleep apnea (6,29,59,60); and changes in upper airway caliber after weight loss (61), uvuloplatopharyngoplasty (UPPP) (31), and while using mandibular repositioning oral appliances (42,62). Nasopharyngoscopy, however, examines only the lumen of the upper airway and does not provide measurements of the surrounding soft tissue or craniofacial structures.

In addition to the standard airway examination, a Müller maneuver can be performed during the nasopharyngoscopy to evaluate collapsibility of the upper airway. The Müller maneuver, a voluntary inspiration against a closed mouth and obstructed nares, is thought to simulate the upper airway collapse that occurs during an apnea. Although the degree of obstruction on negative inspiration with a Müller maneuver does not directly correlate with the site of upper airway collapse during sleep, it provides information on possible anatomic sites of obstruction (11). Studies have suggested that apneics with predominantly retroglossal obstruction identified by a Müller maneuver should not undergo UPPP (5). Surgery directed at advancing the base of the tongue (sliding genioplasty or maxillomandibular advancement) should be considered in these patients. In contrast, apneics with predominantly retropalatal collapse during a Müller maneuver should be considered for a UPPP. However, data demonstrating an improved surgical outcome in patients selected for UPPP, on the basis of findings during nasopharyngoscopy with a Müller maneuver, are not yet compelling.

D. Cephalometry

Cephalometry, a standardized lateral radiograph of the head and neck, primarily evaluates upper airway craniofacial structure. Although cephalometry is widely available and inexpensive, it must be performed in a standardized fashion. During cephalometry, the head needs to be stabilized and the radiograph should be obtained at end-expiration since upper airway size can be affected by respiration (12,13). Cephalometry in patients with sleep apnea has been used primarily for evaluating and quantifying craniofacial structures (mandibular and hyoid position) in patients with retrognathia and/or micrognathia (32,35). In addition, cephalometrics have been utilized to examine craniofacial structure prior to facial surgery (mandibular advancement, bimaxillary advancement, sliding mortis genioplasty) and in the evaluation and efficacy of mandibular repositioning oral appliances (5).

Cephalometrics studies have demonstrated craniofacial differences between patients with obstructive sleep apnea and controls matched for age and gender (25,32–40). In general, these studies have shown that apneics have small retro-posed mandibles, narrow posterior airway spaces, enlargement of the tongue and soft palate, an inferiorly positioned hyoid bones, and retroposition of the maxilla compared with normals (25,32–40). These craniofacial risk factors for sleep apnea are more commonly reported in non-obese apneics than in obese apneics (63). Although differences in craniofacial structure between normals and apneics have been demonstrated in several studies, a meta-analysis found that only mandibular body length demonstrated a clinically significant association in patients with sleep disordered breathing (64). Since only one cephalometric variable was identified that was significantly associated with sleep apnea, the utility of cephalometrics in distinguishing normals from apneics may be called into question.

Other important limitations to cephalometrics include anatomic shortcomings (it is a two-dimensional representation of a three-dimensional structure), its inability to provide volumetric information, or examine upper airway soft tissue structures such as the lateral pharyngeal walls or parapharyngeal fat pads. Moreover, cephalometrics provides limited data about anterior–posterior upper airway structures, provides no information about lateral structures, and cannot be performed dynamically or during sleep (5,57). These limitations have reduced the clinical utility of cephalometry, although its low cost and widespread availability still make it useful, especially in patients undergoing maxillofacial surgery or using an oral appliance.

E. Computed Tomography

Upper airway anatomy can be well delineated with CT scanning, which has excellent resolution for the airway and surrounding craniofacial structures. Standard axial CT images can be reconstructed to demonstrate a three-dimensional representation of upper airway, soft tissue, and craniofacial skeleton (50). Volumetric images can be directly acquired with newer helical CT scanners. Electron beam (ultra-fast) CT has excellent temporal (50 ms) resolution to permit dynamic imaging of the upper airway. CT scanning, has certain limitations since the study is expensive and patients are exposed to radiation. Imaging protocols that require, repeat CT scanning, such as studies during sleep or those examining respiration, can be problematic because of the radiation exposure. CT scanning also has limited resolution for parapharyngeal fat at least compared with MRT. Regardless of these shortcomings, CT upper airway imaging studies have provided important information about the pathogenesis of obstructive sleep apnea (4,13,42,44–56,65).

The majority of these CT upper airway imaging studies have demonstrated narrowing in the retropalatal region of patients with obstructive sleep apnea during both wakefulness (4,13,42,44–56,65) and sleep (4,56). A smaller upper airway and larger tongue volume in obese patients with sleep apnea has been demonstrated with volumetric CT studies (30,50). CT scanning has also been used to examine patients undergoing upper airway surgery (50,52). CT upper airway imaging studies have shown that apneics with retropalatal obstruction have greater improvements in their apnea–hypopnea index following UPPP than those with retroglossal obstruction (52,66). Finally, dynamic changes in upper airway caliber during respiration have been demonstrated with electron beam CT (12,13,47,53). These studies in both normals and apneics have shown that during wakefulness, airway caliber remains relatively constant in inspiration, increases in early expiration, and decreases at the end of expiration (12,13,47,53). Thus CT imaging has provided insight into the pathogenesis of sleep apnea, the changes in upper airway caliber during respiration, and anatomical information that may help to determine the surgical procedure in patients with sleep disordered breathing.

F. Magnetic Resonance Imaging

Magnetic resonance scanning (2,6,18,20,41,67–72) may be the best upper airway imaging modality. MRI has several distinct advantages for studying patients with obstructive sleep apnea: (1) it provides excellent upper airway and soft tissue resolution (including parapharyngeal fat); (2) it provides accurate, reproducible quantification of the upper airway and surrounding soft tissue structure; (3) imaging can be performed in the axial, sagittal, and coronal planes; (4) volumetric data analysis including three-dimensional reconstructions of upper airway soft tissue and craniofacial structures can be performed (see Fig. 25.4); (5) imaging can be accomplished during both wakefulness and sleep; and (6) it does not expose subjects to any radiation, so repeated studies can be performed. Unfortunately MRI also has several limitations: (1) availability is sometimes a problem; (2) it is expensive; (3) studies cannot be performed on patients with ferromagnetic implants (e.g., pacemakers); and (4) achieving sleep in the MR environment is difficult because of noise and arousals (6,73). Nonetheless, MR studies have provided important insights into the pathogenesis of sleep apnea and have significantly advanced our understanding of the mechanisms underlying the efficacy of CPAP, mandibular repositioning appliances, weight loss, and upper airway surgery in patients with sleep apnea (2,6,10,17,18,41,67–72). Airway closure during sleep (6,69,70,73) and the effects of CPAP (10,67,68) have been studied with MRI in patients with obstructive sleep apnea. New ultrafast, spectroscopic, and MR tagging techniques have provided novel information about tissue characteristics and biomechanics of upper airway closure (9,14,69,72). Recent MR studies have demonstrated that the volume to the tongue, lateral pharyngeal walls, and total soft tissue is enlarged in patients with sleep apnea, and this volumetric enlargement increases the risk of sleep apnea. Moreover, MRI may be useful in examining the genetics of sleep apnea

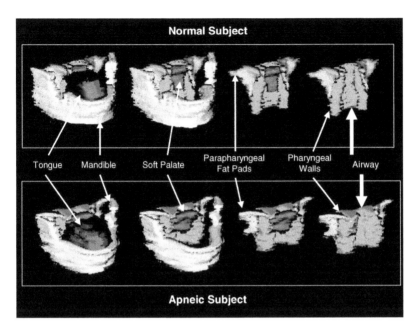

Figure 25.4 (**See color insert**) Volumetric reconstruction of axial MR images in a normal subject and patient with sleep apnea. The mandible is depicted in gray, the tongue in orange/rust, the soft palate in purple, the lateral parapharyngeal fat pads in yellow, and the lateral/posterior pharyngeal walls in green. Both subjects had an elevated body mass index (32.5 kg/m^2). The airway is larger in the normal subject than in the patients with sleep apnea. The tongue, soft palate, and lateral pharyngeal walls are all larger in the apneic than the normal.

by phenotyping upper airway anatomic risk factors [upper airway adipose tissue, soft tissue (soft palate, tongue, lateral pharyngeal walls), and craniofacial structures]. Thus, MRI has become an important imaging modality to study patients with sleep apnea.

IV. Upper Airway Imaging Studies Examining the Pathogenesis of Obstructive Sleep

To better understand the pathogenesis of sleep disordered breathing, the three subsections that follow will review studies examining "static," "dynamic," and state-dependent upper airway imaging in normal subjects and patients with sleep apnea.

A. "Static" Upper Airway Anatomy

During wakefulness, most studies with MRI/CT have shown that the upper airway is smaller in patients with sleep apnea compared with normal controls

(2,4,12,13,15,16,23–25,45,49,69,74). The airway narrowing found in these studies was primarily in the retropalatal region (2,13,47,52). Studies have shown that this reduction in the size of the apneic upper airway compared with the normal airway is secondary to enlargement of the surrounding soft tissues and/or changes to the craniofacial structures (15,16). Cephalometric studies have demonstrated reductions in mandibular body length (which may result in retrognathia), inferiorly positioned hyoid bone, and retropositioning of the maxilla in patients with sleep apnea compared with normals (25,32–40). Reduction in mandibular body length, in particular, has been shown in a meta-analysis to be an important risk factor for obstructive sleep apnea (64). Enlargement of the upper airway soft tissue structures (tongue, lateral pharyngeal walls, soft palate, parapharyngeal fat pads) has also been demonstrated in patients with obstructive sleep apnea compared with normals (15,16). Initially, imaging studies with CT/MRI demonstrated increases in the cross-sectional area and dimensions of the soft palate, tongue, parapharyngeal fat pads, and lateral pharyngeal walls in patients with sleep apnea (2,5,50,65,69,71,75). Figure 25.5 is a mid-sagittal MR image showing narrowing of the upper airway and elongation of the soft palate and tongue in an apneic compared with a normal. Figure 25.6 is an axial MR image in the retropalatal region showing lateral narrowing of the airway in a patient with sleep apnea compared with a normal subject. More recently a case–control study demonstrated that the volume of the upper airway soft tissue structures (tongue, lateral pharyngeal walls, soft palate, parapharyngeal fat pads; see Fig. 25.4) was significantly greater in apneics than in normals and that this enlargement was a significant risk factor for sleep apnea (15). After covariate adjustments for gender, age ethnicity, craniofacial size, and fat surrounding the upper airway, the volume of the lateral pharyngeal walls, tongue, and total soft tissue surrounding the upper airway remained significantly larger in apneics than in normals. Moreover, this investigation showed that increased volume of the lateral pharyngeal walls, tongue, and total upper airway soft

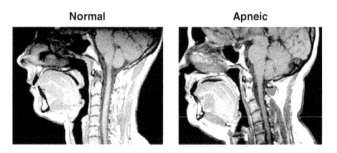

Figure 25.5 Mid-sagittal MRI of a normal subject and a patient with sleep apnea. The upper airway is smaller and soft palate longer in the apneic. The amount of subcutaneous fat (white area at the back of the neck) is greater in the apneic.

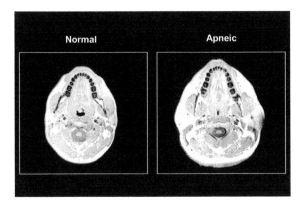

Figure 25.6 Axial MRI in the retropalatal region of a normal subject and a patient with sleep apnea. The upper airway is smaller (laterally narrowed) in the patient with sleep apnea. The amount of subcutaneous fat is greater in the apneic.

tissue significantly increased the risk for sleep apnea even after the covariate adjustments (15).

Why are the upper airway soft tissue structures enlarged and craniofacial structures reduced in size in patients with sleep apnea? Although we do not know the specific answer, there are several possible mechanisms explaining the etiology of the enlargement of the upper airway soft tissue structures in apneics including: (1) edema secondary to negative pressure from airway closure and/or trauma; (2) weight gain; (3) muscle injury; (4) gender; and (5) genetic factors. Each of these mechanisms will be reviewed.

Negative pressure during airway closure or trauma secondary to repeated apneic events may cause edema to the upper airway soft tissue structures, which, in turn, could increase the size of these structures. The soft palate is at particular risk for the development of edema since it can be tugged caudally and traumatized during apneic events. CPAP is thought to reduce upper airway edema (50). Quantitative MR mapping (14,76) has been utilized to study differences in lingual musculature (including evidence for edema) in normal subjects and in patients with sleep apnea. This investigation indicated that there was more edema and/or fat in the genioglossus muscles of apneics compared with normals (14,76). Histologic studies have also shown that patients with sleep apnea have increased edema in the uvula (61). Thus, edema may be an important contributor to the enlargement of the upper airway soft tissue structures.

Although edema may increase the size of the upper airway soft tissue structures in patients with obstructive sleep apnea, obesity is likely to be an even more important contributor. Obesity has become a national epidemic, with >55% of US adults being considered overweight [BMI (body mass index) $>25 \text{ kg/m}^2$] and nearly a quarter being considered obese (BMI $> 30 \text{ kg/m}^2$) (77). Obesity has been shown to be an important risk factor for obstructive sleep apnea

(78,79). In the Wisconsin Sleep Cohort, an increase in BMI by one standard deviation more than tripled the prevalence of sleep apnea (79). Weight gain increases the risk of sleep disordered breathing, and not surprisingly weight loss has been shown to decrease the severity of sleep apnea (80–83) and decrease airway collapsibility (e.g., greater closing pressure) (61). Although obesity is associated with sleep apnea, BMI may not be the best metric to follow since BMI does not specifically evaluate adipose tissue in the neck. Increased neck size, which is a better surrogate than BMI of upper airway fat distribution, has been shown to be an excellent predictor of sleep apnea (79,84,85).

Increased neck size in obese patients with obstructive sleep apnea may be related to fat deposition in the neck. In fact, imaging studies have demonstrated increased adipose tissue surrounding the upper airway (primarily deposited in the lateral parapharyngeal fat pads, see Figs. 25.2, 25.4, 25.7, and 25.8) in obese patients with sleep apnea (2,4,17,18,86,87). These studies (2,4,17,18,86,87) demonstrate that obesity increases fat deposition in the lateral pharyngeal fat pads, which, in turn, has been hypothesized to compress the lateral walls and reduce upper airway caliber. However, it has never been shown that increased fat deposition in the lateral parapharyngeal fat pads actually increases the risk of sleep apnea. Moreover, fat deposition in other anatomic sites could also lead to increased neck size and a narrow upper airway. For instance, fat deposition within the tongue or soft palate or fat deposited under the mandible may also be important in reducing the caliber of the upper airway and may increase

Pre-Weight Loss   Post-Weight Loss

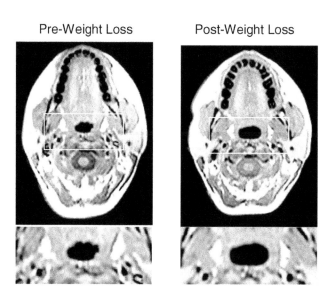

Figure 25.7 Axial retropalatal MRI of a normal subject, pre- and postweight loss. Airway area and lateral airway dimensions increase and the thickness of lateral pharyngeal walls and the size of the parapharyngeal fat pads decrease with weight loss.

Pre-weight loss

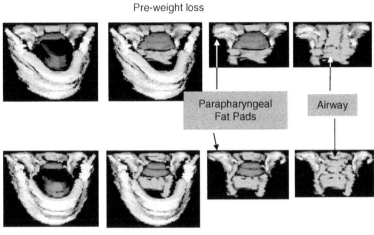

Parapharyngeal Fat Pads

Airway

Post-weight loss

Figure 25.8 (**See color insert**) Upper airway soft tissues [soft palate (purple), the tongue (orange/rust), the lateral pharyngeal walls (green), parapharyngeal fat pads (yellow) and craniofacial mandible (gray)] reconstructions before and after weight loss in a normal subject. The size of the upper airway increases with weight loss. The largest reductions in the size of the upper airway soft tissue structures with weight loss were in the lateral pharyngeal walls and the parapharyngeal fat pads. Mandibular volume did not change with weight loss.

the size of the soft tissue structures. Fat has been demonstrated in the uvula of patients with sleep apnea, which supports the hypothesis that fat deposited outside of the parapharyngeal fat pads may be important in the pathogenesis of sleep apnea (88,89). It has also been suggested, however, that the total amount of fat surrounding the upper airway might be more important than fat localized in a particular anatomic site. Shelton et al. (17) have argued that fat deposition in the space bounded by the mandibular rami would increase tissue pressure and lead to airway narrowing.

In addition to direct fat deposition, weight gain may also directly alter the muscular tissue surrounding the upper airway. Weight gain not only increases adipose tissue but it also increases muscle mass (90,91). Approximately a quarter of the increased weight in obese patients is secondary to fat-free tissue (91,92). In fact, there is a larger percentage of muscle in the uvula of patients with sleep apnea compared with normal subjects (88,93). These data suggest that weight gain may predispose to obstructive sleep apnea by directly increasing the size of the soft tissue structures (tongue, soft palate, lateral pharyngeal walls) surrounding the upper airway, in addition to direct fat deposition in the parapharyngeal fat pads. This hypothesis is supported by data in obese nonapneic women that show that the volume of the lateral pharyngeal walls as well as the parapharyngeal fat pads decrease with weight loss (see Figs. 25.7 and 25.8) (94). Alternatively, obesity may affect upper airway compliance and alter the biomechanical relationships of the upper airway muscles (82). Although obesity is an important risk factor for sleep apnea, the specific effect of weight gain on the upper airway soft tissue structures is not completely understood.

It has also been proposed that patients with obstructive sleep apnea have a primary myopathy, and this myopathy contributes to the enlargement of the upper airway soft tissue structures (57). An increase in type II fast twitch fibers in the genioglossus muscle of apneics has been found in several studies (93,95,96). Since type II fibers are more likely to fatigue than type I fibers, the upper airway muscles in apneics would be more susceptible to fatigue than in normals. Is this remodeling of the upper airway muscles a primary or secondary phenomenon, that is, is it a consequence of sleep apnea rather than being the cause of the apnea? In order to answer this question, Carrera et al. (95) studied the structure and function of the genioglossus in apneics and normals. These investigators also found increased type II fibers in the genioglossus muscle of apneics; however, these changes in the genioglossus muscle were abolished with CPAP. Thus the increased type II fibers in the genioglossus muscle of apneics appears to be a consequence of the sleep apnea and not the cause of the disease, since these finding were reversed by CPAP. Patients with sleep apnea appear to manifest muscle injury (increased type II fibers) that may alter the size, length, and configuration of the upper airway muscles, although these changes may be abolished by CPAP.

Gender may also have an important effect on upper airway soft tissue structures. Several studies (23,97) have demonstrated that upper airway caliber is smaller in women than in men. In addition, studies have shown that women have a smaller neck size (98) than men, so it has been hypothesized that the size of the upper airway soft tissue structures (tongue, soft palate, lateral pharyngeal walls, lateral parapharyngeal fat pads) are smaller in women than in men. Moreover, fat distribution is different in women than in men (99,100). In men, fat is distributed primarily in the upper body and trunk whereas in women it is distributed primarily in the lower body and extremities (99,100). These gender-related differences in fat distribution suggest that the size of the lateral parapharyngeal fat pads may be greater in men than in women. Two studies have examined gender-related differences in upper airway soft tissue structures in normal subjects with MRI (19,20). Both of these studies (19,20) have shown that the size of the tongue, soft palate, and total soft tissue was greater in normal men than in women. Whittle et al. (19) demonstrated that total soft tissue volume, size of the tongue, and soft palate were larger in age- and weight-matched men compared with women. Malhotra et al. (20) demonstrated that airway length, soft palate, and tongue size were greater in men than in women. Surprisingly, both studies found no significant differences in the size of the lateral pharyngeal fat pads between normal men and women (19,20).

These data indicate that gender may not have an impact on the amount of visceral (parapharygneal fat pads) neck fat, but has an important effect on the size of the other upper airway soft tissue structures.

Although it has been hypothesized that genetic factors play a large role in mediating the size of the upper airway soft tissue structures, there are little data as yet to support this hypothesis. Family aggregation of craniofacial structure (reduction in posterior airway space, increase in mandibular to hyoid distance, inferior hyoid placement) has been demonstrated in patients with sleep apnea (98,101). The data from these studies suggest that elements of craniofacial structure in patients with sleep apnea are likely inherited, but studies examining the heritability of upper airway soft tissue structures have not been performed. Macroglossia has been shown to be a risk factor for sleep apnea in children with Trisomy 21 (102), but otherwise the influence of genetic factors on the size of upper airway soft tissue structures has not been well studied. Nonetheless, it seems likely that the size of the tongue, soft palate, and lateral pharyngeal walls should be at least partially genetically determined. Imaging studies need to be performed to determine whether there is family aggregation and heritability of the upper airway soft tissue structures.

The mechanisms discussed for enlargement of the upper airway soft tissue structures have also been proposed to explain the craniofacial abnormalities in patients with sleep apnea. Edema, weight gain, and muscular injury should not directly affect the craniofacial anatomy but gender, ethnicity, and genetic factors are all thought to play an important role in mediating the craniofacial changes in apneics. As discussed, several studies have demonstrated family aggregation of craniofacial morphology (reduction in posterior airway space, increase in mandibular to hyoid distance, inferior hyoid placement) in patients with sleep apnea (101,103). Guilleminault (103) performed a study on first-degree relatives of probands with sleep apnea and demonstrated that family members had retroposed mandibles and inferiorly placed hyoid bones. Mathur et al. (101) also noted cephalometric differences (retroposed maxillae and mandibles, shorter mandibles, longer soft palates, and wider uvulas) in the first-degree relatives of non-obese patients with sleep apnea compared with age-, gender-, height-, and weight-matched controls. In addition to genetic factors, ethnicity (104,105) and gender (104) have been shown to influence craniofacial form. Bimaxillary prognathism has been shown to be more frequent in African-Americans than in Hispanics and Caucasians (105). Gender-related differences in posterior airway space, posterior nasal spine to the soft palate, and mandibular plane to hyoid distance have also been demonstrated (104). Specific craniofacial morphometric characteristics (triangular chin, overjet, a narrow hard palate, and class II malocclusion) have been shown to be more common in women than in men with mild sleep apnea (103). These investigations suggest that ethnicity, gender, and genetic factors play important roles in mediating craniofacial structure.

B. "Dynamic" Upper Airway Imaging

"Static" upper airway imaging studies have provided important insight into the anatomic risk factors for sleep apnea; however, examination of the dynamic behavior of the upper airway is also necessary to completely understand the pathogenesis of sleep disordered breathing. Dynamic evaluation of upper airway narrowing or closure can be performed by examining respiration or during a Müller maneuver. Upper airway imaging studies have shown changes in the airway and surrounding soft tissue structures during respiration and secondary to the negative pressure induced during a Müller maneuver (12,13,106).

CT, MR, and nasopharyngoscopy have all been used to examine dynamic changes in upper airway caliber and the surrounding soft tissue structures during respiration (42,43,53,59,69,107). Electron beam CT has been utilized during wakefulness to evaluate respiratory-related upper airway anatomic changes (12,13). These studies demonstrated that upper airway caliber changes during four distinct phases of the respiratory cycle (Fig. 25.9) (12,13). In early inspiration (phase 1, Fig. 25.9), there is a small increase in upper airway size but during most of inspiration (phase 2, Fig. 25.9) upper airway size is relatively constant. The finding that upper airway caliber is relatively constant in inspiration suggests that there is a balance between the action of the upper airway dilator muscles to increase airway caliber and negative intraluminal pressure to decrease airway caliber. In early expiration, upper airway size increases (phase 3, Fig. 25.9) and this is thought to be secondary to positive intraluminal pressure. Upper airway area was largest in early expiration in these studies (12,13). At the end of expiration (phase 4, Fig. 25.9), there is a significant reduction in upper airway size. It is thought that the end of expiration is a particularly vulnerable time for upper airway narrowing or collapse since the upper airway is no longer maintained open by the phasic action of the upper airway dilator

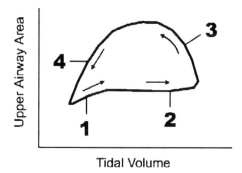

Figure 25.9 Diagram of the changes in upper airway area as a function of tidal volume during the respiratory cycle. Airway caliber is relatively constant in inspiration (phases 1 and 2). Airway size increases in early expiration (phase 3) and decreases in late expiration (phase 4).

muscles (phases 1 and 2, during inspiration) or positive intraluminal pressure (phase 3, early expiration). Upper airway area was smallest at the end of expiration in these investigations (12,13).

The finding that upper airway size is smallest at end expiration may have important implications with regard to the timing of sleep-induced upper airway closure during the respiratory cycle. Apneas are thought to occur during inspiration secondary to negative intraluminal pressure generated by chest wall contraction (108). However, studies (109,110) examining airway resistance have shown that airway closure in apneics can occur during both expiration and inspiration. Studies using nasopharygoscopy also support these observations (29). In these studies airway closure during sleep was noted during expiration and subatmospheric intraluminal pressure was not required for pharyngeal closure (2,29). All these data indicate that the upper airway is vulnerable to collapse at the end of expiration. It has been hypothesized that the delivery of positive airway pressure near the end of expiration could increase airway caliber and help to prevent airway closure during sleep (9,11,13,14).

Dynamic changes in upper airway mechanics can also be examined with nasopharyngoscopy during a Müller maneuver (a forced inspiratory effort with the mouth closed and nose occluded) (106). The Müller maneuver is thought to simulate an apneic event (9,111) and during this maneuver upper airway caliber is reduced. This reduction in upper airway caliber is related to the amount of negative pressure generated during the Müller maneuver, which is effort dependent. Therefore, to accurately interpret upper airway narrowing during a Müller maneuver, it is necessary to simultaneously measure negative intraluminal pressure and airway dimensions. Ritter et al. (106) used such a system to investigate the mechanism of airway closure during a Müller maneuver. In this study changes in upper airway caliber of normal subjects were examined during a Müller maneuver performed at maximal effort and at graded negative intraluminal pressures (-10, -20, -30, and -40 cm H_2O) (106). The data from this study (106) showed that during a Müller maneuver, upper airway narrowing was much greater in the retropalatal region than in the retroglossal region. In the retropalatal region, upper airway area was progressively reduced in a linear fashion as intraluminal pressure became more negative from -10 to -40 cm H_2O (see Fig. 25.10). In addition, airway narrowing was significantly greater in the lateral than in the anterior–posterior dimension at all pressure levels. The findings from this investigation indicate that the reduction in airway caliber during a Müller maneuver in normals is mediated primarily through changes in the lateral pharyngeal walls and that the retropalatal and retroglossal regions respond differently to the generation of negative intraluminal pressure. The latter observation indicates that the upper airway does not collapse as a homogenous tube when exposed to negative intraluminal pressure. Preliminary studies in apneics have demonstrated greater reductions in airway area with the Müller maneuver in patients with sleep apnea apneics than in normal subjects at all pressure levels and in both regions (retropalatal and retroglossal) of the

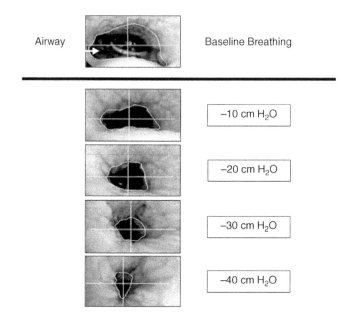

Figure 25.10 Upper airway images in the retropalatal region of a normal subject at baseline and with progressively more negative pressure (-10 to -40 cm H_2O) during a Müller maneuver. The airway is significantly reduced in caliber (lateral narrowing greater than anterior–posterior narrowing) during the submaximal Müller maneuvers.

upper airway. These data suggest that the apneic upper airway is more compliant than the normal upper airway (112).

C. State-Dependent Upper Airway Imaging

Although static and dynamic upper airway imaging during wakefulness has significantly advanced our knowledge about sleep disordered breathing, sleep apnea is a condition that occurs during sleep. Thus the information that can be obtained from state-dependent imaging (studies performed during wakefulness and sleep) is crucial to our understanding of the pathogenesis of sleep apnea. Such studies have shown that the retropalatal region is the most common site of airway narrowing/closure during sleep, although upper airway narrowing can also occur in the retroglossal region (4,6,56,69,73). It has been hypothesized that the upper airway collapses like a homogenous tube during sleep. However, studies have not confirmed this hypothesis. Trudo et al. (73) used MRI to study state-dependent changes in upper airway size in normals and found that the airway was smallest in the retropalatal region in the majority of subjects. In this study, airway volume in the retropalatal region was reduced 19% during sleep; in contrast, airway volume in the retroglossal region increased by 4% (73). These findings indicate that the upper airway does not narrow as a homogenous tube during sleep. These data, which are analogous to the airway findings demonstrated during the Müller maneuver, suggest that factors that control the size of the upper airway are different in the retropalatal and retroglossal regions. Determining why the airway is more likely to collapse in the retropalatal than the retroglossal region during sleep may be fundamental to our understanding of the pathogenesis of sleep apnea.

State-dependent reductions in both anterior–posterior and lateral airway dimensions in the retropalatal region were demonstrated in Trudo's study (73). The state-dependent reduction in the lateral retropalatal airway dimensions was secondary to thickening of the lateral pharyngeal walls (Fig. 25.11), whereas the anterior–posterior airway narrowing was secondary to posterior movement of the soft palate. State-dependent anterior–posterior and lateral airway narrowing during sleep in normals and apneics has also been demonstrated by other investigators (4,6,29,56,59). Horner et al. (4) showed that airway closure during sleep was mediated by both posterior displacement of the soft palate and tongue, and lateral displacement of the pharyngeal walls. Suto et al. (6) performed ultrafast MRI in the sagittal dimension during sleep and demonstrated retropalatal airway closure in both normals and apneics. The airway narrowing in these patients was secondary to reductions in both anterior–posterior and lateral airway dimensions (6). Morrell et al. (59) performed nasopharyngoscopy during

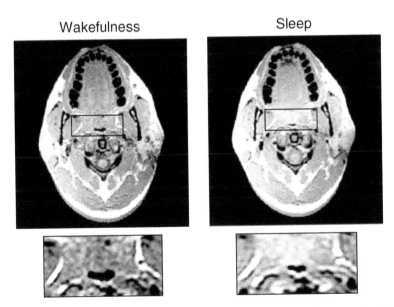

Figure 25.11 State-dependent MRI in the retropalatal region of a normal subject. Airway area is smaller during sleep in this normal subject. The state-dependent change in airway caliber is secondary to reductions in the lateral and anterior–posterior airway dimensions. Thickening of the lateral pharyngeal walls is demonstrated during sleep.

sleep to examine dynamic flow volume relationships in inspiration and expiration over several breaths preceding an apneic event. Similarly to other investigations, they found that the airway closed in both the anterior–posterior and lateral dimensions (59). In addition, Morrell et al. found that the cross-sectional area of the upper airway at the end of expiration was progressively reduced in each successive breath prior to the obstructive apnea. All of these studies examining state-dependent changes in the upper airway demonstrate that airway narrowing during sleep occurs in both the lateral and the anterior–posterior dimensions. In the lateral dimension, state-dependent upper airway narrowing is secondary to thickening and/or motion of the lateral pharyngeal walls. In the anterior–posterior dimension, the soft palate appears to move in the posterior direction. Dynamic and volumetric three-dimensional imaging may be necessary in order to fully understand the biomechanical changes in the configuration/conformation of the lateral pharyngeal walls and soft palate during sleep.

V. Insights into the Treatment of Obstructive Sleep with Upper Airway Imaging

In the following sections, we will review imaging studies that have provided information on the effect of weight loss, CPAP, oral appliances, and surgery on upper airway size and the surrounding soft tissue and craniofacial skeleton.

A. Weight Loss

One of the most important risk factors for obstructive sleep apnea in adults is obesity (78,79,82). Mild to moderate weight loss (5–10%) has been shown in several studies (80–83) to improve obstructive sleep apnea and decrease the collapsibility of the airway (61). However, it is not clear why weight loss decreases the severity of obstructive sleep apnea or how weight loss alters the size and/or configuration of the upper airway soft tissue structures (soft palate, tongue, parapharyngeal fat pads, lateral pharyngeal walls). It has been hypothesized that weight loss reduces the volume of the parapharyngeal fat pads, which, in turn, would increase the size of the upper airway. Welch et al. examined the effects of weight loss on upper airway soft tissue structures in 12 overweight nonapneic women with quantitative three-dimensional MRI (Figs. 25.7 and 25.8). This study demonstrated that a 17.7% weight loss significantly increased the volume of the upper airway and significantly decreased the volume of the lateral pharyngeal walls and parapharyngeal fat pads. The volume of the soft palate and tongue also decreased with weight loss, but these decreases were not statistically significant. Thus structures lateral to the airway (parapharyngeal fat pads and lateral pharyngeal walls) appear to be important in mediating increases in the caliber of the upper airway with weight loss. Further studies are needed to confirm this finding.

B. Continuous Positive Airway Pressure

Although weight loss has been shown to improve sleep disordered breathing, unfortunately it is often difficult to achieve and/or maintain in this population. The best therapeutic option for the treatment of patients with sleep apnea is CPAP therapy since it is noninvasive and highly effective (11). CPAP acts as a pneumatic splint to enlarge the size of the upper airway in both normals and apneics (49,68,113,114). It was thought that CPAP increases the size of the upper airway by anteriorly displacing the tongue and soft palate. However, CT studies found that dilatation of the upper airway with CPAP was greater in the lateral dimension than in anterior–posterior dimension (49). If the tongue and soft palate had been displaced anteriorly with CPAP, the airway dimensional changes should have been greater in the anterior–posterior not in the lateral direction. An MRI study in normals (10) confirmed these findings and showed that increase in the lateral airway dimensions with progressive increases in CPAP (up to 15 cm H_2O) was significantly greater than the increase in the anterior–posterior dimensions (10). In addition, in this investigation CPAP significantly increased airway volume and airway area in the retropalatal and ret-roglossal regions (Figs. 25.12–25.14). The lateral pharyngeal walls were significantly thinned as the airway enlarged with CPAP (Figs. 25.13 and 25.14). There was an inverse relationship between the CPAP setting and the thickness of the lateral pharyngeal walls. However, CPAP had very little effect on the anterior–posterior structures (tongue and soft palate) (10). These data indicate that the effects of CPAP on enlarging the upper airway are primarily mediated through the lateral pharyngeal walls.

C. Oral Appliances

Although CPAP is an excellent treatment option for obstructive sleep apnea, compliance with CPAP remains a significant problem (11). For patients who have difficulty adhering to CPAP, another option is using an oral appliance.

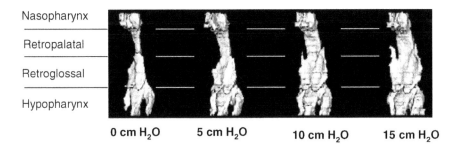

Nasopharynx

Retropalatal

Retroglossal

Hypopharynx

0 cm H_2O 5 cm H_2O 10 cm H_2O 15 cm H_2O

Figure 25.12 Volumetric reconstruction of the upper airway in a normal subject with progressively greater CPAP (0–15 cm H_2O) settings. Upper airway volume increases significantly in the retropalatal and retroglossal regions with higher levels of CPAP.

CPAP - 0 cm H$_2$0   CPAP - 15 cm H$_2$0

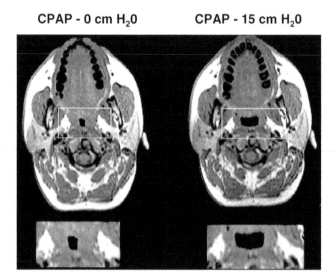

Figure 25.13 Axial retropalatal MRI in a normal subject at two levels of CPAP (0 and 15 cm H$_2$O). Airway area is significantly greater at 15 cm H$_2$O. This airway enlargement is predominantly in the lateral dimension.

The most well studied oral appliances are mandibular repositioning devices. In patients with mild to moderate sleep apnea, mandibular repositioning devices have been found to be an effective, noninvasive alternative to CPAP (11,111,115,116). Mandibular repositioning devices have been shown to increase the posterior airway space (115,117–119). However, the specific biomechanical changes that explain the increase in airway size with these devices are not known. Furthermore there is no "gold standard" oral appliance, and each of them (there are over 50 appliances currently available) may have a different mechanism of action. It has been hypothesized that airway size increases more in the retroglossal than in the retropalatal region with the mandibular repositioning devices since these devices advance the mandible and pull the tongue forward (120,121). It has also been hypothesized that oral appliances increase airway caliber more in the anterior–posterior than in the lateral dimension since these appliances have been shown to increase the posterior airway space. However, more recent studies (117,121) have shown that mandibular repositioning devices increase airway caliber more in the retropalatal than in the retroglossal region. Studies (121) with nasopharyngoscopy in patients with sleep apnea have shown that mandibular repositioning devices increase airway area by 25% in the retropalatal region without a significant increase in the retroglossal region. The increase in retropalatal airway area in this investigation was predominantly in the lateral dimension (121). The increase in the lateral dimensions of the upper airway with oral appliances suggests that the mechanism of action of oral appliances

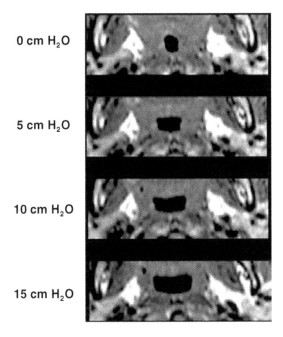

0 cm H$_2$O

5 cm H$_2$O

10 cm H$_2$O

15 cm H$_2$O

Figure 25.14 Axial retropalatal MRI in a normal subject (the same subject as in Fig. 25.12) with CPAP ranging from 0 to 15 cm H$_2$O focusing on the airway, lateral pharyngeal walls, and parapharyngeal fat pads. Airway enlargement with CPAP results in thinning of the lateral pharyngeal walls although the parapharyngeal fat pads are not displaced. The increase in airway size with CPAP is primarily in the lateral dimension the anterior–posterior dimensions of the airway do not change significantly with CPAP.

may be more complex than simply pulling the tongue and soft palate forward. Advancing the mandible may put traction on the lateral walls resulting in an increase in the lateral dimensions of the airway. In order to fully understand the mechanism of action of an oral appliance and how it affects the upper airway structures, we need to perform three-dimensional upper airway imaging studies with and without oral appliances. Such studies may allow us to develop an optimal oral appliance.

D. Upper Airway Surgery

Upper airway surgery is a third line treatment option in patients with obstructive sleep apnea used in patients who are unable to tolerate CPAP or an oral appliance. The most common surgical procedure for patients with sleep apnea is UPPP (11,122). In general, UPPP surgery removes the tonsils (if present), uvula, distal margin of the soft palate, and any excessive pharyngeal tissue. The primary focus of this surgery is on the soft palate. The success rate of UPPP is partially dependent on the site of airway closure (determined by nasopharyngeal pressure catheter measurements or CT scanning during wakefulness); patients with retropalatal obstruction have better results than those with retroglossal obstruction (31,50,52,123). Unfortunately, the success rate in patients undergoing UPPP surgery is 50%, which is an unacceptably high failure rate. A more favorable outcome with UPPP has been demonstrated if the surgery reduces the critical closing pressure (124). Thus far the biomechanical changes that underlie the efficacy or lack of efficacy of UPPP have not been identified. Upper airway imaging studies have not yet been able to determine the pharyngeal anatomic factors that predict surgical success in patients who undergo an UPPP (5,14,66). Preliminary studies with MRI have begun to examine the upper airway anatomic changes in patients undergoing UPPP (125). These MR studies have demonstrated that in patients who have undergone UPPP the airway remains small in the nonresected portion of the soft palate while the airway enlarges in the resected portion of the soft palate (see Figs. 25.15 and 25.16). Studies with CT have also demonstrated increased width of the soft palate after UPPP (115). Upper airway narrowing in the nonresected portion of the soft palate may explain why UPPP has not been more successful in treating patients with obstructive sleep apnea (5,14,66,125).

In patients with craniofacial abnormalities (retrognathia or micrognathia), skeletal surgery such as a sliding genioplasty or a maxillomandibular advancement should be considered. In selected patients maxillomandibular advancement has been shown to be a highly effective treatment option for patients with

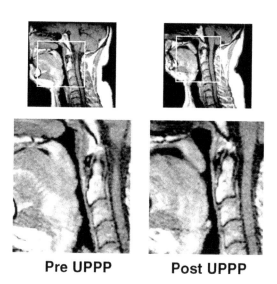

Pre UPPP   **Post UPPP**

Figure 25.15 Mid-sagittal MRI in a patient with sleep apnea before and after UPPP. The uvula is shorter after the UPPP. However, the airway remains narrow in the region of the soft palate that is not resected.

Pre UPPP   Post UPPP

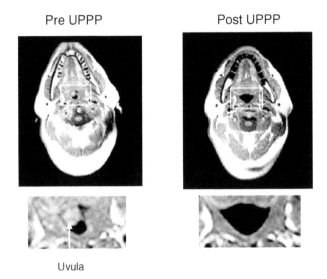

Uvula

Figure 25.16 Axial MRI before and after UPPP in the retropalatal region where the uvula was resected. Airway caliber increases substantially after the UPPP in this region of the airway.

obstructive sleep apnea (11). Nonetheless, the mechanism by which upper airway size is increased by maxillomandibular advancement is not definitively known. In order to understand the mechanisms that mediate the increase in upper airway caliber with maxillomandibular advancement, pre- and postsurgical three-dimensional CT or MR scans should be considered in this population.

VI. Imaging of the Upper Airway in Children

Obstructive sleep apnea syndrome (OSAS) is a common disorder in children. It is estimated that 2% of otherwise normal children are affected with OSAS (126,127). Airway anatomy and nonanatomic factors, including neuromuscular mechanisms and tissue characteristics, could affect airway size and lead to airway collapse during sleep. In adults the incidence of OSAS correlates with age, degree of obesity, and male gender (128). However, in children, OSAS has a different pathophysiology; it is most commonly associated with adenotonsillar hypertrophy and is diagnosed between ages 2 and 8 (129). Interestingly, however, not all children who undergo adenotonsillectomy for OSAS are effectively treated (130–132), suggesting that the enlarged tonsils/adenoids may not be the only cause for the disorder. As in adults, OSAS in children is characterized by recurrent events of partial or complete upper airway obstruction during sleep, resulting in disruption of normal ventilation and sleep patterns

(133,134). Knowledge and recognition of OSAS in children of any age group has a tremendous impact on their quality of life, since OSAS, if untreated, may have profound cardiovascular affects leading to cor-pulmonale in some patients as well as significant neurocognitive consequences affecting behavior and academic performance (135–137).

A. Anatomical Evidence for OSAS

The upper airway of children with OSAS is generally smaller than average. In most cases, large tonsils and/or adenoids (135,138) can explain this finding and removal of these tissues cures or ameliorates the disorder in the majority (135,138,139), but not in all (130–132). Although the importance of adenoidal and tonsillar enlargement in the pathogenesis of pediatric OSAS is unquestioned, much remains to be learned since a weak relationship was found between severity of OSAS and the size of these tissues when assessed by radiographs and physical examination (138,140–142). The role of adenoid and tonsils in pathogenesis of OSAS may be more complex than simply being related to their size. It has been suggested that the three-dimensional orientation of these tissues to the airway is an important factor affecting flow resistance during sleep and determining airway anatomic complexity (143,144).

There is no doubt that craniofacial structures are important in mediating upper airway size, but at the present time, their role is not well understood in children. There are several important reasons why craniofacial structures are thought to be an important risk factor for pediatric OSAS. First, sleep apnea is common and severe in children with distinct craniofacial abnormalities. For instance, sleep apnea occurs commonly in children with craniofacial abnormalities such as Pierre-Robin (145,146), Treacher-Collins (147), Apert (148), and Down syndromes (102,149). Second, there is evidence that in children without these distinct craniofacial anomalies, there are more subtle craniofacial morphologies correlating to OSAS that have been demonstrated using cephalometrics (150–153).

B. Functional Evidence for OSAS

Despite the strong evidence of anatomic abnormalities limiting upper airway size in children with OSAS, several arguments suggest that OSAS is caused by alterations in functional mechanisms (neuromotor tone, tissue properties, etc.) that increase airway collapsibility and predispose to OSAS. First, children with OSAS having large tonsils and adenoids do not obstruct during wakefulness. Second, removal of the adenoid and tonsils in 10–20% of children with OSAS does not cure or resolve OSAS (130–132). Third, not all children with OSAS exhibit enlarged tonsils and adenoids. These arguments suggest that anatomic factors alone cannot be the only cause for OSAS. On the other hand, it is plausible that functional mechanisms may compensate for anatomical vulnerabilities and protect from OSAS. The latter is suggested by the observation that even though children have a smaller upper airway than adults, they are at a lower risk for OSAS. The explanation could be related to the findings of a stiffer upper airway in children compared with adults (97,154).

C. Imaging Modalities for the Upper Airway in Children

Traditional methods used in children to assess the upper airway and surrounding tissues include lateral neck radiographs and cephalometry measurements (142,150,153,155–161). Other methods that have been applied in children for analysis of airway size include nasal pharyngoscopy (162,163), fluoroscopy (135,164), and acoustic reflection (165). However, these methods are two-dimensional and provide little information about lateral structures of the nasopharyngeal and the oropharyngeal regions. CT has been used in adults to quantify the upper airway and surrounding tissues (13,44,50,51,166). However, in children CT has been reserved for selected indications (167–169), because of the radiation involved. MRI is considered useful in evaluating the anatomical properties of the upper airway (2,10,94), and has been recently introduced to study the pediatric airway (143,170).

D. MRI for Upper Airway and Surrounding Tissues in Children

MRI has been recently introduced to study the airway structure in children during growth and development (171) and assess the anatomic role in pathological conditions such as OSAS (143,170). Arens et al. (143) used MRI to study the anatomical relationships between lymphoid, skeletal, and musculature affecting the shape of the upper airway in 18 children with moderate OSAS (age 4.8 ± 2.1 years) with an apnea/hypopnea index of 11.2 ± 6.8, and compared these findings with 18 matched controls. MRI was performed under sedation and axial and sagittal T1 and T2-weighted sequences were obtained (Figs. 25.17 and 25.18). The volume of the upper airway was smaller in OSAS subjects in comparison with controls ($p < 0.005$) and the adenoid and tonsils were larger ($p < 0.005$; $p < 0.0005$, respectively) (Fig. 25.19). In addition, a significant correlation between the percent difference of the combined adenoid and tonsils volume

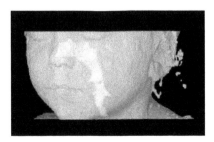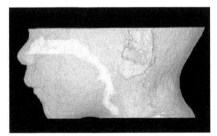

Figure 25.17 Surface rendering and three-dimensional reconstruction of an upper airway in a normal child: anterior and lateral views.

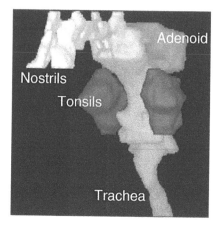

Figure 25.18 (**See color insert**) Three-dimensional construction of an upper airway (light blue), adenoid (orange), and tonsils (red) in a normal child.

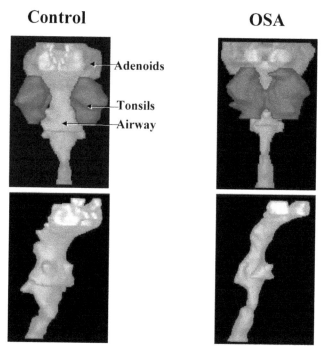

Figure 25.19 (**See color insert**) Three-dimensional construction of an upper airway (light blue), adenoid (orange), and tonsils (red) of normal child and a child with sleep apnea. Note that the tonsils are larger and airway is smaller in the child with sleep apnea.

(OSAS vs. controls) and the apnea/hypopnea index was found ($p = 0.03$, $r = 0.51$), suggesting that volumetric measurements of these tissues may be a useful way of predicting severity of OSAS in these subjects.

Studying 20 children with OSAS and 20 controls (age 3.7 ± 1.4 vs. 3.9 ± 1.7 years, respectively), Arens et al. (171) noted that the upper airway cross-sectional area varies along the airway centerline in a similar form in both normal and in OSAS children, but with the OSAS group being about one-half smaller in the upper two-thirds of the airway. In both groups, from ~20% to 60% along the airway is a region where adenoid and tonsils overlap; this region corresponds to the lowest mean and minimum airway cross-sectional areas and is significantly smaller in OSAS. It is possible that airway obstruction in children with OSAS occurs in this region. These findings are also supported by direct measurements performed in OSAS children using endoscopy and under general anesthesia (162). More recently, Donnelly and co-workers (170,172) have published data using cine MRI showing more dynamic changes in the upper airway of OSAS children than normals. However, future studies are needed to image motion and closure of the airway synchronously with the breathing cycle.

In regard to other soft tissues surrounding the upper airway, Arens et al. (143) noted that the volume of the tongue was similar to controls; however, the soft palate was significantly larger in the children with obstructive sleep apnea, adding further restriction to the upper airway. The soft palate may have been larger in the children with obstructive sleep apnea because of upper airway edema or inflammation. The pterygoid muscles, pharyngeal constrictor muscles, and parapharyngeal fat pads were similar in size in both groups studied. The groups were matched for body mass index. The fact that the size of the parapharyngeal fat pads was similar between the groups suggests that adipose tissue may not be as important a risk factor for sleep disordered breathing children as it is in adults. The primary risk factor for sleep apnea in children appears to be tonsillar size.

In regard to craniofacial measurements, Arens et al. (143) did not find significant lower face skeletal differences in children with obstructive sleep apnea as compared with controls as assessed by mandible volume, width, and length, as well as hard palate length. These findings are in contrast to several studies in children using cephalometry that noted that children with obstructive sleep apnea had retroposed mandible and maxilla, low positioned hyoid bone, and alterations in face length and width (150,151,153,161). It is possible that different measurements and imaging techniques explain these skeletal findings. Future studies need to be performed to determine whether these craniofacial findings are important risk factors for sleep disordered breathing in children.

E. MRI to Assess Developmental Changes of the Upper Airway During Childhood

Using MRI, Arens et al. (171) examined growth of the lower face, airway, and surrounding tissues in 100 normal children. These data indicate that the mid- and lower-face skeleton continue to grow linearly along the sagittal and axial planes throughout childhood, and that the soft tissues defining the upper airway, including the adenoid and tonsils, grow in constant proportion to the skeletal structures during this period. Vogler et al. (173) noted similar findings studying 189 subjects between 1 and 92 years of age. The maintenance of proportional growth among these tissues ensures airway patency throughout childhood and probably contributes to airway stability in normal children, particularly during sleep, as reported by others using functional studies (162,163,174).

F. MRI to Assess the Upper Airway in Children with Craniofacial and Genetic Disorders

MRI could also be useful in assessing the upper airway in children with neuro-logical disorders causing airway hypotonia such as Down syndrome (170,175), and in other genetic disorders associated with craniofacial anomalies involving the mid- and lower-face region, such as Pierre-Robin, Treacher-Collins, Crouzon, and so on. Upper airway obstruction in these children could occur at various sites other than the adenoid or tonsils or at multiple sites with or without involvement of lymphoid tissue. Assessment of the upper airway by MRI in these cases may provide useful information of the region of obstruction and guide in further assessment and therapy.

VII. Clinical Utility of Upper Airway Imaging

At the present time, upper airway imaging is not indicated for the standard diag-nostic evaluation of patients with obstructive sleep apnea nor is it indicated in patients successfully treated with CPAP. However, upper airway imaging should be considered in patients undergoing upper airway surgery and possibly in those patients being fitted for oral appliances. In patients undergoing an UPPP, MRI with a three-dimensional reconstruction (see Fig. 25.4) and/or naso-pharyngoscopy should be considered. As discussed earlier, the success rate in patients undergoing UPPP is related to the site of obstruction, with patients with obstruction in the retropalatal region having greater improvement in their sleep apnea than those with obstruction in the retroglossal region (52). Therefore, in order to identify the location of upper airway narrowing prior to UPPP, naso-pharyngoscopy with a Müller maneuver or MRI of the upper airway should be considered. However, studies need to be performed in order to determine whether UPPP patients selected on the basis of nasopharyngoscopy with a Müller maneuver or MRI have an improved surgical outcome. Another advantage of imaging prior to UPPP is that the imaging studies can be repeated in patients with an unsuccessful UPPP to determine the location of postoperative airway nar-rowing, and this may provide insight into whether further upper airway surgery is required. In patients undergoing maxillomandibular advancement or sliding genioplasty, CT scanning with three-dimensional reconstructions and/or cephalometrics may be indicated. CT is better than MRI in these patients because it is superior for evaluating craniofacial anatomy. If three-dimensional CT scans are unavailable, cephalometrics can be performed prior to maxillomandibular advancement (5). Cephalometric evaluation should also be considered for patients who are being considered for mandibular repositioning devices.

VIII. Conclusions

Upper airway imaging techniques have significantly advanced our understanding of the pathogenesis of obstructive sleep apnea in both children and adults. Static and dynamic upper airway imaging has been utilized to examine the structure and function of the airway during wakefulness and sleep. Upper airway imaging studies have identified the important anatomic risk factors for sleep apnea and these include the volume of the tongue, lateral pharyngeal walls, and total amount of soft tissue surrounding the upper airway. Upper airway imaging studies have also allowed us to understand how upper airway anatomy is modified with weight loss, CPAP, mandibular repositioning devices, and upper airway surgery. At the present time, upper airway imaging should be considered in patients undergoing upper airway surgery and possibly in those patients being fitted for oral appliances. Upper airway imaging has provided important insights into pathogenesis of airway closure, and this, in time, may lead to more effective treatment alternatives for patients with sleep apnea.

Acknowledgments

This chapter was supported by the National Institutes of Health Grants HL-57843, HL-60287, HL-67948, and HL-62408.

References

1. Hudgel DW. The role of upper airway anatomy and physiology in obstructive sleep apnea. Clin Chest Med 1992; 13(3):383–398.
2. Schwab RJ, Gupta KB, Gefter WB, Metzger LJ, Hoffman EA, Pack AI. Upper airway and soft tissue anatomy in normal subjects and patients with sleep-disordered breathing. Significance of the lateral pharyngeal walls. Am J Respir Crit Care Med 1995; 152(5 Pt 1):1673–1689.
3. van Lunteren E. Muscles of the pharynx: structural and contractile properties. Ear Nose Throat J 1993; 72(1):27–29, 33.
4. Horner RL, Shea SA, McIvor J, Guz A. Pharyngeal size and shape during wakefulness and sleep in patients with obstructive sleep apnoea. Q J Med 1989; 72(268):719–735.

5.   Schwab RJ, Goldberg AN. Upper airway assessment: radiographic and other imaging techniques. Otolaryngol Clin North Am 1998; 31(6):931–968.

6.   Suto Y, Matsuo T, Kato T et al. Evaluation of the pharyngeal airway in patients with sleep apnea: value of ultrafast MR imaging. AJR Am J Roentgenol 1993; 160(2):311–314.

7.   van Lunteren E, Strohl KP. The muscles of the upper airways. Clin Chest Med 1986; 7(2):171–188.

8.   Kuna ST, Smickley JS, Vanoye CR. Respiratory-related pharyngeal constrictor muscle activity in normal human adults. Am J Respir Crit Care Med 1997; 155(6):1991–1999.

9.   Schwab RJ. Properties of tissues surrounding the upper airway. Sleep 1996; 19(suppl 10):S170–S174.

10. Schwab RJ, Pack AI, Gupta KB et al. Upper airway and soft tissue structural changes induced by CPAP in normal subjects. Am J Respir Crit Care Med 1996; 154(4 Pt 1):1106–1116.

11. Schwab RJ, Goldberg AN, Pack AI. Sleep apnea syndromes. In: Fishman AP, ed. Pulmonary Diseases and Disorders. 3rd ed. New York: McGraw-Hill Inc., 1998:1617–1637.

12. Schwab RJ, Gefter WB, Pack AI, Hoffman EA. Dynamic imaging of the upper airway during respiration in normal subjects. J Appl Physiol 1993; 74(4):1504–1514.

13. Schwab RJ, Gefter WB, Hoffman EA, Gupta KB, Pack AI. Dynamic upper airway imaging during awake respiration in normal subjects and patients with sleep disordered breathing. Am Rev Respir Dis 1993; 148(5):1385–1400.

14. Schwab RJ. Upper airway imaging. Clin Chest Med 1998; 19(1):33–54.

15. Schwab RJ, Pasirstein M, Pierson R et al. Identification of upper airway anatomic risk factors for obstructive sleep apnea with volumetric MRI. Am J Respir Crit Care Med 2003; 168(5):522–530.

16. Schwab RJ. Pro: sleep apnea is an anatomic disorder. Am J Respir Crit Care Med 2003; 168(3):270–271; discussion 3.

17. Shelton KE, Gay SB, Hollowell DE, Woodson H, Suratt PM. Mandible enclosure of upper airway and weight in obstructive sleep apnea. Am Rev Respir Dis 1993; 148(1):195–200.

18. Shelton KE, Woodson H, Gay S, Suratt PM. Pharyngeal fat in obstructive sleep apnea. Am Rev Respir Dis 1993; 148(2):462–466.

19. Whittle AT, Marshall I, Mortimore IL, Wraith PK, Sellar RJ, Douglas NJ. Neck soft tissue and fat distribution: comparison between normal men and women by magnetic resonance imaging. Thorax 1999; 54(4):323–328.

20. Malhotra A, Huang Y, Fogel RB et al. The male predisposition to pharyngeal collapse: importance of airway length. Am J Respir Crit Care Med 2002; 166(10):1388–1395.

21. Fredberg JJ, Wohl ME, Glass GM, Dorkin HL. Airway area by acoustic reflections measured at the mouth. J Appl Physiol 1980; 48(5):749–758.

22. Bradley TD, Brown IG, Grossman RF et al. Pharyngeal size in snorers, non-snorers, and patients with obstructive sleep apnea. N Engl J Med 1986; 315(21):1327–1331.

23. Brown IG, Zamel N, Hoffstein V. Pharyngeal cross-sectional area in normal men and women. J Appl Physiol 1986; 61(3):890–895.

24. Hoffstein V, Zamel N, Phillipson EA. Lung volume dependence of pharyngeal cross-sectional area in patients with obstructive sleep apnea. Am Rev Respir Dis 1984; 130(2):175–178.

25. Rivlin J, Hoffstein V, Kalbfleisch J, McNicholas W, Zamel N, Bryan AC. Upper airway morphology in patients with idiopathic obstructive sleep apnea. Am Rev Respir Dis 1984; 129(3):355–360.

26. Katsantonis GP, Walsh JK. Somnofluoroscopy: its role in the selection of candidates for uvulopalatopharyngoplasty. Otolaryngol Head Neck Surg 1986; 94(1):56–60.

27. Rojewski TE, Schuller DE, Clark RW, Schmidt HS, Potts RE. Synchronous video recording of the pharyngeal airway and polysomnograph in patients with obstructive sleep apnea. Laryngoscope 1982; 92(3):246–250.

28. Suratt PM, Dee P, Atkinson RL, Armstrong P, Wilhoit SC. Fluoroscopic and computed tomographic features of the pharyngeal airway in obstructive sleep apnea. Am Rev Respir Dis 1983; 127(4):487–492.

29. Badr MS, Toiber F, Skatrud JB, Dempsey J. Pharyngeal narrowing/occlusion during central sleep apnea. J Appl Physiol 1995; 78(5):1806–1815.

30. Fleetham JA. Upper airway imaging in relation to obstructive sleep apnea. Clin Chest Med 1992; 13(3):399–416.

31. Launois SH, Feroah TR, Campbell WN et al. Site of pharyngeal narrowing predicts outcome of surgery for obstructive sleep apnea. Am Rev Respir Dis 1993; 147(1):182–189.

32. Bacon WH, Turlot JC, Krieger J, Stierle JL. Cephalometric evaluation of pharyngeal obstructive factors in patients with sleep apneas syndrome. Angle Orthod 1990; 60(2):115–122.

33. deBerry-Borowiecki B, Kukwa A, Blanks RH. Cephalometric analysis for diagnosis and treatment of obstructive sleep apnea. Laryngoscope 1988; 98(2):226–234.

34. Guilleminault C, Riley R, Powell N. Obstructive sleep apnea and abnormal cephalometric measurements. Implications for treatment. Chest 1984; 86(5):793–794.

35. Lowe AA, Fleetham JA, Adachi S, Ryan CF. Cephalometric and computed tomographic predictors of obstructive sleep apnea severity. Am J Orthod Dentofacial Orthop 1995; 107(6):589–595.

36. Lyberg T, Krogstad O, Djupesland G. Cephalometric analysis in patients with obstructive sleep apnoea syndrome. I. Skeletal morphology. J Laryngol Otol 1989; 103(3):287–292.

37. Lyberg T, Krogstad O, Djupesland G. Cephalometric analysis in patients with obstructive sleep apnoea syndrome: II. Soft tissue morphology. J Laryngol Otol 1989; 103(3):293–297.

38. Partinen M, Guilleminault C, Quera-Salva MA, Jamieson A. Obstructive sleep apnea and cephalometric roentgenograms. The role of anatomic upper airway abnormalities in the definition of abnormal breathing during sleep. Chest 1988; 93(6):1199–1205.

39. Pracharktam N, Hans MG, Strohl KP, Redline S. Upright and supine cephalometric evaluation of obstructive sleep apnea syndrome and snoring subjects. Angle Orthod 1994; 64(1):63–73.

40. Riley R, Guilleminault C, Herran J, Powell N. Cephalometric analyses and flow-volume loops in obstructive sleep apnea patients. Sleep 1983; 6(4):303–311.

41. Rodenstein DO, Dooms G, Thomas Y et al. Pharyngeal shape and dimensions in healthy subjects, snorers, and patients with obstructive sleep apnoea. Thorax 1990; 45(10):722–727.

42. Burger CD, Stanson AW, Daniels BK, Sheedy PF II, Shepard JW Jr. Fast-CT evaluation of the effect of lung volume on upper airway size and function in normal men. Am Rev Respir Dis 1992; 146(2):335–339.

43. Burger CD, Stanson AW, Daniels BK, Sheedy PF II, Shepard JW Jr. Fast-computed tomographic evaluation of the effect of route of breathing on upper airway size and function in normal men. Chest 1993; 103(4):1032–1037.

44. Burger CD, Stanson AW, Sheedy PF II, Daniels BK, Shepard JW Jr. Fast-computed tomography evaluation of age-related changes in upper airway structure and function in normal men. Am Rev Respir Dis 1992; 145(4 Pt 1):846–852.

45. Ell SR, Jolles H, Galvin JR. Cine CT demonstration of nonfixed upper airway obstruction. AJR Am J Roentgenol 1986; 146(4):669–677.

46. Ell SR, Jolles H, Keyes WD, Galvin JR. Cine CT technique for dynamic airway studies. AJR Am J Roentgenol 1985; 145(1):35–36.

47. Galvin JR, Rooholamini SA, Stanford W. Obstructive sleep apnea: diagnosis with ultrafast CT. Radiology 1989; 171(3):775–778.

48. Haponik EF, Smith PL, Bohlman ME, Allen RP, Goldman SM, Bleecker ER. Computerized tomography in obstructive sleep apnea. Correlation of airway size with physiology during sleep and wakefulness. Am Rev Respir Dis 1983; 127(2):221–226.

49. Kuna ST, Bedi DG, Ryckman C. Effect of nasal airway positive pressure on upper airway size and configuration. Am Rev Respir Dis 1988; 138(4):969–975.

50. Ryan CF, Lowe AA, Li D, Fleetham JA. Three-dimensional upper airway computed tomography in obstructive sleep apnea. A prospective study in patients treated by uvulopalatopharyngoplasty. Am Rev Respir Dis 1991; 144(2):428–432.

51. Shepard JW Jr, Garrison M, Vas W. Upper airway distensibility and collapsibility in patients with obstructive sleep apnea. Chest 1990; 98(1):84–91.

52. Shepard JW Jr, Thawley SE. Evaluation of the upper airway by computerized tomography in patients undergoing uvulopalatopharyngoplasty for obstructive sleep apnea. Am Rev Respir Dis 1989; 140(3):711–716.

53. Shepard JW Jr, Stanson AW, Sheedy PF, Westbrook PR. Fast-CT evaluation of the upper airway during wakefulness in patients with obstructive sleep apnea. In: Suratt PM, ed. Proceedings of the First International Symposium on Sleep and Respiration. New York: Alan R. Liss, Inc.; 1990:273–282.

54. Stanford W, Galvin J, Rooholamini M. Effects of awake tidal breathing, swallowing, nasal breathing, oral breathing and the Muller and Valsalva maneuvers on the dimensions of the upper airway. Evaluation by ultrafast computerized tomography. Chest 1988; 94(1):149–154.

55. Stauffer JL, Zwillich CW, Cadieux RJ et al. Pharyngeal size and resistance in obstructive sleep apnea. Am Rev Respir Dis 1987; 136(3):623–627.

56. Stein MG, Gamsu G, de Geer G, Golden JA, Crumley RL, Webb WR. Cine CT in obstructive sleep apnea. AJR Am J Roentgenol 1987; 148(6):1069–1074.

57. Schwab RJ. Imaging for the snoring and sleep apnea patient. Dent Clin North Am 2001; 45(4):759–796.

58. Isono S, Remmers JE, Tanaka A, Sho Y, Sato J, Nishino T. Anatomy of pharynx in patients with obstructive sleep apnea and in normal subjects. J Appl Physiol 1997; 82(4):1319–1326.

59. Morrell MJ, Arabi Y, Zahn B, Badr MS. Progressive retropalatal narrowing preceding obstructive apnea. Am J Respir Crit Care Med 1998; 158(6):1974–1981.
60. Woodson BT, Wooten MR. Comparison of upper-airway evaluations during wakefulness and sleep. Laryngoscope 1994; 104(7):821–828.
61. Schwartz AR, Gold AR, Schubert N et al. Effect of weight loss on upper airway collapsibility in obstructive sleep apnea. Am Rev Respir Dis 1991; 144(3 Pt 1):494–498.
62. Isono S, Tanaka A, Sho Y, Konno A, Nishino T. Advancement of the mandible improves velopharyngeal airway patency. J Appl Physiol 1995; 79(6):2132–2138.
63. Nelson S, Hans M. Contribution of craniofacial risk factors in increasing apneic activity among obese and nonobese habitual snorers. Chest 1997; 111(1):154–162.
64. Miles PG, Vig PS, Weyant RJ, Forrest TD, Rockette HE Jr. Craniofacial structure and obstructive sleep apnea syndrome—a qualitative analysis and meta-analysis of the literature. Am J Orthod Dentofacial Orthop 1996; 109(2):163–172.
65. Caballero P, Alvarez-Sala R, Garcia-Rio F et al. CT in the evaluation of the upper airway in healthy subjects and in patients with obstructive sleep apnea syndrome. Chest 1998; 113(1):111–116.
66. Langin T, Pepin JL, Pendlebury S et al. Upper airway changes in snorers and mild sleep apnea sufferers after uvulopalatopharyngoplasty (UPPP). Chest 1998; 113(6):1595–1603.
67. Abbey NC, Block AJ, Green D, Mancuso A, Hellard DW. Measurement of pharyngeal volume by digitized magnetic resonance imaging. Effect of nasal continuous positive airway pressure. Am Rev Respir Dis 1989; 140(3):717–723.
68. Ryan CF, Lowe AA, Li D, Fleetham JA. Magnetic resonance imaging of the upper airway in obstructive sleep apnea before and after chronic nasal continuous positive airway pressure therapy. Am Rev Respir Dis 1991; 144(4):939–944.
69. Ciscar MA, Juan G, Martinez V et al. Magnetic resonance imaging of the pharynx in OSA patients and healthy subjects. Eur Respir J 2001; 17(1):79–86.
70. Schoenberg SO, Floemer F, Kroeger H, Hoffmann A, Bock M, Knopp MV. Combined assessment of obstructive sleep apnea syndrome with dynamic MRI and parallel EEG registration: initial results. Invest Radiol 2000; 35(4):267–276.
71. Do KL, Ferreyra H, Healy JF, Davidson TM. Does tongue size differ between patients with and without sleep-disordered breathing? Laryngoscope 2000; 110(9):1552–1555.
72. Jager L, Gunther E, Gauger J, Reiser M. Fluoroscopic MR of the pharynx in patients with obstructive sleep apnea. AJNR Am J Neuroradiol 1998; 19(7):1205–1214.
73. Trudo FJ, Gefter WB, Welch KC, Gupta KB, Maislin G, Schwab RJ. State-related changes in upper airway caliber and surrounding soft-tissue structures in normal subjects. Am J Respir Crit Care Med 1998; 158(4):1259–1270.
74. Bohlman ME, Haponik EF, Smith PL, Allen RP, Bleecker ER, Goldman SM. CT demonstration of pharyngeal narrowing in adult obstructive sleep apnea. AJR Am J Roentgenol 1983; 140(3):543–548.
75. Lowe AA, Gionhaku N, Takeuchi K, Fleetham JA. Three-dimensional CT reconstructions of tongue and airway in adult subjects with obstructive sleep apnea. Am J Orthod Dentofacial Orthop 1986; 90(5):364–374.
76. Schotland HM, Insko EK, Schwab RJ. Quantitative magnetic resonance imaging demonstrates alterations of the lingual musculature in obstructive sleep apnea. Sleep 1999; 22(5):605–613.

77. Kuczmarski RJ, Carroll MD, Flegal KM, Troiano RP. Varying body mass index cutoff points to describe overweight prevalence among U.S. adults: NHANES III (1988–1994). Obes Res 1997; 5(6):542–548.

78. Bliwise DL, Feldman DE, Bliwise NG et al. Risk factors for sleep disordered breathing in heterogeneous geriatric populations. J Am Geriatr Soc 1987; 35(2):132–141.

79. Young T, Palta M, Dempsey J, Skatrud J, Weber S, Badr S. The occurrence of sleep-disordered breathing among middle-aged adults. N Engl J Med 1993; 328(17):1230–1235.

80. Loube DI, Loube AA, Mitler MM. Weight loss for obstructive sleep apnea: the optimal therapy for obese patients. J Am Diet Assoc 1994; 94(11):1291–1295.

81. Smith PL, Gold AR, Meyers DA, Haponik EF, Bleecker ER. Weight loss in mildly to moderately obese patients with obstructive sleep apnea. Ann Intern Med 1985; 103(6 Pt 1):850–855.

82. Strobel RJ, Rosen RC. Obesity and weight loss in obstructive sleep apnea: a critical review. Sleep 1996; 19(2):104–115.

83. Wittels EH, Thompson S. Obstructive sleep apnea and obesity. Otolaryngol Clin North Am 1990; 23(4):751–760.

84. Davies RJ, Ali NJ, Stradling JR. Neck circumference and other clinical features in the diagnosis of the obstructive sleep apnoea syndrome. Thorax 1992; 47(2):101–105.

85. Davies RJ, Stradling JR. The relationship between neck circumference, radiographic pharyngeal anatomy, and the obstructive sleep apnoea syndrome. Eur Respir J 1990; 3(5):509–514.

86. Horner RL, Mohiaddin RH, Lowell DG et al. Sites and sizes of fat deposits around the pharynx in obese patients with obstructive sleep apnoea and weight matched controls. Eur Respir J 1989; 2(7):613–622.

87. Mortimore IL, Marshall I, Wraith PK, Sellar RJ, Douglas NJ. Neck and total body fat deposition in nonobese and obese patients with sleep apnea compared with that in control subjects. Am J Respir Crit Care Med 1998; 157(1):280–283.

88. Stauffer JL, Buick MK, Bixler EO et al. Morphology of the uvula in obstructive sleep apnea. Am Rev Respir Dis 1989; 140(3):724–728.

89. Zohar Y, Sabo R, Strauss M, Schwartz A, Gal R, Oksenberg A. Oropharyngeal fatty infiltration in obstructive sleep apnea patients: a histologic study. Ann Otol Rhinol Laryngol 1998; 107(2):170–174.

90. Hill JO, Sparling PB, Shields TW, Heller PA. Effects of exercise and food restriction on body composition and metabolic rate in obese women. Am J Clin Nutr 1987; 46(4):622–630.

91. Wadden TA, Foster GD, Letizia KA, Mullen JL. Long-term effects of dieting on resting metabolic rate in obese outpatients. Jama 1990; 264(6):707–711.

92. Foster GD, Wadden TA, Mullen JL et al. Resting energy expenditure, body composition, and excess weight in the obese. Metabolism 1988; 37(5):467–472.

93. Series F, Cote C, Simoneau JA et al. Physiologic, metabolic, and muscle fiber type characteristics of musculus uvulae in sleep apnea hypopnea syndrome and in snorers. J Clin Invest 1995; 95(1):20–25.

94. Welch KC, Foster GD, Ritter CT et al. A novel volumetric magnetic resonance imaging paradigm to study upper airway anatomy. Sleep 2002; 25(5):532–542.

95. Carrera M, Barbe F, Sauleda J, Tomas M, Gomez C, Agusti AG. Patients with obstructive sleep apnea exhibit genioglossus dysfunction that is normalized after

treatment with continuous positive airway pressure. Am J Respir Crit Care Med 1999; 159(6):1960–1966.

96. Friberg D, Ansved T, Borg K, Carlsson-Nordlander B, Larsson H, Svanborg E. Histological indications of a progressive snorers disease in an upper airway muscle. Am J Respir Crit Care Med 1998; 157(2):586–593.

97. Brooks LJ, Strohl KP. Size and mechanical properties of the pharynx in healthy men and women. Am Rev Respir Dis 1992; 146(6):1394–1397.

98. Guilleminault C, Partinen M, Hollman K, Powell N, Stoohs R. Familial aggregates in obstructive sleep apnea syndrome. Chest 1995; 107(6):1545–1551.

99. Legato MJ. Gender-specific aspects of obesity. Int J Fertil Womens Med 1997; 42(3):184–197.

100. Millman RP, Carlisle CC, McGarvey ST, Eveloff SE, Levinson PD. Body fat distribution and sleep apnea severity in women. Chest 1995; 107(2):362–366.

101. Mathur R, Douglas NJ. Family studies in patients with the sleep apnea–hypopnea syndrome. Ann Intern Med 1995; 122(3):174–178.

102. Marcus CL, Keens TG, Bautista DB, von Pechmann WS, Ward SL. Obstructive sleep apnea in children with Down syndrome. Pediatrics 1991; 88(1):132–139.

103. Guilleminault C, Stoohs R, Kim YD, Chervin R, Black J, Clerk A. Upper airway sleep-disordered breathing in women. Ann Intern Med 1995; 122(7):493–501.

104. Lee JJ, Ramirez SG, Will MJ. Gender and racial variations in cephalometric analysis. Otolaryngol Head Neck Surg 1997; 117(4):326–329.

105. Will MJ, Ester MS, Ramirez SG, Tiner BD, McAnear JT, Epstein L. Comparison of cephalometric analysis with ethnicity in obstructive sleep apnea syndrome. Sleep 1995; 18(10):873–875.

106. Ritter CT, Trudo FJ, Goldberg AN, Welch KC, Maislin G, Schwab RJ. Quantitative evaluation of the upper airway during nasopharyngoscopy with the Muller maneuver. Laryngoscope 1999; 109(6):954–963.

107. Welch KC, Ritter CT, Gefter WB, Schwab RJ. Dynamic respiratory related upper airway imaging during wakefulness in normal subjects and patients with sleep disordered breathing using MRI. Am J Respir Crit Care Med 1998; 157:A54.

108. Suratt PM, Wilhoit SC, Cooper K. Induction of airway collapse with subatmospheric pressure in awake patients with sleep apnea. J Appl Physiol 1984; 57(1):140–146.

109. Sanders MH, Moore SE. Inspiratory and expiratory partitioning of airway resistance during sleep in patients with sleep apnea. Am Rev Respir Dis 1983; 127(5):554–558.

110. Sanders MH, Kern N. Obstructive sleep apnea treated by independently adjusted inspiratory and expiratory positive airway pressures via nasal mask. Physiologic and clinical implications. Chest 1990; 98(2):317–324.

111. Pack AI. Obstructive sleep apnea. Adv Intern Med 1994; 39:517–567.

112. Ritter CT, Trudo FJ, Goldberg AN, Welch KC, Maislin G, Schwab RJ. Quantitative evaluation of the upper airway changes in normals and apneics during Muller maneuver. Am J Respir Crit Care Med 1998; 157:A54.

113. Brown IB, McClean PA, Boucher R, Zamel N, Hoffstein V. Changes in pharyngeal cross-sectional area with posture and application of continuous positive airway pressure in patients with obstructive sleep apnea. Am Rev Respir Dis 1987; 136(3):628–632.

114. Collop NA, Block AJ, Hellard D. The effect of nightly nasal CPAP treatment on underlying obstructive sleep apnea and pharyngeal size. Chest 1991; 99(4):855–860.

115. Schmidt-Nowara W, Lowe A, Wiegand L, Cartwright R, Perez-Guerra F, Menn S. Oral appliances for the treatment of snoring and obstructive sleep apnea: a review. Sleep 1995; 18(6):501–510.
116. Strollo PJ Jr, Rogers RM. Obstructive sleep apnea. N Engl J Med 1996; 334(2):99–104.
117. Liu Y, Zeng X, Fu M, Huang X, Lowe AA. Effects of a mandibular repositioner on obstructive sleep apnea. Am J Orthod Dentofacial Orthop 2000; 118(3):248–256.
118. Schmidt-Nowara WW, Meade TE, Hays MB. Treatment of snoring and obstructive sleep apnea with a dental orthosis. Chest 1991; 99(6):1378–1385.
119. Bonham PE, Currier GF, Orr WC, Othman J, Nanda RS. The effect of a modified functional appliance on obstructive sleep apnea. Am J Orthod Dentofacial Orthop 1988; 94(5):384–392.
120. Bennett LS, Davies RJ, Stradling JR. Oral appliances for the management of snoring and obstructive sleep apnoea. Thorax 1998; 53(Suppl 2):S58–S64.
121. Ryan CF, Love LL, Peat D, Fleetham JA, Lowe AA. Mandibular advancement oral appliance therapy for obstructive sleep apnoea: effect on awake calibre of the velopharynx. Thorax 1999; 54(11):972–977.
122. Sher AE, Schechtman KB, Piccirillo JF. The efficacy of surgical modifications of the upper airway in adults with obstructive sleep apnea syndrome. Sleep 1996; 19(2):156–177.
123. Hudgel DW. Variable site of airway narrowing among obstructive sleep apnea patients. J Appl Physiol 1986; 61(4):1403–1409.
124. Schwartz AR, Schubert N, Rothman W et al. Effect of uvulopalatopharyngoplasty on upper airway collapsibility in obstructive sleep apnea. Am Rev Respir Dis 1992; 145(3):527–532.
125. Welch KC, Goldberg AN, Trudo FJ, Gefter WB, Ritter CT, Schwab RJ. Upper airway anatomic changes with magnetic resonance imaging in uvulopatopharyngoplasty patients. Am J Respir Crit Care Med 1997; 155:A938.
126. Ali NJ, Pitson DJ, Stradling JR. Snoring, sleep disturbance, and behaviour in 4–5 year olds. Arch Dis Child 1993; 68(3):360–366.
127. Redline S, Tishler PV, Schluchter M, Aylor J, Clark K, Graham G. Risk factors for sleep-disordered breathing in children. Associations with obesity, race, and respiratory problems. Am J Respir Crit Care Med 1999; 159(5 Pt 1):1527–1532.
128. Block AJ, Boysen PG, Wynne JW, Hunt LA. Sleep apnea, hypopnea and oxygen desaturation in normal subjects. A strong male predominance. N Engl J Med 1979; 300(10):513–517.
129. Marcus CL. Sleep-disordered breathing in children. Am J Respir Crit Care Med 2001; 164(1):16–30.
130. Rosen GM, Muckle RP, Mahowald MW, Goding GS, Ullevig C. Postoperative respiratory compromise in children with obstructive sleep apnea syndrome: can it be anticipated? Pediatrics 1994; 93(5):784–788.
131. Tal A, Bar A, Leiberman A, Tarasiuk A. Sleep characteristics following adenotonsillectomy in children with obstructive sleep apnea syndrome. Chest 2003; 124(3):948–953.
132. Marcus CL, Ward SL, Mallory GB et al. Use of nasal continuous positive airway pressure as treatment of childhood obstructive sleep apnea. J Pediatr 1995; 127(1):88–94.

133. American Thoracic Society. Standards and indications for cardiopulmonary sleep studies in children. Am J Respir Crit Care Med 1996; 153(2):866–878.
134. The Report of an American Academy of Sleep Medicine Task Force. Sleep-related breathing disorders in adults: recommendations for syndrome definition and measurement techniques in clinical research. Sleep 1999; 22(5):667–689.
135. Brouillette RT, Fernbach SK, Hunt CE. Obstructive sleep apnea in infants and children. J Pediatr 1982; 100(1):31–40.
136. Gozal D. Sleep-disordered breathing and school performance in children. Pediatrics 1998; 102(3 Pt 1):616–620.
137. Amin RS, Kimball TR, Bean JA et al. Left ventricular hypertrophy and abnormal ventricular geometry in children and adolescents with obstructive sleep apnea. Am J Respir Crit Care Med 2002; 165(10):1395–1399.
138. Brodsky L, Adler E, Stanievich JF. Naso- and oropharyngeal dimensions in children with obstructive sleep apnea. Int J Pediatr Otorhinolaryngol 1989; 17(1):1–11.
139. Guilleminault C, Eldridge FL, Simmons FB, Dement WC. Sleep apnea in eight children. Pediatrics 1976; 58(1):23–30.
140. Ahlqvist-Rastad J, Hultcrantz E, Svanholm H. Children with tonsillar obstruction: indications for and efficacy of tonsillectomy. Acta Paediatr Scand 1988; 77(6):831–835.
141. Mahboubi S, Marsh RR, Potsic WP, Pasquariello PS. The lateral neck radiograph in adenotonsillar hyperplasia. Int J Pediatr Otorhinolaryngol 1985; 10(1):67–73.
142. Brooks LJ, Stephens BM, Bacevice AM. Adenoid size is related to severity but not the number of episodes of obstructive apnea in children. J Pediatr 1998; 132(4):682–686.
143. Arens R, McDonough JM, Costarino AT et al. Magnetic resonance imaging of the upper airway structure of children with obstructive sleep apnea syndrome. Am J Respir Crit Care Med 2001; 164(4):698–703.
144. Arens R, McDonough JM, Corbin AM et al. Upper airway size analysis by magnetic resonance imaging of children with obstructive sleep apnea syndrome. Am J Respir Crit Care Med 2003; 167(1):65–70.
145. Spier S, Rivlin J, Rowe RD, Egan T. Sleep in Pierre Robin syndrome. Chest 1986; 90(5):711–715.
146. Abramson DL, Marrinan EM, Mulliken JB. Robin sequence: obstructive sleep apnea following pharyngeal flap. Cleft Palate Craniofac J 1997; 34(3):256–260.
147. Johnston C, Taussig LM, Koopmann C, Smith P, Bjelland J. Obstructive sleep apnea in Treacher-Collins syndrome. Cleft Palate J 1981; 18(1):39–44.
148. Mixter RC, David DJ, Perloff WH, Green CG, Pauli RM, Popic PM. Obstructive sleep apnea in Apert's and Pfeiffer's syndromes: more than a craniofacial abnormality. Plast Reconstr Surg 1990; 86(3):457–463.
149. Donaldson JD, Redmond WM. Surgical management of obstructive sleep apnea in children with Down syndrome. J Otolaryngol 1988; 17(7):398–403.
150. Shintani T, Asakura K, Kataura A. Adenotonsillar hypertrophy and skeletal morphology of children with obstructive sleep apnea syndrome. Acta Otolaryngol Suppl 1996; 523:222–224.
151. Shintani T, Asakura K, Kataura A. Evaluation of the role of adenotonsillar hypertrophy and facial morphology in children with obstructive sleep apnea. ORL J Otorhinolaryngol Relat Spec 1997; 59(5):286–291.

152. Agren K, Nordlander B, Linder-Aronsson S, Zettergren-Wijk L, Svanborg E. Children with nocturnal upper airway obstruction: postoperative orthodontic and respiratory improvement. Acta Otolaryngol 1998; 581–587.
153. Kawashima S, Niikuni N, Chia-hung L et al. Cephalometric comparisons of craniofacial and upper airway structures in young children with obstructive sleep apnea syndrome. Ear Nose Throat J 2000; 79(7):5–6, 499–502.
154. Marcus CL, Lutz J, Hamer A, Smith PL, Schwartz A. Developmental changes in response to subatmospheric pressure loading of the upper airway. J Appl Physiol 1999; 87(2):626–633.
155. Fujioka M, Young LW, Girdany BR. Radiographic evaluation of adenoidal size in children: adenoidal-nasopharyngeal ratio. AJR Am J Roentgenol 1979; 133(3):401–404.
156. Guilleminault C, Pelayo R, Leger D, Clerk A, Bocian RC. Recognition of sleep-disordered breathing in children. Pediatrics 1996; 98(5):871–882.
157. Guilleminault C, Partinen M, Praud JP, Quera-Salva MA, Powell N, Riley R. Morphometric facial changes and obstructive sleep apnea in adolescents. J Pediatr 1989; 114(6):997–999.
158. Fernbach SK, Brouillette RT, Riggs TW, Hunt CE. Radiologic evaluation of adenoids and tonsils in children with obstructive sleep apnea: plain films and fluoroscopy. Pediatr Radiol 1983; 13(5):258–265.
159. Jeans WD, Fernando DC, Maw AR, Leighton BC. A longitudinal study of the growth of the nasopharynx and its contents in normal children. Br J Radiol 1981; 54(638):117–121.
160. Kawashima S, Peltomaki T, Sakata H, Mori K, Happonen RP, Ronning O. Craniofacial morphology in preschool children with sleep-related breathing disorder and hypertrophy of tonsils. Acta Paediatr 2002; 91(1):71–77.
161. Zucconi M, Caprioglio A, Calori G et al. Craniofacial modifications in children with habitual snoring and obstructive sleep apnoea: a case-control study. Eur Respir J 1999; 13(2):411–417.
162. Isono S, Shimada A, Utsugi M, Konno A, Nishino T. Comparison of static mechanical properties of the passive pharynx between normal children and children with sleep-disordered breathing. Am J Respir Crit Care Med 1998; 157(4 Pt 1):1204–1212.
163. Isono S, Tanaka A, Ishikawa T, Nishino T. Developmental changes in collapsibility of the passive pharynx during infancy. Am J Respir Crit Care Med 2000; 162(3 Pt 1):832–836.
164. Donnelly LF, Strife JL, Myer CM III. Glossoptosis (posterior displacement of the tongue) during sleep: a frequent cause of sleep apnea in pediatric patients referred for dynamic sleep fluoroscopy. AJR Am J Roentgenol 2000; 175(6):1557–1560.
165. Monahan KJ, Larkin EK, Rosen CL, Graham G, Redline S. Utility of noninvasive pharyngometry in epidemiologic studies of childhood sleep-disordered breathing. Am J Respir Crit Care Med 2002; 165(11):1499–1503.
166. Shepard JW Jr, Stanson AW, Sheedy PF, Westbrook PR. Fast-CT evaluation of the upper airway during wakefulness in patients with obstructive sleep apnea. Prog Clin Biol Res 1990; 345:273–279; discussion 80–82.
167. Guilleminault C, Heldt G, Powell N, Riley R. Small upper airway in near-miss sudden infant death syndrome infants and their families. Lancet 1986; 1(8478):402–407.

168. Kapelushnik J, Shalev H, Schulman H, Moser A, Tamary H. Upper airway obstruction-related sleep apnea in a child with thalassemia intermedia. J Pediatr Hematol Oncol 2001; 23(8):525–526.

169. Perlyn CA, Schmelzer RE, Sutera SP, Kane AA, Govier D, Marsh JL. Effect of distraction osteogenesis of the mandible on upper airway volume and resistance in children with micrognathia. Plast Reconstr Surg 2002; 109(6):1809–1818.

170. Donnelly LF, Surdulescu V, Chini BA, Casper KA, Poe SA, Amin RS. Upper airway motion depicted at cine MR imaging performed during sleep: comparison between young patients with and those without obstructive sleep apnea. Radiology 2003; 227(1):239–245.

171. Arens R, McDonough JM, Corbin AM et al. Linear dimensions of the upper airway structure during development: assessment by magnetic resonance imaging. Am J Respir Crit Care Med 2002; 165:117–122.

172. Abbott MB, Dardzinski BJ, Donnelly LF. Using volume segmentation of cine MR data to evaluate dynamic motion of the airway in pediatric patients. AJR Am J Roentgenol 2003; 181(3):857–859.

173. Vogler RC, Ii FJ, Pilgram TK. Age-specific size of the normal adenoid pad on magnetic resonance imaging. Clin Otolaryngol 2000; 25(5):392–395.

174. Marcus CL, McColley SA, Carroll JL, Loughlin GM, Smith PL, Schwartz AR. Upper airway collapsibility in children with obstructive sleep apnea syndrome. J Appl Physiol 1994; 77(2):918–924.

175. Uong EC, McDonough JM, Tayag-Kier CE et al. Magnetic resonance imaging of the upper airway in children with Down syndrome. Am J Respir Crit Care Med 2001; 163(3 Pt 1):731–736.

26

Solitary Pulmonary Nodule

YASUYUKI KURIHARA

St. Marianna University School of Medicine,
Kanagawa, Japan

I. Introduction

The solitary pulmonary nodule (SPN) is one of the most common radiologic abnormalities detected in daily practice. In fact, it is estimated that up to one in every 500 chest radiographs demonstrates a lung nodule (1,2). Since the introduction of computed tomography (CT), especially helical CT, the number of incidental findings of SPN has increased.

Although most SPNs prove to be benign, the distinction between benign and malignant lesions can be difficult. A timely and accurate diagnosis of the etiology of an SPN in the least invasive manner is an essential goal of imaging in the assessment of SPN. Evaluation of the specific morphologic features of an SPN with chest radiograph and CT (particularly thin-section CT) is a standard and cost-effective approach and helps to differentiate benign nodules from malignant nodules. Magnetic resonance imaging is being studied as a newer technique to evaluate SPNs. Positron emission tomographic imaging of SPNs will be discussed in depth elsewhere (Chapter 18).

II. Definition of SPN

An SPN is radiologically defined as a single round or oval intraparenchymal lung lesion, no greater than 3 cm in maximum diameter and associated with no other pulmonary abnormality. Lung lesions >3 cm in diameter are more often malignant and defined as a lung mass (3).

The initial step in evaluation of a suspected SPN on chest radiograph is to determine whether the abnormality is a true SPN. This evaluation is essential because up to 20% of suspected nodules are proved to be "pseudo-nodules," such as focal pleural lesions, rib fractures (Fig. 26.1), skin lesions (Fig. 26.2), and artificial devices on the patient's skin surface. In fact, it sometimes is difficult to confirm the intrapulmonary localization of a nodular opacity on a single chest radiograph. Examination of the skin surface usually identifies skin lesions. The use of oblique radiographs, fluoroscopy, or repeated frontal radiographs with localizing metallic markers can avert an extensive costly diagnostic work-up. If a "pseudo-nodule" is not confirmed with these additional procedures,

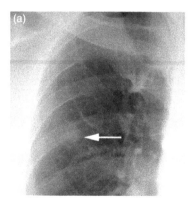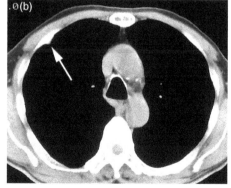

Figure 26.1 Rib fracture mimicking a solitary pulmonary nodule. (a) Frontal chest radiograph shows a round increased opacity projecting over the third rib. (b) Chest CT scan shows an old rib fracture with prominent callus formation (arrow) causing a focal round opacity.

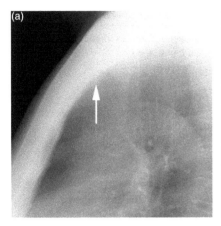
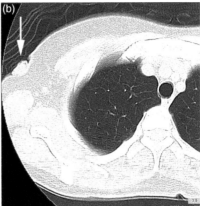

Figure 26.2 Skin lesion mimicking a solitary pulmonary nodule. (a) Lateral chest radiograph shows a well-defined nodule behind the sternum (arrow). (b) Chest CT shows a verruca at the right axilla (arrow).

CT should be used to confirm the location and further characterize the nodular abnormality.

It is also important to determine whether a suspected SPN is truly solitary, because as many as 50% of patients with suspected SPNs detected on chest X-ray turn out to have multiple nodules on CT evaluation (4). The presence of multiple lung nodules is suggestive of metastatic or granulomatous disease and requires a different approach than that for the assessment of a true SPN.

III. Differential Diagnosis of the SPN

The differential diagnosis of SPN is extensive and includes neoplastic, infectious, inflammatory, vascular, and congenital disorders (Table 26.1). Other benign etiologies of SPNs are rheumatoid necrobiotic nodules, intrapulmonary lymph nodes, inflammatory myofibroblastic tumors, amyloidosis, hyalinizing granuloma, and sarcoidosis. Though most SPNs are benign (5), primary malignancy may be found in ~30–40% of SPNs (6). In areas where granulomatous infection (such as tuberculosis) is endemic, nodules identified by radiography are more likely to be benign.

Clinical features such as the patient's age, a history of cigarette smoking, previous history of malignancy, and presenting symptoms are useful and increase the probability that an SPN is malignant. A combination of clinical features and imaging characteristics provides a precise evaluation of SPNs and can influence the diagnostic accuracy and choice of therapy. Bayesian analysis, logistic regression models, and neural network analysis can be useful in a more precise determination of the probability of malignancy in SPNs. Bayesian analysis

Table 26.1 Differential Diagnosis of a Solitary Pulmonary Nodule

Neoplastic	Malignant	Bronchogenic carcinoma
		Carcinoid tumor
		Lymphoma
		Metastasis
	Benign	Hamartoma
		Sclerosing hemangioma (pneumocytoma)
Inflammatory	Infectious	Mycobacteria (tuberculosis, non-tuberculous mycobacteria)
		Fungi
		Bacterial pneumonia
		Dirofilariasis
	Noninfectious	Rheumatoid (bionecrotic) nodule
		Wegener's granulomatosis
		Sarcoidosis
		Amyloidosis
		Inflammatory myofibroblastic tumor
		Intrapulmonary lymphnode
Vascular		Arteriovenous malformation
		Pulmonary arterial aneurysm
		Pulmonary infarction
		Hematoma
Congenital		Bronchogenic cyst
		Bronchial atresia
		Sequestration

uses likelihood ratios for numerous radiographic findings and clinical features associated with SPNs to estimate the probability of malignancy (7,8). Although Bayesian analysis and neural network analysis are the most sophisticated approaches for the assessment and management of SPN, these techniques have been of little practical use to the clinician evaluating a patient with an SPN.

IV. Morphologic Evaluation of SPNs

A. Distribution of SPNs

Although primary lung carcinoma may occur anywhere in the lung without a predominant distribution, some SPNs tend to localize to specific areas of the lung. Most granulomatous diseases (sarcoidosis, tuberculosis) have upper lobe predominance due to delayed lymphatic clearance in the upper lung (9). In contrast, arteriovenous malformation (10) and pulmonary infarctions are usually seen in the lower lobes, possibly because pulmonary perfusion predominates in the dependent lung. Intralobar sequestration is common in the medial–basal segment of the lower lobe, probably related to the ligamental artery. Sclerosing hemangioma (pneumocytoma) and intrapulmonary lymph

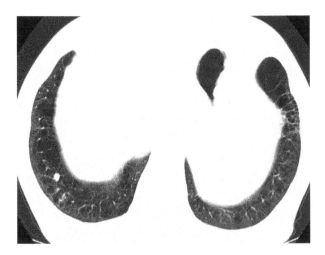

Figure 26.3 Intrapulmonary lymph node in a 75-year-old man. Chest CT scan shows a well-defined small nodule at the periphery of right lower lobe.

nodes (11) (Fig. 26.3) usually occur in the lower lungs. Peripheral or subpleural predominace is seen in pulmonary infarction and dirofilariasis, which is caused by embolism of dead larvae in the peripheral arteries. Some neoplastic conditions have subpleural predominance for unknown reasons. They include inflammatory myofibroblastic tumor (12), rheumatoid necrobiotic nodules, amyloidosis (13), and intrapulmonary lymph nodes (14).

B. Size

The size of an SPN is a good indicator of the likelihood of malignancy. The vast majority (97%) of SPNs >3 cm in size (by strict definition, therefore, these would be considered masses) are malignant (15) while a smaller SPN is more likely to be benign. However, small size alone cannot exclude lung cancer. Fifteen percent of malignant nodules are <1 cm in diameter and ~42% are <2 cm in diameter (16). The size of an SPN provides helpful information but does not allow a definitive distinction of benign from malignant SPNs, especially for nodules <2 cm in diameter.

C. Growth Rate

A comparison of a current chest image with a prior image must be the first step in determining the benignity or malignancy of an SPN. It is generally agreed that an SPN that does not grow over a 2 year period is benign and does not require resection (2 year rule) (17). However, slow growing malignant tumors, such as bronchioloalveolar carcinoma, may grow after this time period. Many authors have evaluated the "doubling time" of a nodule to help determine whether it is malignant. This is defined as the time required for a nodule to double in volume, which corresponds to a 26% increase in diameter for a spherical lesion. Benign lesions typically have a doubling time of <1 month or >16 months. Malignant nodules often have a doubling time between 30 and 400 days (18).

Clinical management of patients with SPNs may be challenging as clinicians often do not have access to prior radiographic images in patients with SPNs, and a 2 year follow-up is a relatively long time to confirm the benignity of a lesion. In fact, the assumption that 2 year stability implies benignity has recently come into question. In one study, lack of growth of a nodule had a predictive value for benignity of only 65% (47), suggesting that 2 year stability is not a reliable sign of benignity. Furthermore, it can be difficult to reliably detect minimum growth in small nodules <1 cm, because a smaller nodule will show a smaller increase in diameter, even though its proportional change in volume is identical to that of a larger nodule. For example, after one doubling, a nodule with a diameter of 4 mm will only increase to 5 mm, which is difficult to detect even on CT, whereas a nodule with a diameter of 3 cm will increase to 3.75 cm. To overcome this limitation, it has been proposed that the growth rate of small SPNs be evaluated with volumetric measurements on repeated CT with three-dimensional isotropic voxels rather than simple measurement of the diameter. According to volumetric measurement on repeated CT, malignant SPNs had doubling times <177 days and showed an asymmetric growth pattern, whereas benign SPNs had doubling times ≥396 days (19). This measurement is very accurate and sensitive since a single repeated CT obtained only 30 days after the initial CT scan may depict growth in most malignant tumors as small as 5 mm (20).

Furthermore, patients with an acute process, such as focal pneumonia or pulmonary infarction, can present with what appears to be an SPN on chest radiography. In such patients, a follow-up radiograph after 1–2 weeks may show a decrease in the size of a nodule. In a CT study of patients with acute symptoms, 92/108 (85%) of benign nodules demonstrated resolution, or decreased in size or density at the time of the first follow-up CT within 3 months, while the remaining 15% (16/108) showed evidence of improvement of the nodule within the following 15 months (21). A population-based CT mass screening study concluded that the criterion specific to benign lesions showing the greatest sensitivity (45%) was attained with a combination of lesion regression or polygonal shape (22). Therefore, nodular regression is a strong indicator of benignity. However, if there is a high suspicion of cancer, it is not advisable to obtain follow-up radiographs hoping that the SPN will decrease in size (3).

D. Margins, Contours, and Marginal Changes

A careful observation of the contour and marginal changes of an SPN as depicted on thin-section CT provides useful information for differentiation between malignancy and benignity, although the exact contour of an SPN may be modified by underlying pulmonary disease such as emphysema, pulmonary fibrosis, or bullous lung disease (Fig. 26.4). The margins and contours of SPNs are classified as smooth, lobulated, irregular, or spiculated. Smooth and well-defined margin usually indicates benignity, but is not diagnostic. This appearance is observed with almost equal frequency among malignant and benign SPNs using high-resolution CT (23) and 21–38% of SPNs with a smooth margin are malignant and could represent metastatic disease (15,16) (Fig. 26.5). A lobulated margin, or scalloped-shaped border, implies uneven growth of an SPN and can indicate malignancy, although lobulation also occurs in 27% of benign SPNs (23). A polygonal shaped SPN usually indicates that the contour is marginated with interlobular septae and is a strong diagnostic indicator of benignity (22,24) (Fig. 26.6), because most infectious diseases develop along with airways and finally involve intra-alveolar airspaces which are separated by interlobular septae. Lesions showing bronchogenic spread are usually marginated by interlobular septae or pulmonary veins, although involvement of the pulmonary veins is usually noted in malignancy rather than in benignity (100% and 13%, respectively) (25,26). Most (88.5%) SPNs with an irregular or spiculated margin are malignant (16). Spiculated margins result from cicatrization (scarring) of the lung interstitium surrounding a lesion.

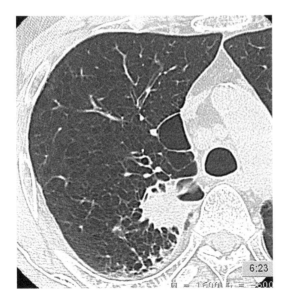

Figure 26.4 A 58-year-old man with primary lung carcinoma and emphysema. Chest CT reveals an irregularly nodule in the right upper lobe. The contour of the nodule is modified with marginal air cysts and bulla associated with emphysema.

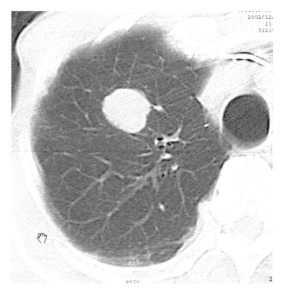

Figure 26.5 Metastatic tumor originating from renal pelvic carcinoma in an 85-year-old man. Thin-section chest CT shows a well-defined nodule at the right apex.

Further fibrotic changes in the surrounding tissue and collapse of the marginal alveoli and secondary lobules cause convergence of marginal pulmonary structures (such as vessels, interlobular septae, pleura) and result in perinodular linear opacities. The pleural tail or pleural indentation is a linear opacity seen extending from the edge of a peripherally situated SPN that indents the visceral pleural (Fig. 26.7) and may be caused by inward retraction and apposition of the visceral pleura. Although these findings can be associated with malignancies such as adenocarcinoma and peripheral squamous cell carcinoma, they are also seen in benign inflammatory processes, such as tuberculoma, organizing pneumonia, and progressive massive fibrosis seen in silicosis. Their presence is of limited diagnostic value.

The presence of small satellite nodules surrounding the periphery of an SPN is strongly suggestive of a granulomatous infection such as tuberculosis (27). These small satellite lesions have a centrilobular distribution due to the bronchogenic spread of granulomatous lesions (Fig. 26.8). Associated findings such as focal bronchiectasis and localized pleural thickening close to the SPN usually indicate the healing process of focal infection or granulomatous diseases.

A halo sign is characterized by the presence of ground-glass opacity surrounding an SPN and is suggestive of hemorrhagic SPNs such as angioinvasive infection (aspergillosis), hemorrhagic infarction, and tumors that may present with marginal hemorrhage (angiosarcoma, sclerosing hemangioma).

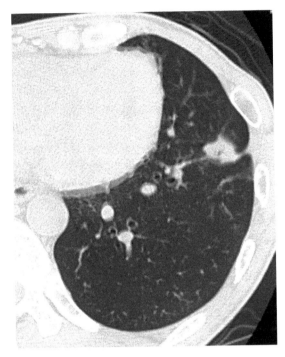

Figure 26.6 Focal pneumonia in a 56-year-old man. Thin-section CT scan shows a nodule with polygonal shape indicating that the contour is marginated with interlobular septi.

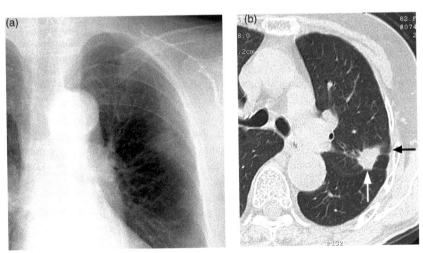

Figure 26.7 Adenocarcinoma in an 82-year-old woman. (a) Frontal chest radiograph shows an irregular nodule in the left upper lung. (b) Thin-section CT reveals a spiculated nodule with pleural indentation (black arrow) and deviated major fissure (white arrow).

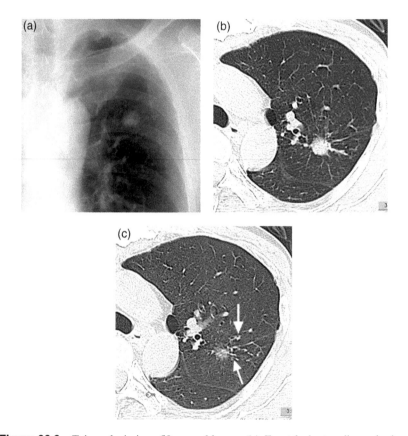

Figure 26.8 Tuberculosis in a 50-year-old man. (a) Frontal chest radiograph shows a compact nodule in the left upper lung. (b) Thin-section CT shows irregular nodule with long speculations. (c) CT scan just above B shows the top of the nodule with several satellite lesions (arrows) suggesting a history of bronchogenic spread.

A few types of SPNs have such characteristic morphologic features that one may make a diagnosis on its CT features alone. These include arteriovenous malformations with feeding and draining vessels (Fig. 26.9), rounded atelectasis with a "comet tail" sign, mucoid impaction with a globe sign, pseudo-alveolar sarcoidosis with a galaxy sign (Fig. 26.10), aspergillosis with a mycetoma, and pulmonary infarction characterized as a wedge shape abutting the pleura with air bronchograms.

E. Cavitation

Cavitation implies necrotic change in the SPN and can occur in both benign and malignant SPNs including lung carcinoma (especially squamous cell carcinoma),

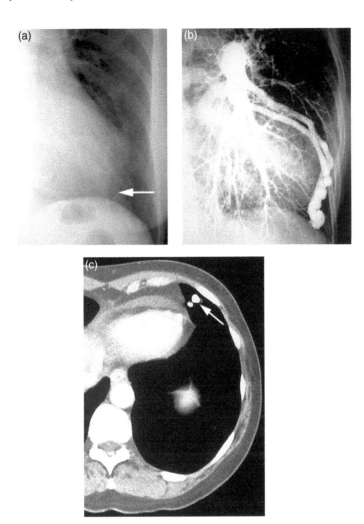

Figure 26.9 Arteriovenous malformation. (a) Frontal chest radiograph shows a well-defined small nodule just above the left diaphragm with a connecting dilated vessel (arrow). (b) Pulmonary angiogram shows arteriovenous malformation with a tortuous and dilated feeding artery and a drainage vein. (c) CT scan shows well-enhancing vascular structures (arrow).

abscess, tuberculosis, fungal infection (Fig. 26.11), atypical mycobacterium infection, Wegener's granulomatosis, and pulmonary infarction.

Wall thickness and shape have been touted as methods to determine whether a cavitary nodule is malignant. Benign cavitary SPNs generally have smooth, thin walls; however, malignant SPNs typically have thick, irregular walls. Studies have suggested that most cavitary SPNs with thin walls (1 mm

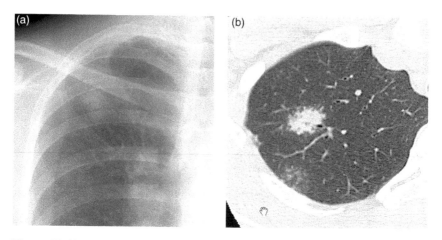

Figure 26.10 Pseudoalveolar sarcoidosis in a 26-year-old man. (a) Frontal chest radiograph shows an irregular nodule in the right upper lobe. Note the right hilar lymphadenopathy. (b) Thin-section chest CT scan shows "sarcoid galaxy" composed of numerous small granulomas. Fine nodular opacities are seen around the large nodule.

thickness) are benign. Of the cavitary SPNs with a maximum wall thickness ≤4 mm, 92–95% were benign. Of cavities that were 5–15 mm in their thickest part and considered indeterminant, 51% were benign and 49% malignant. Of those >15 mm thick, 84–95% were malignant (28,29).

A further detailed assessment of the internal characteristics of SPNs may provide useful information. The presence of air bronchograms (usually air

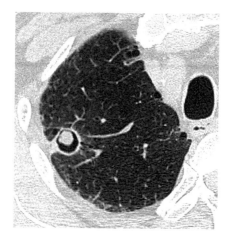

Figure 26.11 Aspergilloma in a 73-year-old man. Chest CT scan shows a thin wall cavitary lesion with an intramural mycetoma.

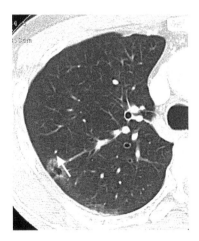

Figure 26.12 Bronchioloalveolar cell carcinoma in a 54-year-old man. Thin-section CT scan shows a focal ground-glass density with pseudocavitation (bubbly lucencies) (arrow), which is common in the disease entity.

bronchiolograms) and pseudocavitation (small, bubbly lucencies) within the SPNs are suggestive of a localized form of bronchioloalveolar cell carcinoma (30) (Fig. 26.12) or lymphoma. However, these internal characteristics are also seen in benignities, including organizing pneumonia, pulmonary infarction, and sarcoidosis.

F. Fat

The presence of fat attenuation (-40 to -120 HU) in an SPN is a pathognomonic finding of a hamartoma (Fig. 26.13), which is the most common benign neoplasm of the lung and the third most common cause of an SPN following granuloma and carcinoma. Most investigators have estimated that 50% of hamartomas contain significant fat deposits, with 30% showing calcification or ossification that often resembles popcorn in appearance. One of the diagnostic problems is small air cysts or pseudocavitation, which could be manifested by zones with density numbers in the negative range that can mimic fat density. The use of thin-section CT is useful to eliminate this partial volume effect.

G. Calcification

The presence and specific patterns of calcification within SPNs have been historically used to differentiate a benign from a malignant nodule. Classically, there are four benign patterns of calcification: dense central, diffuse solid, laminar, and popcorn calcification. The first three are usually indicative of prior granulomatous infection, particularly tuberculosis (Fig. 26.14) and histoplasmosis. Popcorn calcification usually represents chondroid calcification

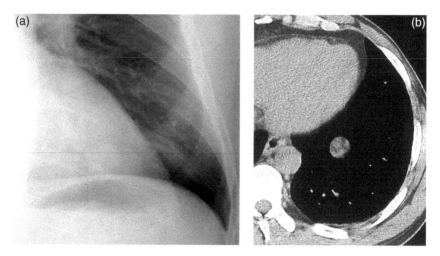

Figure 26.13   Hamartoma. (a) Frontal chest radiograph shows a well-defined nodule behind the heart. (b) Thin-section CT scan shows the presence of fat attenuation in the nodule, which is a pathognomonic finding of hamartoma.

of a pulmonary hamartoma (Fig. 26.15), because the cartilaginous matrix is generally the dominant mesenchymal component of the benign tumor and exhibits a variable degree of calcification and ossification (31). Calcification in lung carcinoma is rarely seen on chest radiographs, but is seen on CT in 6–9% of cases (32,33), and such calcification is typically diffuse and amorphous. Other patterns

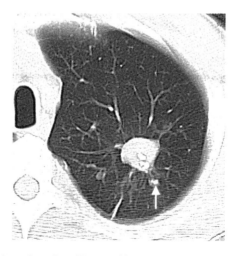

Figure 26.14   Tuberculoma in a 67-year-old man. CT scan shows a well-defined nodule with dense-central calcifications. Note satellite lesions with calcification (arrow).

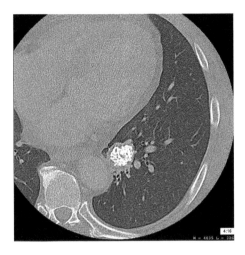

Figure 26.15 Hamartoma in a 57-year-old man. Bony window of the chest CT scan shows marked "popcorn" calcifications of pulmonary hamartoma in the left lower lobe.

of calcification such as eccentric or stippled calcifications are radiologically inde-terminant and seen in both benign and malignant lesions.

Although the identification of calcium on chest radiograph is thought to be one of the reliable indicators of benignity of SPNs, the overall ability of chest radiograph to detect calcification in an SPN is low. Of the "definitely calcified" nodules on chest radiograph, up to 7% may not be calcified and may be potentially malignant (34). Therefore, a low threshold for recommending CT may be appropriate for evaluation of an SPN. Definitive identification of calcification requires thin-section CT using 1–3 mm collimated scans recon-structed with a high spatial frequency algorithm (5).

Quantitative CT densitometry was introduced for better detection of calci-fication in SPN and differentiation between benign and malignant nodules (35). It was founded that calcification which was invisible on plain radiographs could be detected using thin-section CT. On the basis of an initial report, benign SPNs have relatively high CT numbers ($\geq$164 HU), presumably because of diffuse calcification, whereas malignant SPNs have comparatively low CT numbers (mean CT number of 92 HU). Historically, there was considerable variation in CT densitometry among scanners because of partial volume averaging, altered imaging location, different chest wall thicknesses, and different patient sizes. Subsequently, the proposed approach to solve this problem was the development of a phantom, which simulated CT measurements in patients and permitted a comparison of the CT density of each nodule (36). Presently, most thoracic radiologists no longer use the reference CT phantom for this purpose and instead calculate the average CT number through the central portion of the nodule (5). A CT number of $\geq$200 HU is a reliable indicator of microscopic calcification and indicates benignity. However, in order to reduce the risk of misjudging a calcified carcinoma as benign, patients with SPNs >2 cm or appear spiculated on chest radiographs should not undergo CT densitometry as CT densitometry may be of less value in these cases (3).

H. MR Signal Intensity

To date, the role of MR imaging for evaluation of SPNs has been limited, because of its rather limited spatial resolution due to respiratory and cardiac motion and the low signal-to-noise ratio of the normal lung parenchyma. According to

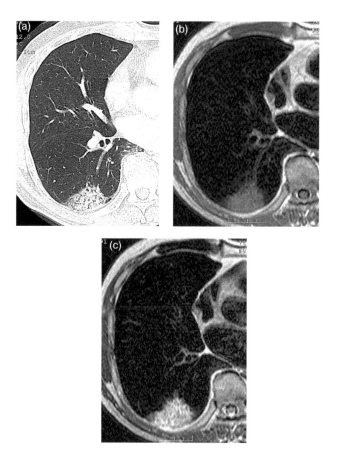

Figure 26.16   Mucin-producing bronchioloalveolar cell carcinoma in a 74-year-old man. (a) Chest CT shows a focal ground-glass density with air-bronchiolograms. (b) T1-weighted image shows a slightly hyperintense focal lesion. (c) T2-weighted image shows a very high signal intensity of the lesion suggesting the presence of mucinous materials.

previous studies, most masses in the lung displayed relatively long T1 and T2 relaxation times and tissue type predictions based on these measurements were not possible because of the wide overlap in the T1 and T2 value (37). However, the tissue-contrast resolution of MR imaging is generally superior to that of CT, and MR has been expected to serve as a complementary modality in differentiating SPNs by predicting the internal composition of nodules. The quality of MR imaging has recently been improved in the chest because of technical developments including suppression of thoracic, cardiac and respiratory motion artifacts, spatial presaturation, and capability of a higher scan speed (38).

Presently, MR imaging can demonstrate tissue characteristics in SPNs, such as mucinous, fibrotic, necrotic, vascular, and cellular components (39) and there may be characteristic signal intensity patterns in a few pulmonary lesions. T2-weighted images were reported to be useful to distinguish tuberculomas from malignant lung tumors, because most tuberculomas are relatively hypointense, whereas malignant tumors are hyperintense on T2-weighted imaging (40). A signal intensity comparable with that of static fluid on heavily T2-weighted MR imaging (MR white lung sign) is characteristic of mucinous bronchioloalveolar carcinoma (41) (Fig. 26.16). Most progressive massive fibrosis lesions show a characteristic signal intensity pattern of isointensity on T1-weighted images and hypointensity on T2-weighted images when compared

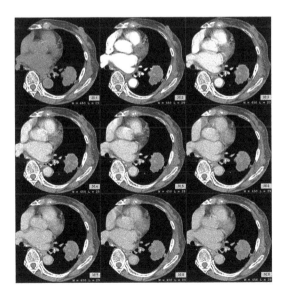

Figure 26.17 Metastatic pulmonary tumor from a carcinoma of the appendix in a 79-year-old woman. Contrast enhanced serial scans (scan interval: 30 s) show that maximum enhancement of the nodule is >40 HU, suggestive of malignancy.

with skeletal muscle (42). Further studies will be necessary to determine the utility and ability of MR imaging to differentiate various lesions.

V. Flow and Perfusion of SPNs

A. CT and MR Nodular Enhancement

The blood supply and metabolism of malignant neoplasms are known to be qualitatively and quantitatively different from those of benign nodules. Many investigators have confirmed a hypothesis that the degree of contrast material enhancement of an SPN, measured with CT, may indicate the vascularity of the SPN, and thus the likelihood of malignancy (43,44). The technique involves thin-section CT scans through an SPN before and after administration of 100 mL of nonionic contrast material with a power injector (Fig. 26.17). Scans obtained at a 1 min interval for 5 min after contrast injection are compared with a baseline unenhanced scan. Attenuation of the SPN is measured in a centrally located region of interest. A nodular enhancement value of <15 HU is strongly indicative of a benign nodule (43). The rare exception is a tumor with central necrosis or a mucin-producing malignancy such as a bronchioloalveolar cell carcinoma. A maximum enhancement of >20 HU appears to be a good predictor of malignancy (44), and a larger enhancement is actually nonspecific, because inflammatory lesions such as focal organizing pneumonia and malignancy may enhance. Dynamic MR imaging using gradient echo sequences also demonstrate similar findings (45,46).

References

1. Holin SN, Dwork RE, Glaser S, Rickli AE, Sticklen JB. Solitary pulmonary nodules found in a community-wide chest roentgenographic survey. Am Tuberc Pulm Dis 1959; 79:427–439.
2. Swensen SJ, Silverstein MD, Edell ES, Trastek VF, Aughenbaugh GL, Ilstrup DM, Schleck CD. Solitary pulmonary nodules: clinical prediction model versus physicians. Mayo Clinic Proc 1999; 74(4):319–329.
3. Webb WR. Radiologic evaluation of the solitary pulmonary nodule. AJR 1990; 154:701–708.
4. Costello P, Anderson W, Blume D. Pulmonary nodule: evaluation with spiral volumetric CT. Radiology 1991; 179:875–876.
5. Leef JL, Klein JS. The solitary pulmonary nodule. Radiol Clin North Am 2002; 40:123–143.
6. Erasmus JJ, Connolly JE, McAdams HP, Roggli VL. Solitary pulmonary nodules: Part I. Morphologic evaluation for differentiation of benign and malignant lesions. RadioGraphics 2000; 20:43–58.
7. Gurney JW. Determining the likelihood of malignancy in solitary pulmonary nodules with Bayesian analysis. Radiology 1993; 186:405–413.
8. Matsuki Y, Nakamura K, Watanabe H, Aoki T, Nakata H, Katsuragawa S, Doi K. Usefulness of an artificial neural network for differentiating benign from malignant

pulmonary nodules on high-resolution CT: evaluation with receiver operating characteristic analysis. AJR 2002; 178:657–663.

9. Gurney JW, Schroeder BA. Upper lobe lung disease: physiologic correlates. Radiology 1988; 167:359–366.

10. Moyer JH et al. Pulmonary arteriovenous fistulas: physiologic and clinical considerations. Am J Med 1962; 32:417.

11. Yokomise H, Mizuno H, Ike O, Wada H, Hitomi S, Itoh H. Importance of intrapulmonary lymph nodes in the differential diagnosis of small pulmonary nodular shadow. Chest 1998; 113:703–706.

12. Agrons GA, Rosado-de-Christenson ML, Kirejczyk WM, Conran RM, Stocker JT. Pulmonary inflammatory pseudotumor: radiologic features. Radiology 1998; 206:511–518.

13. Pickford HA, Swensen SJ, Uts JP. Thoracic cross-sectional imaging of amyloidosis. AJR 1997; 168:351–355.

14. Bankoff MS, McEniff NJ, Bhadelia RA, Garcia-Moliner M, Daly BD. Prevalence of pathologically proven intrapulmonary lymph nodes and their appearance on CT. AJR 1996; 167:629–630.

15. Zerhouni EA, Stitik FP, Siegelman SS, Naidich DP, Sagel SS, Proto AV, Muhm JR, Walsh JW, Martinez CR, Heelan RT. CT of the pulmonary nodule: a cooperative study. Radiology 1986; 160:319–327.

16. Siegelman SS, Khouri NF, Leo FP, Fishman EK, Braverman RM, Zerhouni EA. Solitary pulmonary nodules: CT assessment. Radiology 1986; 160:307–312.

17. Good CA, Wilson TW. The solitary circumscribed pulmonary nodule; study of seven hundred five cases encountered roentgenologically in a period of three and one-half years. J Am Med Assoc 1958; 166:210–215.

18. Lillington GA, Caskey CI. Evaluation and management of solitary pulmonary nodules. Clin Chest Med 1993; 14:111–119.

19. Yankelevitz DF, Reeves AP, Kostis WJ, Zhao B, Henschke CI. Small pulmonary nodules: volumetrically determined growth rates based on CT evaluation. Radiology 2000; 217:251–256.

20. Yankelevitz DF, Gupta R, Zhao B, Henschke CI. Small pulmonary nodules: Evaluation with repeat CT-preliminary experience. Radiology 1999; 212:561–566.

21. Li F, Sone S, Takashima S, Maruyama Y, Hasegawa M, Yang ZG, Kawakami S, Wang JC. Roentgenologic analysis of 108 Non-cancerous focal lung lesions detected in screening CT for lung cancer. Jpn J Lung Cancer 1999; 39:369–380.

22. Takashima S, Sone S, Li F, Maruyama Y, Hasegawa M, Kadoya M. Indeterminate solitary pulmomonary nodules revealed at population based CT screening of the lung: using first follow-up diagnostic CT to differentiate benign and malignant lesions. AJR 2003; 180:1255–1263.

23. Zwirewich CV, Vedal S, Miller RR, Muller NL. Solitary pulmonary nodule: high-resolution CT and radiologic–pathologic correlation. Radiology 1991; 179:469–476.

24. Takashima S, Sone S, Li F, Maruyama Y, Hasegawa M, Matsushita T, Takayama F, Kadoya M. Small solitary pulmonary nodules (<1 cm) detected at population based CT screening for lung cancer: reliable high resolution CT features of benign lesions. AJR 2003; 180:955–964.

25. Mori K, Saitou Y, Tominaga K, Yoki K, Miyazawa N, Okuyama A, Sasagawa M. Small nodular lesions in the lung periphery: new approach to diagnosis with CT. Radiology 1990; 177:843–849.

26. Shiotani S, Yamada K, Oshima F, Nomura I, Noda K, Tajiri M, Ishibashi M, Kameda Y, Kaneko M, Sugimura K. Evaluation of benign pulmonary lesions less than 20 mm in diameter by thin-section computed tomography. Jpn J Lung Cancer 1997; 37:47–54.
27. Carucci LR, Maki DD, Miller WT. Clustered pulmonary nodules: highly suggestive of benign disease. J Thorac Imaging 2001; 16:103–105.
28. Woodring JH, Fried AM, Chuang VP. Solitary cavities of the lung: diagnostic implications of cavity wall thickness. AJR 1980; 135:1269–1271.
29. Woodring JH, Fried AM. Significance of wall thickness in solitary cavities of the lung: a follow-up study. AJR 1983; 140:473–474.
30. Weisbrod GL, Towers MJ, Chamberlain DW, Herman SJ, Matzinger FR. Thin-wall cystic lesions in bronchioalveolar carcinoma. Radiology 1992; 185:401–405.
31. Bateson EM. Relationship between intrapulmonary and endobronchial cartilage containing tumor (so-called hamartoma). Thorax 1965; 20:447–461.
32. Mahoney MC, Shipley HL, Corcoran HL, Dickson BA. CT demonstration of calcification in carcinoma of the lung. AJR 1990; 154:255–258.
33. Kurihara Y, Nakajima Y, Ishikawa T, Kurisu S, Taira Y, Yokote K, Osada H, Koike M, Nakamura T. The prevalence and pattern of calcification in primary lung carcinoma as demonstrated by computed tomography. Jpn J Lung Cancer 1993; 33:1037–1044.
34. Berger WG, Erly WK, Krupinski EA, Standen JR, Stern RG. The solitary pulmonary nodule on chest radiography: can we really tell if the nodule is calcified? AJR 2001; 176:201–204.
35. Siegelman SS, Zerhouni EA, Leo FP et al. CT of the solitary pulmonary nodule. AJR 1980; 135:1–13.
36. Zerhouni EA, Boukadoum M, Siddiky MA, Newbold JM, Stone DC, Shirey MP, Spivey JF, Hesselman CW, Leo FP, Siegelman SS. A standard phantom for quantitative CT analysis of pulmonary nodule. Radiology 1983; 149:767–773.
37. Webb WR, Gamsu G, Stark DD, Moon KL, Moore EH. Evaluation of magnetic resonance sequences in imaging mediastinal tumors. AJR 1984; 143:723–727.
38. Low RN, Sigeti JS, Song SY, Shimakawa A, Pelc NJ. Dynamic contrast-enhanced breath-hold MR imaging of thoracic malignancy using cardiac compensation. J Magn Reson Imaging 1996; 6:625–631.
39. Awaya H, Matsumoto T, Honjo K, Miura G, Emoto T, Matsunaga N. A preliminary study of discrimination among the components of small pulmonary nodules by MR imaging: correlation between MR image and histologic appearance. Radiat Med 2000; 18:29–38.
40. Chung MH, Lee HG, Kwon SS, Park SH. MR imaging of solitary pulmonary lesion: emphasis on tuberculomas and comparison with tumors. J Magn Reson Imaging 2000; 11:629–637.
41. Gaeta M, Minutoli F, Ascenti G, Vinci S, Mazziotti S, Pandolfo I, Blandino A. MR white lung sign: incidence and significance in pulmonary consolidations. J Comput Assist Tomogr 2001; 25:890–896.
42. Matsumoto S, Mori H, Miyake H, Yamada Y, Ueda S, Oga M, Takeoka H, Anan K. MRI signal characteristics of progressive massive fibrosis in silicosis. Clin Radiol 1998; 53:510–514.
43. Swensen SJ, Brown LR, Colby TV, Weaver AL, Midthun DE. Lung nodule enhancement at CT: prospective findings. Radiology 1996; 201:447–455.

44. Yamashita K, Matsunobe S, Tsuda T, Nemoto T, Matsumoto K, Miki H, Konishi J. Solitary pulmonary nodule: preliminary study of evaluation with incremental dynamic CT. Radiology 1995; 194:399–405.
45. Guckel C, Schnabel K, Deimling M, Steinbrich W. Solitary pulmonary nodules: MR evaluation of enhancement patterns with contrast-enhanced dynamic snapshot gradient-echo imaging. Radiology 1996; 200:681–686.
46. Ohno Y, Hatabu H, Adachi S, Kono M, Sugimura K. Solitary pulmonary nodules: potential role of dynamic MR imaging in management—initial experience. Radiology 2002; 224:503–511.
47. Yankelevitz DF, Henschke CI. Does 2-year stability imply that pulmonary nodules are benign? AJR AM J Roentgenol 1997; 168:325–328.

27

Cystic Fibrosis: Radiologic Considerations

DAVID A. LIPSON

University of Pennsylvania Medical Center,
Philadelphia, Pennsylvania, USA

EDWIN J. R. VAN BEEK

University of Iowa,
Iowa City, Iowa, USA

University of Sheffield,
Sheffield, UK

I. Introduction

Cystic fibrosis (CF) is the most common lethal genetic disease among Caucasians, with an estimated incidence of 1:2500 live births in the United States. Formally described in the 1930s, CF causes a spectrum of disease characterized by rhinosinusitis, pancreatic insufficiency, malabsorption, and bronchiectasis (1). Presently, there are over 33,000 patients with CF in the United States, and it is estimated that approximately 1:25 Caucasians are heterozygous carriers of the autosomal recessive disease.

II. CF Genetics

CF is caused by a mutation in a gene on chromosome 7 that encodes for a trans-membrane protein termed the "cystic fibrosis transmembrane conductance regulator" (CFTR) (2). Over 1000 different mutations of the gene have been described which determine disease severity. The gene encoding for CFTR contains >250 kb of DNA with 27 exons. The protein that it encodes contains over 1480 amino acids that contain two hydrophobic membrane spanning domains and two cytoplasmic nucleotide-binding folds (NBF) that are joined by a regulatory (R) domain with multiple potential phosphorylation sites. Six classes of protein mutations have been identified (Table 27.1). The most common CFTR genetic mutation is a deletion (Δ) of phenylalanine (F) at position 508 (ΔF508 homozygosity), which causes a DNA frame shift and subsequent defective maturation of the CFTR protein.

III. CF Pathophysiology

CFTR, ubiquitously distributed in the human body, functions as a kinase regulated chloride channel and likely regulates other ion channels, as well. While the exact pathogenesis of the disease is debated, abnormal ion transport in the airways of persons with CF lead to altered pulmonary secretions early in life. Pulmonary secretions are typically thickened and difficult to expectorate. Over time, failure to clear this mucus allows for bacterial colonization of the airways, typically with *Staphylococcus aureus*, and later *Pseudomonas aeruginosa*. Over time, an enormous neutrophil response in the airways of patients with CF produces a large amount of intraluminal DNA, which promotes inflammation. Leukocytes and bacteria produce large amounts of elastase that exceed airway antiprotease activity causing airway damage. Eventually, a "vicious cycle" of altered secretions, infection, and inflammation begins. This cycle leads to progressive pulmonary tissue destruction, bronchiectasis, respiratory insufficiency, and death.

Table 27.1   Six Genetic Class Mutations have been Described in CF

CF class mutations	
I	Defective synthesis
II	Defective maturation
III	Blocked activation
IV	Decreased conductance
V	Decreased abundance and/or incorrect splicing
VI	Defective regulation

In the gastrointestinal tract, steatorrhea is a common clinical finding as >90% of patients are pancreatic insufficient. In fact, a clue to the disease in infants is often failure to thrive because of fat malabsorption. Subsequently, patients may develop CF-related diabetes mellitus, fat-soluble vitamin deficiency (typically vitamins A, D, E, and K), biliary cirrhosis, and rarely recurrent pancreatitis. Thickened bowel secretions, similar to what is observed in the lung, may predispose patients with CF to small bowel obstruction. This complication is typically found in the terminal ileum and is termed the distal intestinal obstruction syndrome (DIOS). It is commonly the presenting feature in neonates with CF, who develop meconeum ileus due to impacted faecoliths, which may require surgical intervention.

In the lung, the earliest sign of disease may be chronic cough, first intermittent, and then becoming continuous. Patients may suffer from recurrent respiratory infections, recurrent bouts of bronchitis and bronchiolitis, airflow obstruction, and reactive airways disease. Radiographically, patients may exhibit signs of hyperinflation with diaphragmatic flattening or an increased retrosternal airspace. As the disease progresses, patients develop severe bronchiectatic changes (Fig. 27.1) and may develop recurrent pneumothoraces, massive or submassive hemoptysis, or allergic bronchopulmonary aspergillosis.

Over 98% of males with CF are infertile due to bilateral absence of the vas deferens and obstructive azospermia. Women with the disorder may have some decreased fertility due to thickened cervical secretions, but this is debated. Sweat gland dysfunction is common with evidence of elevated sweat chloride concentrations (>60 mEq/L) on the skin of patients with CF.

IV. Predicting Natural History in CF

If a baby is born with CF, today it has an estimated expected survival of >33 years. In fact, CF is no longer considered a disease only of children, as 40.2% of patients with CF are >18 years of age. This is due, in part, to the development of broad spectrum antipseudomonal antibiotics, and CF care centers in the 1960s and 1970s. Additionally, there has been an increase in the number of adult diagnoses with recognition of more mild CF phenotypes. The median age of death has increased from 18.7 years in 1987 to 25.1 years in 2002 (3).

However, predicting the natural history of a patient with the disease has been difficult. Kerem et al. (4) found that a FEV_1 of <30% was associated with predicted median survival of 2 years; survival was decreased in younger and female patients. Because of this study, a value of 30% is now commonly quoted as the level of lung function when one must consider lung transplantation (5–7). However, Milla and Warwick (8) found that patients with a predicted FEV_1 of <30% had a median survival of 3.9 years and that the annual rate of decline of lung function is an important predictor in determining outcome.

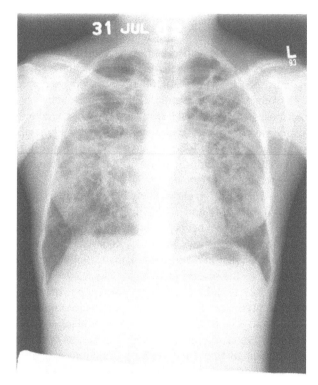

Figure 27.1 PA chest radiograph revealing diffuse bronchiectasis in a patient with advanced CF.

Subsequently, in 1999 Doershuk and Stern (9) reported that a predicted FEV$_1$ of <30% was associated with median survival of 4.6 years. In fact, one quarter of the patients lived for >9 years with severely impaired lung function. It is clear from this data that the FEV$_1$ alone is not sufficient to predict the natural history of patients with CF. In 2001, Liou et al. (10) developed a 5-year survivorship model that included age, percent predicted FEV$_1$, gender, weight, presence of pancreatic sufficiency, CF-related diabetes mellitus, presence of either *Staphylococcus* or *Burkholderia cepacia* infection, and annual number of acute exacerbations. It is unclear whether this model will become a standard tool to help predict survival in the disease.

V. Radiography

A. Conventional Chest Radiography

The absolute role for routine chest imaging in monitoring adults with CF is controversial (11–13). Several standardized scoring systems have been developed, and these have been shown to be helpful in evaluating disease progression and responses to medical therapies (14–16). However, annual routine chest radiographs do not seem to significantly alter medical management in adult patients with CF. It is generally recommended that routine posterior/anterior and lateral chest radiographs be obtained every 2–4 years in otherwise clinically stable patients. New or changing symptoms, consistent with an exacerbation or complication of CF (i.e., hemoptysis, pneumothorax) should prompt radiographic evaluation (11).

B. Computed Tomography

Thin-section computed tomography (CT) scanning is superior to conventional chest radiographs for monitoring anatomic aspects of lung disease in CF (17). It is also clear that CT has increased the sensitivity for detection of mucus plugging, bronchiectasis, and hilar lymphadenopathy in CF compared with routine conventional chest radiography. In a comparison of CT with plain radiographs, Jacobsen et al. (18) showed that CT increased detection of mucus plugging from 33% to 58%, increased detection of bronchiectasis from 50% to 90%, and increased detection of hilar lymphadenopathy from 8% to 75%. CT is also useful in detecting complications in advanced CF, such as the development of an aspergilloma (Fig. 27.2), for evaluating the efficacy of airway

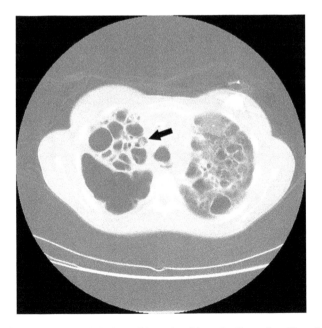

Figure 27.2 Severe upper lobe bronchiectasis with cavity formation. Note the aspergilloma in the right upper lobe (arrow).

clearance, and for assessing the severity of bronchiectasis (Figs. 27.3 and 27.4). For HRCT the Bhalla score is most commonly employed (Table 27.2), but other scoring systems also exist and are based on similar features (19).

Helbich et al. (20) compared a global CT-based scoring system in 117 children and young adults with CF and correlated their CT findings with pulmonary function testing results, clinical status measurements, and serum immunoglobulin levels within 2 weeks of the CT. They found that the most common CT abnormalities in patients with CF were bronchiectasis (80.3%), peribronchial wall thickening (76.1%), mosaic perfusion (63.9%), and mucus plugging (51.3%). Not surprisingly, they found that as the patients aged, there was an increase in the overall number of CT findings. Interestingly, CT scores correlated with pulmonary function testing results, serum immunoglobulin levels, as well as clinical disease severity scores.

In children, CT imaging can be problematic because of respiratory motion. Long et al. (21) developed an imaging protocol with the use of a step-wise increase in positive pressure ventilation using a noninvasive facemask. They described the acquisition of motion-free, thin slice, inspiratory and expiratory images during 8–12 s respiratory pauses.

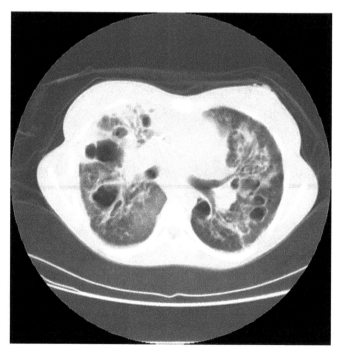

Figure 27.3 Bronchiectasis and cavity formation in advanced CF.

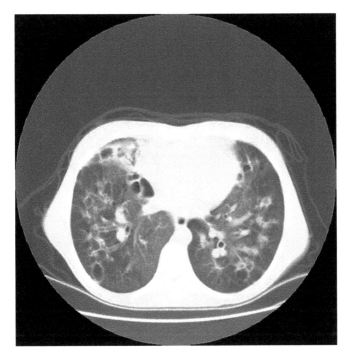

Figure 27.4 Bronchiectasis and inspissated secretions in a patient with CF.

Thin-section CT has also been used to determine bronchial and arterial dimension measurements and studies have been performed to assess the additional benefit of obtaining these values. De Jong et al. (22) evaluated five CT scoring systems and correlated the CT scores with bronchial and arterial dimensions and with the results of pulmonary function testing. They found that CT scoring was reproducible and correlated with disease severity as measured by pulmonary function testing. The ratio of bronchial diameter to its accompanying pulmonary artery diameter was also correlated with thin-section CT scores, but not correlated with pulmonary function tests. The ratio of bronchial wall thickness to the accompanying pulmonary arterial diameter was correlated neither to the thin-section CT scores nor to the pulmonary function test results.

While CT is clearly more beneficial than chest radiography in the anatomic localization and detection of lung disease in CF, concern has grown over the years about radiation exposure, especially in young children or women of child bearing potential. Some CF centers perform these examinations sparingly because of radiation concerns (23,24).

Table 27.2 Bhalla Scoring System for HRCT in Patients with CF (Maximum Score = 27)

Category	0	1	2	3
Severity of bronchiectasis	Absent	Mild: luminal diameter slightly greater than adjacent blood vessel	Moderate: lumen 2 or 3× diameter of adjacent vessel	Severe: lumen >3 × diameter adjacent vessel
Severity of peribronchial thickening	Absent	Mild: wall thickness equal to diameter of adjacent blood vessel	Moderate: wall thickness greater than up to twice diameter of adjacent vessel	Severe: wall thickness >2× diameter adjacent vessel
Extent bronchiectasis	Absent	1–5	6–9	>9
Extent mucus plugging	Absent	1–5	6–9	>9
Extent sacculations or abscesses	Absent	1–5	6–9	>9
Generations bronchial divisions involved	Absent	Up to fourth generation	Up to fifth generation	Up to sixth generation and distal
Severity of bullae	Absent	Unilateral (1–4)	Bilateral (1–4)	>4
Severity of emphysema	Absent	1–5	>5	
Severity of mosaic perfusion	Absent	1–5	>5	
Severity of collapse or consolidation	Absent	Subsegmental	Segmental or lobar	

C. Magnetic Resonance Imaging

Hyperpolarized helium-3 magnetic resonance imaging (MRI) has been shown to be a useful, nonradioactive, tool in detecting gas distribution defects and altered ventilation in patients with a variety of lung diseases (25,26). The technique has been proposed for imaging of pediatric lung diseases, including asthma and CF (27).

Donnelly et al. (28) were the first to demonstrate the use of hyperpolarized helium-3 MRI in four young adult patients with moderate to severe CF. Ventilation defects were consistently demonstrated and they introduced a scoring system for ventilation MR images.

Using this scoring system the Sheffield group was also able to demonstrate ventilation defects in children with CF (29). The defects proved much less pronounced early in life and correlated well with general well-being as assessed clinically (based on body mass index) and with spirometry. Furthermore, the hyperpolarized helium-3 findings showed abnormalities much earlier than corresponding chest X-rays (Figs. 27.5 and 27.6). These findings support the notion that hyperpolarized helium-3 MR imaging is capable of detecting early lung changes.

VI. Conclusions

Although radiography may help detect disease at an earlier time, it is not clear that early detection of disease can prevent or even delay progressive pulmonary

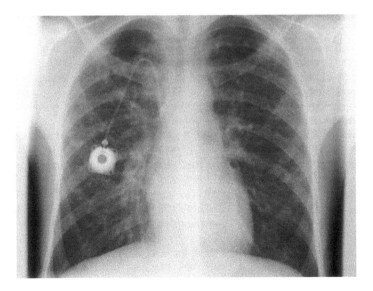

Figure 27.5   Chest X-ray of a 12-year-old child with moderate CF, demonstrating mild bronchiectatic changes in the upper lung zones.

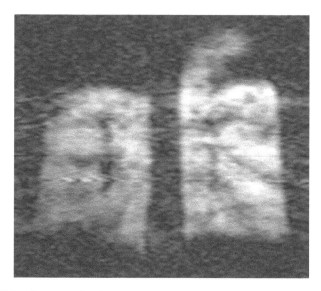

Figure 27.6   Corresponding hyperpolarized helium-3 MRI of subject in Fig. 27.5.

disease in patients with CF (30). Novel imaging methods may be useful in clinical studies or as surrogates to pulmonary function testing in patients with CF in clinical trials.

References

1. Anderson DH. Cystic fibrosis of the pancreas and its relation to celiac disease: a clinical and pathologic study. Am J Dis Child 1938; 56:344–399.
2. Kerem B, Rommens JM, Buchanan JA et al. Identification of the cystic fibrosis gene: genetic analysis. Science 1989; 245:1073–1080.
3. Cystic Fibrosis Foundation Patient Registry 2002 Annual Data Report to the Center Directors. Bethesda, Maryland, September 2003.
4. Kerem E, Reisman J, Corey M et al. Prediction of mortality in patients with cystic fibrosis. N Engl J Med 1992; 326(18):1187–1191.
5. Yankaskas JR, Mallory GB Jr, for the Consensus Committee. Lung transplantation in cystic fibrosis. Chest 1998; 113:217–226.
6. Maurer JR, Frost AE, Glanville AR et al. International guidelines for the selection of lung transplant candidates. Am J Respir Crit Care Med 1998; 158:335–339.
7. Arcasoy SM, Kotloff RM. Lung transplantation. N Engl J Med 1999; 340(14): 1081–1091.
8. Milla CE, Warwick WJ. Risk of death in cystic fibrosis patients with severely compromised lung function. Chest 1998; 113(5):1230–1234.
9. Doershuk CF, Stern RC. Timing of referral for lung transplantation for cystic fibrosis: overemphasis on FEV1 may adversely affect overall survival. Chest 1999; 115(3):782–787.

10. Liou TG, Adler FR, Fitzsimmons SC et al. Predictive 5-year survivorship model of cystic fibrosis. Am J Epidemiol 2001; 153(4):345–352.

11. Yankaskas JR, Marshall BC, Sufian B et al. Cystic fibrosis adult care. Consensus conference report. Chest 2004; 125:1S–39S.

12. Wood BP. Cystic fibrosis. Radiology 1997; 204:1–10.

13. Brody AS. Scoring systems for CT in cystic fibrosis: who cares? Radiology 2004; 231:296–298.

14. Brasfield D, Hicks G, Soong S et al. The chest roentgenogram in cystic fibrosis: a new scoring system. Pediatrics 1979; 63:24–29.

15. Weatherly MR, Palmer CG, Peters ME et al. Wisconsin cystic fibrosis chest radiograph scoring system. Pediatrics 1993; 91488–91495.

16. (a) Shwachman H, Kulczycki LL. Long term study of 105 patients with CF. Am J Dis Child 1958; 96:6–15. (b) Chrispin AR, Norman AP. The systematic evaluation of a chest radiograph in CF. Pediatr Radiol 1974; 2:101–106.

17. Taccone A, Romano L, Marzoli A et al. High-resolution computed tomography in cystic fibrosis. Eur J Radiol 1992; 15:125–129.

18. Jacobsen LE, Houston CS, Habbick BF et al. Cystic fibrosis: a comparison of computed tomography and plain chest radiographs. Can Assoc Radiol J 1986; 37:17–21.

19. Bhalla M, Turcios N, Aponte V et al. Cystic fibrosis: scoring system with thin-section CT. Radiology 1991; 179:783–788.

20. Helbich TH, Heinz-Peer G, Wunderbaldinger P et al. Radiology 1999; 213:537–544.

21. Long FR, Castile RG, Brody AS et al. Lungs in infants and young children: improved thin-section CT with a noninvasive controlled-ventilation technique — initial experience. Radiology 1999; 212:588–593.

22. De Jong PA, Ottink MD, Robben SGF et al. Pulmonary disease assessment in cystic fibrosis: comparison of CT scoring systems and value of bronchial arterial dimension measurements. Radiology 2004; 231:434–439.

23. DiMarco AF, Briones B. Is chest CT performed too often? Chest 1993; 103:985–986.

24. Van der Bruggen-Bogaarts BA, Broerse JJ, Lammers JW et al. Radiation exposure in standard and high-resolution chest CT scans. Chest 1995; 107:113–115.

25. Kauczor HU, Chen XJ, van Beek EJ et al. Pulmonary ventilation imaged by magnetic resonance: at the doorstep of clinical application. Eur Respir J 2001; 17(5):1008–1023.

26. Van Beek EJR, Wild JM, Kauczor HU, Schreiber W, Mugler III JP, de Lange EE. Functional MRI of the lung using hyperpolarized helium-3 gas. J Magn Reson Imaging 2004; 20:540–554.

27. Altes TA, de Lange EE. Applications of hyperpolarized helium-3 gas magnetic resonance imaging in pediatric lung disease. Top Magn Reson Imaging 2003; 14(3):231–236.

28. Donnelly LF, MacFall JR, McAdams HP et al. Cystic fibrosis: combined hyperpolarized ^{3}He-enhanced and conventional proton MR imaging in the lung—preliminary observation. Radiology 1999; 212:885–889.

29. Van Beek EJR, Hill C, Woodhouse N, Fichele S et al. Assessment of cystic fibrosis in children using hyperpolarized helium-3 MRI: comparison with Shwachman score, Chrispin–Norman score and spirometry. Proceedings of the 12th scientific meeting of ISMRM, Kyoto, Japan 2004:165.

30. Accurso FJ. Early pulmonary disease in cystic fibrosis. Curr Opin Pulm Med 1997; 3(6):400–403.

28

Lung Transplantation: Radiographic Considerations

ROBERT M. KOTLOFF and DAVID A. LIPSON

University of Pennsylvania Medical Center,
Philadelphia, Pennsylvania, USA

I. Introduction

Human lung transplantation was first attempted in 1963 but it was not until two decades later that extended survival was achieved. Further refinements in patient selection, surgical technique, immunosuppression, and post-operative care have led to the successful application of lung transplantation to a wide variety of advanced disorders of the airways, lung parenchyma, and pulmonary vasculature (1). There has been a marked proliferation of lung transplant centers worldwide and by the end of 2001, ~14,000 procedures had been performed (2).

Although lung transplantation offers the prospect of vastly improved quality of life, long-term survival remains an elusive goal for the majority of recipients. The surgical procedure itself is rigorous, imperfect, and performed on a debilitated and often marginally nourished patient population. Not surprisingly, the perioperative period is a precarious time and mortality is highest during the initial three post-operative months. Beyond this period, there is a reduced but nonetheless inexorable attrition of patients, culminating in 5 and 10 years actuarial survival rates of 45% and 23%, respectively (2). These late deaths are predominantly due to chronic rejection and infection.

In order to optimize outcomes in the face of significant and ever-present risk, it is essential that both the selection of candidates and the care of recipients be conducted in a meticulous and highly vigilant fashion. Radiographic assessment plays a vital role in both pretransplant screening and post-transplant care and is the focus of this chapter.

II. Screening of Transplant Candidates

Given the considerable risks associated with lung transplantation and the extreme scarcity of donor organs, criteria employed in the selection of suitable candidates are necessarily stringent. Transplantation is offered only to patients who are deemed to be at high risk of dying from their disease and for whom alternative therapies have failed or are unavailable. Patients should be functionally disabled but still ambulatory and free of significant co-morbidities, especially cardiac, renal, and hepatic disease. In recognition of the somewhat inferior outcomes achieved in association with advanced recipient age and the rigors of the more extensive surgical procedures, the following age limits have been recommended: 55 years for heart–lung, 60 years for bilateral lung, and 65 years for single-lung transplantation (3). Standard selection criteria, reflecting the input of an international consensus panel, are listed in Table 28.1.

Radiographic assessment, typically involving chest radiography, computed tomography (CT), and quantitative perfusion scintigraphy, constitutes an integral component of the evaluation of potential lung transplant candidates. This assessment provides information on the severity of the primary disease

Table 28.1   General Guidelines for Recipient Selection

Indications
- Advanced obstructive, fibrotic, or pulmonary vascular disease with a high risk of death within 2–3 years
- Alternative therapies unsuccessful or unavailable
- Ambulatory but with severe functional limitation (NYHA class III or IV)
- Age ≤55 years for heart lung; ≤60 years for bilateral lung; ≤65 years for single-lung

Absolute contraindications
- Severe extrapulmonary organ dysfunction including:
  - Renal insufficiency with creatinine clearance <50 mL/min
  - Hepatic dysfunction with biopsy-proven cirrhosis, coagulopathy, or portal hypertension
  - Left ventricular dysfunction or severe coronary artery disease (consider heart–lung transplantation)
- Acute, critical illness
- Active malignancy or recent history of malignancy with significant likelihood of recurrence (except for basal and squamous cell carcinoma of the skin)
- Chronic hepatitis B or C infection with biopsy-proven cirrhosis
- Infection with the human immunodeficiency virus
- Severe psychiatric illness; drug or alcohol dependence
- Active or recent (past 6 months) cigarette smoking, alcohol, or percent of ideal body weight)
- Nonambulatory with poor rehabilitation potential
- Extremes of weight (<70% or >130% of ideal body weight)

Relative contraindications (considered on an individual basis)
- Chronic medical conditions that are poorly controlled or associated with end-organ damage
- History of noncompliance with medical care
- Daily corticosteroid requirements in excess of 20 mg of prednisone (or equivalent)
- Mechanical ventilation (excluding noninvasive ventilation)
- Prior thoracic surgery
- Aspergilloma, especially when associated with significant pleural reaction
- Active collagen vascular disease, particularly with extrapulmonary manifestations
- Preoperative colonization of the airways with pan-resistant bacteria (presence of *Burkholderia cepacia* considered an absolute contraindication by some centers)[a]

[a]Applies to patients with cystic fibrosis.
Source: Maurer JR, Frost AE, Estenne M, Higenbottam T, Glanville AR. International guidelines for the selection of lung transplant candidates. J heart Lung Transplant 1998; 17:703.

process as well as on its distribution, which is of particular importance in determining the specific lung targeted for replacement by single-lung transplantation. In addition, radiographic evaluation can detect previously unsuspected lung cancers, the presence of which would preclude further consideration of transplantation. This is of obvious concern in the large population of former smokers who present for evaluation, but is also germane to patients with widespread pulmonary fibrosis, a condition that may enhance the risk of lung cancer as well (4). Demonstration by the Early Lung Cancer Action Project of the superiority of CT over chest radiography in detecting malignant lung nodules in a high risk population has provided the impetus for routine application of this screening procedure to transplant candidates (5). However, the potential pitfalls and economic inefficiencies of this approach must be acknowledged. In the Early Lung Cancer Action Project, CT imaging detected solitary or multiple lung nodules in nearly one-quarter of the study population but only 12% of those with nodules (2.7% of the total population) were ultimately shown to have a malignancy. Similarly, in a study exclusively involving lung transplant candidates, only 3 of 66 nodules demonstrated by chest CT proved to be bronchogenic carcinomas (6). Thus, although CT scanning is capable of identifying a substantial number of patients with asymptomatic nodules, only a small fraction of these nodules are malignant. In order to establish the exact nature of the nodule, it has been recommended that patients undergo either serial radiographic surveillance for evidence of growth over a 2 year period or, in the case of nodules exceeding 10 mm, a biopsy procedure (7). This strategy is problematic among lung transplant candidates as the need for radiographic surveillance could unduly delay transplantation for a considerable number of patients with benign disease and these patients are often too tenuous to safely undergo biopsy procedures that might otherwise provide a more expeditious means of excluding malignancy.

Chest radiography and CT are also useful in assessing the magnitude of pleural thickening that can arise as a result of prior invasive chest procedures or in association with the presence of mycetomas (Fig. 28.1). When severe,

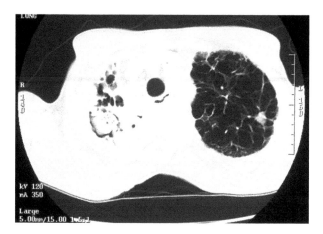

Figure 28.1   CT scan demonstrating a large right upper lobe mycetoma in a patient with underlying chronic obstructive pulmonary disease. The patient was deemed unsuitable for lung transplantation on the basis of the extensive degree of associated pleural thickening.

pleural thickening results in obliteration of normal tissue planes, rendering anatomic dissection and explantation of the native lung technically difficult, time-consuming, and potentially bloody. In those with mycetomas, difficult dissection also runs the risk of violating the fungal cavity and spreading organisms into the pleural space. The presence of a mycetoma has been associated with excessive post-transplantation mortality (8). The degree of pleural disease and mycetoma formation that precludes transplantation is a matter of judgment that is likely to be influenced by the experience and aggressiveness of the particular transplant team.

III. Complications in the Transplant Recipient

A. Reperfusion Pulmonary Edema/Primary Graft Failure

Mild, transient pulmonary edema ("reimplantation response," "reperfusion pulmonary edema") is a nearly universal feature of the freshly transplanted allograft. It is presumed to be a consequence of ischemia–reperfusion injury and the attendant increase in microvascular permeability, but surgical trauma and lymphatic disruption may be contributing factors. In ∼15% of cases, injury is sufficiently severe to cause a form of acute respiratory distress syndrome termed primary graft failure (9). Histologically, a pattern of diffuse alveolar damage is present. The diagnosis of primary graft failure rests on the development of widespread radiographic infiltrates and markedly impaired oxygenation within the initial 72 h following transplantation, and the exclusion of other causes of early graft dysfunction such as volume overload, pneumonia, rejection, atelectasis, and pulmonary venous outflow obstruction. Treatment is supportive, relying on conventional mechanical ventilatory techniques as well as on the use of such adjunct measures as inhaled nitric oxide, independent lung ventilation, and extracorporeal life support for those who cannot be stabilized by other means. With a mortality rate of up to 60%, primary graft failure ranks second only to infection as a leading cause of early deaths among transplant recipients. Recovery in survivors is often protracted and incomplete, though attainment of normal lung function and exercise tolerance is possible (9). Results of emergent retransplantation in this setting have been poor (10).

Radiographic Considerations

In cases of mild reperfusion edema, the chest radiograph typically demonstrates perihilar or basilar interstitial or airspace opacities [Fig. 28.2(a)] that appear within the first day or two post-operatively and peak in severity by day 4. Findings on CT scan include septal thickening, ground glass opacities, and focal consolidation. In the setting of single-lung transplantation, the native lung is radiographically uninvolved while involvement may be asymmetric following bilateral lung transplantation. Patients with primary graft failure initially demonstrate similar radiographic features, but progress within hours to

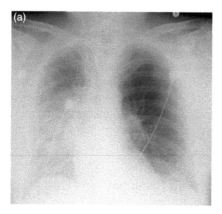 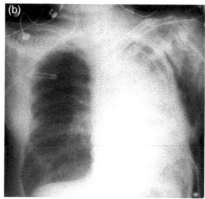

Figure 28.2 Chest radiographs from two patients who underwent single-lung transplantation for emphysema, demonstrating (a) mild reperfusion pulmonary edema in a right lung allograft and (b) primary graft failure in a left lung allograft.

several days to a state of complete or near-complete opacification of the allograft(s) [Fig. 28.2(b)].

B. Airway Complications

At the time of allograft implantation, no attempt is made to re-establish the bronchial arterial supply. Consequently, the anastomosis and the donor bronchus are precariously dependent upon retrograde blood flow through low pressure pulmonary venous to bronchial vascular collaterals, placing them at considerable risk for ischemic injury. Because lethal dehiscense of the bronchial anastomosis was initially a common complication, surgical techniques have evolved to buttress the bronchial anastomosis and provide a nurturing blood supply. A telescoping technique is currently employed that intussuscepts the donor bronchus within that of the recipient (or vise versa), overlapping by one to two cartilaginous rings. As a result, life-threatening dehiscence is now a rare occurrence. Partial dehiscence is still occasionally encountered in the early post-transplant period but typically heals with expectant management only. The most common form of airway complication that remains is anastomotic narrowing, which may result from ischemia-induced stricture or bronchomalacia, or from the formation of excessive granulation tissue. Independent of the mechanism, anastomotic narrowing typically develops within several weeks following transplantation. Clues to its presence include focal wheezing on the involved side, recurrent bouts of pneumonia or purulent bronchitis, and suboptimal pulmonary function studies demonstrating significant airflow obstruction. Diagnosis is based on direct bronchoscopic visualization. Techniques employed to address anastomotic narrowing include balloon dilatation, laser debridement, and stent placement, all readily performed through a flexible bronchoscope (11).

Radiographic Considerations

Detection on chest radiography of a new spontaneous pneumothorax or abrupt worsening of a preexistent small post-operative pneumothorax should prompt the performance of bronchoscopy to evaluate for bronchial dehiscence (Fig. 28.3). In single-lung transplant recipients, pneumothorax due to bronchial dehiscence develops ipsolateral to the allograft; a contralateral pneumothorax is likely related to problems involving the native lung. Following bilateral lung transplantation, a single continuous pleural space often results. This can create confusion as unilateral dehiscence of the bronchial anastomosis may lead to bilateral pneumothoraces.

CT imaging is touted to be far more sensitive than chest radiography in detecting airway dehiscence. In one study, CT visualization of a bronchial defect was found to be 100% sensitive and 94% specific for airway dehiscence, whereas detection of extraluminal air (Fig. 28.4) was 100% sensitive and 72% specific (12). Although these performance statistics are impressive, further corroboration by other groups is required before CT can be viewed as a pivotal tool in diagnosing dehiscence. It is important to note that the widely employed telescoping bronchial anastomotic technique can appear on CT images as an endobronchial flap under which a linear air collection can develop; these normal findings may be confused with the findings associated with bronchial dehiscence (13). Furthermore, small extraluminal air collections can be seen with bronchoscopically intact anastomoses in the early post-operative period (12).

McAdams et al. investigated the utility of helical CT as a noninvasive means of detecting and assessing bronchial anastomotic stenosis (14). These

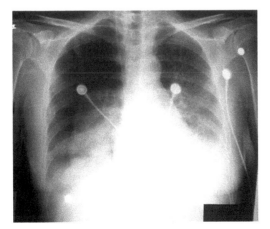

Figure 28.3 Chest radiograph demonstrating a spontaneous right pneumothorax in a bilateral lung transplant recipient. On bronchoscopy, partial dehiscence of the right bronchial anastomosis was documented.

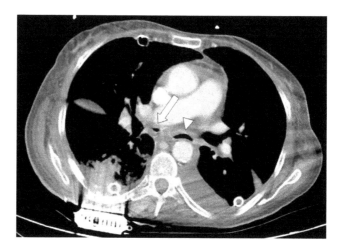

Figure 28.4 CT scan demonstrating a small collection of air in the mediastinum (arrow) lateral to the esophagus (arrowhead) in a patient with documented right bronchial anastomotic dehiscence.

investigators compared the accuracy of conventional axial CT images with that of "virtual bronchoscopy" (i.e. 3-dimensional endobronchial reconstruction images), using direct bronchoscopic inspection as the gold standard. The accuracy of virtual bronchoscopy and axial CT images in detecting bronchial stenosis was 97% and 80%, respectively, for the right bronchial anastomosis and 92% and 75%, respectively, for the left. Accuracy of virtual bronchoscopy and axial images in determining stenosis length was 72% and 68%, respectively, for the right anastomosis and 81% and 69%, respectively, for the left. Although promising, the information provided by virtual bronchoscopy falls short of that gleaned from conventional bronchoscopic inspection. It is anticipated that its major role in the future will be in excluding significant airway stenosis and thus sparing the patient the need for a more invasive procedure (for detailed discussion of virtual bronchoscopy in Chapter 2).

C. Native Lung Hyperinflation

Patients with emphysema were initially deemed to be physiologically unsuitable for single-lung transplantation based on concerns that the highly compliant native lung would be preferentially ventilated, leading to progressive hyperinflation and detrimental encroachment on the allograft. Subsequent experience has demonstrated that most recipients do well, with the predominance of both ventilation and perfusion directed towards the allograft (15), but clinically significant native lung hyperinflation does develop in a minority of patients. Acute hyperinflation leading to respiratory and hemodynamic compromise in the immediate post-operative period has been reported in 15–30% of emphysema patients undergoing single-lung transplantation (16,17). Although risk factors remain poorly defined, the combination of positive pressure ventilation and significant allograft edema serves to magnify the compliance differential between the two lungs and may predispose to this complication. Acute hyperinflation can be rapidly addressed by the initiation of independent lung ventilation, ventilating the native lung with a low respiratory rate, and prolonged expiratory time to facilitate complete emptying (Fig. 28.5).

Beyond the perioperative period, some patients with emphysema demonstrate exaggerated or progressive native lung hyperinflation associated with suboptimal or deteriorating pulmonary function due to extrinsic compression of the allograft (Fig. 28.6). It is important to recognize that native lung hyperinflation may at times be the consequence, rather than the cause, of allograft dysfunction. In this regard, development of bronchiolitis obliterans within the allograft can result in secondary hyperinflation of the native lung, presumably due to a combination of volume loss and diminished ventilation of the diseased allograft. The distinction between these two clinical situations is critical (but often difficult) as surgical volume reduction of the native lung is likely to result in meaningful and sustained improvement in pulmonary function only in the setting of an intrinsically normal but compressed allograft (18,19).

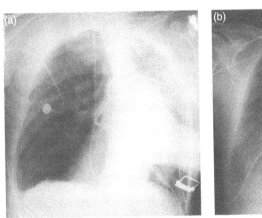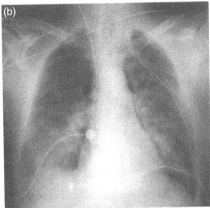

Figure 28.5 (a) Chest radiograph, taken shortly after completion of a left single-lung transplant in a patient with underlying emphysema, demonstrating acute native lung hyperinflation with contralateral shift of the mediastinum and crowding of the allograft (partially obscured by the patient's hand). The radiograph was obtained after the patient, who was being mechanically ventilated, developed high peak airway pressures, hypotension, hypoxemia, and hypercapnia. (b) A second radiograph obtained within 1 h of the first, demonstrating the resolution of native lung hyperinflation after insertion of a double lumen endotracheal tube and the initiation of independent lung ventilation.

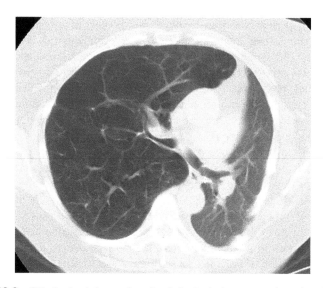

Figure 28.6 CT obtained 6 months after left single-lung transplantation for emphysema, demonstrating chronic, persistent native lung hyperinflation with marked mediastinal shift and crowding of the left lung allograft. The radiographic findings were associated with suboptimal pulmonary function parameters attributed to the compression of the allograft. The patient was being considered for right lung volume reduction surgery to correct the problem.

Radiographic Considerations

Among single-lung transplant recipients with underlying emphysema, native lung hyperinflation is a common chest radiographic finding in the immediate post-operative period. Unless associated with respiratory or hemodynamic compromise, however, this radiographic finding does not warrant specific intervention and often will improve when the patient is removed from mechanical ventilation. In one series of 51 patients with emphysema, 31% developed radiographic evidence of acute native lung hyperinflation but in only half of these patients was this clinically significant (16).

For patients who develop late, progressive native lung hyperinflation associated with declining lung function, imaging may sometimes assist in distinguishing between an intrinsically normal and abnormal allograft. In this regard, demonstration by high resolution CT (HRCT) of air trapping or bronchiectasis within the allograft suggests the presence of bronchiolitis obliterans and argues against the consideration of surgical volume reduction.

D. Infectious Complications

Infection is an ever-present threat to the well-being of the lung transplant recipient and is a leading cause of both early and late mortality. Infection rates among lung transplant recipients appear to be higher than those encountered in other solid organ transplant populations, likely related to the unique exposure of the lung allograft to the external environment and to the greater magnitude of immunosuppression employed (20,21).

Bacterial infections of the lower respiratory tract constitute the majority of infectious complications. Bacterial pneumonia is most frequently encountered in the first post-transplant month, with an incidence of 16% reported in a recent series (22). In addition to the immunosuppressed status of the recipient, other factors that predispose to early bacterial pneumonias include the need for prolonged mechanical ventilatory support, blunted cough due to post-operative pain and weakness, disruption of lymphatics, impaired mucociliary clearance due to ischemic injury to the bronchial mucosa, and passive transfer of occult infection in the transplanted organ. Bacterial infections, in the form of purulent bronchitis, bronchiectasis, and pneumonia, reemerge as a late complication among patients who develop bronchiolitis obliterans syndrome (BOS). Gram-negative pathogens, in particular *Pseudomonas aeruginosa*, are most frequently isolated in association with both early and late infectious events (20,21).

Cytomegalovirus (CMV) is the most common viral pathogen encountered in the post-transplant period. Although the availability of effective antiviral therapy has significantly reduced the risk of death as a direct consequence of CMV infection, this virus continues to cause frequent, troubling infections, is associated with an increased risk of bacterial and fungal superinfections, and has been implicated as a risk factor in the development of BOS (23,24). Infection in the recipient can occur following passive transmission of latent virus from the lung allograft or transfused blood products or from the reactivation of endogenous virus remotely acquired by the recipient. Those with primary infection (i.e. seronegative recipients who acquire infection from seropositive donors) are at the greatest risk for developing severe, organ-invasive disease, particularly pneumonia (25).

CMV infection typically emerges 1–3 months following transplantation, though onset may be delayed in patients receiving antiviral prophylaxis. Infection is often subclinical, evidenced only by silent viremia or shedding of virus in the respiratory tract or urine. Clinical disease may present as a mononucleosis-like syndrome of fever, malaise, and leukopenia or as organ-specific invasion of the lung, gastrointestinal tract, central nervous system, or retina. A diagnosis of CMV pneumonia, the most common manifestation of invasive disease in the lung transplant recipient, is unequivocally established only by the demonstration of characteristic viral cytopathic changes on lung biopsy or on cytologic specimens obtained by bronchoalveolar lavage but, unfortunately, the sensitivity of these findings is relatively low. A positive rapid CMV culture of bronchoalveolar lavage fluid or identification of CMV antigen in the bloodstream provides circumstantial support for the diagnosis of CMV pneumonia in the appropriate clinical context but asymptomatic replication of virus in the absence of tissue invasion confounds interpretation of these tests. Treatment of CMV disease with a course of ganciclovir is usually effective though relapses may occur.

Although a number of opportunistic and endemic fungi have been reported to cause pulmonary infections in lung transplant recipients, *Aspergillus* species are by far the most frequently encountered. Invasive aspergillosis is the most serious and life-threatening form of aspergillus infection to plague the lung transplant recipient. An overall incidence of 5% has been calculated from pooled studies (26,27). The majority of cases occur within the first post-transplant year. Most patients present with pneumonia, occasionally associated with disseminated infection. Symptoms of invasive aspergillosis are nonspecific and include fever, cough, pleuritic chest pain and hemoptysis. Treatment options include amphotericin B and the triazoles itraconazole and voriconazole. Surgical resection of localized infection should be considered in cases refractory to antifungal therapy. Despite a multitude of treatment options, the composite mortality rate associated with invasive disease in published series involving lung transplant recipients approaches 60% (27).

Bronchial infection is a less morbid but equally prevalent form of aspergillosis. The devitalized cartilage and foreign suture material of the fresh bronchial anastomosis create a nurturing environment for localized infection at the anastomotic site. A more diffuse ulcerative bronchitis, with the formation of pseudomembranes, is occasionally seen and likely follows severe ischemic injury to the bronchial mucosa. Clustered within the first 6 months post-transplantation, these bronchial infections are usually asymptomatic and detected on surveillance bronchoscopy. Although usually responsive to antifungal therapy, airway infections due to aspergillus can rarely progress to invasive pneumonia or lead to fatal erosion into the adjacent pulmonary artery (27–29).

Radiographic Considerations

The medical literature is replete with descriptions of the "classic" radiographic features of various types of pneumonia, with the implied message that radiographic patterns can be used to pinpoint the etiologic agent. In reality, information provided by chest radiography and CT is ultimately nonspecific and often fails not only to differentiate among various infectious possibilities but also to distinguish infectious from noninfectious entities like acute rejection and reperfusion injury (Fig. 28.7). In a review of 45 episodes of pneumonia in lung transplant recipients, Collins et al. (30) found that the most common CT findings were consolidation, ground glass opacities, septal thickening, and multiple nodules. Overall, there was no characteristic pattern of findings in this series that permitted distinction among the cases of bacterial, CMV, and aspergillus pneumonia. Others have suggested that the finding of nodular opacities with associated cavitation or with a circumferential rim of ground glass attenuation (halo sign) is highly suggestive of aspergillosis and "may obviate the need for further investigation" (31). In the Collins series, cavitation was

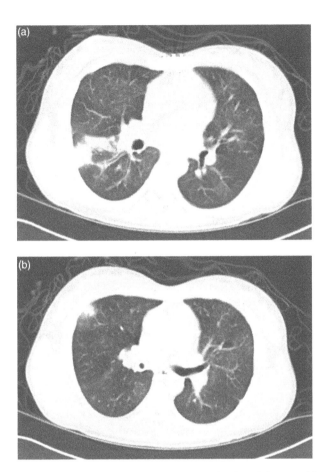

Figure 28.7 Two CT images demonstrating multifocal nodular opacities in a lung transplant recipient with *Staphylococcal aureus* pneumonia. The radiographic differential diagnosis included invasive aspergillosis and post-transplantation lymphoproliferative disease.

seen exclusively in association with aspergillus infection but was present in only 25% of cases. In contrast, the halo sign was encountered in 3 of 16 cases of bacterial pneumonia and has been reported by others in association with post-transplant lymphoproliferative disease (PTLD) (32) and lung cancer (33).

Despite the nonspecific nature of the findings, the utility of radiographic studies should not be underestimated. Assessment for the presence of infection in transplant recipients with fever or respiratory-related signs and symptoms invariably begins with a standard chest radiograph, a universally available low-cost technique. CT has emerged as a valuable companion procedure, offering greater sensitivity, superior resolution of parenchymal abnormalities, and better definition of mediastinal structures and the pleural space. Together, these studies are extremely valuable in documenting the presence of abnormalities and in guiding the clinician in the selection of diagnostic procedures.

E. Post-transplant Lymphoproliferative Disease

PTLD is a term applied to a spectrum of abnormal B cell proliferative responses ranging from benign polyclonal hyperplasia to more commonly encountered malignant lymphomas. The incidence of PTLD in the lung transplant population ranges from 1.8% to 7.9% in single-center case series, with an overall pooled incidence of 4.9% (34–36). Among the myriad neoplasms that arise following transplantation, PTLD is second in frequency only to nonmelanoma skin cancers.

Epstein-Barr virus (EBV) has been identified as the stimulus for B cell proliferation, which proceeds in an unchecked fashion due to the muted cytotoxic T cell response in the immunosuppressed host. EBV-naïve recipients who acquire primary infection at the time of organ transplantation are at greatest risk of developing PTLD. In one series, the incidence of PTLD was 33% among recipients who were seronegative prior to transplant, compared with only 1.7% for those who were previously exposed (34). The use of antilymphocyte antibodies has also been associated with an increased risk of PTLD, likely reflecting the profound impact of these agents on intrinsic T cell activity (37).

The incidence of PTLD is greatest within the first post-transplantation year and the mode of presentation of these early-onset cases is distinct from that of late-onset cases (36,38). In this regard, the majority of early-onset cases involve the pulmonary allograft while intra-abdominal and disseminated forms of disease predominate in cases presenting beyond the first year. The diagnosis of PTLD is most firmly established by tissue biopsy though fine needle aspiration may occasionally yield sufficient material to make a cytologic diagnosis. Demonstration of the presence of EBV-infected cells by immunohistochemical staining or in situ hybridization techniques can help to confirm a diagnosis in difficult cases.

Initial treatment centers on reduction in the magnitude of immunosuppression to permit partial restoration of host cellular immunity directed toward EBV. Patients whose disease is confined to the allograft are most likely to respond to this measure but there is an attendant risk of precipitating acute or chronic rejection with this approach. Use of rituximab, a chimeric human–mouse monoclonal antibody directed against the B-cell marker CD20 has been associated with complete tumor regression and minimal side effects (39–41). It offers an attractive option for patients with more aggressive disease and those who fail or cannot tolerate a reduction in immunosuppression. Standard chemotherapy has been employed for refractory cases, but the associated neutropenia is poorly tolerated by an already profoundly immunosuppressed patient population. There is no proven role for antiviral therapy in the setting of established PTLD, though there is preliminary evidence that the prophylactic use of antiviral agents initiated prior to the rapid replication phase of infection may reduce the subsequent risk of developing PTLD (35,42).

Mortality related to PTLD has been reported in the range of 37–50% (36,38). Early-onset disease and disease restricted to the allograft are associated with a more benign course. In contrast, disseminated disease carries a much graver prognosis (36,43).

Radiographic Considerations

PTLD most commonly presents as single or multiple pulmonary nodules that may have smooth or irregular margins (Fig. 28.8). Nodules may be surrounded by a rim of ground glass density (halo sign), mimicking the features of invasive aspergillosis (32). Other intrathoracic findings seen in a minority of patients include hilar and mediastinal adenopathy, and pleural effusions. Cavitation is distinctly unusual and its presence should prompt consideration of alternative etiologies.

F. Lung Cancer

The development of lung cancer following lung transplantation has been reported exclusively in patients with underlying chronic obstructive pulmonary disease or pulmonary fibrosis, both of which predispose to lung cancer (4,44). Additionally, the majority of these patients have significant smoking histories. The reported incidence of lung cancer following transplantation is 2.0–3.7% in patients with chronic obstructive lung disease and 3.4–4.0% in the pulmonary fibrosis population (33,45). Data are conflicting on whether transplantation confers an increased likelihood of developing this form of cancer or whether the incidence is comparable to that of the general population with similar risk factors (46). Lung cancer may complicate the transplant course in several ways. Most commonly, cancer may arise *de novo* in the remaining native lung

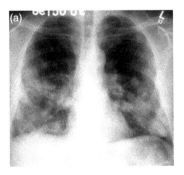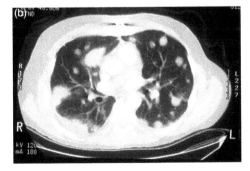

Figure 28.8 Chest radiograph and CT scan demonstrating multiple nodular opacities in a patient with PTLD.

following single-lung transplantation. Additionally, previously unsuspected cancer may be incidentally detected in the explanted lung at the time of transplantation, placing the recipient at risk for subsequent recurrence (45). On occasion, lung transplantation has been performed as definitive treatment for underlying bronchioloalveolar carcinoma; a high rate of recurrence in the allografts has been documented in these circumstances (47). Finally, a case of lung cancer of donor origin transmitted with the allograft has been documented (48).

Lung cancer in the transplant recipient can progress in a rapid fashion over a short period of time (Fig. 28.9), mimicking an infectious process (45). This aggressive behavior may reflect loss of antitumor immune surveillance in the immunosuppressed host or may be due to a more specific effect of cyclosporine in promoting tumor growth (49).

Radiographic Considerations

The radiographic features of bronchogenic carcinoma were best described in a recent multicenter case series of 24 lung transplant recipients (33). All cancers developed in the native lung. The vast majority of patients presented with one or more nodules or masses. Not surprisingly, CT was superior to chest radiography in detecting nodules and in assessing for accompanying intrathoracic adenopathy and pleural effusions. By CT imaging, all nodules and all but one mass were noncalcified and most had irregular borders. Atypical features seen

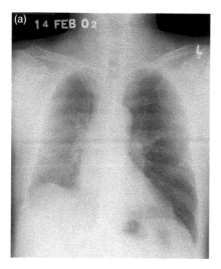 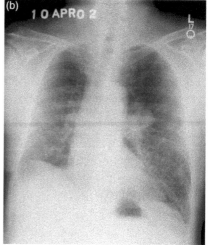

Figure 28.9 Serial chest radiographs taken ~8 weeks apart in a patient who had undergone a right single-lung transplant for emphysema. The latter study demonstrates a new left perihilar mass with associated reticular interstitial opacities involving the native lung. On biopsy, this was proven to represent a primary adenocarcinoma of the lung with lymphangitic spread.

in a minority of nodules included surrounding ground glass attenuation (halo sign) and an associated air bronchogram. Pleural effusions were visualized by CT scan in nearly half of the patients and one-quarter had accompanying hilar or mediastinal adenopathy.

G. Acute Allograft Rejection

Most transplant recipients experience at least one episode of acute rejection within the first several months following transplantation. Beyond this initial period, the risk of acute rejection steadily declines, reaching a low but not negligible rate by the end of the first year. Episodes of acute rejection may be clinically silent; surveillance biopsies from asymptomatic and functionally stable recipients have demonstrated evidence of acute rejection in up to one third of cases (50). When present, clinical manifestations are nonspecific and include malaise, low-grade fever, dyspnea, cough, and leukocytosis. Radiographic infiltrates, a decline in arterial oxygenation at rest or with exercise and an abrupt fall of > 10% in spirometric values are important clues to the possible presence of rejection but similar findings accompany infectious episodes. Transbronchial lung biopsy has emerged as the gold standard for diagnosis of acute rejection. The procedure is safe, can be performed in serial fashion over time, and has a sensitivity and specificity in excess of 90% for the diagnosis of acute rejection. The histologic hallmark of acute rejection is the presence of perivascular lymphocytic infiltrates that, in more severe cases, spill over into the adjacent interstitium and alveolar airspaces. A lymphocytic bronchitis or bronchiolitis may accompany the parenchymal involvement. Treatment of acute rejection consists of a three-day pulse of high dose intravenous methylprednisolone. In most cases, this results in rapid improvement in symptoms, pulmonary function, and radiographic abnormalities but follow-up biopsies show persistent histologic evidence of rejection in 25–50% of episodes (51,52).

Radiographic Considerations

A variety of radiographic findings have been described in association with acute rejection; although raising suspicion of this complication, none are pathognomonic. Radiographic manifestations include interstitial opacities, consolidation, ground glass attenuation (best seen on CT), septal thickening, and pleural effusions (Fig. 28.10). As similar features may be seen in association with pneumonia and reperfusion injury, other clues must be sought to distinguish among these possibilities. This is particularly true within the first month following transplantation, when all three of these complications occur commonly. The temporal course of the process can provide helpful clues; onset of radiographic abnormalities within the first several days following transplantation argues strongly against acute rejection while rapid resolution following a corticosteroid pulse is virtually diagnostic (Fig. 28.10).

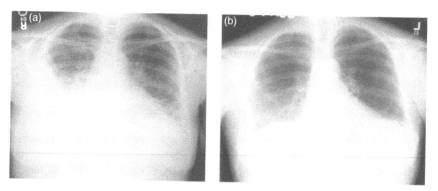

Figure 28.10 (a) Chest radiograph demonstrating a large loculated right pleural effusion and bilateral interstitial opacities occurring 4 weeks following bilateral lung transplantation. Transbronchial lung biopsies demonstrated acute cellular rejection. (b) Follow-up chest radiograph obtained 1 week after the patient received high-dose intravenous methylprednisolone for treatment of rejection demonstrates marked improvement in the right effusion and complete resolution of interstitial opacities.

Kundu et al. (53) examined 100 chest radiographs taken <24 h before performance of transbronchial biopsy in order to investigate the utility of chest radiographic abnormalities in diagnosing acute rejection. Overall, the sensitivity and specificity of chest radiography were only 50% and 69%, respectively. Sensitivity was higher during the first 3 months post-transplantation than beyond this period (65% vs. 32%), whereas specificity trended in the opposite fashion (43% vs. 77%). As the authors point out, the higher sensitivity and lower specificity within the first 3 months may simply reflect the confounding presence of reperfusion pulmonary edema during this initial time period.

The enhanced sensitivity and detail provided by HRCT in detecting lung disease has prompted a number of investigations into its role in diagnosing acute allograft rejection. Loubeyre et al. (54) examined 190 paired biopsies and HRCT scans among 32 heart–lung and lung transplant recipients. The most common finding associated with biopsy-proven acute rejection was ground glass attenuation, present in 65% of cases compared to 14% of cases of CMV pneumonitis and only 9% of cases in which biopsies were normal. Ground glass opacities were detected in 85% of cases of acute rejection occurring within the first month, but in only 54% thereafter. Although the numbers in each group were small, ground glass opacities were seen in all cases of grades 3 and 4 rejection, but in only a minority of those with grades 1 and 2. The overall sensitivity, specificity, positive and negative predictive value of ground glass attenuation in the diagnosis of acute rejection were 65%, 85%, 54%, and 90%, respectively.

Gotway et al. (55) examined the utility of a broader array of HRCT findings in diagnosing acute rejection, excluding studies obtained within the first post-transplant month in order to minimize the confounding impact of reperfusion edema. Individually, none of the typical features attributed to acute rejection—ground glass opacities, consolidation, pleural effusion, or septal thickening—was present in >50% of patients with biopsy-proven acute rejection. The specificity of both ground glass opacities and consolidation approximated 75% whereas that of septal thickening and pleural effusions fell far short of this mark. The radiographic combination of volume loss and septal thickening, with or without associated pleural effusion, was unique to patients with acute rejection (i.e. 100% specificity) but was present in only 20% of cases.

Taken in sum, these and other studies suggest that chest radiography and HRCT possess limited performance characteristics that compromise their ability to screen for and definitively diagnose acute rejection. In most cases, transbronchial lung biopsy serves as the final arbiter.

H. Bronchiolitis Obliterans Syndrome

Despite current immunosuppressive strategies, the majority of lung transplant recipients develop BOS, a disorder characterized by progressive, irreversible airflow obstruction. BOS is the functional corollary of obliterative bronchiolitis, a fibroproliferative process characterized by submucosal inflammation and fibrosis of the bronchiolar walls ultimately leading to complete obliteration of the airway lumen. In contrast to acute cellular rejection, obliterative bronchiolitis is difficult to diagnose by transbronchial biopsy, with reported sensitivity as low as 17% (56). By convention, therefore, diagnosis rests on the demonstration of physiologic rather than histologic criteria. The term "BOS" has thus evolved, defined as an otherwise unexplained and sustained decline in FEV1 of at least 20% below the peak post-transplant baseline (24). Although presumed to represent chronic rejection, the pathogenesis of BOS remains poorly understood. Acute rejection, particularly when recurrent or severe, has been consistently identified as the major risk factor for development of BOS, supporting the view that BOS reflects an immunologically mediated injury (57,58). Other risk factors that have been more variably identified include CMV and other viral infections, lymphocytic bronchiolitis, older donor age, prolonged ischemic time, HLA-mismatching, and gastroesophageal reflux with occult aspiration (24).

BOS is rarely encountered in the first post-transplant year but its incidence increases steadily beyond that point, involving approximately two-thirds of recipients by the fifth year. Onset of disease is typically insidious and heralded by dyspnea and cough. Recurrent bouts of purulent tracheobronchitis, with recovery of *Pseudomonas aeruginosa* from sputum cultures, are highly characteristic. Progressive airflow obstruction documented by spirometry is the rule, though the pace of decline is highly variable and the course may be interrupted by periods of functional stability. A wide range of therapies have been employed, all of which center on augmentation of immunosuppression. At best, treatment appears to slow the rate of decline rather than to fully arrest or reverse the process. The prognosis is generally poor, with a 40% mortality rate within 2 years of onset (59). The only definitive treatment is retransplantation but this strategy remains highly controversial in the context of a scarce donor organ pool (60).

Radiographic Considerations

The allograft typically appears normal on chest radiography until the very late stages of BOS, when pruning of the pulmonary vasculature, volume loss, irregular linear opacities, and bronchiectasis may occasionally be seen. In contrast, HRCT reveals evidence of air trapping on expiratory images (Fig. 28.11) in a large percentage of patients with BOS. Studies examining the diagnostic utility of this finding have documented a sensitivity of 74–91% and specificity of 67–94% (61–64). To some extent, the variability in performance between studies reflects differences in the "gold standard" chosen for diagnosis of bronchiolitis obliterans (biopsy vs. pulmonary function) and in the radiographic scoring system utilized to define clinically significant air trapping. Limited data suggest that the finding of bronchiectasis on HRCT is relatively specific for BOS but is encountered in only 15–36% of patients (63,64).

The studies discussed above suggest that HRCT can provide corroborating evidence of the presence of bronchiolitis obliterans in patients with established disease. As the current gold standard for diagnosis—spirometry—is noninvasive, easily performed in serial fashion, highly reproducible, and relatively inexpensive, HRCT offers no distinct diagnostic advantages for patients who meet

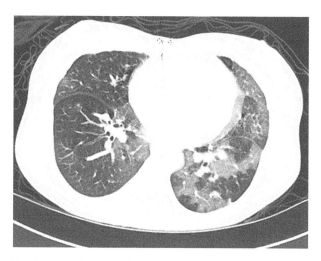

Figure 28.11 HRCT taken at full expiration in a patient with severe bronchiolitis obliterans syndrome demonstrates air trapping in a patchwork distribution throughout the left lung and more diffusely on the right.

physiologic criteria for BOS. However, reliance on the current spirometric definition requiring a significant and sustained decline in lung function results in the
detection of disease at a relatively advanced stage poorly responsive to therapeutic interventions. Consequently, there has been tremendous interest in developing noninvasive imaging modalities capable of detecting abnormalities in the
small airways prior to onset of full-blown BOS and, therefore, at a stage more
amenable to treatment. Miller et al. (65) examined the value of HRCT in predicting onset of BOS within 1 year in a group of 50 lung transplant recipients imaged
at a time when they had stable, peak post-transplant lung function. The presence
of air trapping on expiratory images was the best predictor, with a sensitivity and
specificity of 56% and 76%, respectively. None of the other CT findings
examined (mosaic perfusion pattern, bronchiectasis, tree-in-bud opacities)
proved to be of value in predicting subsequent onset of BOS. Among 49 lung
transplant recipients free of BOS, Knollmann et al. (66) found that "mean lung
attenuation" at end expiration, determined by computer analysis, was significantly lower in patients who subsequently developed BOS within the next year
than in those who maintained stable lung function. After defining an optimal
diagnostic threshold for lung attenuation, the sensitivity and specificity of this

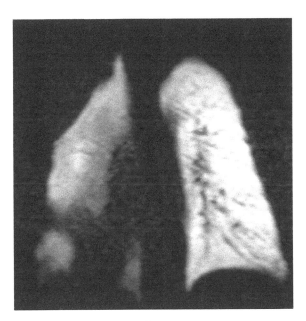

Figure 28.12   Coronal hyperpolarized ^{3}He MR anterior image of a patient with
COPD following successful left lung transplantation. The lung allograft demonstrates
homogeneous distribution of the hyperpolarized ^{3}He gas. The native right emphysematous
lung reveals multiple large ventilation defects. (Image courtesy of Eduard E. de Lange,
University of Virginia.)

parameter in predicting the development of BOS were 69% and 71%, respectively. By logistic regression analysis that incorporated the more conventional visual CT findings of air trapping, bronchiectasis, and mosaic perfusion, only mean lung attenuation was an independent MR predictor of BOS. Taken in sum, the studies by Miller et al. and Knollmann et al. suggest that HRCT holds promise as a screening tool but has not yet achieved the level of performance necessary to justify early and aggressive therapeutic intervention based on CT findings.

A potential screening tool still in a nascent stage of development is magnetic resonance imaging (MRI) using inhaled hyperpolarized [3]He gas (for more extensive description in Chapter 7). When used as an exogenous contrast agent, hyperpolarized [3]He MR can provide unparalleled, high-resolution gas distribution images of the lung (67–69). Traditional proton MRI of the lung is limited by low-signal intensity due to low-proton density as well as by inhomogeneities in the magnetic field. These problems may be overcome with the use of inhaled hyperpolarized [3]He gas, which is capable of detecting subtle changes in gas distribution in the lung. Imaging following successful lung

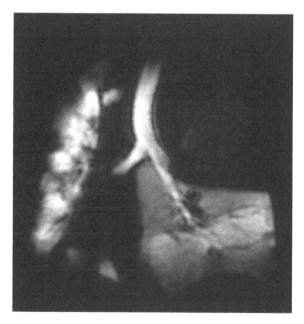

Figure 28.13 Coronal hyperpolarized [3]He MR anterior image of a patient with bullous emphysema following right lung transplantation. The patient has developed severe BOS in the transplanted allograft. Numerous ventilation defects are present. The native emphysematous left lung demonstrates a large area of diminished [3]He ventilation in the upper lung zone consistent with extensive bullous destruction. (Image courtesy of Eduard E. de Lange, University of Virginia.)

transplantation reveals homogeneous gas distribution throughout the lung allograft (Fig. 28.12) (15,70). Preliminary evidence in lung transplant recipients suggests that ventilatory defects detected by MRI using hyperpolarized ^{3}He correlate with the presence of BOS (Fig. 28.13) (70–72).

Traditional nuclear ventilation/perfusion scans in patients with BOS reveal diminished ventilation of the peripheral lung as well as nonspecific perfusion abnormalities (73). While these static images are too insensitive to reliably diagnose bronchiolitis obliterans, they suggest that abnormalities in ventilation and perfusion matching may be a cardinal feature of this disease. Analysis of pulmonary perfusion may be performed using MR techniques based on the dynamic observation of pulmonary magnetization after bolus injection of paramagnetic contrast agents, direct magnetic labeling of blood, or alternative approaches that exploit differences in signal intensity between different cardiac phases (these techniques are described in more detail in Chapters 6, 10, and 11). In addition, in contrast to other available airspace tracers, the signal intensity of hyperpolarized ^{3}He decays measurably in the distal airspaces over a period of seconds at a rate that is highly dependent on local levels of alveolar oxygen, allowing for the determination of regional lung oxygen concentrations (74,75). When combined, these noninvasive and nonradioactive techniques have been utilized as an integrated method for analyzing ventilation and perfusion distributions in the lung and may be useful in the future as a means of detecting subtle derangements associated with early bronchiolitis obliterans.

Acknowledgment

This work was supported by the Craig and Elaine Dobbin Pulmonary Research Fund of the University of Pennsylvania.

References

1. Arcasoy SM, Kotloff RM. Lung transplantation. N Engl J Med 1999; 340:1081–1091.
2. Trulock EP, Edwards LB, Taylor DO, Boucek MM, Mohacsi PJ, Keck BM, Hertz MI. The registry of the international society for heart and lung transplantation: twentieth official adult lung and heart-lung transplant report-2003. J Heart Lung Transplant 2003; 22:625–635.
3. Maurer JR, Frost AE, Estenne M, Higenbottam T, Glanville AR. International guidelines for the selection of lung transplant candidates. Am J Respir Crit Care Med 1998; 158:335–339.
4. Hubbard R, Venn A, Lewis S, Britton J. Lung cancer and cryptogenic fibrosing alveolitis. A population-based cohort study. Am J Respir Crit Care Med 2000; 161:5–8.

5. Henschke CI, McCauley DI, Yankelevitz DF, Naidich DP, McGuinness G, Miettinen OS, Libby DM, Pasmantier MW, Koizumi J, Altorki NK, Smith JP. Early Lung Cancer Action Project: overall design and findings from baseline screening. Lancet 1999; 354:99–105.

6. Kazerooni EA, Chow LC, Whyte RI, Martinez FJ, Lynch JP. Preoperative examination of lung transplant candidates: value of chest CT compared with chest radiography. Am J Roentgenol 1995; 165:1343–1348.

7. Henschke CI, Yankelevitz DF, Libby D, McCauley D, Pasmantier M, Smith JP. Computed tomography screening for lung cancer. Clin Chest Med 2002; 23:49–57.

8. Hadjiliadis D, Sporn TA, Perfect JR, Tapson VF, Davis RD, Palmer SM. Outcome of lung transplantation in patients with mycetomas. Chest 2002; 121:128–134.

9. Christie JD, Bavaria JE, Palevsky HI, Litzky L, Blumenthal NP, Kaiser LR, Kotloff RM. Primary graft failure following lung transplantation. Chest 1998; 114:51–60.

10. Novick RJ, Stitt LW, Al-Kattan K, Klepetko W, Schafers HJ, Duchatelle JP, Khaghani A, Hardesty RL, Patterson GA, Yacoub MH. Pulmonary retransplantation: predictors of graft function and survival in 230 patients. Pulmonary Retransplant Registry. Ann Thorac Surg 1998; 65:227–234.

11. Chhajed PN, Malouf MA, Tamm M, Spratt P, Glanville AR. Interventional bronchoscopy for the management of airway complications following lung transplantation. Chest 2001; 120:1894–1899.

12. Semenkovich JW, Glazer HS, Anderson DC, Arcidi JM Jr, Cooper JD, Patterson GA. Bronchial dehiscence in lung transplantation: CT evaluation. Radiology 1995; 194:205–208.

13. McAdams HP, Murray JG, Erasmus JJ, Goodman PC, Tapson VF, Davis RD. Telescoping bronchial anastomoses for unilateral or bilateral sequential lung transplantation: CT appearance. Radiology 1997; 203:202–206.

14. McAdams HP, Palmer SM, Erasmus JJ, Patz EF, Connolly JE, Goodman PC, Delong DM, Tapson VF. Bronchial anastomotic complications in lung transplant recipients: virtual bronchoscopy for noninvasive assessment. Radiology 1998; 209:689–695.

15. Lipson DA, Roberts DA, Hansen-Flaschen J, Gentile TR, Jones G, Thompson A, Dimitrov IE, Palevsky HI, Leigh JS, Schnall M, Rizi RR. Pulmonary ventilation and perfusion scanning using hyperpolarized helium-3 MRI and arterial spin tagging in healthy normal subjects and in pulmonary embolism and orthotopic lung transplant patients. Magn Reson Med 2002; 47:1073–1076.

16. Weill D, Torres F, Hodges TN, Olmos JJ, Zamora MR. Acute native lung hyperinflation is not associated with poor outcomes after single-lung transplant for emphysema. J Heart Lung Transplant 1999; 18:1080–1087.

17. Yonan NA, el-Gamel A, Egan J, Kakadellis J, Rahman A, Deiraniya AK. Single-lung transplantation for emphysema: predictors for native lung hyperinflation. J Heart Lung Transplant 1998; 17:192–201.

18. Schulman LL, O'Hair DP, Cantu E, McGregor C, Ginsberg ME. Salvage by volume reduction of chronic allograft rejection in emphysema. J Heart Lung Transplant 1999; 18:107–112.

19. Venuta F, De Giacomo T, Rendina EA, Della Rocca G, Flaishman I, Guarino E, Ricci C. Thoracoscopic volume reduction of the native lung after single-lung transplantation for emphysema. Am J Respir Crit Care Med 1997; 156:292–293.

20. Maurer JR, Tullis E, Grossman RF, Vellend H, Winton TL, Patterson GA. Infectious complications following isolated lung transplantation. Chest 1992; 101:1056–1059.
21. Kramer MR, Marshall SE, Starnes VA, Gamberg P, Amitai Z, Theodore J. Infectious complications in heart–lung transplantation. Analysis of 200 episodes. Arch Intern Med 1993; 153:2010–2016.
22. Weill D, Dey GC, Hicks RA, Young KR Jr, Zorn GL Jr, Kirklin JK, Early L, McGiffin DC. A positive donor gram stain does not predict outcome following lung transplantation. J Heart Lung Transplant 2002; 21:555–558.
23. Duncan SR, Paradis IL, Yousem SA, Similo SL, Grgurich WF, Williams PA, Dauber JH, Griffith BP. Sequelae of cytomegalovirus pulmonary infections in lung allograft recipients. Am Rev Respir Dis 1992; 146:1419–1425.
24. Estenne M, Maurer JR, Boehler A, Egan JJ, Frost A, Hertz M, Mallory GB, Snell GI, Yousem S. Bronchiolitis obliterans syndrome 2001: an update of the diagnostic criteria. J Heart Lung Transplant 2002; 21:297–310.
25. Ettinger NA, Bailey TC, Trulock EP, Storch GA, Anderson D, Raab S, Spitznagel EL, Dresler C, Cooper JD. Cytomegalovirus infection and pneumonitis: impact after isolated lung transplantation. Am Rev Respir Dis 1993; 147:1017–1023.
26. Gordon SM, Avery RK. Aspergillosis in lung transplantation: incidence, risk factors, and prophylactic strategies. Transpl Infect Dis 2001; 3:161–167.
27. Mehrad B, Paciocco G, Martinez FJ, Ojo TC, Iannettoni MD, Lynch JP III. Spectrum of *Aspergillus* infection in lung transplant recipients: case series and review of the literature. Chest 2001; 119:169–175.
28. Kessler R, Massard G, Warter A, Wihlm JM, Weitzenblum E. Bronchial-pulmonary artery fistula after unilateral lung transplantation: a case report. J Heart Lung Transplant 1997; 16:674–677.
29. Birsan T, Taghavi S, Klepetko W. Treatment of aspergillus-related ulcerative tracheobronchitis in lung transplant recipients. J Hear Lung Transplant 1998:437–438.
30. Collins J, Muller NL, Kazerooni EA, Paciocco G. CT findings of pneumonia after lung transplantation. Am J Roentgenol 2000; 175:811–818.
31. Ward S, Muller NL. Pulmonary complications following lung transplantation. Clin Radiol 2000; 55:332–339.
32. Rappaport DC, Chamberlain DW, Shepherd FA, Hutcheon MA. Lymphoproliferative disorders after lung transplantation: imaging features. Radiology 1998; 206:519–524.
33. Collins J, Kazerooni EA, Lacomis J, McAdams HP, Leung AN, Shiau M, Semenkovich J, Love RB. Bronchogenic carcinoma after lung transplantation: frequency, clinical characteristics, and imaging findings. Radiology 2002; 224:131–138.
34. Aris RM, Maia DM, Neuringer IP, Gott K, Kiley S, Gertis K, Handy J. Post-transplantation lymphoproliferative disorder in the Epstein-Barr virus-naive lung transplant recipient. Am J Respir Crit Care Med 1996; 154:1712–1717.
35. Levine SM, Angel L, Anzueto A, Susanto I, Peters JI, Sako EY, Bryan CL. A low incidence of posttransplant lymphoproliferative disorder in 109 lung transplant recipients. Chest 1999; 116:1273–1277.
36. Paranjothi S, Yusen RD, Kraus MD, Lynch JP, Patterson GA, Trulock EP. Lymphoproliferative disease after lung transplantation: comparison of presentation and outcome of early and late cases. J Heart Lung Transplant 2001; 20:1054–1063.

37. Swinnen LJ, Costanzo-Nordin MR, Fisher SG, O'Sullivan EJ, Johnson MR, Heroux AL, Dizikes GJ, Pifarre R, Fisher RI. Increased incidence of lymphoproliferative disorder after immunosuppression with the monoclonal antibody OKT3 in cardiac-transplant recipients. N Engl J Med 1990; 323:1723–1728.

38. Armitage JM, Kormos RL, Stuart RS, Fricker FJ, Griffith BP, Nalesnik M, Hardesty RL, Dummer JS. Posttransplant lymphoproliferative disease in thoracic organ transplant patients: ten years of cyclosporine-based immunosuppression. J Heart Lung Transplant 1991; 10:877–886.

39. Reynaud-Gaubert M, Stoppa AM, Gaubert J, Thomas P, Fuentes P. Anti-CD20 monoclonal antibody therapy in Epstein-Barr virus-associated B cell lymphoma following lung transplantation. J Heart Lung Transplant 2000; 19:492–495.

40. Verschuuren EA, Stevens SJ, van Imhoff GW, Middeldorp JM, de Boer C, Koeter G, The TH, van Der Bij W. Treatment of posttransplant lymphoproliferative disease with rituximab: the remission, the relapse, and the complication. Transplantation 2002; 73:100–104.

41. Niedermeyer J, Hoffmeyer F, Hertenstein B, Hoeper MM, Fabel H. Treatment of lympho-proliferative disease with rituximab. Lancet 2000; 355:499.

42. Malouf MA, Chhajed PN, Hopkins P, Plit M, Turner J, Glanville AR. Anti-viral prophylaxis reduces the incidence of lymphoproliferative disease in lung transplant recipients. J Heart Lung Transplant 2002; 21:547–554.

43. Tsai DE, Hardy CL, Tomaszewski JE, Kotloff RM, Oltoff KM, Somer BG, Schuster SJ, Porter DL, Montone KT, Stadtmauer EA. Reduction in immunosuppression as initial therapy for posttransplant lymphoproliferative disorder: analysis of prognostic variables and long-term follow-up of 42 adult patients. Transplantation 2001; 71:1076–1088.

44. Skillrud DM, Offord KP, Miller RD. Higher risk of lung cancer in chronic obstructive pulmonary disease. A prospective, matched, controlled study. Ann Intern Med 1986; 105:503–507.

45. Arcasoy SM, Hersh C, Christie JD, Zisman D, Pochettino A, Rosengard BR, Blumenthal NP, Palevsky HI, Bavaria JE, Kotloff RM. Bronchogenic carcinoma complicating lung transplantation. J Heart Lung Transplant 2001; 20:1044–1053.

46. Penn I. Posttransplant malignancies. Transplant Proc 1999; 31:1260–1262.

47. Garver RI Jr, Zorn GL, Wu X, McGiffin DC, Young KR Jr, Pinkard NB. Recurrence of bronchioloalveolar carcinoma in transplanted lungs. N Engl J Med 1999; 340:1071–1074.

48. de Perrot M, Wigle DA, Pierre AF, Tsao MS, Waddell TK, Todd TR, Keshavjee SH. Bronchogenic carcinoma after solid organ transplantation. Ann Thorac Surg 2003; 75:367–371.

49. Hojo M, Morimoto T, Maluccio M, Asano T, Morimoto K, Lagman M, Shimbo T, Suthanthiran M. Cyclosporine induces cancer progression by a cell-autonomous mechanism. Nature 1999; 397:530–534.

50. Trulock EP, Ettinger NA, Brunt EM, Pasque MK, Kaiser LR, Cooper JD. The role of transbronchial lung biopsy in the treatment of lung transplant recipients. Chest 1992; 102:1049–1054.

51. Sibley RK, Berry GJ, Tazelaar HD, Kraemer MR, Theodore J, Marshall SE, Billingham ME, Starnes VA. The role of transbronchial biopsies in the management of lung transplant recipients. J Heart Lung Transplant 1993; 12:308–324.

52. Aboyoun CL, Tamm M, Chhajed PN, Hopkins P, Malouf MA, Rainer S, Glanville AR. Diagnostic value of follow-up transbronchial lung biopsy after lung rejection. Am J Respir Crit Care Med 2001; 164:460–463.

53. Kundu S, Herman SJ, Larhs A, Rappaport DC, Weisbrod GL, Maurer J, Chamberlain D, Winton T. Correlation of chest radiographic findings with biopsy-proven acute lung rejection. J Thorac Imaging 1999; 14:178–184.

54. Loubeyre P, Revel D, Delignette A, Loire R, Mornex JF. High-resolution computed tomographic findings associated with histologically diagnosed acute lung rejection in heart–lung transplant recipients. Chest 1995; 107:132–138.

55. Gotway MB, Dawn SK, Sellami D, Golden JA, Reddy GP, Keith FM, Webb WR. Acute rejection following lung transplantation: limitations in accuracy of thin-section CT for diagnosis. Radiology 2001; 221:207–212.

56. Chamberlain D, Maurer J, Chaparro C, Idolor L. Evaluation of transbronchial lung biopsy specimens in the diagnosis of bronchiolitis obliterans after lung transplantation. J Heart Lung Transplant 1994; 13:963–971.

57. Bando K, Paradis IL, Similo S et al. Obliterative bronchiolitis after lung and heart–lung transplantation: an analysis of risk factors and management. J Thorac Cardiovasc Surg 1995; 110:4–14.

58. Heng D, Sharples LD, McNeil K, Stewart S, Wreghitt T, Wallwork J. Bronchiolitis obliterans syndrome: incidence, natural history, prognosis, and risk factors. J Heart Lung Transplant 1998; 17:1255–1263.

59. Date H, Lynch JP, Sundaresan S, Patterson GA, Trulock EP. The impact of cytolytic therapy on bronchiolitis obliterans syndrome. J Heart Lung Transplant 1998; 17:869–875.

60. Kotloff RM. Lung retransplantation: all for one or one for all? Chest 2003; 123:1781–1782.

61. Worthy SA, Park CS, Kim JS, Muller NL. Bronchiolitis obliterans after lung transplantation: high-resolution CT findings in 15 patients. Am J Roentgenol 1997; 169:673–677.

62. Bankier AA, Van Muylem A, Knoop C, Estenne M, Gevenois PA. Bronchiolitis obliterans syndrome in heart–lung transplant recipients: diagnosis with expiratory CT. Radiology 2001; 218:533–539.

63. Lee ES, Gotway MB, Reddy GP, Golden JA, Keith FM, Webb WR. Early bronchiolitis obliterans following lung transplantation: accuracy of expiratory thin-section CT for diagnosis. Radiology 2000; 216:472–477.

64. Leung AN, Fisher K, Valentine V, Girgis RE, Berry GJ, Robbins RC, Theodore J. Bronchiolitis obliterans after lung transplantation: detection using expiratory HRCT. Chest 1998; 113:365–370.

65. Miller WT Jr, Kotloff RM, Blumenthal NP, Aronchick JM, Gefter WB, Miller WT. Utility of high resolution computed tomography in predicting bronchiolitis obliterans syndrome following lung transplantation: preliminary findings. J Thorac Imaging 2001; 16:76–80.

66. Knollmann FD, Ewert R, Wundrich T, Hetzer R, Felix R. Bronchiolitis obliterans syndrome in lung transplant recipients: use of spirometrically gated CT. Radiology 2002; 225:655–662.

67. Middleton H, Black RD, Saam B, Cates GD, Cofer GP, Guenther R, Happer W, Hedlund LW, Johnson GA, Juvan K et al. MR imaging with hyperpolarized ^{3}He gas. Magn Reson Med 1995; 33:271–275.

68. Ebert M, Grossmann T, Heil W, Otten WE, Surkau R, Leduc M, Bachert P, Knopp MV, Schad LR, Thelen M. Nuclear magnetic resonance imaging with hyperpolarised helium-3. Lancet 1996; 347:1297–1299.
69. Saam BT. Magnetic resonance imaging with laser-polarized noble gases. Nat Med 1996; 2:358–359.
70. de Lange EE, Altes TA, Jones DR, Daniel T, Salerno M, Brookeman JR, Mugler JP. Bronchioliotis obliterans following lung transplantation: evaluation with hyperpolarized helium-3 MR imaging. Proceedings of 10th Annual Scientific Meeting of the International Society of Magnetic Resonance in Medicine (abstract #2024) 2002.
71. Palmer SM, McAdams HP, MacFall JR, Donnelly L, Davis RD, Tapson VF. Hyperpolarized helium-3 magnetic resonance imaging of bronchiolitis obliterans syndrome in lung transplant patients. Am J Respir Crit Care Med 1999; 159:A276.
72. McAdams HP, Palmer SM, Donnelly LF, Charles HC, Tapson VF, MacFall JR. Hyperpolarized ^{3}He-enhanced MR imaging of lung transplant recipients: preliminary results. AJR Am J Roentgenol 1999; 173:955–959.
73. Halverson RAJ, DuCret RP, Kuni CC, Olivari MT, Tylen U, Hertz MI. Obliterative bronchiolitis following lung transplantation: utility of aerosol ventilation lung scanning and high resolution CT. Clin Nuclear Med 1991; 16:256–258.
74. Eberle B, Weiler N, Markstaller K, Kauczor H, Deninger A, Ebert M, Grossmann T, Heil W, Lauer LO, Roberts TP, Schreiber WG, Surkau R, Dick WF, Otten EW, Thelen M. Analysis of intrapulmonary O_2 concentration by MR imaging of inhaled hyperpolarized helium-3. J Appl Physiol 1999; 87:2043–2052.
75. Deninger AJ, Eberle B, Ebert M, Grossmann T, Heil W, Kauczor H, Lauer L, Markstaller K, Otten E, Schmiedeskamp J, Schreiber W, Surkau R, Thelen M, Weiler N. Quantification of regional intrapulmonary oxygen partial pressure evolution during apnea by ^{3}He MRI. J Magn Reson 1999; 141:207–216.

Index

Index

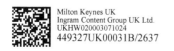
Milton Keynes UK
Ingram Content Group UK Ltd.
UKHW020003071024
449327UK00031B/2637